CALCIUM AND PHOSPHORUS IN HEALTH AND DISEASE

MODERN NUTRITION

Edited by Ira Wolinsky and James F. Hickson, Jr.

Published Titles

Calcium and Phosphorus in Health and Disease, John J.B. Anderson and Sanford C. Garner
Manganese in Health and Disease, Dorothy Klimis-Tavantzis
Nutrition and AIDS: Effects and Treatment, Ronald R. Watson

Forthcoming Titles

Zinc in Health and Disease, Mary E. Mohs

Edited by Ira Wolinsky

Published Titles

Advanced Nutrition: Macronutrients, Carolyn D. Berdanier
Childhood Nutrition, Fima Lifshitz
Handbook of Dairy Foods and Nutrition, Gregory D. Miller, Judith K. Jarvis and Lois D. McBean
Nutrition and Health: Topics and Controversies, Felix Bronner
Nutritional Care for HIV-Positive Persons: A Manual for Individuals and Their Caregivers, Saroj M. Bahl and James F. Hickson, Jr.
Practical Handbook of Nutrition in Clinical Practice, Donald F. Kirby and Stanley J. Dudrick

Forthcoming Titles

Laboratory Tests for the Assessment of Nutritional Status, 2nd Edition, H. E. Sauberlich
Nutrition and Cancer Prevention, Ronald R. Watson and Siraj I. Mufti
Nutrition and Hypertension, Michael B. Zemel
Nutrition: Chemistry and Biology, 2nd Edition, Julian E. Spallholz and L. Mallory Boylan
Nutritional Concerns of Women, Ira Wolinsky and Dorothy Klimis-Tavantzis

CALCIUM AND PHOSPHORUS IN HEALTH AND DISEASE

Edited by
John J. B. Anderson
Sanford C. Garner

CRC Press
Boca Raton New York London Tokyo

Library of Congress Cataloging-in-Publication Data

Calcium and phosphorus in health and disease / edited by John J.B.
Anderson and Sanford C. Garner.
p. cm. -- (Modern nutrition)
Includes bibliographical references and index.
ISBN 0-8493-7845-1
1. Calcium--Metabolism. 2. Phosphorus--Metabolism. 3. Bones--Metabolism. I. Anderson, John J. B. (John Joseph Baxter), 1934- . II. Garner, Sanford C. III. Series: Modern nutrition (Boca Raton, Fla.)
QP535.C2C2622 1995 95-3188
612.3'924--dc20 CIP

Direct all inquiries to CRC Press, Inc., 2000 Corporate Blvd., N.W., Boca Raton, Florida 33431.

International Standard Book Number 0-8493-7845-1
Library of Congress Card Number 95-3188
Printed in the United States of America 1 2 3 4 5 6 7 8 9 0
Printed on acid-free paper

SERIES PREFACE FOR MODERN NUTRITION

The CRC Series in Modern Nutrition is dedicated to providing the widest possible coverage to topics in nutrition. Nutrition is an interdisciplinary, interprofessional field par excellence. It is noted by its broad range and diversity. We trust that the titles and authorship in this series will reflect that range and diversity.

Published for a scholarly audience, the volumes of the CRC Series in Modern Nutrition are designed to explain, review, and explore present knowledge and recent trends, developments, and advances in nutrition. As such, they will also appeal to the educated layman. The format for the series will vary with the needs of the author and the topic, including, but not limited to, edited volumes, monographs, handbooks, and texts.

Contributors from any bona fide area of nutrition, including the controversial, are welcome.

We welcome the contribution *Calcium and Phosphorus in Health and Disease* to the series. As a nutrition scientist who started his career in bone and calcium research, I can appreciate the expert roster of authors and editors, the timeliness, and the comprehensiveness of this volume.

Ira Wolinsky, Ph.D.
Series Editor

PREFACE

This volume has evolved from several decades of teaching and research in the areas of calcium and bone metabolism. The role of nutrition, especially the adequate supply of dietary calcium, phosphorus, vitamin D and other nutrients, has become much more important in understanding perturbations of calcium and bone metabolism in recent years because of the increasing numbers of elderly women (and surviving men) who suffer hip fractures. Therefore, this book has focused on the major topics of calcium and bone metabolism as applied to human function. We hope that this approach will benefit particularly the new graduate students and research fellows in medicine who are entering these areas of investigation.

The long-standing efforts of several research groups at the University of North Carolina at Chapel Hill have served as the impetus for compiling and editing this work. Two research groups, in particular, have been instrumental in fostering research at UNC-CH in the areas of calcium and bone metabolism, namely those of Paul Munson and Roy Talmage. Many researchers have been trained in these groups, and most of them remain active investigators today. Through the leadership of Talmage and Munson, new information and concepts have been advanced by many different individuals. The legacy of these two outstanding scientists, both retired, continues at many major research institutions throughout the world.

The invited contributors consist primarily of colleagues at UNC-CH and Duke University, with one participant from the Karolinska Institute in Stockholm. As this volume is designed to be a teaching source rather than a research compendium, the authorship has been kept rather limited and in close proximity. The latter point has made the final editing steps much easier.

A few features used in the text need emphasis. First, many commonly used terms are abbreviated; the reader should refer to the list provided on page XV. Secondly, most of the text figures have been designed so that slides or overheads can be reproduced from them for use in teaching and in other presentations. We also think that the detailed index should be helpful to readers of this book. Finally, we anticipate that errors will have crept into the text, and we apologize in advance for these noisome incursions.

In concluding this preface, we invite comments from other researchers/teachers about the content of this volume and any use of the chapters by colleagues in their teaching of young investigators. We would welcome suggestions for the inclusion of additional topics, references, or illustrations. We hope that this book will encourage incipient researchers to enter the areas of calcium and bone metabolism and to use nutritional approaches in their work.

John J. B. Anderson
Sanford C. Garner
Chapel Hill and Durham, NC — October 1994

FOREWORD

Axiom: "Calcium is the axis around which all life revolves, and phosphate supplies the energy to turn the axis."

The statement above may appear to be much too strong, except to the dedicated calcium researcher. It emphasizes the importance of calcium (Ca) and phosphate (Pi) to all life. The role of Pi in energy transport and utilization is well known, as are its other metabolic activities, such as the control of pH. As will be discussed below, Pi is also very important in its relationship to Ca.

Why is Ca so important? The element has two properties, one or both of which affect almost every metabolic function of living forms. One property is the ability of Ca ions to complex with organic compounds, particularly proteins, thereby affecting the activity of the compounds. The other is the solubilities of Ca salts that range from completely soluble to almost insoluble. Many errors in the interpretation of experimental results in Ca research have been made by failing to keep foremost in mind these two properties. These properties are so important to life that they are worth further elaboration.

The first property refers to the ability of Ca ions to complex with organic compounds, primarily proteins. Intracellularly, when Ca ions attach to proteins, a change in the conformation of the molecule usually results. For example, the net result of the conformation change with muscle proteins is the contraction of muscle fibers. For intracellular enzymes the net result is the control of the activity of the enzyme. In both cases the process is reversible, and the degree of complexing is, thus, proportional to the Ca ion concentration of the medium. For intracellular function, the optimum Ca ion concentration is of the order of 10^{-7} M. An increase to 10^{-5} M is usually lethal. In summary, then, the control of the intracellular concentration of Ca ion is of major importance in the regulation of both intracellular and extracellular functions.

Our purpose here is not to discuss the intracellular functions of Ca, but to point out the problem faced by mammals, including man, whose extracellular Ca ion concentration is 10^{-3} M, approximately 10,000 times higher than that of the intracellular fluid. Cell membranes also complex Ca, the binding of which is proportional to the ion concentration of extracellular fluids. Either extremely high or low concentrations of Ca ions bound to cell membranes can be disastrous to the cell, and such differences in the amount of Ca bound may be factors in hormone-related diseases. One unresolved question relates to the process by which Ca is transported across cellular membranes, such as through the intestinal mucosa or across renal tubules. The approximately 10,000-fold difference in the Ca ion concentrations between the cell media and the extracellular fluids must be maintained while Ca passes through the cells. Obviously when considering the actions of Ca-regulating hormones, the differential between extracellular and intracellular Ca concentrations and the reversibility of the Ca complexed to cell membranes must be kept in mind.

The second property, i.e., the widely varying solubilities of phosphate salts of Ca, is of equal importance to the ability of Ca to complex with proteins. The contrasting solubilities of the calcium phosphate salts made it possible for land vertebrates to develop a living internal skeleton. While it is well known that these salts are important in regulating blood pH, the role of their solubilities in regulating bone metabolism is often overlooked. Primary calcium phosphate ($Ca(H_2PO_4)_2$) is extremely soluble. Secondary calcium phosphate ($CaHPO_4$) has a solubility of around 2×10^{-3} M. Tertiary calcium phosphate ($Ca_3(PO_4)_2$) has a solubility only slightly greater than 10^{-4} M. Approximately 85% of the Ca in solution in the extracellular fluid of mammals is secondary calcium phosphate. In contrast, bone of all mammals contains tertiary calcium phosphate which, after precipitation, becomes crystallized. And therein lies the problem.

If a low solubility Ca salt is added to a solution containing ionic Ca and Pi, the concentrations of both the cation and anion of that salt are reduced to the solubility of the added salt. The precipitation of Ca and Pi can be easily demonstrated by adding tertiary calcium phosphate, apatite crystals, or bone (living or dead) to mammalian plasma. Both Ca and Pi will be removed. Thus, a second axiom must also be true: "Mammalian extracellular fluid is undersaturated with calcium phosphate in respect to itself; however, this same fluid is supersaturated in respect to bone."

The Ca ion concentration of the extracellular fluids of mammals is one of nature's constants. How can the Ca concentration be maintained, when every time the extracellular fluid passes over bone surfaces, both Ca and Pi are removed? Many studies have demonstrated the rapidity with which Ca is taken up by bone. It has been calculated that, in humans, Ca equivalent to its total content in extracellular fluids is removed by bone many times an hour. This continuous loss of extracellular Ca raises the issue of how plasma Ca is maintained at a constant concentration; i. e., the problem of Ca homeostasis. The only answer is that Ca must be returned to fluids by bone through the utilization of metabolic energy. Mechanisms that maintain Ca homeostasis must act in relation to the terms of the two characteristics of Ca discussed above. Unfortunately, these concepts are often ignored in interpreting research data or providing theories explaining Ca homeostasis.

Any discussion of the control of plasma Ca concentrations must begin with parathyroid hormone (PTH). PTH is known to play a major role in Ca homeostasis. In the absence of this hormone, plasma Ca levels fall, and Ca is removed from cell membranes, changing the nature of their function. While all cells may be affected, the first obvious affect is on muscle cells (including cardiac). The loss of Ca from these cell membranes allows Ca ions to flow freely down the gradient into the intracellular compartment, causing muscle fiber contraction, tetany, and death. While the action of PTH has a long history of controversy, it is now generally agreed that the hormone exercises its control of plasma Ca concentrations by its action on bone. Somehow PTH is able to counterbalance the continuous effects of a supersaturated fluid flowing over the very low solubility salt.

One of the known actions of PTH is to increase the activity of osteoclasts, those bone cells dedicated to resorbing bone. Since the hormone raises plasma Ca levels, it was naturally assumed that the increased osteoclastic activity raised plasma Ca concentrations. Indeed osteoclastic destruction of bone does add Ca to extracellular fluids, but only in extreme situations can this addition counterbalance the enormous effect of a supersaturated solution passing over acres of bone surfaces. To put it simply, if a change in osteoclastic activity were required to maintain normal plasma Ca, mammals with osteopetrosis (limited number of functional osteoclasts) would have low plasma Ca concentrations, and conversely humans with highly developed Paget's disease (excess number of functional osteoclasts) would have hypercalcemia.

An enormous amount of additional research has demonstrated that osteoclastic activity could not, in itself, maintain a normal plasma Ca concentration. Reference is made to only one report, which provides references to earlier studies.[1] In this study, two substances that increase osteoclastic activity (prostaglandin E_2 [PGE_2] and PTH) were administered to parathyroidectomized rats. Both substances stimulated osteoclast production and activity and moved minute amounts of Ca from bone to extracellular fluid, but only PTH was able to maintain normal plasma Ca concentrations. While increased osteoclastic activity, as well as increased renal reabsorption of Ca, are important actions of PTH, the actual setting of plasma Ca concentrations by PTH is dependent upon its action on cells lining bone surfaces and related osteoblast-derived cells, including active osteoblasts and bone-lining cells, which are in communication with underlining osteocytes. The question is "how does cellular action at bone surfaces counterbalance the rapid effect of a supersaturated fluid coming into constant contact with a very low solubility salt?" A complete answer has not been elucidated. However, a plausible explanation can be derived based on the following ten statements, all of which have experimental support.

1. Receptor sites for PTH exist on bone-lining cells, osteocytes, and osteoblasts.
2. Administration of PTH into living mammals produces ultrastructural changes in bone lining cells and in underlying osteocytes within minutes.

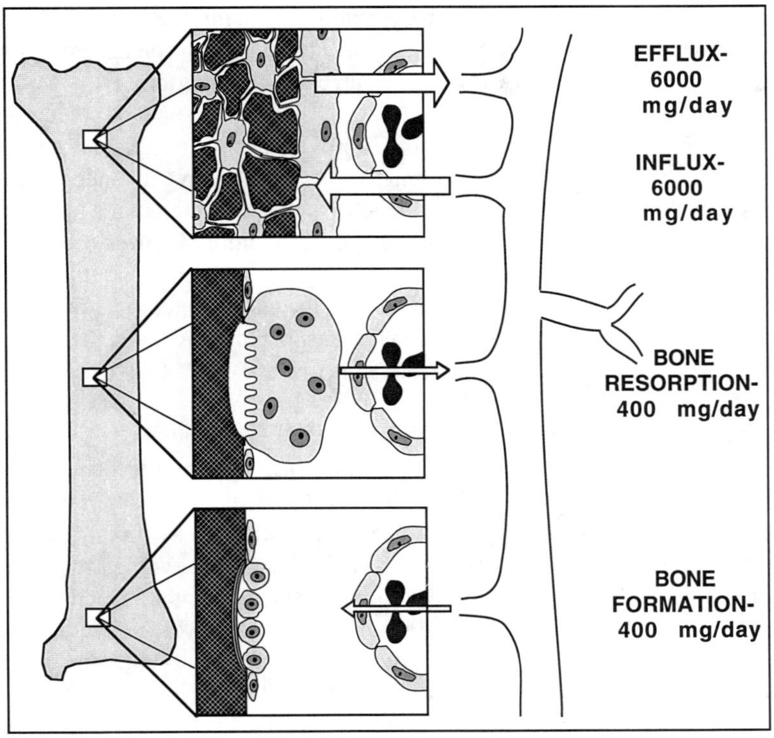

FIGURE 1. Exchange of calcium between bone and blood. The Ca in blood (and all extracellular fluid) is constantly depleted (Ca influx) as Ca and Pi precipitate onto the surface of hydroxyapatite (calcium phosphate) crystals as blood passes through bone. The tremendous influx of Ca (and Pi) into bone is balanced by an equal amount of Ca (and Pi) ion returned to blood (Ca efflux) by the action of the bone-lining cells and other osteoblast-derived bone cells. The amount of Ca and Pi ions entering bone from blood through bone formation is at least an order of magnitude less that the influx of these ions that results from the extracellular fluid Ca-Pi solubility product in relation to bone mineral. Similarly, the amount of Ca and Pi that can be returned from bone to blood by osteoclastic resorption is quite small and should equal the amount of ions required for bone formation in an individual whose skeleton is undergoing no net change in bone mass.

3. Following PTH administration there is a rapid entry of Ca and related elements into bone-lining cells and underlying osteocytes. This effect of PTH has been demonstrated by electron microscopy of stained bone surfaces.
4. Utilizing radioisotopes of Ca, PTH has been shown to return to extracellular fluids the last Ca to enter the bone fluid compartment, followed later by the removal of previously deposited Ca salts.
5. In the absence of circulating PTH, the ionic Ca concentration of extracellular fluid falls but equilibrates well above the solubility value for apatite crystals or tertiary calcium phosphate.
6. Channels between cells covering bone surfaces allow rapid movement of extracellular fluid over bone surfaces.
7. All bone surfaces studied have been shown to contain a variety of proteins, many of which are unique in their ability to reversibly complex Ca.
8. Several independent calculations have been made indicating that in humans, Ca enters and leaves bone at a rate exceeding 6400 mg/day. In contrast, the calculated transfer of Ca from bone to ECF by osteoclasts is less than 400 mg/day (Figure 1).
9. In mammals, an exchangeable Ca compartment exists that is larger than the extracellular fluid compartment. Its size varies with changing physiological conditions. It has been defined as the fluid volume with which any isotope of Ca, when injected intravenously, rapidly equilibrates.

10. Bone surface cells synthesize specific Ca-binding proteins that vary in their capacity to complex Ca as well as the avidity with which they bind. These proteins have an impact on the exchangeability of the attached Ca with the surrounding medium.

From these ten items and the characteristics of Ca provided above, a postulate can be derived that explains in part the action of PTH in maintaining a constant plasma Ca concentration.

The first action of PTH has been postulated to be to increase or maintain a high rate of Ca entry into bone cells. (Cells in other parts of the body may also be similarly affected.) In bone cells, the entry of Ca is primarily from the bone surface side. Through normal and specialized protective mechanisms, Ca is rapidly transported to the exterior of the cell. The removal of Ca could either be by a metabolic pump (not yet demonstrated) or via transport of the Ca complexed to intracellular membranes, or both. The net result is an increase in the return of Ca to extracellular fluid against a strong gradient.

It appears obvious that if the only method by which PTH could enhance Ca movement were by metabolic pump or membrane-bound transport, the utilization of energy would be excessive and impossible to maintain. Thus, it is postulated that PTH-induced Ca entry into these bone cells slightly increases the intracellular Ca concentration. This subtle increase in intracellular ionic Ca is sufficient to increase or change the nature of specific proteins that are synthesized by these cells and then secreted onto bone surfaces. For example, it has been demonstrated that changes in the rate of Ca entry into osteoblasts changes the rate of collagen synthesis. The proteins synthesized have a high affinity for Ca, and when secreted, sequester Ca onto bone surface, thus enlarging the exchangeable Ca compartment. The Ca so sequestered equilibrates with its fluid medium and elevates the Ca concentration of the extracellular fluid. The existence of some form of these proteins, even in the absence of PTH, could explain why, in PTX animals, the ionic plasma Ca level equilibrates at a lower concentration but the Ca concentration is still maintained much higher than the solubility of bone crystals would explain. Also, under normal conditions, when circulating PTH is always present, only minimal amounts of metabolic energy would be required to transfer Ca from bone in order to correct small errors in the Ca ion concentration of extracellular fluid.

While the evidence is not detailed here, it is postulated that the fundamental action of the hormone, calcitonin, is also related to the system described above. It differs from PTH in that calcitonin causes Pi to react with the Ca complexed onto surface proteins. The result is that Ca is bound in a less exchangeable form, thereby reducing the Ca concentration of the extracellular fluid. Unlike PTH, the primary function of calcitonin is not to influence extracellular fluid Ca level but to store Ca temporarily on bone surfaces. This temporary storage conserves Ca for use in bone formation when dietary Ca is not available.

These comments are written here in the hope that they will provide a new insight for those who use this volume, either as a text or a reference source. The entire volume attests to the importance of Ca and Pi. This foreword is an attempt to provide the basic building blocks as to why Ca plays such a major role in normal human physiology and nutrition.

Roy V. Talmage, Ph.D.
Emeritus Professor
Departments of Surgery and Pharmacology
University of North Carolina
School of Medicine

REFERENCE

Vander Wiel, C. J. and Talmage, R. V., Comparison of the effects of prostaglandin E_2 and parathyroid hormone on plasma calcium concentration and osteoclast function, *Endocrinology*, 105, 588, 1979.

CONTRIBUTORS

Erik Allander, M.D.
Department of Social Medicine
Huddinge University Hospital
Karolinska Institute
Huddinge, Sweden
and
Director
WHO Collaborating Centre for the Epidemiology of Rheumatic Diseases
Karolinska Institute
Stockholm, Sweden

Wallace W. Ambrose, M.S.
Dental Research Center
School of Dentistry
University of North Carolina at Chapel Hill
Chapel Hill, North Carolina

John J.B. Anderson, Ph.D.
Department of Nutrition
Schools of Public Health and Medicine
University of North Carolina at Chapel Hill
Chapel Hill, North Carolina

Connie W. Bales, Ph.D.
Department of Medicine
Sarah W. Stedman Center for Nutritional Studies
Duke University Medical Center
Durham, North Carolina

James W. Bawden, D.D.S., Ph.D.
Department of Pediatric Dentistry
School of Dentistry
University of North Carolina at Chapel Hill
Chapel Hill, North Carolina

Agna Boass, Ph.D.
Dental Research Center
School of Dentistry
University of North Carolina at Chapel Hill
Chapel Hill, North Carolina

Marc K. Drezner, M.D.
Departments of Medicine and Cell Biology
Sarah W. Stedman Center for Nutritional Studies
Duke University Medical Center
Durham, North Carolina

Sanford C. Garner, Ph.D.
Department of Surgery
Duke University Medical Center
Durham, North Carolina

Brian Herman, Ph.D.
Laboratories for Cell Biology
Department of Cell Biology and Anatomy
Lineberger Comprehensive Cancer Center
University of North Carolina at Chapel Hill
School of Medicine
Chapel Hill, North Carolina

Philip F. Hirsch, Ph.D.
Department of Pharmacology
School of Medicine and
Dental Research Center
School of Dentistry
University of North Carolina at Chapel Hill
Chapel Hill, North Carolina

Gayle E. Lester, Ph.D.
Division of Orthopedic Surgery
School of Medicine
University of North Carolina at Chapel Hill
Chapel Hill, North Carolina

Bruce Lobaugh, Ph.D.
Departments of Medicine and Cell Biology
Duke University Medical Center
Durham, North Carolina

Dexter S. Louie, Ph.D.
Department of Nutrition
Schools of Public Health and Medicine
University of North Carolina at Chapel Hill
Chapel Hill, North Carolina

Charles P. McKay, M.D.
Department of Pediatrics
Division of Nephrology
Duke University Medical Center
Durham, North Carolina

Robert G. McMurray, Ph.D.
Departments of Physical Education, Exercise and Sport, Science and Nutrition
University of North Carolina at Chapel Hill
Chapel Hill, North Carolina

David A. Ontjes, M.D.
Departments of Medicine and Pharmacology
School of Medicine
University of North Carolina at Chapel Hill
Chapel Hill, North Carolina

Tai-Chan Peng, M.D.[†]
Department of Pharmacology
School of Medicine
University of North Carolina at Chapel Hill
Chapel Hill, North Carolina

[†] Died, September 2, 1991.

Svein U. Toverud, D.M.D., Ph.D.
Department of Pharmacology
School of Medicine
Dental Research Center
School of Dentistry
University of North Carolina at Chapel Hill
Chapel Hill, North Carolina

Mitsuo Yamauchi, D.D.S., Ph.D.
Department of Periodontics
School of Dentistry
Dental Research Center
University of North Carolina at Chapel Hill
Chapel Hill, North Carolina

TABLE OF CONTENTS

TABLE OF COMMON ABBREVIATIONS USED IN THIS BOOK

$1\alpha(OH)D_3$	1-alpha-hydroxyvitamin D
^3H	tritium
25(OH)D	25-hydroxyvitamin D
^{45}Ca	45-calcium radioisotope
$1,25(OH)_2D$	1,25-dihydroxyvitamin D
$24,24(OH)_2D$	24,25-dihydroxyvitamin D
APUD	amine precursor uptake and decarboxylation
ATP	adenosine triphosphate
ATPase	adenosine triphosphatase
ATPR	adenosine triphosphate receptor
BAG-75	bone acidic glycoprotein-75
BBMV	brush border membrane vesicles
BLMV	basolateral membrane vesicles
BGP	bone GLA-protein (osteocalcin)
BMC	bone mineral content
BMD	bone mineral density
BMI	body mass index
BMU	bone multicellular unit
BSP	bone sialoprotein
Ca	calcium
Ca^{++}	calcium ion
Ca_i^{2+}	intracellular ionized calcium
CaBP	calcium-binding protein
cAMP	cyclic adenosine monophosphate
CBG	corticosteroid-binding globulin
CCM	calcium citrate malate
cDNA	complementary deoxyribonucleic acid
CGRP	calcitonin gene-related peptide
CICR	calcium-induced calcium release
CLD	control liquid diet
COL	collagenous domains
COOH	carboxy terminal (applied to protein molecules)
CSF-1	colony stimulating factor-1
CT	calcitonin
D1	duodedum (initial segment)
DAG	diacylglycerol
DBP	vitamin D-binding protein
deH-HHMD	dehydro-histidinohydroxymerodesmosine
deH-HLNL	dehydro-hydroxylysinonorleucine
DEXA	dual X-ray absorptiometry
DHP	dihydropyridine
DHT	dihydrotestosterone
DPA	dual-photon absorptiometry
dPP	dentin phosphophyryn
Dpyr	deoxypyridinoline
ECF	extracellular fluid
EDTA	ethylenediaminetetraacetic acid
EFCa	endogenous fecal excretion of calcium
EGF	epidermal growth factor

ELD	ethanol liquid diet
ERD	end-stage renal disease
ERT	estrogen replacement therapy
FACIT	Fibril Associated Collagen with Interrupted Triple Helices
G-protein (N_s)	guanine nucleotide regulatory protein (stimulatory)
GFR	glomerular filtration rate
GGHYL	glucosyl-galactosyl-hydroxylysine
GHYL	galactosyl-hydroxylysine
GI	gastrointestinal
GLA	γ-carboxylated glutamine residue
Gly	glycine
H^+	hydrogen ion
HDL	high density lipoprotein
hER	human estrogen receptor
hGR	human glucocorticoid receptor
HHL	histidinohydroxylysinonorleucine
HHM	humoral hypercalcemia of malignancy
hMR	human mineralocorticoid receptor
HPLC	high-performance liquid chromatography
hPR	human progestin receptor
HTOP	high-turnover osteoporosis
hTR	human thyroid hormone receptor
Hyl	hydroxylysine
Hyl^{ald}	2-hydroxy-5-amino-5-carboxypentanal (hydroxyallysine)
Hyp	hydroxyproline
^{125}I	^{125}iodine radioisotope
ICMA	immunochemiluminescent assay
IGF-1	insulin-like growth factor-1
IGF-2	insulin-like growth factor-2
IL-1	interleukin-1
IL-4	interleukin-4
IL-6	interleukin-6
IP_3	inositol trisphosphate
iPTH	immunoreactive PTH
IRMA	immunoradiometric assay
It	terminal ileum
IU	international units
J	jejunum
K^+	potassium ion
Kcal	kilocalorie
Kd	kilodalton
Km	Michaelis-Menten constant (enzymatic reaction)
LBM	lean body mass
LDL	low-density lipoprotein
LH	luteinizing hormone
LHRH	luteinizing hormone-releasing hormone
Lys	lysine
Lys^{ald}	5-amino-5-carboxypentanal (allysine)
M	molar concentration
m->s	mucosal to serosal transfer
MCT	medullary carcinoma of the thyroid

MEDOS	Mediterranean Osteoporosis Study
MEN (IIA and IIB)	multiple endocrine neoplasia, types IIA and IIB
Mg^{2+}	magnesium ion
MLCK	myosin light chain kinase
mM	millimolar concentation
MOC	mechanically operated calcium channels
mRNA	messenger RNA
MV	matrix vesicle
Na^{+}	sodium ion
NADP	nicotinamide adenine dinucleotide phosphate
NC	noncollagenous domains
NH_2	amino terminal (applied to protein molecules)
NHANES	National Health and Nutrition Examination Survey
NM	nonmated
nM	nanomolar concentration
NMDAR	N-methyl-D-aspartate receptors
NMR	nuclear magnetic resonance
OCA	oral contraceptive agents
OI	osteogenesis imperfecta
OPN	osteopontin
ORSA	osteoclast resorption-stimulating activity
P	phosphorus, both inorganic and organic
PBM	peak bone mass
PDGF	platelet-derived growth factor
pg	picogram
PHP	pseudohypoparathyroidism
Pi	inorganic phosphate(s)
PICP	carboxy-terminal segment of type I procollagen
PINP	amino-terminal segment of type I procollagen
PIP_2	phosphoinositol bisphosphate
PLC	phospholipase C
PQQ	pyrroloquinoline quinone (methoxatin)
preproPTH	proPTH with 25 amino acid leader sequence
Pro	proline
proPTH	PTH with 6 N-terminal amino acids
PSP-I	parathyroid secretory protein-I
PTH	parathyroid hormone
PTH_{1-34}	parathyroid hormone 1-34 (N-terminal fragment)
PTH_{1-84}	parathyroid hormone 1-84 (intact)
PTHrP	parathroid hormone-related peptide
PTX	parathroidectomy
Pyr	pyridinoline
QCT	quantitative computed tomography
RA	radiographic absorptiometry
RDAs	recommended daily allowances
RER	rough endoplasmic reticulum
RGD	arginine-glycine-aspartic acid (integrin binding site)
RIA	radioimmunoassay
RNA	ribonucleic acid
ROC	receptor-operated channels
RR	relative risk ratio

s->m	serosal to mucosal transfer
SD	standard deviation
SE	standard error
SEM	scanning electron microscopy (or micrograph)
Ser	serine
SHBG	sex-hormone-binding globulin
SIMS	secondary ion mass spectrometry
SMOC	second messenger-operated calcium channels
SPA	single photon absorptiometry
SPX	single photon X-ray
SR	sarcoplasmic reticulum
SR/ER	sarcoplasmic reticulum/endoplasmic reticulum
SRE	steroid response element
TBG	thyroxine-binding globulin
TF:GF	concentration ratio, tubular fluid to glomerular filtrate
TGF-α	transforming growth factor α
TGF-β	transforming growth factor β
Tm	transport maximum (renal)
TmP	transport maximum for phosphate
TNF	tumor necrosis factor
TRAP	tartrate-resistant acid phosphatase
UV	ultraviolet light
VDR	vitamin D receptor
VDRE	vitamin D response element
VGCC	voltage-gated calcium channel
V_{max}	maximum velocity (enzymatic reaction)
V_o^+	increase in bone resorption rate
V_o^-	increase in bone accretion rate
w/v	weight per volume
WHO	World Health Organization

DEDICATION

This volume is dedicated to the many researchers and teachers who have contributed and continue to contribute to our knowledge of calcium and phosphorus metabolism. We also dedicate this book to our late colleague, Tai-Chan Peng, M.D. (February 28, 1928–September 2, 1991).

Chapter 1

CALCIUM AND PHOSPHORUS NUTRITION IN HEALTH AND DISEASE: INTRODUCTION

John J. B. Anderson, Ph.D. and Sanford C. Garner, Ph.D.

TABLE OF CONTENTS

I. INTRODUCTION

Calcium (Ca) and phosphorus (P) are essential elements in the maintenance of bodily functions, but only a small portion, approximately 0.1%, of total body Ca is in solution in the blood, extracellular fluids, and cell cytoplasmic fluid at any time. A slightly larger percentage of P is soluble in the form of inorganic P (Pi), which is essential for cellular functions, such as nucleic acid synthesis, and energy storage molecules, such as ATP. Bone tissue contains about 97% of the Ca and 70% of the P in the body. These elements combine chemically to form the mineralized component of bone tissue, which provides the rigidity to bone structures.

The absolute requirements for Ca at different stages of the life cycle have been reasonably well established only in the last century as our understanding of Ca-deficiency diseases has advanced.

II. CALCIUM-DEFICIENCY DISEASES

Historically, deficiencies of Ca intakes have been associated with bone defects, particularly rickets, and with a concurrent dietary deficiency of vitamin D. Thus, the inadequate supply of Ca associated with a deficiency of vitamin D was marked by bone abnormalities in young children. The necessity for adequate Ca nutrition in women of reproductive age was not always recognized, but the effects of the maternal demands for Ca for fetal bone calcification and milk production for suckling infants were recognized in the adage, "For each child, a tooth is lost."

The possible effects of insufficient Ca intakes are being considered today because of the dramatic increases in the number of individuals, mainly women, suffering from osteoporotic fractures as the population ages. Much emphasis has been given to enhancement of Ca intakes of people in the age groups at risk for osteoporosis. Although food fortification and supplementation with Ca may have a small benefit in these individuals, a need exists for greater acceptance of the role of lifelong Ca

0-8493-7845-1/95/$0.00+$.50

nutrition in allowing the genetic potential of individuals for maximal peak bone mass development to be expressed in adolescence or early adulthood. The impact of adequate mineral intake is potentially much greater in a preventative role by enhancing peak bone mass development in early life and maintaining the bone mass of individuals in later decades than in retarding bone loss in those who already have decreased bone mass and osteoporotic fractures.

Demographic data indicate that the largest growing segment of the United States population is among the elderly. The National Center for Health Statistics has estimated that by the year 2030, those Americans over age 65 will represent almost 24% of the entire population! Osteoporosis, now a major health concern for this segment of the population, will be an even greater problem because of the anticipated increase in the numbers of hip fractures each year. In 1988, the Surgeon General's Report on Nutrition and Health indicated that approximately 15–20 million Americans were affected by osteoporosis. The total costs of osteoporosis to the U.S. economy were estimated to be $7 to $10 billion in 1986.[1] Ca and P are the two main minerals associated with osteoporosis, although other micronutrients as well as macronutrients are clearly required for optimal bone health at any age. Understanding of the needs for dietary Ca and P have largely been derived from the functional changes observed in individuals or animals with obvious deficiencies.

III. FUNCTIONS OF CALCIUM AND PHOSPHORUS

Ca ions serve as essential cofactors in many enzyme reactions, such as the blood clotting cascade; they are necessary for muscle contraction, and they regulate the permeability of sodium ions across cell membranes, including those of nerve cells. Due primarily to this last function, the plasma Ca concentration is tightly regulated, and it varies only slightly over time for a given individual. Pi ions are required for the entry of glucose into the glycolytic pathway, and they are components of nucleic acids and many other biomolecules. Due to the role of phosphate-containing compounds (e.g., ATP and creatine phosphate) in energy production in cells, the fluxes of Pi ions across cell membranes are much greater than those of Ca ions. In addition, the Pi concentration of extracellular fluids is not as tightly regulated as that of Ca, and the Pi concentration may vary widely for an individual, depending on dietary intake. Of these two important and essential inorganic ions, blood Ca concentration is the one that is maintained under rigorous homeostatic regulation.

IV. CALCIUM HOMEOSTASIS

Cellular life developed in primordial oceans that were relatively rich in Ca but deficient in P. When more advanced lifeforms eventually moved onto land, the availability of minerals in the environment was reversed. Organisms living on land needed to conserve Ca ions, while P was present in excess. A need exists for a constant dietary intake of Ca, as this ion is lost through urinary excretions, sweat, cell desquamation, intestinal secretions, and other secretions. The homeostatic mechanisms for maintaining a constant Ca concentration of extracellular fluid are functions of three organ systems: (1) bone, which serves as a reservoir for Ca and P, (2) the gastrointestinal tract, which is the only source of new Ca and Pi ions, and (3) the kidney, which assists in regulating whole body Ca and P by reabsorption of the urinary filtrate. The Ca-related functions of these organ systems are controlled by three major hormones: parathyroid hormone (PTH), vitamin D, and calcitonin (CT). PTH is the primary regulator of plasma Ca, responding rapidly to minor changes in Ca concentration. Vitamin D, in the 1,25-dihydroxyvitamin D ($1,25(OH)_2D$) form, functions as a hormone, with its production regulated by plasma PTH and Pi concentrations. Vitamin D is essential for the maintenance of adequate Ca absorption from dietary sources and must be present for mineralization of bone to proceed normally. CT is a potent agent in lowering plasma Ca and in inhibiting resorption of bone. However, the physiologic function of CT as a regulator of plasma Ca appears to be relatively minor compared to the actions of PTH and vitamin D.

The skeleton contains approximately 1000 times as much Ca as is present in blood and soft tissue combined. During intermeal periods, the need for a constant transfer of Ca between bone and blood to maintain a blood Ca concentration that is optimal for cellular function contributes to a very dynamic environment in bone. The structure of bone itself undergoes dynamic renewal or remodeling throughout life as the shapes of bones change with growth and as minor defects in bone structure are corrected before they accumulate to weaken bone mechanically.

Although Ca is present in relatively large amounts in the foods available to most people in the Western world, the failure of many people to consume adequate amounts of Ca-rich foods presents a potential problem in maintaining adequate supplies of dietary Ca for bone building early in life and for preserving bone structure throughout the remainder of life. This problem may be compounded in non-Western cultures where little or no intake of dairy products greatly reduces the potential food sources for obtaining the recommended amounts of Ca in the diet. Coupled with inadequate intakes of vitamin D and limited exposure to sunlight, a low Ca diet also contributes to development of rickets in the young or osteomalacia in adults. Although the incidence of these conditions has been reduced dramatically in Western countries by fortification of dairy products with vitamin D, they are still widespread in many areas of the world today.

Rickets is characterized by disordered growth and mineralization of the growth plate in childhood or adolescence before the growth plates have closed. In mature bone, abnormalities related to vitamin D deficiency include reduced mineralization, which is termed osteomalacia. Both rickets and osteomalacia represent defects in bone health that are potentially preventable with improved nutritional status.

Ca and P availability to pregnant and lactating women is essential for the proper skeletal development of fetuses and infants who are totally dependent on their mothers for all nutrients. The potential for loss of mineral from the mother's skeleton during these periods is minimal in women consuming amounts of Ca and P similar to recommended dietary intakes. However, as with rickets, reduced consumption of these nutrients may result from diverse cultural dietary patterns or lack of available Ca-rich foods. Poverty may also place mothers at risk for greater loss of bone mineral during pregnancy and lactation. Inadequate Ca intake may be particularly acute in young women who become pregnant before they have attained their peak bone mass.

At the other end of the age spectrum, the major skeletal problem is osteoporosis in older individuals. The osteopenia associated with aging in both men and women is a likely prerequisite for osteoporosis. Osteoporosis, the increased risk of fractures resulting from loss of bone mass, is manifest primarily in women after the menopause when the protective effects of estrogen are lost. Although the potential for treatment of osteoporosis with nutritional supplementation with Ca, vitamin D, or any other nutrient remains controversial, it is likely that improved nutrition during growth could aid in delaying or preventing the onset of this condition. When adequate nutrition allows for the attainment of maximum peak bone mass in adolescence and young adulthood, bone mass will remain above a hypothetical "fracture risk threshold" until later in life, even if bone loss with aging is inevitable.

Other diseases, such as abnormalities in the secretion of PTH, also affect Ca and bone metabolism.

V. DISEASES AFFECTING CALCIUM METABOLISM

The concentration of plasma Ca is tightly regulated for each individual, and the range of normal values is relatively narrow for the population at large. Although the reference range for total plasma Ca varies slightly among clinical laboratories, the range of normal values is usually between 2.1 and 2.6 m*M* (8.5–10.5 mg/dL). Routine laboratory analyses for admission to hospitals frequently include measurement of total Ca, and patients with deviations above or below the normal range for Ca are often discovered before other symptoms of hyper- or hypocalcemia are evident. Hyperparathyroidism, or excessive secretion of PTH, which was once found only after chronically elevated PTH had caused excessive resorption of bone mineral or long-term hypercalcemia had led to the development of kidney stones, is routinely diagnosed today by elevated serum Ca.

As diagnoses of individuals with hypercalcemia have been increasing in recent decades, many causes of this condition have been uncovered. In addition to the response to oversecretion of PTH, increased plasma Ca may also result from other circulating factors secreted by tumors, particularly the PTH-related protein (PTHrP) that has been identified in many cases of humoral hypercalcemia of malignancy (HHM). Direct resorption of bone and release of Ca into the circulation may occur when metastases of cancers are established within bone. Other cases of hypercalcemia may be linked to ingestion of drugs prescribed for other conditions. For example, hypercalcemia has been found to result from excessive vitamin D consumption, but vitamin A, thiazide diuretics, lithium, and estrogens and androgens also have been linked to the elevation of plasma Ca when they are taken chronically.

A decrease in plasma Ca below the normal range, or hypocalcemia, is less common than hypercalcemia because the body defends against it. Hypocalcemia can have such serious consequences that the body has developed its defense system against this situation in a nearly fail-safe manner. The most common endocrine condition leading to hypocalcemia is inadequate or nonexistent secretion of PTH. Although the total absence of parathyroid tissue from birth is an exceedingly rare condition, the parathyroid glands may be removed anytime after birth during excision of the thyroid or parathyroid as a consequence of secondary hyperparathyroidism.

Nutritionally, the most likely cause of hypocalcemia is an inadequate intake of vitamin D coupled with a lack of exposure to sunlight and insufficient consumption of Ca from foods. This topic, and others in this introductory chapter, are covered in greater detail in subsequent chapters.

VI. PHILOSOPHY OF THIS VOLUME

This volume takes a "life cycle" approach to issues of Ca and P homeostasis and the role of these nutrients in health and disease. As the preceding discussion shows, the potential for reducing the severity of osteoporosis as our population ages in the next few decades is greatest during the early part of the life cycle when peak bone mass is being attained. Lifelong attention to the proper maintenance of bone health through adequate nutrition is more likely to be effective than attempts to restore bone that has already been lost as a result of menopause or as a consequence of aging.

Chapter 2 continues the presentation of introductory information, discusses the availability of Ca and P in the diet (particularly the foods consumed by Americans), and shows how the availability, intake, and absorption of Ca and P impact on issues of health and maintenance of bone strength throughout the life cycle.

In Section I, the issues of Ca and P homeostasis are introduced (Chapter 3), and specific details of intestinal absorption (Chapter 4) and renal handling (Chapter 5) of Ca and P are discussed. In addition, the specific circumstances of intracellular Ca regulation are covered (Chapter 6).

In Section II, the structure and function of the skeletal (Chapter 7) and dental (Chapter 8) tissues are described. Special emphasis is given to the organic matrix of calcified tissue (Chapter 9) and to the markers of bone turnover (Chapter 10) that are of potential benefit for diagnostic and investigational purposes.

Section III contains specific information on the endocrine regulation of blood Ca and P by PTH (Chapter 11), vitamin D (Chapter 12), calcitonin (Chapter 13), and the estrogens and corticosteroids (Chapter 14).

In Section IV the changing demands on Ca and P metabolism across the life cycle are discussed from pregnancy (Chapter 15) and lactation (Chapter 16) through the remainder of life (Chapter 17). The special topics of the potential deleterious effects of alcohol on bone and Ca metabolism (Chapter 18) and the benefits of physical activity (Chapter 19) in promoting bone mass are covered. In the concluding chapter of this section the declining bone mass in the elderly population is highlighted (Chapter 20).

Osteoporosis is covered in Section V with chapters on osteoporosis and its treatment (Chapter 21) and on the worldwide epidemiology of this condition (Chapter 22).

The volume concludes with a summation (Chapter 23) of the topics included in this work. Brief discussions of critical gaps in our understanding of Ca and P metabolism are provided, and the critical roles of these minerals in the maintenance of skeletal integrity and overall health of individuals in our society are underscored.

GENERAL REFERENCES

1. **Avioli, L. V. (ed.),** *The Osteoporotic Syndrome: Detection, Prevention, and Treatment,* 3rd ed., Wiley-Liss, New York, 1993.
2. Committee on Diet and Health, Food and Nutrition Board, Commission of Life Sciences, National Research Council, *Diet and Health: Implications for Reducing Chronic Disease Risk,* National Academy Press, Washington, D.C., 1989.
3. **Favus, M. J. (ed.),** *Primer on the Metabolic Bone Diseases and Disorders of Mineral Metabolism,* 2nd ed., Raven Press, New York, 1993.
4. **Garn, S. M.,** The earlier gain and the later loss of cortical bone, In: *Nutritional Perspective,* Charles C Thomas, Springfield, IL, 1970.
5. **Marcus, R.,** *Osteoporosis,* Blackwell Scientific Publications, Boston, 1994.
6. **Nordin, B. E. C. (ed.),** *Calcium,* Springer-Verlag, New York, 1988.
7. **Riggs, B. L. and Melton, L. J., III (eds.),***Osteoporosis: Etiology, Diagnosis, and Management,* Raven Press, New York, 1988.
8. **Shils, M. E., Olson, J. A., and Shike, M. (eds.),** *Nutrition in Health and Disease,* 2 volumes, 8th ed., Lea and Febiger, Philadelphia, 1994.
9. Subcommittee on Dietary Allowances, Food and Nutrition Board, Commission on Life Sciences, U.S. Dept. of Health and Human Services, PHS, Washington, D.C., National Research Council, *Recommended Dietary Allowances,* 10th ed., National Academy Press, Washington, D. C., 1989.
10. *Surgeon General's Report on Nutrition and Health,* U.S. Government Printing Office, 1988.
11. U.S. Department of Health and Human Services, PHS, *Healthy People 2000: National Health Promotion and Disease Prevention Objectives,* HHS Publication No. (PHS) 91-50213, U.S. Government Printing Office, Washington, D.C., 1990.

REFERENCE

1. **Schneider, E. L. and Guralnik, J. M.,** The aging of America, *J. Am. Med. Assoc.,* 263, 2335, 1990.

Chapter 2

DIETARY ISSUES OF CALCIUM AND PHOSPHORUS

John J. B. Anderson, Ph.D. and Sanford C. Garner, Ph.D.

TABLE OF CONTENTS

I. INTRODUCTION

Calcium (Ca) and phosphorus (P) are discussed together in dietary terms because of their coexistence in dairy foods. In addition, Ca and P, in the form of phosphate ion (Pi), function together as the inorganic mineral component of bone and other calcified tissues, and their plasma and extracellular fluid concentrations are regulated through bone, kidney, and intestines by a common set of hormonal mechanisms (see Chapter 4). Dietary recommendations (RDAs) have traditionally stressed an equivalence in consumption of these two nutrients. The presence of significant amounts of P in almost all foods, however, reduces the ratio of Ca to P (Ca:P) to less than 1 when considering all foods consumed.

Recently, as the prevalence of osteoporosis increases with the aging of the American population, greater attention has been focused on the role of lifelong Ca intakes in development and prevention

0-8493-7845-1/95/$0.00+$.50

TABLE 1
Female RDAs for Calcium, Phosphorus, and Vitamin D through the Lifecycle

Age Years	Calcium mg	Phosphorus mg	Vitamin D µg
0–0.5	400	300	7.5
0.5–1.0	600	500	10
1–10	800	800	10
11–24	1200	1200	10
25–50	800	800	5
51+	800	800	5
Pregnancy	1200	1200	10
Lactation	1200	1200	10

Recommended Dietary Allowances, (10th edition, 1989).[31]

of this condition. However, decreased consumption of dairy products by many teenagers and young adults, coupled with the increasing prevalence of Pi-containing additives in food preparation along with the common substitution of Pi-containing carbonated drinks for milk, is shifting the ratio of Ca to P in the diet even farther away from unity. This common pattern of low Ca intake coupled with high P consumption has critical implications for Ca availability during periods of bone consolidation because of the potential long-term detrimental effect of high P on parathyroid hormone (PTH) secretion (see Chapter 11). (Vitamin D, an important nutrient for Ca absorption, will be covered in Chapter 12.)

II. CALCIUM AS A NUTRIENT

Ca, a mineral required by the body for a variety of physiological functions and for the maintenance of bone tissues throughout life, needs to be consumed in adequate amounts each day, preferably from foods rather than supplements (*Foods First, Supplements Second*). The best available estimates of daily amounts needed by males and females, according to age or state of pregnancy and lactation, have been provided in the Recommended Dietary Allowances, or RDAs (see Table 1). Implicit in setting the RDAs is an understanding that the adult RDAs for Ca and other nutrients consist of two components: (1) a basic requirement of approximately 550 mg per day, and (2) a safety factor of approximately 250 mg per day, which should ensure that almost 100% (actually an estimated 97.5%) of the adult population should satisfy their requirements. (Allowances for males and females are estimated in the same way, so that no differences exist in RDAs according to gender). Males, however, are more likely to have higher requirements than females because of greater average body size and skeletal mass.[1] For example, the average adult male skeleton contains 1200 g of Ca compared to 900 g for a female. The adult RDAs are set as follows: 800 mg per day for those over age 24, and 1200 mg per day for those between 19 and 24. RDAs for infants, children, adolescents, and adults, along with P and vitamin D RDAs, are given in Table 1.

The Ca RDAs during pregnancy and lactation are now set at 1200 mg per day, with no additional increment for adolescent girls and young adult women (younger than 25 years of age). Females who do not have an adequate Ca intake during lactation, however, can lose significant amounts of bone mass for use in milk production, i.e., Ca and P content, which will not be replaced unless the females eat high-Ca foods or take supplements. Research data are now supporting the importance of consuming adequate amounts of Ca during these critical reproductive periods of life.

Ca behaves as a "threshold nutrient" because of its limited absorption at high dietary intake (see Figure 1). This phenomenon has long been established for agricultural and experimental animals, but it has only recently been described for humans.[2] In essence, high intakes of Ca yield little

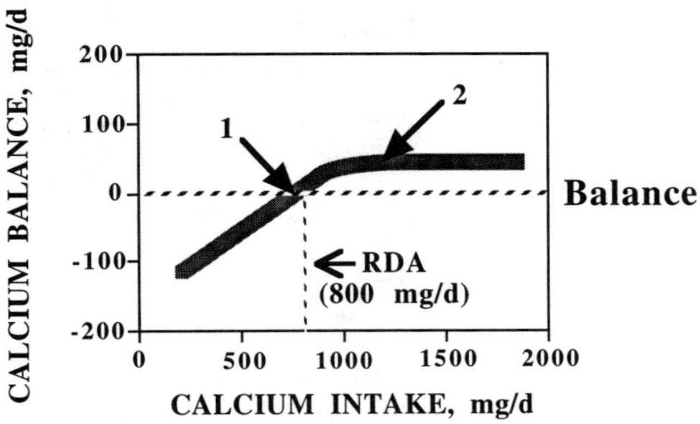

FIGURE 1. Calcium as a "Threshold Nutrient." As daily Ca intake increases, Ca balance increases until output equals input (1). Further increases in Ca intake result in positive balance, but eventually, Ca intakes reaches a level at which no further increase in balance is seen (2), i.e., the "threshold" level for Ca consumption. (Based on data from Matkovic and Heaney.[2])

additional absorption of Ca ions beyond a threshold value. In the example given in Figure 1 for young adult females, an intake of approximately 700 mg per day provides for a positive Ca balance, and no further increase in Ca balance is achieved above approximately 1000 mg per day.

III. PHOSPHORUS AS A NUTRIENT

Phosphorus is also an essential nutrient that must be consumed in amounts that support both extracellular and cellular functions, but which are not so excessive compared to Ca as to adversely alter the Ca homeostatic mechanisms. Too much dietary P relative to Ca contributes to persistent losses of Ca, which over an extended period of time must negatively affect bone mass. The mechanism for this loss relates to a persistently elevated PTH concentration in blood (see following). Thus, an abnormally high P intake may decrease bone mass and increase the risk of osteoporosis-associated fractures.

In contrast to Ca, P is present in nearly all foods in good amounts, especially in food from animal sources, so that a deficiency is difficult to produce. Thus, little nutritional concern exists for P. The RDAs for P across the life cycle are identical to those for Ca. In practice adult dietary Ca:P ratios range between 1:1.3 and 1:2. Thus, a healthy adult intake pattern would contain approximately 800 mg Ca and 1150 mg P. The Ca and P contents and Ca:P ratios of common food items are shown in Table 2.

The RDAs for P have been set the same as those for Ca since the first edition of the U.S. RDA was published in the early 1940s. No rationale for the P RDA has been provided by the RDA committees for the last 50 years. Information on typical intakes of P by Americans over the last few decades shows that the mean amounts of dietary P always exceed mean Ca intakes in adult eating patterns. Furthermore, the mean intake of P by males is always greater than that of females. Thus, when compared to mean Ca intakes, the Ca:P ratios never reach 1:1, as predicated by the RDAs. Also, females tend to have lower Ca:P ratios than males at all adult stages of the life cycle. The RDAs of P probably need to be based on the significant difference in body size between the genders, especially the lean compartment of body composition that distinguishes the two sexes. Similarly, the RDAs for Ca should also be specifically set for each sex because of threshold differences in the Ca balance for each sex.

For these reasons, the P RDAs are unrealistically set and thus serve little purpose. In fact they have been ignored by nutritionists since the inception of the RDAs. The Ca RDAs are much more appropriately set. Therefore, the recommendations regarding P should be based on the typical consumption patterns of Ca, so that the Ca:P ratio remains in the healthy range of about 1:1.2 to 1:1.4. These ratios are consumed by the healthiest adult populations, whose measurements of bone mass or density have been found typically to be the highest.

TABLE 2
Calcium and Phosphorus Composition of Selected Foods in Standard Portion Sizes

Source:	Calcium mg/serving	Phosphorus mg/serving	Ca:P Ratio
Baked Goods			
White bread, 1 slice	35	30	1:0.9
Whole wheat, 1 slice	20	74	1:3.7
English muffin, 1	96	67	1:0.7
Pancake, plain, 1	27	71	1:2.6
Waffle, frozen, 1	29	134	1:4.6
Toaster type pastry, 1	104	104	1:1
Hamburger bun, 1	61	50	1:0.8
Yellow cake, chocolate frosting, 1/16th cake	63	122	1:1.9
Dairy and Dairy Products			
American processed cheese, 1 oz	174	211	1:1.2
Cheddar cheese, 1 oz	204	146	1:0.7
Cottage cheese, 1% fat, 1 C	138	302	1:2.2
Mozzarella, part skim, 1 oz	207	149	1:0.7
Skim milk, 1 c	302	247	1:0.8
Whole milk, 1 c	291	228	1:0.8
Evaporated skim milk, 1 c	738	497	1:0.7
Vanilla ice cream, regular 1 c	176	134	1:0.8
Ice milk, regular hard, 1 c	176	129	1:0.7
Chocolate pudding, canned, 5 oz	74	117	1:1.6
Yogurt, plain, 1 c	415	326	1:0.8
Egg, whole, raw, 1	25	86	1:3.4
Egg substitute, frozen, 1/4 c	43	43	1:1
Fruit			
Apple, 2.75″ diam, with peel, 1	10	10	1:1
Banana, 1	7	22	1:3.1
Grapefruit, 1/2 pink, 1	13	11	1:0.8
Orange, 1	52	18	1:0.3
Strawberries, fresh, 1 c	21	28	1:1.3
Grains			
Oatmeal, regular, 1/2 c	9	89	1:9.9
Grits, 1/2 c	0	15	0
Corn flour, 1 c	8	318	1:40
Egg noodles, enriched, cooked, 1/2 c	10	55	1:5.5
Wheat germ, toasted, 1/4 c	13	324	1:24.9
Flour, all purpose, white, 1 c		135	1:7.1
Meats, Fish, Poultry			
Perch, baked, 3.5 oz	137	277	1:2.0
Tuna, water pack, 3 oz	10	103	1:10.3
Ground beef, cooked, regular, 3 oz	8	135	1:16.9
T-bone steak, cooked, 3 oz	7	150	1:21.4
Pork chop, center loin, broiled, 1	8	184	1:23
Chicken, drumstick, roasted, 1	13	81	1:6.2
Turkey, roasted, white meat, 3 oz	16	186	1:11.6
Frankfurter, beef and pork, 1	6	49	1:8.2
Vegetables			
Baked beans, canned, vegetarian, 1/2 c	64	132	1:2.1
Green beans, cooked from frozen, 1/2 c	30	16	1:0.5
Broccoli, cooked from frozen, 1/2 c	47	50	1:1.1
Carrots, raw, 1	19	32	1:1.7
Corn, cooked from frozen, 1/2 c	2	39	1:19.5
Peas, green, cooked/frozen, 1/2 c	19	72	1:3.8
Potatoes, baked, flesh and skin, 1	21	115	1:5.5
Sweet potatoes, baked, 1	32	63	1:2.0
Tomatoes, fresh, whole, 1	6	30	1:5.0

Data are taken from Hands.[20]

IV. CALCIUM INTAKES BY AMERICANS

The concern for obtaining sufficient amounts of Ca in the diet is for both the maintenance of the skeleton as a functional reserve of essential minerals, including Ca, Pi, Mg, and others, and as a source of Ca ions (Ca^{++}) for various cellular activities. A cup (8 oz) of milk of any kind, including skim milk, provides approximately 290 mg of Ca. This value is the standard to which other foods are compared.

A. CALCIUM FROM FOODS

Consistency of Ca intake every day at a level approaching or meeting the RDA should satisfy the requirements for this essential element for an estimated 97.5% of the population. Long-term or lifetime consumption at the gender- and age-specific RDAs can best be accomplished by eating the recommended number of servings of foods rich in Ca every day. If adequate Ca cannot be met from the consumption of foods, then supplements will be needed to bring the daily intake up to the RDA. Foods are recommended as the first approach to meeting daily needs because foods provide many nutrients, and often non-nutrients, in addition to Ca (see Figure 2).

Ca is found in relatively few foods in the amounts needed to meet age-specific RDAs (see Table 1). The majority of Ca in the American diet is contributed by food groups including milk and other dairy products (except butter), breads and baked goods that use Ca in processing, dark green leafy vegetables (except spinach, which contains Ca-binding oxalates), fortified orange juices, and a few other foods (see Figure 3 & Table 2). Mixed food dishes containing cheese or milk solids are usually also good sources of Ca (see Figure 2). Examples of mixed foods include cheese casseroles and pizza. In addition to providing Ca, dark green vegetables are also sources rich in non-nutrients, such as dietary fiber. Low-fat milk and yogurt contain not only Ca, but also P, vitamin D, protein, and several other essential micronutrients in good amounts.

The RDAs for Ca are now considered to be somewhat underestimated with respect to young girls between 6 and 11 years of age, and they are probably set too high for young adult women between ages 19 and 25. The explanations for these statements relate to the earlier prepubertal skeletal development and, hence, incorporation of Ca by girls than in previous generations, and the threshold behavior of Ca at any age of the lifecycle.[2] The result of these two facts is that many females fail to incorporate enough Ca in their daily eating habits.

B. CALCIUM FROM SUPPLEMENTS

Many health providers recommend Ca supplementation as a method for counterbalancing low intakes of the nutrient in individual diets; however, several points need to be considered about Ca supplementation and the effect it may have on the nutritional status of girls and young adult women.

First, a three-year longitudinal study of pubertal twins failed to demonstrate a positive association between increased Ca supplementation and bone measurement values. Healthy pubertal boys and girls consuming Ca at less than the RDA had almost identical bone measurement values after three years as those receiving Ca at approximately 180% of the age-specific RDA.[3] Secondly, the Ca intake of an individual must be considered in relation to the total diet, including several micronutrients closely linked to Ca, such as P, magnesium, trace minerals, riboflavin, and vitamin D, as well as fat and other macronutrients. The usage of Ca supplements as a major contributor of Ca tends to diminish the importance of foods supplying Ca and the other nutrients just mentioned, as well as the non-nutrient molecules found in plant foods. Several investigators have shown that adequate Ca intakes from dairy foods correlate well with the provision of healthy amounts of most other nutrients.[4] Thus, foods supply a broad range of nutrients in reasonable amounts that are difficult to duplicate with supplements. For this reason, food fortification with Ca in small amounts (100–250 mg) per serving to improve the intakes of typically low-Ca consumers may be a better approach than supplementation of the diet with a single nutrient.[5]

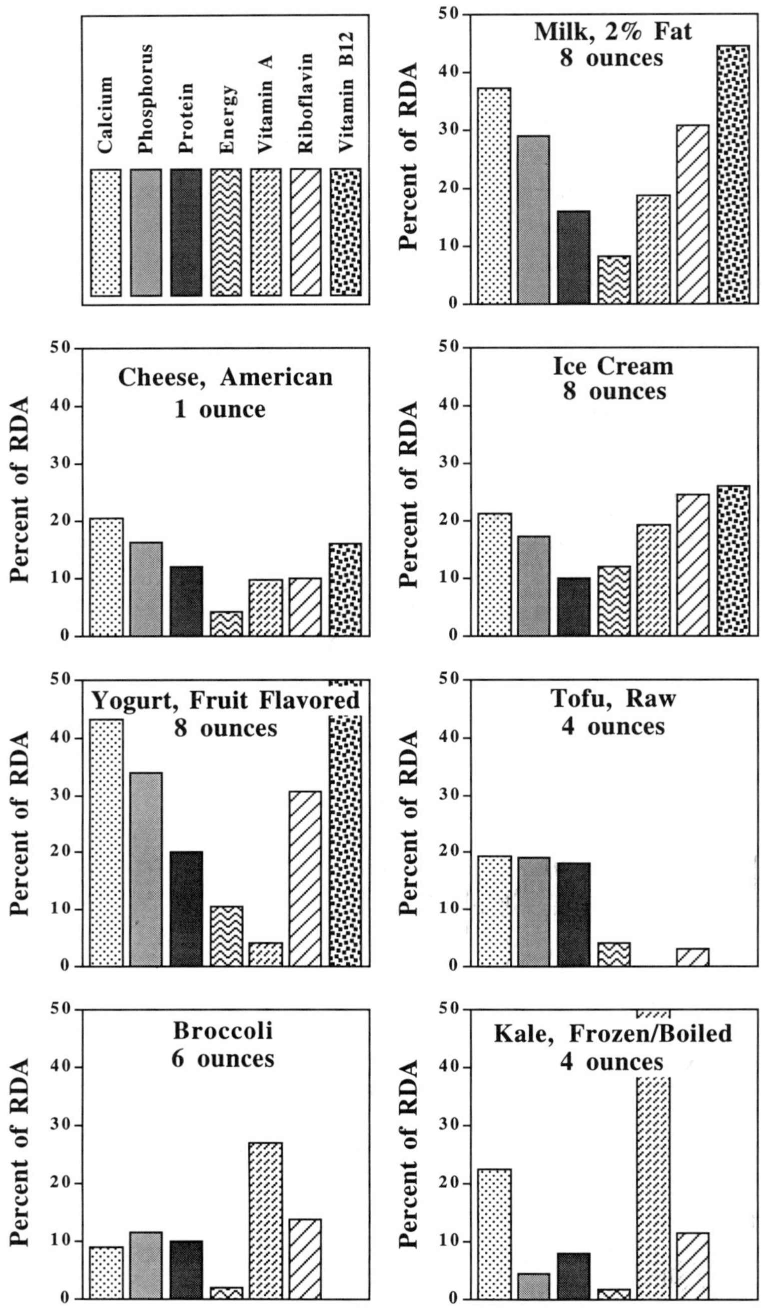

FIGURE 2. (A & B): Contribution of a Serving of a Representative Sample of Food Items to Daily Calcium Intake. All RDAs are based on recommended levels for women 25 years and older. The RDAs/RDIs are as follows: calcium = 800 mg; phosphorus = 800 mg; protein = 50 g; energy = 2000 kcal; vitamin A = 800 RE; riboflavin = 1.3 mg; and vitamin B_{12} = 2 µg. (Data are taken from Smolin and Grosvenor.[32])

If supplements need to be taken to assure that RDA amounts of Ca are consumed each day, the specific supplement must be readily dissolved in the stomach so that absorption of the Ca by the small intestine can occur efficiently. Some supplements in the past have been found to dissolve poorly, which means that the Ca they contain is not bioavailable in the gastrointestinal tract. Some Ca supplements have been found to be highly unavailable because of the compacting technique used to make the pills.

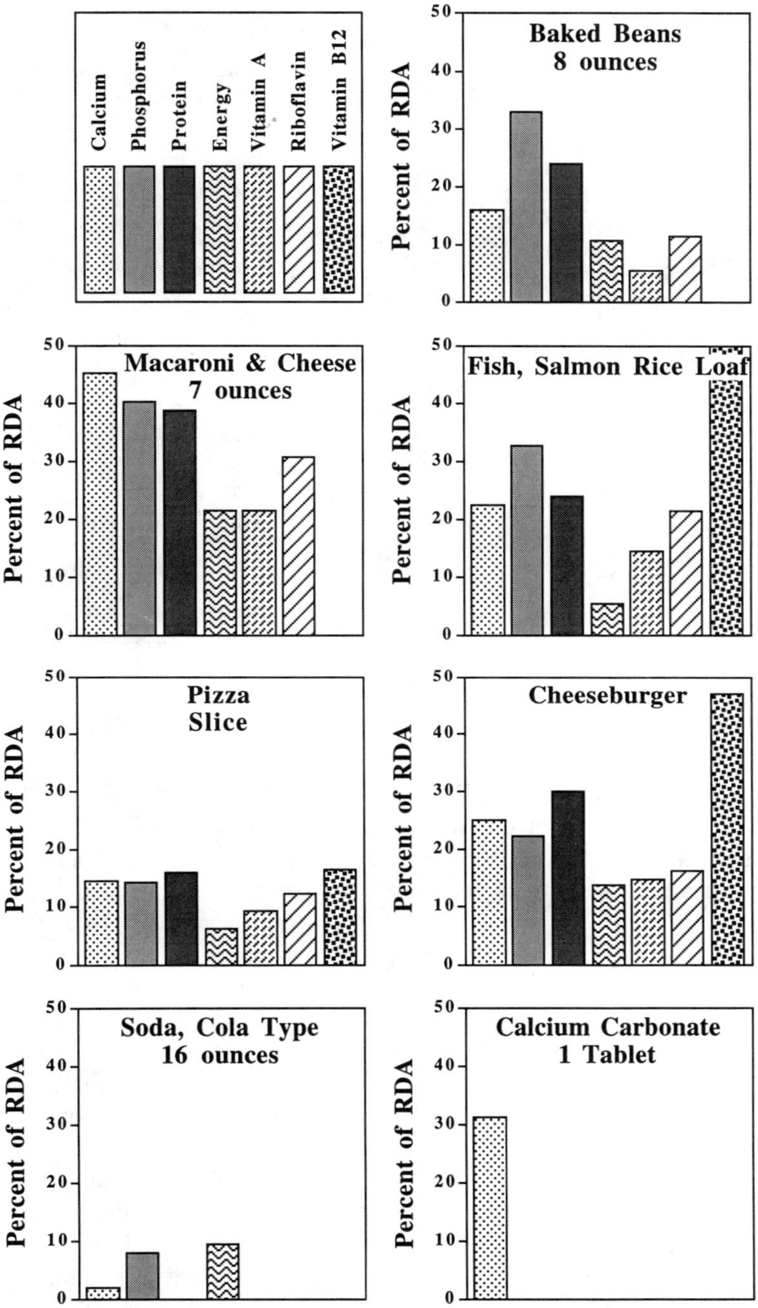

FIGURE 2B.

The Ca supplements with the highest bioavailability are Ca citrate malate (CCM), Ca citrate, and Ca lactate. However, the weight of the anion portion of these compounds requires a much larger supplement pill to provide a given amount of Ca compared to Ca carbonate (see Figure 4). Ca phosphate supplements have been administered in some clinical research studies.

Research on Ca-nutrient interactions has not been extensive. A few studies of Ca:Fe and Ca:Zn interactions at high Ca intake levels suggest that Ca may depress the absorption of divalent mineral cations. Further work is needed to establish any major adverse effect of Ca supplementation on the absorption of other minerals.

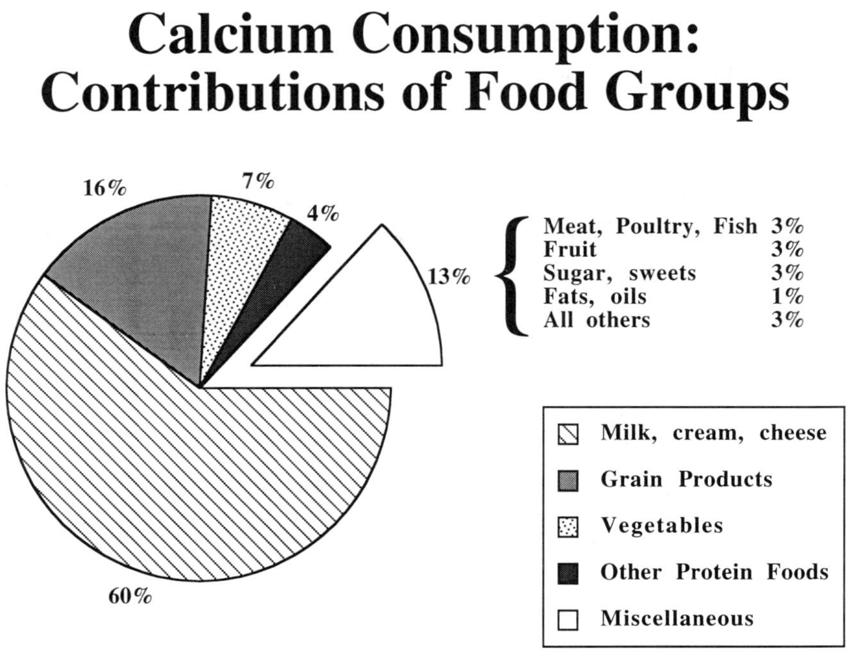

FIGURE 3. Contributions of Food Groups to Calcium Consumption. (Data taken from the USDA data for U.S. food supply historical series and 1955, 1965, and 1977–78 food consumption surveys.[33])

C. INTESTINAL ABSORPTION AND BIOAVAILABILITY OF CALCIUM

Bioavailability refers to the chemical state of Ca within the luminal contents of the small intestine; if too much Ca, as Ca ions, is bound to oxalates or other anions that precipitate Ca in the gut, then much of the Ca will not be bioavailable. Only oxalates and a few other anions have a significant adverse impact on Ca bioavailability. In general, Ca is readily bioavailable from nearly all foods, with the exceptions of oxalate-rich spinach and rhubarb (see Chapter 4).

Ca absorption from nearly all foods (including plants and milk products) and supplements occurs at an almost identical efficiency in adults and, presumably, in children and adolescents, even though age-related differences in absorption efficiency exist. Adult absorption efficiencies from foods and supplements average 30 to 32%, but from CCM complexes used in fortifying orange juices, the average absorption efficiency is closer to 35%. The reason for the enhanced absorption with CCM has not been established. Ca absorption occurs by the following two routes (see Chapter 4): (1) a transcellular pathway requiring active transport at the basolateral membrane, which is enhanced by the vitamin D hormone, i.e., 1,25-dihydroxyvitamin D, and (2) a paracellular passive route, which operates primarily in the ileum. The paracellular Ca entry, which is not dependent on vitamin D, may allow greater absorption of Ca from CCM, but the mechanism has not been established. Large doses of Ca supplements can effectively "push" quantitatively more Ca across the gut barrier by this passive route, but at a low efficiency. Thus, the modest increase in absolute amounts of absorbed Ca are not likely to be toxic.

Finally, Ca intakes need to be high enough to counterbalance the potentially negative effects of the high amounts of P that are consumed in the diets of virtually everyone in the U.S., and the presumed adverse effects of excessive intakes of protein by practically all omnivorous Americans. Because of the generally high bioavailability and, therefore, absorption of P as Pi, the serum concentration of this element rises quite rapidly following the ingestion of food. The serum Pi concentration peaks at approximately 1 hour, and the rise in Pi over this brief period has a modest Ca-lowering effect because of the action of calcitonin on osteoclasts.[6] Thus, the declines of the serum concentrations of each mineral following the intake of food result from their transfer into

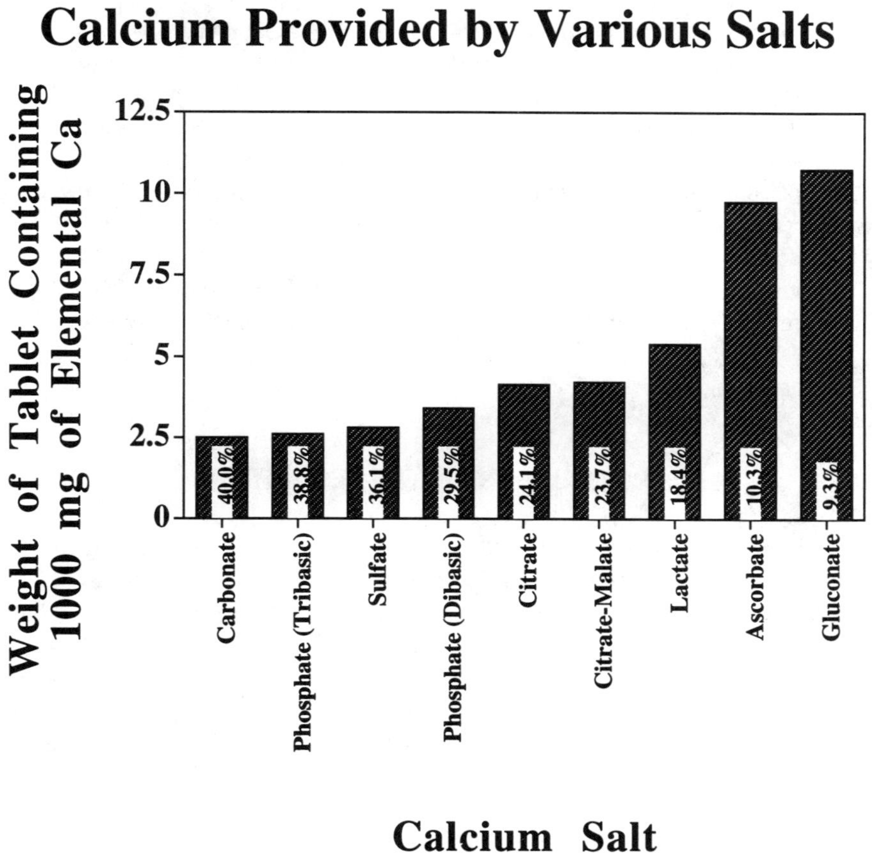

FIGURE 4. Amount of Elemental Calcium Provided by Various Salts. The weight of a tablet containing 1000 mg of elemental Ca is indicated by the height of the bar above each salt. The percentage of Ca by weight is shown in the label at the base of each bar.

bone. The return of Pi to its premeal fasting level occurs within 2–3 hours. The depression of serum Ca following a meal stimulates parathyroid hormone (PTH) secretion. A few reports have shown that low-Ca and high-P diets fed to women for several weeks led to persistently elevated PTH levels in the blood, which presumably remove mineral from bone,[4,7] Calvo[8] has put forth convincing evidence that the current consumption of P by Americans may be underestimated because of the increased addition of phosphates to processed foods, especially to carbonated beverages, and the preference of the American population for these foods and drinks.

The adverse effects of high-protein intakes on Ca retention have been known for several decades. High-protein intakes may contribute to low bone mass through mechanisms that increase urinary losses of Ca. Only in recent years has it been suggested that regular protein consumption at high levels may negatively impact on bone mineral density and potentially contribute to increased fracture rates of the hip.[9] The acute and short-term effects of protein in increasing urinary Ca losses in human subjects have been demonstrated under diverse experimental conditions.[10-14] Many of the human studies have been re-analyzed in a type of meta-analysis by Kerstetter and Allen,[15] who concluded that, with the exception of one report, all investigations showed adverse effects of high-protein intakes on Ca through hypercalciuria. Human experimental evidence using a long-term prospective design has not yet shown that excessive dietary protein leads to osteopenia and osteoporotic fractures.[16] Because such long-term experimental human investigations with sufficient statistical power are not likely to be undertaken in the future, data from observational epidemiologic studies must be utilized in trying to determine the magnitude of the effect of protein-rich diets, if any, on bone mineral density. A report on the effects of high-protein intakes in young adult women suggests that this protein consumption pattern does contribute to lower bone measurements.[17]

D. CALCIUM TOXICITY

The upper level of Ca intake that produces toxic symptoms has not been well documented, but 2000–3000 mg of additional Ca as supplements may be toxic or contribute to kidney stones. FDA documents state that a total of 2500 mg of Ca per day is the toxic level, beyond which safety cannot be assured. In fact, however, no increase in the incidence of renal stones has been reported since the use of Ca supplements accelerated after the 1984 NIH Consensus Conference on Osteoporosis. Although supplemental Ca has not been shown to affect bone mass appreciably in several prospective trials,[3,18] the limited toxicity of this nutrient suggests that supplemental Ca is generally safe. Little concern about toxic effects of Ca exists, but some concern remains about Ca interactions with other minerals.

V. PHOSPHORUS INTAKES BY AMERICANS

Because of the wide availability of P in foods, it is easy to ingest large amounts of P, which is quite different from the limited distribution of Ca among the basic food groups. Most foods in all food groups contain plentiful amounts of P. Extra P from cola-type soft drinks (including the diet cola drinks) and from food additives adds to the high intake of P from unprocessed foods in the diet without providing sufficient Ca. As a result a dietary imbalance between Ca and P may occur. An optimal dietary ratio of Ca to P for adults ranges from 1:1 to 1:2 with a value of 1:1.4 being good. Adults who consume little milk or other dairy products have ratios that exceed 1:2 and may even approximate 1:4.

A. PHOSPHORUS FROM FOODS

All food groups, including miscellaneous foods, contribute P to the diet, since P occurs naturally in all cells. Milk products, meat products, and grains contribute approximately 80% of the P consumed by Americans of all ages[19] (see Figure 5). Infants, by nature of their diet have a greater percentage of their P intake from milk and milk products (66%).[19] Table 2 illustrates both the Ca and P composition and the Ca-to-P (Ca:P) ratio of selected foods from the basic food groups.[20] Except for most dairy products and a very few other foods, the Ca:P ratio varies greatly from 1:1.

The typical consumption patterns of P in the American population have been documented in national surveys, but the relationship of Ca to P in typical diets has been examined only cursorily. Greger and Krystofiak summarized the data on P intake of Americans from three different surveys. Whereas the surveys differed in the estimates of the quantities of P consumed by Americans, when expressed as ratios, the figure comes to about 450–620 mg/1000 kilocalories, 15 mg/g protein or 1.5–1.6 mg P/mg Ca.[19]

The United States Department of Health and Human Services (USDHHS) reported that the P intake of the U.S. population is adequate and averaged 136% of the Recommended Dietary Allowances (RDA).[21] Children under 1 year of age consumed the most P daily while females 9–18 years consumed the lowest amount. Males consumed more than females, individuals above the poverty level consumed more than those below the poverty level, and the white population group consumed more than the black population group.

Also of concern today is the accuracy of the data on P consumption that has been reported in the past because of the large increase in the ingestion of processed foods. Comparison of estimated amounts (either hand or computer calculations from nutrient composition tables) of P to chemical analyses of P contents of foods taken from daily menus demonstrated significant underestimation of P content by indirect methods. Estimates from composition tables were lower than the chemical analyses, i. e., actual intakes of P, by 250–350 mg/day, depending on the amount of processed, convenience, or restaurant food actually consumed.[22] Other investigators estimated that P intakes

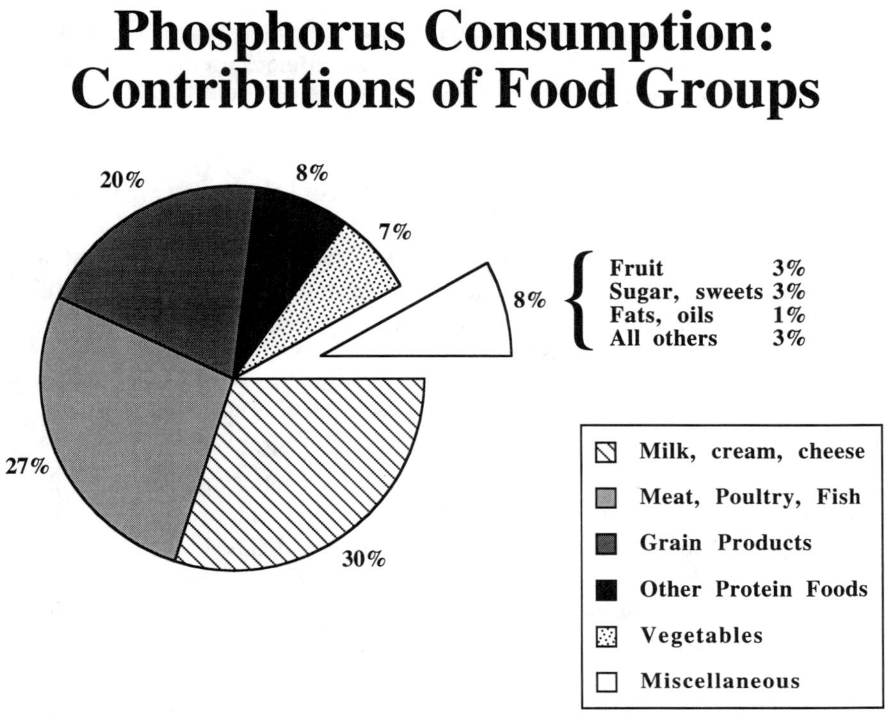

FIGURE 5. Contributions of Food Groups to Phosphorus Consumption. (Data taken from the USDA data for U.S. food supply historical series and 1955, 1965, and 1977–78 food consumption surveys.[33])

could be as great as 2.5 times the RDA for individuals who preferred processed or convenience foods (Bell, et al.[22a]). Such intakes would result in Ca:P ratios of 1:3 to 1:4 and contribute to elevated PTH levels as shown by Calvo et al.[7] Concern has been raised about the high intakes of P by Americans, because of its potential induction of secondary hyperparathyroidism.

Another contribution to the total intake of P is the use of carbonated beverages, which has increased over the last 20 years. Since dairy foods contribute significantly to the consumption of both Ca and P, soft drink consumption could directly affect Ca:P balance by replacing milk as a beverage. Phosphoric acid is used as an acidulent and flavoring agent for all colas and some root beers. Colas, both regular and diet, contain P in varying amounts from 44 to 70 mg per 12 oz serving.[23] This information is important when you consider the increased use of carbonated beverages among the U.S. population. Most carbonated beverages are consumed by individuals between the ages of 19 and 44 years.[24] Nineteen to 24-year-old men consume the most regular soft drinks (13.0 ± 12.1 oz daily), whereas women aged 35 to 44 consume the most diet soft drinks (9.5 ± 12.2 oz daily).

The ready supply of phosphorus from foods coupled with the generally high bioavailability of P makes it highly unlikely that a deficiency will occur. Therefore, P supplements are not recommended for the general population. However, for individuals with chronic gastrointestinal problems necessitating the use of antacids, P can be bound and rendered unavailable by aluminum hydroxide antacids causing secondary P depletion.[25]

B. PHOSPHORUS FROM PHOSPHATE ADDITIVES

The different types of phosphate food additives used by industry to enhance food quality or other properties amounts to over an estimated 400 mg per person per day,[19] and this staggering quantity may be an underestimation. Recent data from the International Food Additive Council suggest that Americans may actually be ingesting significantly greater amounts, perhaps as much as 500 mg per day,[26] but laboratory analyses of the phosphate content of foods with these intentional additives have not been made available to nutrition researchers. Better and more up-to-date measurements are needed of the American food supply that is consumed by individuals, not simply disappearance data, before truly good estimates of P intakes are available.

C. INTESTINAL ABSORPTION AND BIOAVAILABILITY OF PHOSPHORUS

Although both organic and inorganic forms of P are widely distributed in foods, 75% or so of the P in foods is converted to inorganic P (Pi) following the various digestive steps in the stomach and upper small intestine. The organic P usually remains associated with the fat-soluble dietary molecules that are absorbed without digestion of the phosphate groups from these molecules, such as is the case with phosphatidylcholine (lecithin).

The net absorption of Pi is highly efficient; and the Pi efficiency is more than twice that of Ca absorption, which is usually stated as being between 25% and 30% in adults. The efficiency of Pi absorption by infants has been reported to be as high as 80–90%. Typical meals that contain representative items from all food groups, including dairy, have ratios of Ca:P approaching 1:1.4 to 1:1. If the actual amount of Ca in the meal is 350 mg and the amount of P is 500 mg, then 75% of the P, or 375 mg is absorbed, most of it within the first postprandial hour, but only 30% or 105 mg of Ca is absorbed, and this process usually takes several hours to be completed.[6]

The bioavailability of P is generally high from typical American diets, but it is apparently adversely affected both by high phytate consumption from whole grains and legumes and by phosphate additives in processed foods.[27] The P absorption efficiencies of adults range between 50 and 70%, depending on other dietary factors, but they are always much higher than the absorption efficiencies of Ca. In fact, there appears to be a proportionality between the absorption of these two macrominerals. When P absorption is low, Ca absorption is also reduced, according to analyses of balance studies made by Franz. Therefore, high P intakes from a diet containing large amounts of foods processed with phosphates are likely to depress Ca absorption because of lowered bioavailability.

The mechanism for the reduced bioavailability of each mineral in human experiments examining high phosphate intakes is presumed to be the formation of ionic complexes in the gut luminal fluid, because stool content of P under these conditions is considerably elevated, as is Ca content of feces in these studies.[28]

D. ALTERATIONS OF CALCIUM HOMEOSTASIS BY HIGH PHOSPHORUS INTAKES

The experimental observation of abnormally altered Ca homeostasis, and the sequela of bone mineral loss as a result of high P intake compared to Ca has been known for almost 40 years. Research on laboratory animal models and farm animals by many different investigators has shown that low Ca:P ratios in the dietary rations fed to these animals produced enlargements of the parathyroid glands, low serum Ca and elevated serum Pi concentrations, and loss of bone mineral mass. The greater the reduction in Ca, i.e., lower Ca:P ratio, the more serious the effects. When assays for parathyroid hormone (PTH) became more sensitive and accurate, significant elevations in PTH also were documented, as were increased concentrations of the hormonal form of vitamin D, i.e., 1,25-dihydroxyvitamin D.

Human experimental observations on this diet-induced secondary hyperparathyroidism have been reported only in recent years. Calvo and co-workers[7] have reported that consumption of a diet containing a low Ca:P ratio (1:4) for a month led to persistent elevation of serum PTH concentrations compared to the same subjects on a diet with a normal Ca:P ratio. These investigations of healthy young adult women suggest that nutritional secondary hyperparathyroidism may be a more serious problem than previously recognized.

Cross-sectional human observations that examined the associations between dietary P intake and bone measurements of the radius in young adult women by regression analyses have also demonstrated an adverse effect of high P intakes on bone mineral content and density at both the distal (wrist) and mid-shaft sites, which represent more trabecular and more cortical bone tissue, respectively. In the study of Metz and colleagues from our laboratory,[17] the consistent adverse effect of high P was found when the Ca:P ratio of the diet fell below 0.5 (1:2), i.e., in the lower 50% of the females who were consuming approximately 50–65% of their age-specific RDA.

In summary, the overall meaning of these diverse experimental observations adds up to a consensus that too much P in the diet relative to Ca will increase the loss of bone from the skeleton and contribute to low bone mass (osteopenia) at some later time in life, which predisposes individuals to osteoporotic fractures. Only longitudinal studies on the order of decades are lacking to provide the final conclusive evidence of the adverse effects of nutritional secondary hyperparathyroidism.

VI. INTERACTIONS OF CALCIUM AND PHOSPHORUS WITH VITAMIN D

Three potential interactions among these nutrients may occur. Each of these interactions could be of major significance for the conservation of Ca when typical dietary intakes of Ca are not adequate to meet physiological needs. In general, the influence of vitamin D (really its hormonal form, 1,25-$(OH)_2D$) on both minerals is positive when vitamin D intakes are not excessive (See Chapter 12 for toxic effects of excessive vitamin D intakes). For example, vitamin D enhances the intestinal absorption of both Ca and P, but presumably this vitamin-D-mediated intestinal absorption has its maximal effect only at low dietary levels and, conversely, benefits little when intakes of Ca are adequate, i. e., approximately at RDA amounts. Vitamin D at normal intakes also has limited effects on bone metabolism, but the presence of normal circulating concentrations of 1,25-$(OH)_2D$ apparently favors bone formation. At the kidney, normal serum concentrations of vitamin D may enhance Ca reabsorption by renal tubules and thereby conserve Ca in the body, but this effect is not well substantiated (see Chapter 5). If vitamin D has an effect on P retention or excretion at the renal level, it has not been adequately documented. Finally, the hormonal form of vitamin D may enhance Ca transfer across the placenta for fetal skeletal development.

In summary, the action of the hormonal metabolite of vitamin D at normal circulating concentrations tends to support the retention, i.e., conservation, of both Ca and P. High vitamin D intakes over extended periods, however, can have adverse effects on Ca metabolism, as can inadequate intakes of this essential fat-soluble vitamin. Inadequate intakes of vitamin D may have little or no adverse effects if dietary Ca and P are sufficient, but if both Ca and vitamin D intakes are well below RDAs, then rachitic symptoms are likely to occur. Rickets typically results from low Ca intakes coupled with a deficiency of both dietary and skin biosynthesized vitamin D. Typical vitamin D contents of foods are listed in Table 3.

VII. CALCIUM AND PEAK BONE MASS DEVELOPMENT

On average, bone growth in length ceases by age 18 in females and by age 22 in males, but bone consolidation, i.e., mineral accumulation at all skeletal sites, continues for approximately five or more additional years. Thus, peak bone mass, i.e., the maximal amount of bone mass accrued in the skeleton, is attained by age 35 (see Chapter 17 for additional discussion of peak bone mass). After that time bone mass remains fairly constant, although a slight decline in bone mass from the age of 35 to the time of menopause occurs in most women. At menopause, the rate of bone loss substantially increases in almost all women unless they receive estrogen replacement therapy. The rate of loss for the immediate decade following menopause ranges from 1 to 2% per year. For the high losers, the loss can amount to 20% of their skeletal mass existent at the start of menopause. If these same women had developed a low peak bone mass by the middle of their third decade of life, they would be, in general, at an even greater risk for fractures.

The benefit of Ca intakes at or closely approximating the age-specific RDAs for women during adolescence and early adulthood is that these women can optimize their peak bone mass. Regular

TABLE 3
Vitamin D Content of Foods

Food	Serving Size	Vitamin D, IU/svg.
Cheese and Cheese Products		
American cheese food	1 oz (28 g)	8
Cheddar	1 oz (28 g)	3
Cheese Whiz	1 oz (28 g)	1
Cottage (all)	1 cup (226 g)	5
Cream cheese	1 oz (28 g)	2
Swiss	1 oz (28 g)	28
Cream, Dairy		
Sweet, heavy, fluid	1 T (15 g)	15
Sweet, light, fluid	1 T (15 g)	8
Sour cream	1 T (15 g)	1
Milk:		
Fluid (cow):		
All milks, fortified	1 c (244 g)	100
Canned, evaporated	1/2 c (126 g)	110
Goat milk	1 c (244 g)	5
Human milk	1 c (244 g)	1–24
Milk Desserts:		
Pudding, prepared	1/2 c (130 g)	50
Eggs (Vitamin D is in yolk)		
Cooked, whole egg	1 (50 g)	23
Raw, whole egg	1 (50 g)	27
Fats and Spreads		
Butter	1 tsp (4.7 g)	1.4
Cod liver oil	1 tsp (4.7 g)	400
Margarine	1 tsp (4.7 g)	15
Fish and Shellfish		
Eel, smoked	1 oz (28 g)	1814
Herring, raw	1 oz (28 g)	255
Oysters, raw, medium	4 (57 g)	2.9
Salmon, Atlantic, canned	1 oz (28 g)	142
Sardines, canned	1 oz (28 g)	85
Shrimp, canned	1 oz (28 g)	30
Meats		
Bacon, cooked:		
Regular, medium	1 pce (6.3 g)	3
Canadian	1 oz (28 g)	10
Ham	3 oz (85 g)	21.3
Liver, cooked:		
Calf, fried	3 oz (85 g)	11.9
Chicken, simmered	1 ea (20 g)	10
Lunchmeats and Sausages:		
Bologna, beef	1 pce (23 g)	7
Brauschweiger	1 oz (28 g)	9–12
Frankfurter, 10/pkg	1 ea (45 g)	11–16
Pork sausage, cooked	1 patty (27 g)	23
Salami	1 pce (23 g)	8–10
Summer sausage	1 pce (23 g)	11–15
Turkey breast meat	1 oz (28 g)	5.3

Data are taken from Hands.[20]

physical activity over this same time frame also helps significantly in maximizing bone mass at a time when it counts (see Chapter 19). Maintaining both adequate Ca intakes and regular activity later in adulthood take on increasing importance for retaining bone mass in postmenopausal women and, hopefully, for preventing or delaying osteoporotic fractures of the hip. Keep in mind that in women two types of bone loss occur: (1) bone loss due to estrogen deficiency or cessation of production by the ovaries (natural or surgical menopause), and (2) bone loss due to age and presumably reduced activity. Males basically are affected only by age-related bone loss. The age-related bone loss in both males and females may, in fact, be related to the decline in adrenal-cortical production of androgenic and anabolic steroids, such as androstenedione. These hormones are generally thought to promote tissue growth in both sexes.

Thus, adequate dietary Ca intakes probably have their greatest impact early in the life cycle in contributing to an optimal peak in bone mass and thereby preventing osteoporosis.

VIII. OTHER NUTRIENTS OF IMPORTANCE IN CALCIUM METABOLISM

All nutrients are required for normal bone development and growth, but adequate energy and protein are especially critical. Many micronutrients, including vitamin D, are also needed.

Important issues of Ca also relate to usual protein consumption from animal (meat) sources,[29] and to lactose intake from unfermented dairy products. Intakes high in animal protein are considered hazardous to bone mass because of increased urinary Ca losses with high-protein diets. Lactose intolerance and milk allergy also can mean a severe restriction in milk consumption and, hence, low bone mass in children and adolescents compared to healthy peers.[30] Nowadays, this restriction can be overcome with the use of lactase-modified milk products or yogurt and Ca supplements.

Balanced dietary intakes that supply the minimum numbers of servings from each of the basic food groups should provide adequate amounts of Ca and other nutrients each day. One cup of milk (8 oz) contains approximately 290 mg of Ca; a cup of yogurt has somewhat greater amounts of Ca, depending on its contents (see Table 2). Recall that plant foods also supply the non-nutrients now considered important for health. However, strict vegetarians may have problems getting adequate amounts of Ca unless they include Ca-precipitated tofu and other Ca-rich foods in adequate amounts in their meals almost every day.

IX. SUMMARY

The diets of most American women are low or deficient in Ca. This long-term low nutritional status, which typically starts in adolescence, puts females at a disadvantage in developing an optimal peak bone mass and in preventing osteoporotic fractures (Additional discussion of diseases resulting from Ca deficiency is included in Chapter 1). Males in general, do not have the same problem early in life, because they consume more Ca-rich foods and more food energy. Asian ethnic populations have similar difficulties getting adequate dietary Ca as Americans and Western Europeans do. Black ethnic groups throughout the world also usually have low Ca intakes, but they also have greater bone mass than other ethnic groups, i.e., Caucasian and oriental. These genetic differences in bone mass tend to have more significance than usual dietary patterns of Ca intake.

Evidence is accumulating from different investigative approaches that adults need to consume P in amounts that do not compromise Ca retention by the skeleton. Intakes of P exceed the adult age-specific RDAs in practically 100% of the population, but Ca is consumed in amounts well below the RDAs by almost 50% of women and by approximately 25% of men. Therefore, abnormal intake ratios of Ca:P exist for roughly 35–40% of the American population. Recent research findings using human subjects demonstrate that circulating parathyroid hormone concentrations are consistently elevated in individuals with ratios of 1:4 or slightly higher. This secondary (nutritional) hyperparathyroidism may result in significant bone loss if sustained for a long period. Animal studies show similar effects, and cross-sectional human bioepidemiologic data support an adverse effect of high P intakes on measurements of bone mass. Whether this situation has a major prominence in the U.S. is not established, but typical diets with ratios of 1:4 (Ca:P) are considered bone unhealthy!

Based on the different approaches to the problem of excess consumption of this essential element, recommendations can be made that adults, especially females, consume P in amounts that produce a Ca:P ratio of approximately 1:1.2 to 1:1.4, but no lower than 1:2. In essence, then, P intakes need to be indexed on the basis of the typical pattern of Ca consumption in order to avoid mild nutritional secondary hyperparathyroidism.

The public consciousness of the role of Ca intake in bone health has increased dramatically in the last decade because of the attention focused on osteoporosis and the increased number of people living into their 70s, 80s and beyond as life expectancy has increased. However, the balance between Ca and P intakes and the potential impact of other nutrients on Ca bioavailability should be addressed on a lifelong basis to maximize bone health and minimize the impact of age-related losses of bone mass.

REFERENCES

1. **Anderson, J. J. B., Bennett, L., Curtis, R. C., Metz, J. A., Adeleke, V. M., Tylavsky, F. A., Taft, T. N. and Koch, G. G.,** Radial bone mass in healthy young adult white males: effects of calcium intake and exercise. (manuscript in preparation)
2. **Matkovic, V. and Heaney, R. P.,** Calcium balance during human growth: evidence for threshold behavior, *Am. J. Clin. Nutr.*, 55, 992, 1992.
3. **Johnston, C. C., Jr., Miller, J. Z., Slemenda, C. W., Reister, T. K., Christian, J. C. and Peacock, M.,** Calcium supplementation and increases in bone mineral density in children, *New Engl. J. Med.*, 327, 82, 1992.
4. **Barger-Lux, M. J. and Heaney, R. P.,** Effects of calcium restriction on metabolic characteristics of premenopausal women, *J. Clin. Endocrinol. Metab.*, 76, 103, 1993.
5. **Anderson, J. J. B. and Allen, J. C.,** Nutrition of macrominerals and trace elements, in *Functional Foods*, Goldberg, I. eds., Chapman and Hall, New York, 1994.
6. **Anderson, J. J. B.,** Nutritional biochemistry of calcium and phosphorus, *J. Nutr. Biochem.*, 2, 300, 1991.
7. **Calvo, M. S., Kumar, R. and Heath, H.,** Persistently elevated parathyroid hormone secretion and action in young women after four weeks of ingesting high phosphorus, low calcium diets, *J. Clin. Endocrinol. Metab.*, 70, 1334, 1990.
8. **Calvo, M. S.,** Dietary phosphorus, calcium metabolism and bone, *J. Nutr.*, 123, 1627, 1993.
9. **Abelow, B. J., Holford, T. R. and Insogna, K. L.,** Cross-cultural association between animal protein and hip fracture: a hypothesis, *Calcif. Tissue Int.*, 50, 14, 1992.
10. **Hegsted, M. and Linkswiler, H. M.,** Long-term effects of level of protein intake on calcium metabolism in young adult women, *J. Nutr.*, 251, 244, 1981.
11. **Schuette, S. A. and Linkswiler, H. M.,** Effects of Ca and P metabolism in humans by adding meat, meat plus milk, or purified proteins plus Ca and P to a low protein diet, *J. Nutr.*, 112, 338, 1982.
12. **Anderson, J. J. B., Thomsen, K. and Christiansen, C.,** High protein meals, insular hormones and urinary calcium excretion in human subjects, in *Osteoporosis 1987*, Christiansen, C., Johansen, J. and Riis, B. J., Eds., Osteopress ApS, Copenhagen, 1987.
13. **Breslau, N. A., Brinkley, L., Hill, K. D. and Pak, C. Y. C.,** Relationship of animal protein-rich diet to kidney stone formation and calcium metabolism, *J. Clin. Endocrinol. Metab.*, 66, 140, 1988.
14. **Geddie, M. K. and Anderson, J. J. B.,** Meal-associated homeostatic changes in calcium metabolism. (manuscript in preparation)
15. **Kerstetter, J. E. and Allen, L. H.,** Dietary protein increases urinary calcium, *J. Nutr.*, 120, 134, 1990.
16. **Orwoll, E. S.,** The effects of dietary protein insufficiency and excess on skeletal health, *Bone*, 13, 343, 1992.
17. **Metz, J. A., Anderson, J. J. B. and Gallagher, P. N., Jr.,** Intakes of calcium, phosphorus, and protein, and physical-activity level are related to radial bone mass in young adult women, *Am. J. Clin. Nutr.*, 58, 537, 1993.
18. **Dawson-Hughes, B., Dallal, G. E., Krall , E. H., Harris, S., Sokoll, L. J. and Falconer, G.,** Effect of vitamin D supplementation on wintertime and overall bone loss in healthy postmenopausal women, *Ann. Int. Med.*, 115, 505, 1991.
19. **Greger, J. L. and Krystofiak, M.,** Phosphorus intake of Americans, *Food Technol.*, 36, 78, 1982.
20. **Hands, E. S.,** FOOD Finder: Food Sources of Vitamins and Minerals, 2nd Edition, ESHA Research, Salem, OR, 1990.
21. Nutrition-monitoring, Phosphorus, in *Nutrition Monitoring in the United States: A Progress Report of the Joint Nutrition Monitoring Evaluation Committee*, eds., U.S. Department of Health and Human Service, U. S. Department of Agriculture, Washington, D.C., 1986.

22. **Oenning, L. L., Vogel, J. and Calvo, M. S.,** Accuracy of methods estimating calcium and phosphorus intake in daily diets, *J. Am. Diet. Assoc.*, 88, 1076, 1988.
22a. **Bell, R. R., Draper, H. H., Tzeung, D. Y. M., Shin, H. K. and Schmidt, G. R.,** Physiological responses of adults to foods containing phosphate additives, *J. Nutr.*, 107, 42, 1977.
23. **Massey, L. K. and Strang, M. M.,** Soft drink consumption, phosphorus intake and osteoporosis, *J. Am. Diet. Assoc.*, 80, 581, 1982.
24. **Morgan, K. J., Stults, V. J. and Stampley, G. L.,** Soft drink consumption patterns of the U.S. population, *J. Am. Diet. Assoc.*, 85, 352, 1985.
25. Anonymous, Chemical forms and bioavailability of dietary minerals, *World Rev. Nutr. Diet*, 46, 15, 1985.
26. Anonymous, Disappearance of Phosphorus in US Food Applications, International Food-Additives Council, Atlanta, 1992.
27. **Franz, K. B.,** Influence of phosphorus on intestinal absorption of calcium and phosphorus, in *Magnesium in Health and Disease*, Itokawa, Y. and Durlach, J. eds., John Libbey, London, 1988.
28. **Zemel, M. B. and Linkswiller, H. M.,** Calcium metabolism in the young adult as affected by level and form of phosphorus intake and level of calcium intake, *J. Nutr.*, 111, 315, 1981.
29. **Anderson, J. J. B.,** The role of nutrition in the functioning of skeletal tissue, *Nutr. Rev.*, 50, 388, 1992.
30. **Henderson, R. C. and Hayes, P. R. L.,** Bone mineralization in children and adolescents with a milk allergy, *Bone Miner.*, 27, 1, 1994.
31. Subcommittee on the Recommended Dietary Allowances, Food and Nutrition Board, Commission on Life Sciences, National Research Council, *Recommended Dietary Allowances*, 10th edition, National Academy Press, Washington, D.C., 1989.
32. **Smolin, L. A. and Grosvenor, M. B.,** *Nutrition: Science and Applications*, Saunders, Fort Worth, TX, Food Composition Tables, 1994.
33. U.S. Department of Health and Human Services, Public Health Service, National Center for Health Statisitics and U.S. Department of Agriculture, Food and Consumer Services, *Nutrition Monitoring in the United States*, Hyattsville, MD, DHHS Publication No. (PHS) 86-1255, 356, 1986.

Section I.

CALCIUM AND PHOSPHORUS METABOLISM

This section introduces the concept of homeostasis as it applies to the regulation of both calcium (Ca) and phosphorus (P) concentrations in blood. The overview chapter (Chapter 3) introduces the organs most critically involved in the control of these two mineral ions, namely the small intestine and the kidney, which are covered in this section along with the intracellular regulation of Ca concentrations, and the skeleton (covered in the next section). The role of the gut in the intestinal absorption of Ca ions and, to a lesser extent, that of inorganic phosphate (Pi) anions, is the focus of Chapter 4, which also provides background information on Ca bioavailability and the interactions between Ca and other nutrients or food components in the gut lumen and in the body. The chapter on renal regulation of Ca and P reabsorption (Chapter 5) highlights the critical role of the kidney in conserving Ca for body uses and eliminating typically unneeded Pi anions. (Recall from Chapter 2 that the Western diet generally provides more than enough P but insufficient amounts of Ca.) The final chapter of this section (Chapter 6) deals with the cellular regulation of Ca and, to a limited extent, P. The ionic cytosolic concentration of Ca is highly controlled because Ca ions serve as essential activators of several critical enzymes. Actually, increases in Ca ions, if chronic, can wreak havoc on cellular functions.

The content of this section on the regulation, both extracellular and intracellular, of Ca ions provides the background for subsequent sections in this text.

Chapter 3

BLOOD CALCIUM AND PHOSPHORUS REGULATION

Bruce Lobaugh, Ph.D.

TABLE OF CONTENTS

0-8493-7845-1/95/$0.00+$.50

I. INTRODUCTION

Calcium (Ca) and phosphorus (P) are mineral ions important as both structural and functional elements in an impressive diversity of biological processes and systems. A wide variety of pathologic conditions is associated with either deficiency or excess of one or both of these minerals. In extreme situations, the life of the organism can be threatened if appropriate steps are not taken to resolve the abnormality. Consequently, it is not surprising that homeostatic systems have evolved to insure regulation of the concentrations of Ca and Pi (inorganic phosphorus) within narrow limits appropriate to the function of each ion. Details regarding the biological significance of Ca and P, the mechanisms governing regulation of these ions in the blood, and the hormones that modulate those regulatory systems are reviewed in this chapter.

A. PHYSIOLOGIC SIGNIFICANCE OF CALCIUM

Ca is the fifth most abundant chemical element in the human body and the most ubiquitous mineral ion[1] (see Table 1). It plays two major physiologic roles: structural and functional.[2] As a structural component, Ca combines with Pi to comprise the mineral portion of bone and teeth and with phospholipids and proteins, where it plays an essential role in maintaining the integrity of cell membranes. As a functional element of both the extracellular fluid and cytosol, Ca has critical roles in a variety of biochemical and physiologic processes, including neuromuscular excitability, blood coagulation, transfer of other inorganic ions across membranes, hormone secretion, release of cellular enzymes, signal transduction, and reproductive functions such as sperm motility and fertilization of the ovum. The activities of numerous enzymes are affected by Ca either acting alone (e.g., glyceraldehyde phosphate dehydrogenase, pyruvate dehydrogenase, α-ketoglutarate dehydrogenase) or through its activation of calmodulin (e.g., adenylate cyclase, cyclic nucleotide phosphodiesterase, Ca-magnesium ATPase, myosin light chain kinase, phosphorylase b kinase, NAD kinase, ornithine decarboxylase). These enzymes control such crucial intracellular functions as cyclic nucleotide metabolism, glycogen metabolism, microtubule and microfilament function, and cell division. These and other specific functions of Ca are summarized in Table 2.

TABLE 1
Elemental Composition of the Human Body

Element	% of Total Atoms
H	63
O	25.5
C	9.5
N	1.4
Ca	0.31
P	0.22
Cl	0.08
K	0.06
S	0.05
Na	0.03
Mg	0.01

(Modified from Lehninger 1975[1])

TABLE 2
Biological Functions of Calcium

Molecular Level
Component of skeletal hydroxyapatite
Regulation of certain enzymes (as a cofactor)
Insolubilizing agent
Intracellular electrolyte balance

Cellular Level
Decreased membrane permeability to Na, K
Maintenance of neuromuscular irritability
Intercellular cement
Activator of muscle contraction
Enzyme catalyst — Mitochondrial granules
Mitotic stimulant
Universal regulator (via Calmodulin)

Organismal Level
Blood clotting
Maintenance of muscle contractility
Hormone secretion
Major structural component of bone and teeth
Maintenance of neural transmission
Homeostasis of vasculature and heart
Maintenance of electrolyte balance
Energy metabolism
Phosphorus homeostasis

(Modified from Kutsky, 1981[42])

Marked disturbances in Ca homeostasis can be associated with a number of serious or catastrophic events including irritability, drowsiness, disorientation, coma, nephrolithiasis, kidney failure, bronchospasm, intestinal cramping, and loss of skeletal integrity.[3,4]

B. PHYSIOLOGIC SIGNIFICANCE OF PHOSPHORUS

Phosphorus is the sixth most prevalent chemical element in the human body[1] (Table 1). Like Ca, P is of both structural and functional significance to the organism.[2] The majority of the mineral is located in the skeleton where it largely plays a structural role. However, a significant fraction is also present in extracellular fluids, primarily in the form of inorganic Pi ions, and in the soft tissues as Pi esters. Pi is a basic component of many biological macromolecules and smaller intermediates including membrane phospholipids, nucleic acids, phosphoproteins, energy-storing organophosphate compounds (e.g., ATP, creatine phosphate), and enzyme cofactors (e.g., NADP, phosphoinositides). As part of these compounds, Pi plays a role in many fundamental physiologic processes including gene regulation, modulation of enzyme activity, and maintenance of cellular membrane integrity. Moreover, Pi is a crucial constituent of the Pi buffer system, one of several major mechanisms that function to ensure that systemic pH remains within limits compatible with life. These and other specific functions of P are summarized in Table 3.

Disturbances in Pi metabolism that severely depress extracellular concentrations of the ion may be manifested by neuromuscular weakness, cardiac ventricular dysfunction, defective renal tubular reabsorption of other ions, hemolysis, and rickets/osteomalacia.[5]

II. DISTRIBUTION OF CALCIUM AND PHOSPHORUS IN THE HUMAN BODY

In order to fully comprehend the mechanisms underlying blood Ca and P homeostasis, it is necessary to first understand how these two mineral ions are distributed in the body. The following paragraphs provide a brief review of these concepts.

TABLE 3
Biological Functions of Phosphorus

Molecular Level
Component of skeletal hydroxyapatite
B-complex vitamins — Cofactor
High-energy bonds
Structural component of RNA, DNA
Component of phosphoproteins and phospholipids

Cellular Level
Component of membrane phospholipids
Buffering of intracellular fluids
Carbohydrate and energy metabolism
Mitochondrial respiration

Organismal Level
Buffering of extracellular fluids
Major structural component of bone and teeth
Genetics of RNA and DNA
Energy metabolism (via ATP, Krebs cycle, etc.)
Muscle contraction (via ATP)
Calcium homeostasis

(Modified from Kutsky, 1981[42])

A. DISTRIBUTION OF CALCIUM AND PHOSPHORUS

An adult human contains about 1000–1300 g of Ca and 500–800 g of P. Although the majority of both minerals is stored in the skeleton as the mineral component of bone, soluble Ca has essential roles in cellular metabolism, and both soluble P and organic P are essential for maintaining body functions.

1. Distribution of Calcium and Phosphorus in Adult Humans

Almost 99% of the Ca is located in the skeleton, another 0.5% in the teeth, and the remainder is found in the soft tissues, extracellular fluid, and plasma (Table 4). Total body Ca is about 25 g/kg of lean-body weight. Whereas less than 1% is present in soluble form in the extra- and intracellular fluid compartments, another 1% has been shown by ^{45}Ca kinetic analysis to be freely exchangeable with extracellular fluid.[6]

Unlike Ca, P is widely distributed in unmineralized tissues that account for about 15% of total body P (Table 4).

2. Distribution of Calcium and Phosphorus in Plasma

There are at least three distinct fractions of both Ca and Pi in normal human plasma: ionized, protein-bound, and complexed (see Figure 1). The ionic and complexed forms of each mineral are diffusible through membranes and are sometimes collectively referred to as ultrafilterable. Whereas only about 50% of plasma Ca is ultrafilterable, almost 90% of inorganic Pi can be so classified.[7]

Total plasma Ca in adults is ordinarily between about 8.7 and 10.2 mg/dL, and ionized Ca ranges from 4.7 to 5.3 mg/dL (1.17 to 1.33 mmol/L). Albumin is the major Ca-binding protein by far, accounting for 70–90% of the bound mineral. Globulins provide sites for most of the remaining protein-bound Ca. The binding of Ca to protein is pH-sensitive (i.e., increased under alkaline conditions), and marked changes in total Ca concentration may be associated with protein abnormalities (e.g., hyper- and hypoalbuminemia). Such changes may occur in the absence of a parallel effect on ionized Ca, the physiologically significant fraction and the Ca species that is subject to precise endocrine regulation. The least prevalent fraction consists of complexes between Ca and other ions (primarily citrate, Pi, or bicarbonate).

The plasma typically contains about 14 mg/dL of elemental phosphorus, of which 8 to 9 mg occurs within phospholipids. An additional trace exists as an anion of pyrophosphoric acid, and the

TABLE 4
Distribution of Calcium and Phosphorus in a 70 kg man

Tissue	Calcium (mmol)	Calcium % of Total	Phosphorus (mmol)	Phosphorus % of Total
Bone	31,350.00	99.50	19,000	85.60
Muscle	48.00	0.15	1,900	8.60
ECF	35.00	0.11	17	0.08
RBC	0.04	0.00	40	0.18
Other	66.96	0.24	1,243	5.60
Total	31,500.00	100.00	22,200	100.00

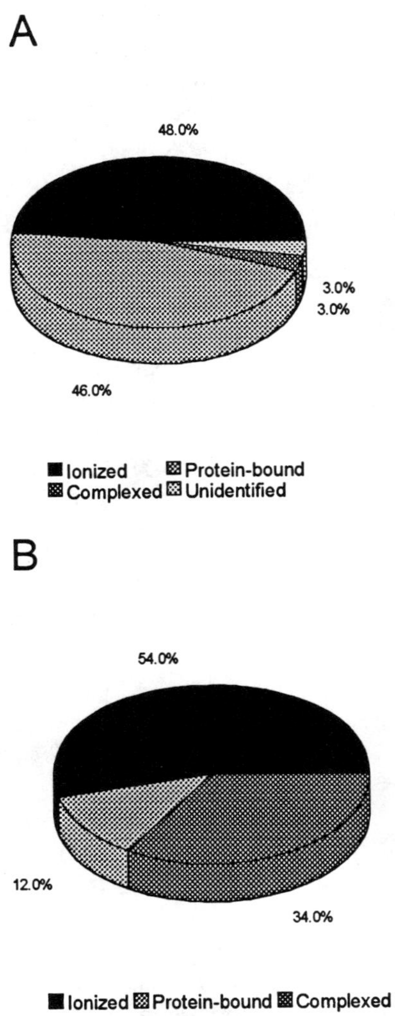

A

	mmol/L	mg/dL
Ionized	1.18	4.72
Protein-bound	1.14	4.56
Complexed	0.08	0.32
Unidentified	0.08	0.32
Total	2.48	9.92

B

	mmol/L	mg/dL
Ionized	0.61	1.89
Protein-bound	0.14	0.43
Complexed	0.40	1.24
Total	1.15	3.56

FIGURE 1. Distribution of Calcium (A) and Phosphate (B) in Human Plasma. About half of the total calcium (ionized and complexed) is ultrafilterable and participates directly in the regulation of physiological processes. (Adapted from Reference 43)

remainder is in the form of inorganic (ortho)phosphate. Total plasma inorganic Pi exhibits considerably more variation than Ca and can be affected by age, sex, diet, and pH. In addition, a circadian rhythm has been described which can be associated with changes in plasma Pi of as much as 50% throughout the day.[8]

Total plasma inorganic Pi ranges from about 2.5 to 4.5 mg/dL in fasting adults. Protein binding is relatively insignificant for Pi, but complexes between Pi and sodium, Ca and magnesium account for almost 35% of the total inorganic ion.

B. CALCIUM AND PHOSPHORUS POOLS AT BALANCE

Plasma Ca and inorganic Pi exist as pools in dynamic balance with three major input/output components: intestine, bone, and kidney. The homeostatic mechanisms operate at these sites to maintain the concentrations of both ions within tolerable limits.

1. Calcium

A simplified schematic of Ca fluxes into and out of the plasma is shown in Figure 2A. The numbers provided are for illustration rather than definition and vary according to numerous factors including individual age, body weight, and Ca content of the diet. The extracellular pool of Ca (i.e., that of the blood and interstitial fluids) is in equilibrium with Ca entering the pool via the intestine, bone, and renal tubule.[9] At balance, the output of Ca (via losses in the urine and sweat) is equivalent to input of the mineral (net gastrointestinal absorption defined as the amount consumed minus fecal output). Moreover, loss of mineral from the skeleton (resorption) equals incorporation of Ca into bone (accretion). An uncompensated change in any of the three input/output components will result in a Ca imbalance (hypocalcemia when output exceeds input, hypercalcemia when input exceeds output). Hormonal modulation of the processes of gastrointestinal absorption, renal tubular reabsorption, and bone resorption and accretion provides a system through which appropriate responses to hypo- or hypercalcemic challenges can be directed.

2. Phosphorus

The control system for Pi (see Figure 2B) features the same three components as those involved in Ca homeostasis (i.e., intestine, bone, and kidney). In addition, the plasma Pi pool is in equilibrium with the soft tissues (not shown in the diagram). The primary regulatory site is the kidney, which excretes the ion in amounts necessary to balance the excess typically absorbed via the gut. The calciotropic hormones, parathyroid hormone (PTH), and 1,25-dihydroxyvitamin D (1,25$(OH)_2$D), which are important in Ca homeostasis, also play key roles in the regulation of plasma Pi concentrations.

III. BLOOD CALCIUM AND PHOSPHORUS HOMEOSTASIS

The homeostatic system, which has evolved to hold blood Ca and Pi within their respective tolerance limits, is a classic endocrine feedback loop system consisting of several hormones (PTH, 1,25$(OH)_2$D, and, possibly, calcitonin (CT)) and three major target organs (intestine, kidney, and bone). A neuroendocrine link has not been demonstrated to date.

A. ELEMENTARY MODEL OF THE CALCIUM AND PHOSPHORUS HOMEOSTATIC SYSTEM

The basic model of the blood Ca and P homeostatic system can be broken down into two parts:[10] (1) the controlled subsystem (i.e., plasma ionized Ca and plasma Pi concentrations), and (2) the controlling subsystem (hormones and target organs) (see Figure 3). This simple representation does not fully reflect the true state of nature, however. Indeed, there are many other components that could be included in a comprehensive scheme (e.g., other ions [pH, sodium, potassium, chloride, bicarbonate, sulfate], hormones [growth hormone, prolactin, insulin, glucocorticoids, cytokines], and target organs for the biochemical modulators). A full discussion of all these factors is beyond the scope of this chapter. Interested readers should consult one of the general reviews listed at the end of the chapter for additional information.

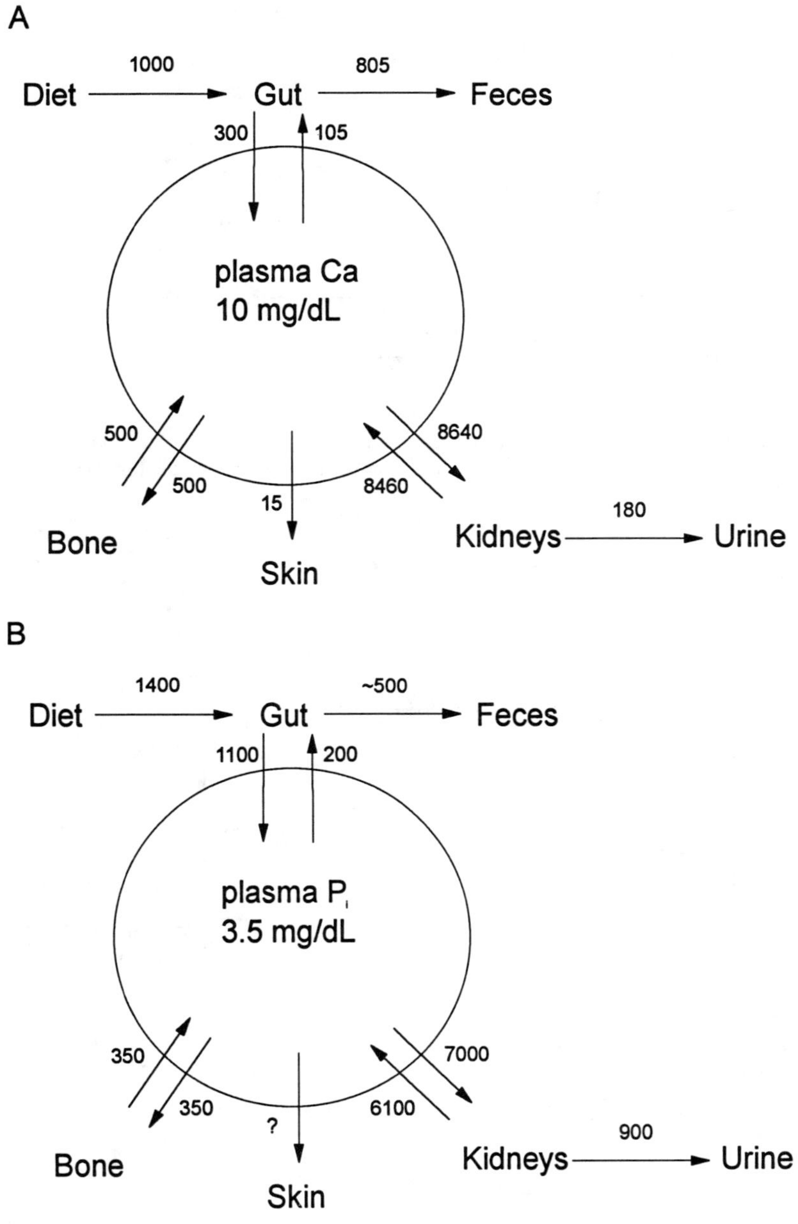

FIGURE 2. Schematic Representation of Calcium (A) and Phosphate (B) Metabolism in an Adult Human. The greatest part of total body calcium and phosphate resides in the skeleton, a dynamic organ that exchanges both minerals with the extracellular fluid (plasma) pool. Since systemic input=output for each mineral, the individual is in calcium and phosphate balance. (Adapted from Reference 9)

B. MECHANISMS OF HOMEOSTASIS

A simple tank model of blood Ca/Pi homeostasis (see Figure 4) illustrates in schematic fashion how the input/output components are integrated into the overall regulatory framework.[11] The level of fluid in the tank corresponds to the blood concentration of Ca or Pi, whereas the inlet and outlet tubes represent primarily the intestine and kidney, respectively, when a state of balance is manifest. The height of the outlet tube reflects the renal transport maximum (Tm) above which excretion is a linear function of concentration. The diameter of the outlet tube corresponds to the glomerular

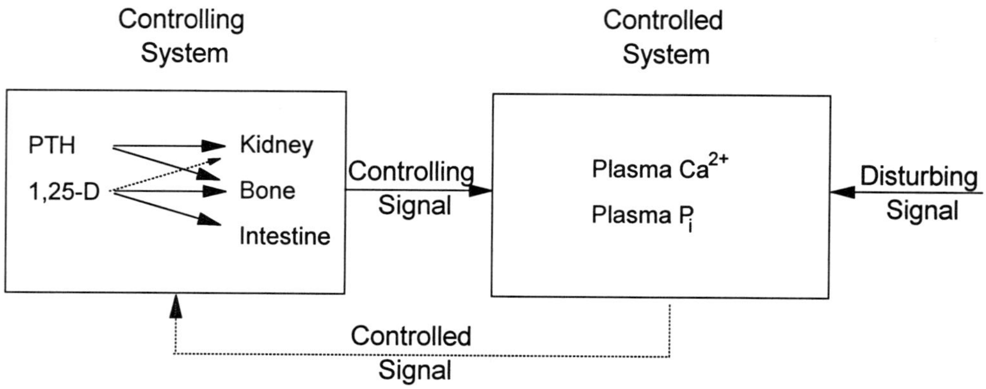

FIGURE 3. Components of the Blood Calcium and Phosphate Homeostatic System. The ions under the control of this system feed back negatively on hormone secretion to maintain the plasma concentration of each within narrow limits. (Modified from Reference 10)

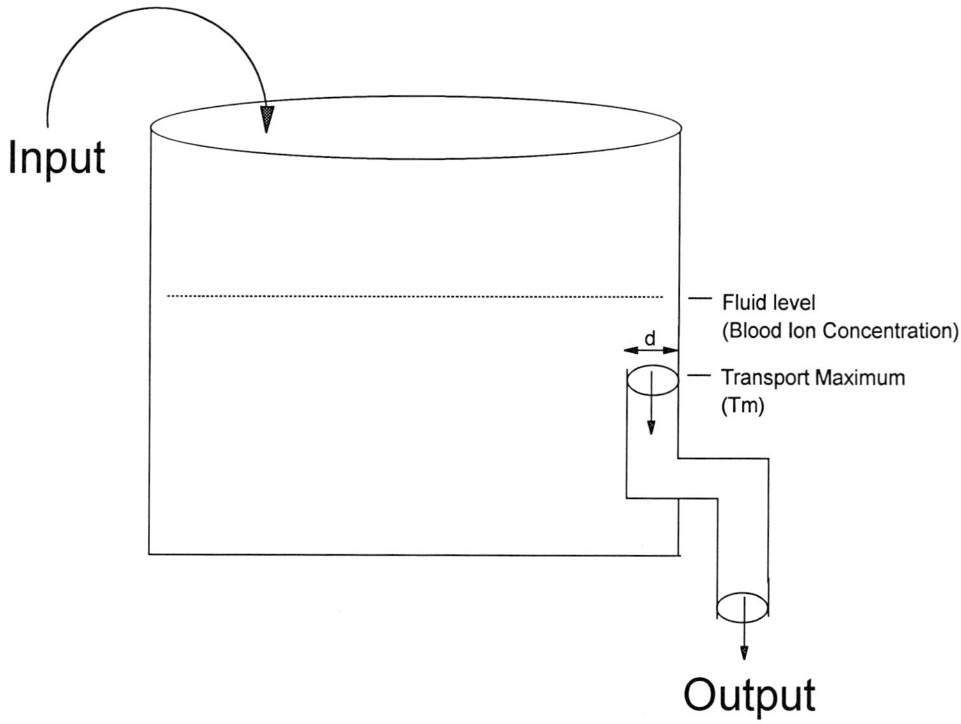

FIGURE 4. Simple Tank Analogy of Blood Calcium and Phosphate Regulation. In this diagram, "d" represents the glomerular filtration rate and the height of the outlet tube corresponds to the transport maximum (Tm) for the ion. When the blood ion concentration exceeds the Tm, the ion is excreted as a linear function of concentration. (Modified from Reference 11)

filtration rate, a general index of the filtering capacity of the kidneys. Each of these mechanisms is subject to complex regulation by a variety of hormonal and metabolic factors (detailed later).

1. Gastrointestinal Absorption

The intestinal absorption of Ca and P supplies the material necessary to maintain the critical functions of these two elements (see Chapter 1). The amounts of the minerals absorbed depend ultimately on two factors: the bioavailability of each in the diet and the capacity of the gut to absorb that which is available. Two absorptive processes operate under normal conditions: physiologically-regulated transcellular active transport, which is a saturable process; and nonsaturable passive (diffusional) transport, which depends on the intraluminal concentration of Ca or Pi.[12,13]

The dietary intake of Ca varies widely in the U.S. population and ranges from 300 to 1500 mg/day. The level of Ca consumed tends to decline with age and is frequently lower in women than in men.[14] At the lower region of the range, daily intake falls below the Recommended Dietary Allowance (RDA) for Ca in adults (800 mg/day) and is far less than the recommended adult female allowances of 1000–1500 mg/day that were announced at the 1984 NIH Consensus Conference on Osteoporosis.[15] At extremely low intakes (i.e., <200–300 mg/day), influx cannot match losses in urine and sweat, and a negative Ca balance ensues.

Ingested Ca is absorbed variably along the different intestinal segments.[16] Absorption appears to be most efficient in the duodenum and cecum. Net Ca secretion may occur in the other regions (i.e., jejunum, ileum, and distal colon). However, the bioavailability of fecal Ca in the cecum is uncertain, and the ileum may be a significant site of absorption during dietary Ca restriction or during times when passage of luminal contents through the more proximal segments is accelerated.[17]

Unlike Ca, the average adult dietary intake of P (1200–1500 mg/day) substantially exceeds the RDA (800 mg/day) for the mineral. About 60–80% of dietary Pi is absorbed over a wide range of intakes, and net absorption is directly proportional to the amount consumed. At extremely low intake levels, the intestine is capable of greater absorptive efficiency (80–90%).[18]

The jejunum is the most active intestinal segment for absorption of dietary Pi, but absorption also occurs throughout the small intestine.[19] An age-related decline in net Pi uptake has been demonstrated in experimental animals. In addition, formation of nonabsorbable salts with Ca, aluminum, or magnesium can significantly reduce the amount of dietary Pi available for assimilation.[20]

2. Kidney Filtration and Reabsorption

The kidneys are the primary excretory organs for both Ca and Pi in man and are thus essential in preventing the systemic development of hypercalcemia and hyperphosphatemia (see Chapter 5). Further, since tubular reabsorption ordinarily plays an important part in the conservation of both Ca and Pi, a reduction in the number of functional nephrons, or in their capacity to reabsorb normally, may result in hypocalcemia/hypophosphatemia. The significance of the kidneys to the homeostatic regulation of both minerals is amply demonstrated by the wide range of clinically serious consequences associated with marked loss of renal function (as in chronic dialysis or acute renal failure patients).

Kidneys filter about 10 grams of Ca per day in normocalcemic individuals regardless of the dietary intake of the mineral. More than 98% of this filtered load (i.e., ultrafilterable Ca concentration times the glomerular filtration rate) is reabsorbed in the various segments throughout the nephron. Thus, only 150–200 mg of the total filtered Ca is lost in the urine each day, and this renal excretion counterbalances in large measure the daily influx of Ca from the gut.[21]

Unlike Ca almost 90% of total blood Pi is ultrafilterable. Thus, the Pi concentration of the glomerular filtrate is very similar to that of plasma. In healthy individuals about 80–90% of the filtered Pi load is reabsorbed. A majority (60–75%) of this reabsorption occurs in the proximal tubule, but Pi is also reabsorbed in the distal tubule and/or cortical collecting duct. In man, tubular Pi reabsorption is characterized by a transport maximum (TmP) above which conservation of the ion does not occur.[19]

3. Exchange of Calcium and Phosphate between Blood and Bone

Under ideal conditions of Ca and Pi balance, excretion via the urine (but also to a considerably lesser degree through the sweat and feces) is matched precisely by influx into the extracellular fluid compartment. Intestinal absorption of ingested mineral is ordinarily the mechanism through which excreted Ca and Pi are replaced. However, if dietary content is inadequate or a malabsorptive disorder is manifest, Ca and Pi can be mobilized from bone to maintain blood concentrations (at the expense of skeletal homeostasis). Movement of mineral from bone is facilitated by two distinct processes: a low magnitude, high capacity, slow-acting system (osteoclastic resorption); and the high magnitude, low capacity, rapidly responsive transfer of mineral from the skeletal surface to bone fluid via osteocytes and bone-surface cells.[19]

The skeleton may also act as a buffer in instances when influx exceeds efflux through the accretion of mineral into bone. A different cell (the osteoblast) plays a significant role in bone mineralization. The role of bone formation in blood mineral homeostasis is not well understood, however, and may depend primarily on the concentrations of Ca and Pi both systemically and locally.

C. HORMONES AND METABOLIC FACTORS INVOLVED IN CALCIUM AND PHOSPHORUS HOMEOSTASIS

The calcemic hormones PTH and $1,25(OH)_2D$ are essential for maintenance of Ca and P homeostasis through their actions in bone, kidney, and gastrointestinal tract.

1. Parathyroid Hormone

Bioactive (intact) PTH is secreted by the chief cells of the parathyroid glands as an 84-amino acid polypeptide hormone (see Chapter 11). Circulating intact PTH has a half-life of less than 4 minutes.[22] Hormone secretion (but not synthesis) is governed primarily by the extracellular fluid-ionized Ca concentration (mediated by a cell surface Ca receptor). A host of other agents (e.g., biogenic amines, magnesium, aluminum, vitamin D metabolites, and CT) have also been shown to affect PTH release, particularly in pathologic conditions. However, their relevance in "normal" Ca and Pi homeostasis remains unclear.[23]

The major actions of PTH are directed toward preservation of the blood-ionized Ca concentration within a narrow physiologic range. These include (1) increasing renal tubular Ca reabsorption, (2) mobilizing Ca from the skeleton, and (3) increasing gastrointestinal Ca absorption (via its stimulation of $1,25(OH)_2D$ biosynthesis). The hormone also exerts important phosphatemic effects including (1) reducing renal tubular Pi reabsorption, (2) mobilizing Pi (together with Ca) from the skeleton, and (3) enhancing the influx of Pi from the gut (again through stimulation of $1,25(OH)_2D$ production).

2. 1,25-Dihydroxyvitamin D

1,25-Dihydroxyvitamin D is more appropriately classified as a hormone than as a vitamin. Vitamin D can be synthesized in skin after exposure to ultraviolet light, even in the absence of dietary intake (see Chapter 12). Following a series of hydroxylation steps in the liver (to 25-hydroxyvitamin D [25-(OH)D]) and kidney (to $1,25(OH)_2D$), the hormonal metabolite is produced. The renal hydroxylation of $1,25(OH)_2D$ is precisely regulated by a variety of factors including PTH, Ca, Pi, CT, and $1,25(OH)_2D$ itself.[24-26] Whereas many of the intermediates possess calciotropic activity, $1,25(OH)_2D$ is the most potent naturally occurring compound. Circulating $1,25(OH)_2D$ has a half-life of about 1.5 days, a period considerably in excess of that for PTH.

The classically recognized effects of $1,25(OH)_2D$ on Ca and Pi homeostasis include (1) enhancing gastrointestinal absorption of Ca and Pi, and (2) acting in synergism with PTH to promote the release of Ca and Pi from bone.

3. Other Hormones and Metabolic Factors

Ca and P homeostasis is primarily dependent on PTH and $1,25(OH)_2D$, but other metabolic factors and hormones, including Ca and P themselves, CT, and other hormonal and local factors may play a role.

a. Calcium and Phosphate

Ca and Pi participate in regulating their own and each other's absorption from the intestine. Each ion can act to inhibit uptake of the other. The nature of this effect is physicochemical, involving the formation of nonabsorbable calcium phosphate salts. In addition, aluminum and magnesium can retard Pi absorption through a similar mechanism.

Autoregulation by Ca of renal tubular reabsorption occurs in the ascending loop of Henle and collecting duct. Hypercalcemia increases the filtered load and impairs reabsorption of the ion at these sites. This phenomenon can overwhelm the stimulatory effect of PTH on tubular Ca reabsorption and accounts for the hypercalciuria observed in hyperparathyroidism. Ample experimental evidence also exists to suggest that similar autoregulatory adaptations can occur in the kidney to counter phosphatemic challenges.[27,28]

Both Ca and Pi also act indirectly in their own homeostasis by modulating the biosynthesis, secretion, or both of PTH and 1,25$(OH)_2$D. These effects are described in the following discussion.

b. Other Nutritional Factors

Dietary protein exerts a hypercalciuric effect irrespective of the level of dietary Ca intake.[29] The renal clearance of Ca is closely and directly linked to that of sodium.[30] Caffeine induces hypercalciuria in dose-dependent fashion.[31] Lactose stimulates intestinal Ca absorption through an effect on the nonsaturable component,[32] whereas phytic acid (from plant products), uronic acids (from cereals), oxalic acids (from vegetables), and long-chain fatty acids may reduce absorption by complexing Ca in the gut.[33]

c. Calcitonin

Calcitonin (CT) is a 32-amino acid peptide produced by the C-cells of the thyroid gland (see Chapter 13). Secretion of the hormone is directly stimulated (or inhibited) by acute increases (or decreases) of the blood Ca concentration. Its half-life in the circulation is on the order of 10 minutes. The most recognized biological action of CT is inhibition of osteoclastic bone resorption. As such, the hormone would seem a natural antagonist for PTH, but the importance of CT in "normal" mineral and skeletal metabolism is in doubt. Indeed, total thyroidectomy without CT replacement does not result in any demonstrable derangement of Ca or Pi homeostasis. It has been suggested that CT may play a significant role in mineral metabolism during periods of heightened calcemic challenge to the organism (e.g., growth, pregnancy, and lactation), but experimental data supporting this hypothesis remain equivocal.

d. Parathyroid Hormone-Related Protein

Parathyroid hormone-related protein (PTHrP) is a polypeptide with limited sequence homology to PTH (confined to 8 of the first 13 amino-terminal amino acids) that exists in at least three isoforms (139, 141, and 173 amino acid residues). PTHrP shares a common receptor with PTH and binds to this receptor with equal affinity.[34] Consequently, the range of biological activities PTHrP elicits is very similar to those of PTH. PTHrP was initially characterized as a major cause of the humoral hypercalcemia of malignancy syndrome, a nonparathyroid hypercalcemic disorder seen in cancer patients. PTHrP normally circulates at considerably lower concentration than PTH and probably has no major role in the day-to-day maintenance of blood Ca and Pi. However, like CT, PTHrP may be important in certain special processes such as placental and/or neonatal Ca transport, possibly as an autocrine or paracrine agent.

e. Other Hormonal Factors

Many other hormones not directly involved in Ca and Pi homeostasis can nonetheless affect skeletal and/or mineral balance under some circumstances. Among these are growth hormone, adrenal glucocorticoids, thyroid hormone, and the sex steroids (see Chapter 14). The exact cellular mechanisms of action relating to the skeletal effects of these hormones are generally not well understood. Nonetheless, states of deficiency or excess of these hormonal modulators can result in predictable disturbances of mineral metabolism either directly or indirectly through changes in the circulating concentrations of the major Ca-regulating hormones.

f. Local Factors

Local factors may be more important than systemic hormones for some aspects of skeletal homeostasis. The skeleton is a dynamic structure that undergoes growth, maturation, and constant remodeling. The observation that bone remodeling occurs at discrete foci throughout the skeleton suggests that many of the basic cellular events are likely controlled by factors generated in the microenvironment of bone. A number of potent local stimulators and inhibitors of bone cell activity have recently been described. Immune cell products associated with osteoclast activation include interleukin-1 (IL-1), lymphotoxin, tumor necrosis factor (TNF), and colony stimulating factor-1 (CSF-1). In addition, vitamin A, transforming growth factor-α (TGF-α, a tumor product) and E-series prostaglandins have been shown to stimulate bone resorption. Osteoclast inhibitors include γ-interferon and transforming growth factor-β (TGF-β, also a potent osteoblast activator).

D. RESPONSE OF THE HOMEOSTATIC SYSTEM TO PHYSIOLOGIC AND PATHOLOGIC PERTURBATIONS

The homeostatic system for Ca, and to a lesser extent for Pi, are able to minimize the perturbations to the normal concentrations of these ions in the extracellular fluids. These systems must be capable of preventing both wide swings of Ca or Pi in the face of the normal fluctuations that occur physiologically, and the potentially more dangerous changes accompanying pathologic perturbations.

1. Physiologic Perturbation

Ca and Pi concentrations may be expected to vary during the day as the potential supply of the ions from intestinal absorption increases following meals and decreases during periods of fasting, including sleep. These normal fluctuations in extracellular ion concentrations are kept to a minimum by the homeostatic systems described in the following section.

a. Calcemic Stimuli

Changes in blood Ca are sensed by Ca receptors on the parathyroid gland cell surfaces. Within minutes, reciprocal changes in parathyroid hormone secretion can be measured, and the circulating concentration of PTH increases or falls. The hormone secreted in response to hypocalcemic stimuli exerts its effects on target cells in the kidney and skeleton, whereas hypercalcemic challenges result in a reduction (but never a complete cessation) of PTH released and a consequent diminution of target organ effects. The paragraphs that follow outline the normal homeostatic responses to a hypocalcemic stress.

In bone, PTH-mediated release of Ca from a readily-exchangeable pool is evident within minutes of hormone exposure, and a second, slower release follows after hours or days from a skeletal pool that turns over less rapidly. The resorptive effects of PTH on bone are, at least in part, dependent on the presence of 1,25$(OH)_2$D. Interestingly, when PTH concentrations are low (hypoparathyroid states), the hormone facilitates uptake of mineral into the skeleton. Thus, the PTH-mediated balance between skeletal uptake and release appears to be a dose-dependent phenomenon.

In the kidney, PTH increases the tubular reabsorption of Ca (and reduces Pi reabsorption) within minutes of exposure. Additionally, the hormone stimulates biosynthesis of 1,25$(OH)_2$D through its modulation of 25-hydroxyvitamin D-1α-hydroxylase activity. This effect occurs much more slowly. Thus, the concentration of 1,25$(OH)_2$D increases over hours or days, and the effects of this newly synthesized, slowly cleared hormone can persist for several days thereafter.

1,25Dihydroxyvitamin D acts synergistically with PTH in bone to promote release of Ca and Pi to the circulation. Like PTH, 1,25$(OH)_2$D also may be important to the process of Ca deposition into bone under certain poorly understood conditions. This function of 1,25$(OH)_2$D has been deduced on the basis of the abnormal bone development and Ca deposition observed in vitamin D-deficiency states.

In the gut, 1,25$(OH)_2$D acts through both genomic and nongenomic mechanisms to promote enhanced absorption of Ca and Pi. The hormone induces the formation of a specific Ca binding protein (calbindin-D_{28K}) and increases the concentration, turnover, and/or activity of several other proteins including an alkaline phosphatase, Ca ATPase, and brush-border actin. Although it remains unclear exactly how the flux of Ca and Pi across the cells is modulated, one or more of these proteins is likely to be important. Recently, a novel "transcaltachic" effect of $1{,}25(OH)_2D$ has been described.[35] This action, which may rely on voltage-dependent Ca channels, results in measurable uptake of luminal $^{45}Ca^{2+}$ into blood within minutes of hormone exposure and is not blocked by inhibitors of protein synthesis.

In the parathyroid gland, $1{,}25(OH)_2D$ suppresses PTH gene transcription.[36] Although this appears to be an element of negative feedback regulation, the impact of this effect on actual secretion of PTH under normal physiologic conditions has not been firmly established. However, the increase in blood-ionized Ca brought about through the homeostatic adjustments described earlier does provide a powerful negative feedback signal to PTH secretion (direct) and $1{,}25(OH)_2D$ biosynthesis (both direct and indirect through diminished circulating PTH).

A multicompartmental analysis of Ca kinetics in adult males revealed that short-term homeostatic adjustments to calcemic challenge rely more heavily on the rapid exchange of Ca between extracellular fluid and the skeleton than on influx/efflux from kidney or gut.[6] The latter mechanisms can only elicit major changes in overall blood Ca more gradually (weeks). Nonetheless, all three control points (i.e., gut, bone, and kidney) are crucial to the precise regulation of Ca concentration. For example, balance studies in young women have demonstrated that the intestine is the primary defense against hypercalcemia secondary to very high dietary Ca intake (accounting for up to 90% of the overall homeostatic buffering capacity), but the skeleton (~9%) and kidney (~1%) each play vital roles in handling the extra Ca that cannot be fully buffered by the gut.[37] On the other hand, if the stability of ionized Ca is threatened endogenously (e.g., by an intravenously infused load), the protective influence of the intestine is bypassed, and greater demands are placed on the renal and/or skeletal components. Under such frank hypercalcemic challenge, urinary output and skeletal uptake are linear functions of blood Ca. Indeed, up to 50% of the filtered Ca load can be excreted, and the skeletal clearance rate may approach that of the kidneys.[38]

Extreme dietary Ca deprivation also overwhelms or bypasses the intestines' capacity to adapt, leaving the skeleton and/or kidney responsible for the maintenance of normocalcemia. However, Ca is lost to the urine even in the face of Ca deficiency. Thus, the skeleton is the major reservoir of mineral under such conditions, and the blood-Ca concentration can be preserved even during prolonged starvation. The above discussion serves to emphasize that the relative significance of the intestines, kidneys, and skeleton in the preservation of normocalcemia depends upon the degree, direction, and source (dietary versus endogenous) of the calcemic stress.

In summary, the major net effects of the homeostatic response to hypocalcemic stress are increased Ca mobilization from bone, decreased renal Ca excretion, increased gastrointestinal Ca absorption and increased Pi excretion (which may lead to a modest reduction in blood Pi). All of these actions serve to increase blood-Ca concentration. Conversely, hypercalcemia is associated with decreased skeletal release (i.e., net skeletal uptake), increased urinary output, reduced dietary absorption, and increased renal retention of Pi.

b. Phosphatemic Stimuli

The kidney is the principal regulatory organ for Pi homeostasis. This can be deduced from several observations: (1) the blood Pi concentration is maintained at or near the renal transport maximum for the ion (TmP);[39] (2) hypophosphatemia (acting independently of the Ca/PTH axis but through an incompletely characterized mechanism) affects the renal biosynthesis of $1{,}25(OH)_2D$, which in turn, leads to enhanced gastrointestinal absorption of the mineral;[25] and (3) since dietary P (unlike Ca) usually exceeds the body's nutritional requirement, and intestinal absorption is, in large part, a function of the amount consumed, it is through excretion rather than absorption that Pi balance is preserved.

No Pi "sensors" have been identified that are analogous to the Ca receptors of the parathyroid gland. Rather, hyperphosphatemic challenges are met through Pi excretion (governed by the TmP), enhanced excretion (e.g., a reduction of the TmP by PTH), and inhibition of $1{,}25(OH)_2D$ production.

Hypophosphatemia triggers a sequence of compensatory events which include (1) stimulation of $1,25(OH)_2D$ production in the kidney, (2) enhanced mobilization of P (and Ca) from bone, and (3) a PTH-independent decrease in TmP.

Although these homeostatic responses are able to handle most phosphatemic stimuli, chronic, extremely high dietary Pi loads present a challenge to a system characterized by essentially unregulated gastrointestinal absorption. Deposition of calcium phosphate in soft tissues can be a consequence of the unrestricted influx of Pi under such conditions.

Thus, hypophosphatemia produces a net increase in P from bone, reduced loss of mineral in the urine and, over time, additional intestinal absorption. In contrast, acute hyperphosphatemia is associated with enhanced phosphaturia and diminished entry via the intestine.

2. Pathologic Perturbation

Extremes of Ca and Pi concentrations in the extracellular fluids are not compatible with life. Therefore, the homeostatic systems for these ions must be able to minimize the extreme serum levels that may result from pathologic perturbation of mineral metabolism.

a. Hypercalcemia

The great majority of pathologic hypercalcemia cases can be attributed to one of two sources: primary hyperparathyroidism or malignancy. Together these disorders account for about 90% of presenting patients.[40] Primary hyperparathyroidism is characterized by either frankly supranormal PTH concentration or by an inappropriately high level of the hormone in the face of overt or borderline hypercalcemia. Thus, some aspect of the negative feedback relationship between ionized Ca and PTH secretion is aberrant. Malignancy-associated hypercalcemia is the most common hypercalcemic syndrome among hospitalized patients.[41] It is frequently the result of PTHrP secretion by the tumor, but other malignant mechanisms can also occur (e.g., ectopic $1,25(OH)_2D$ production, and bone resorption stimulated by other local or systemic tumor-related factors). Less common hypercalcemic disorders involve other elements of the homeostatic system and include vitamin D intoxication, familial hypocalciuric hypercalcemia (enhanced tubular reabsorption), sarcoidosis (abnormal $1,25(OH)_2D$ production), and conditions that can be associated with increased bone turnover (e.g., hyperthyroidism, and immobilization).

b. Hypocalcemia

Adequate parathyroid function and end-organ responsiveness to PTH normally ensure the maintenance of ionized Ca within normal limits when hypocalcemic challenges are encountered. However, inadequate PTH secretion or a primary or acquired (secondary to vitamin D deficiency, resistance or hypomagnesemia) resistance to the action of PTH can result in chronic, pathologic hypocalcemia. Idiopathic hypoparathyroidism is a hypocalcemic disorder characterized by insufficient PTH secretion or the congenital absence of the parathyroid glands. Acquired forms of hypoparathyroidism can also occur secondary to hypomagnesemia (reversible) or result from irradiation, neoplastic infiltration of the glands, or from surgical removal of or damage to the parathyroids. Pseudohypoparathyroidism refers to a heterogeneous group of diseases which all feature end-organ unresponsiveness to PTH.

c. Hyperphosphatemia

The pathologic development of hyperphosphatemia can, in general, be attributed to two basic mechanisms. First (and more common), Pi retention occurs as a consequence of reduced renal excretion. The reduction may reflect a decreased glomerular filtration rate (e.g., chronic renal failure), an increased tubular reabsorption secondary to either a hormonal influence (e.g., hypoparathyroidism), or a genetic defect in tubular function (e.g., tumoral calcinosis). Secondly, hyperphosphatemia can occur after a dramatic, prolonged increase in Pi intake or in conditions associated with massive cell destruction and the subsequent release of soft tissue Pi stores.

d. Hypophosphatemia

In rare instances, negative Pi balance may be due to inadequate dietary intake or defective gastrointestinal absorption (e.g., vitamin D deficiency, malabsorption syndromes, or antacid abuse). More commonly, however, hypophosphatemia results from inadequate renal conservation of the ion (e.g., hyperparathyroidism, renal tubular defects, X-linked hypophosphatemic rickets, or tumor-induced osteomalacia). Finally, a shift of Pi from extracellular to intracellular compartments can occur (e.g., nutritional repletion, respiratory alkalosis, or acute gout).

IV. SUMMARY AND CONCLUSIONS

A detailed model that schematically illustrates all major components of the Ca/Pi homeostatic system is presented in Figure 5. The intestine is the gateway for entry of mineral into the circulation, and the kidneys are the principal excretory organs. Bone acts as the primary reservoir for the storage of Ca and Pi in the body. PTH is the major regulator of renal reabsorption of the minerals, whereas $1,25(OH)_2D$ holds a similar role with respect to gastrointestinal absorption. Both hormones exhibit significant effects on bone.

Disturbances of ionized Ca homeostasis are detected by receptors for the mineral on the parathyroid gland surface. The interaction of Ca with these sensors continuously updates the parathyroids with information concerning how much bioactive parathyroid hormone is needed systemically to maintain the blood Ca concentration at its set point. The hormone exerts direct effects on bone (where it stimulates either short- and long-term release of Ca from the skeleton [resorption] or

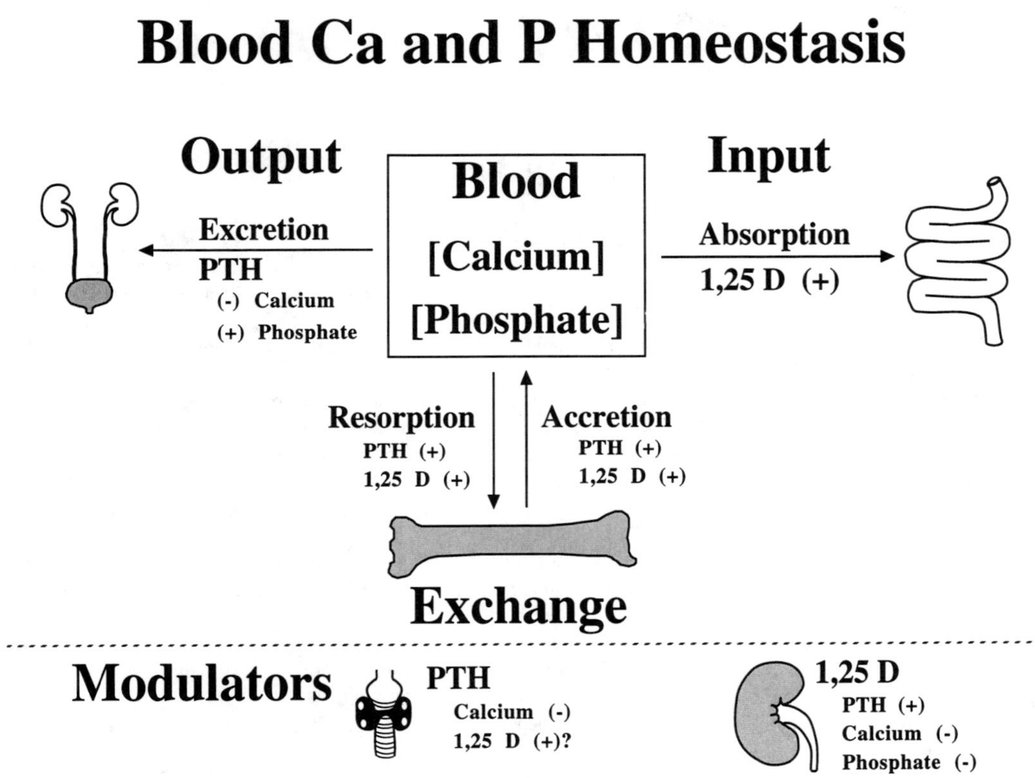

FIGURE 5. Integrated Summary of Blood Calcium and Phosphate Homeostasis. Under equilibrium conditions, input from intestinal absorption equals output in the urine. PTH and 1,25-dihydroxyvitamin D function to keep the system in balance or to adapt to special needs (e.g., lactation, calcium deprivation, etc.). Each hormone stimulates both skeletal resorption and accretion, probably through different mechanisms. Since resorption and accretion are coupled processes, the actions of these hormones on both the mineralization and demineralization components of skeletal remodeling/homeostasis are not surprising. Note: (+) symbolizes stimulation, (–) indicates inhibition of a process.

incorporation of mineral into bone [accretion]) and kidney (where it affects the degree to which Ca is reabsorbed from the glomerular filtrate). PTH also acts indirectly on the entry of dietary Ca into the organism via the intestine through its regulatory influence on the biosynthesis of $1,25(OH)_2D$. This vitamin D hormone stimulates gastrointestinal absorption of Ca through both genomic and nongenomic mechanisms. It also functions in concert with PTH in modulating the release of Ca from bone. The net effect of these responses is either (1) increased entry or recycling of Ca into the extracellular fluid compartment when relative hypocalcemia is manifest, or (2) net Ca efflux (via calciuria, skeletal accretion, and diminished gastrointestinal absorption) when the system senses hypercalcemia.

The same hormones and target organs are the cornerstones of blood Pi homeostasis. However, since gastrointestinal absorption of this mineral is normally so efficient, systemic input of Pi from the diet is usually neither a limiting factor nor a particularly useful control point. Rather, the dominant organ in Pi homeostasis is the kidney, and alterations in TmP present most of the homeostatic challenges to the organism. To counteract hypophosphatemia, the production of $1,25(OH)_2D$ is increased, intestinal Ca (and Pi) absorption is enhanced, Pi (and Ca) are mobilized from bone, bioactive PTH secretion is reduced, and the TmP is increased. Conversely, hyperphosphatemia is associated with a transient fall in blood Ca, a subsequent increase of PTH, a PTH-induced reduction of TmP, and phosphaturia. $1,25(OH)_2D$ production and its target organ effects are inhibited.

It must be emphasized that the acute regulatory objective of this elaborate network of hormones, target organs, and compartments is the preservation of blood concentrations of Ca and Pi (i.e., mineral homeostasis) even if this requires a sacrifice of bone integrity (i.e., skeletal homeostasis). These two processes, though intricately associated, are indeed distinct and of different priority to the short-term well-being of the organism.

REFERENCES

1. **Lehninger, A. L.,** *Biochemistry*, 2nd ed., Worth, New York, 1975.
2. **Broadus, A. E.,** Physiological functions of calcium, magnesium and phosphorus and mineral ion balance, in *Primer on the Metabolic Bone Diseases and Disorders of Mineral Metabolism.*, 2nd ed., Favus, M. J., ed., Raven Press, New York, 1993.
3. **Habener, J. F. and Potts, J. T., Jr.,** Primary hyperparathyroidism: clinical features, in *Endocrinology*, Vol. 2, 2nd ed., DeGroot, L. J., ed., W.B. Saunders, Philadelphia, 1989.
4. **Parfitt, A. M.,** Surgical, idiopathic, and other varieties of parathyroid hormone-deficient hypoparathyroidism, in *Endocrinology*, Vol. 2, 2nd ed., DeGroot, L. J., Ed., W.B. Saunders, Philadelphia, 1989.
5. **Bringhurst, F. R.,** Calcium and phosphate distribution, turnover and metabolic actions, in *Endocrinology*, Vol. 2, 2nd ed., DeGroot, L. J., Ed., W.B. Saunders, Philadelphia, 1989.
6. **Neer, R., Berman, M., Fisher, L. and Rosenberg, L. E.,** Multicompartmental analysis of calcium kinetics in normal adult males, *J. Clin. Invest.*, 46, 1365, 1967.
7. **Parfitt, A. M. and Kleerekoper, M.,** The divalent ion homeostatic system-physiology and metabolism of calcium, phosphorus, magnesium and bone, in *Clinical Disorders of Fluid and Electrolyte Metabolism*, 3rd ed., Maxwell, M. H. and Kleeman, C. R., eds., McGraw-Hill, New York, 1980.
8. **Portale, A. A., Halloran, B. P. and Morris, R. C., Jr.,** Dietary intake of phosphorus modulates the circadian rhythm in serum concentration of phosphorus: implications for the renal production of 1,25-dihydroxyvitamin D, *J. Clin. Invest.*, 80, 1147, 1987.
9. **Schaafsma, G.,** Calcium in extracellular fluid: homeostasis, in *Calcium in Human Biology*, Nordin, B. E. C., ed., Springer-Verlag, London, 1988.
10. **Neer, R. M.,** Calcium and inorganic phosphate homeostasis, in *Endocrinology*, Vol. 2, 2nd ed., DeGroot, L. J., ed., W.B. Saunders, Philadelphia, 1989.
11. **Nordin, B. E. C.,** Plasma calcium and plasma magnesium homeostasis, in *Calcium, Phosphate and Magnesium Metabolism*, Nordin, B. E. C., ed., Churchill Livingstone, Edinburgh, 1976.
12. **Bronner, F., Pansu, D. and Stein, W. D.,** An analysis of intestinal calcium transport across the rat intestine, *Am. J. Physiol.*, 250, G561, 1986.

13. **Pansu, D., Bellaton, C. and Bronner, F.**, Effect of Ca intake on saturable and nonsaturable components of duodenal Ca transport, *Am. J. Physiol.*, 240, G32, 1981.
14. **Heaney, R. P., Gallagher, J. C., Johnston, C. C., Neer, R. M., Parfitt, A. M. and Whedon, G. D.**, Calcium nutrition and bone health in the elderly, *Am. J. Clin. Nutr.*, 36, 986, 1982.
15. NIH Consensus Development Conference, Osteoporosis, *J. Am. Med. Assoc.*, 252, 799, 1984.
16. **Bruns, M. E., Boass, A. and Toverud, S. U.**, Regulation by dietary calcium of vitamin D-dependent calcium binding protein and active calcium transport in the small intestine of lactating rats, *Endocrinology*, 121, 278, 1987.
17. **Marcus, C. S. and Lengemann, F. W.**, Absorption of Ca^{45} and Sr^{85} from solid and liquid food at various levels of the alimentary tract of the rat, *J. Nutr.*, 77, 155, 1962.
18. **Wilz, D. R., Gray, R. W., Dominguez, J. H. and Lemann, J., Jr.**, Plasma 1,25-$(OH)_2$-vitamin D concentrations and net intestinal calcium, phosphate and magnesium absorption in humans, *Am. J. Clin. Nutr.*, 32, 2052, 1979.
19. **Bales, C. W. and Drezner, M. K.**, Divalent ion homeostasis: calcium and phosphorus metabolism, in *Textbook of Internal Medicine*, 2nd ed., Kelly, W. N., ed., J.B. Lippincott, Philadelphia, 1992.
20. **Spencer, H., Kramer, L., Norris, C. and Osis, D.**, Effect of small doses of aluminum-containing antacids on calcium and phosphorus metabolism. *Am. J. Clin. Nutr.*, 36, 32, 1982.
21. **Lemann, J., Jr.**, Urinary excretion of calcium, magnesium and phosphorus, in *Primer on the Metabolic Bone Diseases and Disorders of Mineral Metabolism*, 2nd ed., Favus, M. J., ed., Raven Press, New York, 1993.
22. **Segre, G. V., Niall, H. D., Habener, J. F. and Potts, J. T., Jr.**, Metabolism of parathyroid hormone: physiological and clinical significance, *Am. J. Med.*, 56, 774, 1974.
23. **Mallette, L. E. and Gagel, R. F.**, Parathyroid hormone and calcitonin, in *Primer on the Metabolic Bone Diseases and Disorders of Mineral Metabolism*, 2nd ed., Favus, M. J., ed., Raven Press, New York, 1993.
24. **Nesbitt, T., Drezner, M. K. and Lobaugh, B.**, Abnormal parathyroid hormone stimulation of 25-hydroxyvitamin D 1α-hydroxylase activity in the hypophosphatemic mouse, *J. Clin. Invest.*, 77, 181, 1986.
25. **Lobaugh, B. and Drezner, M. K.**, Abnormal regulation of renal 25-hydroxyvitamin D 1α-hydroxylase activity in the X-linked hypophosphatemic mouse, *J. Clin. Invest.*, 71, 400, 1983.
26. **Nesbitt, T., Lobaugh, B. and Drezner, M. K.**, Calcitonin stimulation of renal 25-hydroxyvitamin D-1-hydroxylase activity in *Hyp* mice: evidence that the regulation of calcitriol production is not universally abnormal in X-linked hypophosphatemia, *J. Clin. Invest.*, 79, 15, 1987.
27. **Trohler, U., Bonjour, J. P. and Fleisch, H.**, Renal tubular adaptation to dietary phosphorus, *Nature*, 261, 145, 1976.
28. **Goldfarb, S., Westby, G. R., Goldberg, M. and Agus, Z. S.**, Renal tubular effects of chronic phosphate depletion, *J. Clin. Invest.*, 59, 770, 1977.
29. **Linkswiler, H. M., Joyce, C. L. and Arnaud, C. R.**, Calcium retention of young adult males as affected by level of protein and calcium intake, *Trans. NY Acad. Sci.*, 36, 333, 1974.
30. **Kleeman, C. R., Bohannon, J., Bernstein, D., Ling, S. and Maxwell, M. H.**, Effect of variations in sodium intake on calcium excretion in normal humans, *Proc. Soc. Exp. Biol. Med.*, 115, 29, 1964.
31. **Heaney, R. P. and Recker, R. R.**, Effects of nitrogen, phosphorus and caffeine on calcium balance in women, *J. Lab. Clin. Med.*, 99, 46, 1982.
32. **Pansu, D., Bellaton, C., and Bronner, F.**, Effect of lactose on duodenal calcium-binding protein and calcium absorption, *J. Nutr.*, 109, 508, 1979.
33. **Kies, C.**, *Nutritional Bioavailability of Calcium*, American Chemical Society, (ACS Symposium Series 275), Washington, D.C., 1985, 105.
34. **Orloff, J. J., Wu, T. L., and Stewart, A. F.**, Parathyroid hormone-like proteins: biochemical responses and receptor interactions, *Endocr. Rev.*, 10, 476, 1989.
35. **Nemere, I., Yoshimoto, Y. and Norman, A. W.**, Studies on the mode of action of calciferol. LIV. Calcium transport in perfused duodena from normal chicks: enhancement with 14 minutes of exposure to 1,25-dihydroxyvitamin D_3, *Endocrinology*, 115, 1476, 1984.
36. **Silver, J., Russell, J. and Sherwood, L. M.**, Regulation by vitamin D metabolites of messenger RNA for preproparathyroid hormone in isolated bovine parathyroid cells, *Proc. Natl. Acad. Sci. USA*, 82, 4279, 1985.
37. **Phang, J. M., Berman, M., Finerman, G. A., Neer, R. M., Rosenberg, L. E. and Hahn, T. J.**, Dietary perturbation of calcium metabolism in normal man: compartmental analysis, *J. Clin. Invest.*, 48, 67, 1969.
38. **Nordin, B. E. C. and Peacock, M.**, Role of kidney in regulation of plasma calcium, *Lancet*, 2, 1280, 1969.
39. **Harris, C. A., Baer P. G., Chirito, E. and Dirks, J. H.**, Composition of mammalian glomerular filtrate, *Am. J. Physiol.*, 227, 972, 1974.
40. **Stewart, A. F. and Broadus, A. E.**, Mineral metabolism, in *Endocrinology and Metabolism*, Felig, P., Baxter, J. P., Broadus, A. E. and Frohman, L. A., eds., McGraw-Hill, New York, 1987.
41. **Lobaugh, B. and Drezner, M. K.**, Evaluation of hypercalcemia and hypocalcemia, in *Textbook of Internal Medicine*, 2nd ed., Kelly, W. N., ed., J.B. Lippincott, Philadelphia, 1992.
42. **Kutsky, R. J.**, *Handbook of Vitamins, Minerals and Hormones*, 2nd ed., Van Nostrand Reinhold, New York, 1981.
43. **Walser, M.**, Ion association. VI. Interaction between calcium, magnesium, inorganic phosphate, citrate and protein in normal human plasma, *J. Clin. Invest.*, 40, 723, 1961.

Chapter 4

INTESTINAL BIOAVAILABILITY AND ABSORPTION OF CALCIUM

Dexter Louie, Ph.D.

TABLE OF CONTENTS

0-8493-7845-1/95/$0.00+$.50

I. INTRODUCTION

Calcium (Ca) is a major mineral component of the vertebrate skeleton, which holds 99% of the Ca in the body, with the remaining 1% mainly in extracellular fluid (see Chapter 3). Nonskeletal Ca has many vital bodily functions including nerve conduction, blood clotting, muscle contraction, and intracellular signal transduction. Long-term maintenance of proper extracellular Ca concentration requires both adequate dietary intake and proper absorption of Ca. Blood Ca concentrations are regulated within a narrow range by a number of hormones (see Chapters 11, 12, and 13). If Ca derived from the diet is insufficient, bone mineral is removed to maintain Ca levels. Thus, adequate intake and absorption of Ca ensures optimal mineralization during periods of rapid growth, maintains bone mass and density during the later stages of the life cycle, and prevents reduced bone strength.

This chapter focuses on the physiologic control of Ca absorption and on the mechanisms by which Ca ions are transferred across the intestinal barrier. Various methods used to study Ca absorption are covered. The mechanisms for Ca transport in the intestine, either through the cell (transcellular and saturable) or around the cell (paracellular and nonsaturable) are examined. The extent to which Ca is absorbed from food depends on Ca bioavailability. Several components of foods enhance or decrease Ca absorption because of various types of binding to Ca ions within the lumen of the small bowel. The ways in which these factors in food alter Ca absorption and homeostasis are examined.

II. HUMAN CALCIUM ABSORPTION — OVERVIEW

The amount of Ca absorbed by humans depends on a variety of factors including the length of the intestinal segment, transit time of the chyme, Ca bioavailability from foods, and the intraluminal Ca concentration. The jejunum absorbs a larger amount of Ca than the duodenum, due mainly to the greater length of the jejunum.[1,2] The duodenum, however, has the greatest active absorptive capacity per unit length. The longer the chyme resides in a particular intestinal segment, the greater the chance for movement of ions across the "water barrier" to the intestinal mucosa for greater absorption. The ileum has lower Ca absorption per unit length than the jejunum,[2,3] and vitamin D-induced absorption is similar in both segments. However, given the slightly greater length of the ileum and its ability to absorb more Ca through a paracellular route, the ileum still absorbs a larger amount of Ca than other intestinal segments.

The availability of Ca for absorption from foods is an important consideration when recommending Ca intake. If Ca is complexed to different food components, the amount of Ca absorbed is decreased. This reduction in absorption efficiency is especially important for vegan diets, which may contain several factors that inhibit absorption of Ca. Thus, the type of diet must be considered when recommending Ca intakes to meet daily needs. Dietary interactions that affect Ca absorption are covered in detail in the section on Ca bioavailability.

Increasing dietary Ca induces a proportional increase in the amount of Ca absorbed by diffusion via the paracellular route, but there is no increase in the active saturable process of absorption. The fraction of dietary Ca absorbed decreases with increased dietary Ca, although the absolute amount of Ca absorbed actually increases.[4] Ca loads between 15–500 mg result in absorption averaging 64.0% at the lowest loads and 28.6% at the highest.

Since Ca requirements change throughout the life cycle, it is important to know the concomitant efficiency of Ca absorption. Infants need to absorb 125 mg Ca daily to meet growth needs of skeletal Ca deposition with absorptive efficiency up to 60%. The efficiency of absorption in younger children remains high (up to 60% or so), but teenagers past the growth spurt have an absorptive efficiency of Ca similar to that of adults, i.e., 25–30%. During pregnancy there are changes in Ca absorption and metabolism. Absorption changes from the normal 27% efficiency to 54% at 5 or 6 months of gestation and 42% at term.[5] Ca absorption decreases with increasing age, particularly in

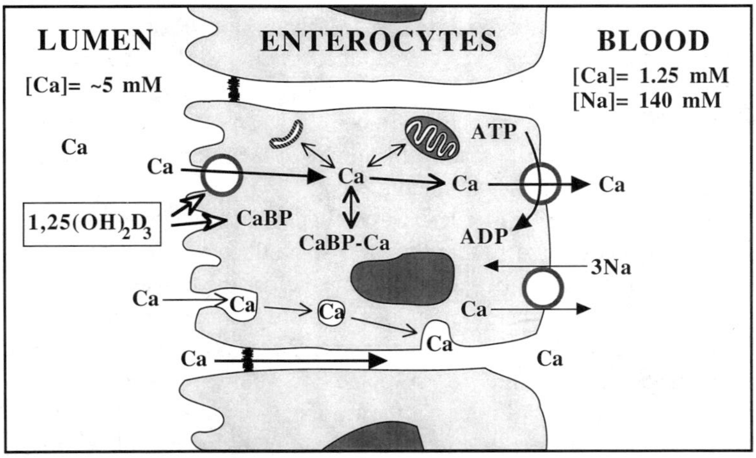

FIGURE 1. Diagram of Pathways for Calcium Absorption from the Intestinal Lumen to the Blood. The paracellular pathway for calcium movement occurs between cells, can occur in both directions, and is influenced by both luminal calcium concentration and transepithelial electrical gradient. Transcellular movement of calcium begins with binding of calcium to the luminal brush border. Calcium entry can be stimulated by vitamin D. Calcium is then equilibrated within the cell by the cytosolic pool, mitochondria, or endoplasmic reticulum. Transport of calcium across the cytosol has been attributed to vitamin D-inducible calcium-binding proteins (CaBP) and also to endosomes and lysosomes. Calcium extrusion from the cell occurs via an ATP-dependent calcium pump and to a lesser extent by a Na^+-Ca^{++} exchange port. Calcium, contained within endosomes or lysosomes, exits by fusion with the basolateral membrane.

the saturable component. This decrease is greater in women than in men. A variety of physiologic and endocrine factors, including estrogen, affect Ca metabolism, which in turn affects the signals within the body that regulate Ca absorption.[6]

III. PATHWAYS OF CALCIUM ABSORPTION

Ca absorption occurs by two major pathways, paracellular (absorption between the intestinal cells) and transcellular (absorption through the intestinal cells). This section covers the various mechanisms and influences on absorption through both pathways.

Ca is absorbed from the intestinal lumen, where Ca concentrations are in the millimolar range. Ultimately Ca is released into the blood, which contains an ionized, or free, Ca concentraton of approximately 1.25 m*M*. One method for studying Ca entry is by using rightside-out brush border membrane vesicles (BBMV). Under different bathing concentrations of Ca, the measured movement of Ca in BBMV can be described as the sum of saturable and nonsaturable steps.[7-9]

Other methods of studying Ca transport are by *in vivo* perfusion, *in situ* loops, and everted gut sacs. These techniques also describe saturable and nonsaturable Ca absorption kinetics. The nonsaturable portion is attributed to movement of Ca between cells, or paracellular movement (see Figure 1). The saturable step has been well studied and represents transcellular or transepithelial transport. This transport has three separate phases: (1) Ca entry into the enterocyte across the brush border membrane, (2) Ca movement across the intracellular space, and (3) Ca exit from the cell across the basolateral membrane (see Figure 1). The main physiologic regulator of intestinal Ca absorption is vitamin D, which can enhance active transcellular movement of Ca by 30%.

A. PARACELLULAR CALCIUM MOVEMENT

Paracellular transport of Ca occurs between the cells of the intestinal epithelium. A tight junction joins the cells, and Ca passes through these junctions to enter the circulation. The amount of paracellular transport of Ca depends on the concentration of luminal Ca, i.e., the greater the level of Ca, the greater the amount of Ca fluxes across the tight junction. Different dietary factors probably work to loosen these tight junctions to promote Ca absorption. Passive absorption of Ca via a paracellular route accounts for a large percentage of total Ca absorbed, perhaps as high as 90% in animal models.[10]

Paracellular flux of Ca can occur in both the mucosal to serosal (m $\rightarrow$ s) and serosal to mucosal (s $\rightarrow$ m) direction. Paracellular flux of Ca differs among the segments of the intestine, being lowest in the duodenum and higher in the jejunum and ileum.

To differentiate between transcellular and paracellular Ca transport, two critical measurements must be made: (1) simultaneous paracellular flux of ^{3}H-mannitol, which is a measure of permeability of the tight junction; and (2) voltage-dependent Ca flux across the tissue preparation. To meet these criteria, investigators mount intestinal preparations in Ussing chambers and manipulate the electrochemical gradient. The electromotive drive to enhance Ca transport can be short-circuited (eliminated) by changing the potential difference between the two sides of the membrane with the voltage clamped. One can compare the amount of Ca moved from one side to the other by measuring the changes in current under different concentrations of Ca or other treatments. In this way, the amount of Ca flux over time can be calculated. This Ca flux can be compared with ^{3}H-mannitol absorption, which occurs only through a paracellular pathway. In this experimental setup, if one measures the concentration-dependent Ca flux, the m $\rightarrow$ s flux has components of both saturable and nonsaturable pathways. In contrast the s $\rightarrow$ m flux can be calculated as a linear function throughout all gut segments.

By plotting results of voltage-clamp Ca flux studies, one can separate the voltage-independent (transcellular) Ca flux and quantify the diffusive or paracellular transport. Voltage-independent Ca flux is 30% of the total in the duodenum and ileum and is 40% in the jejunum.[11] The m $\rightarrow$ s flux is greater than the s $\rightarrow$ m flux in the duodenum, while the s $\rightarrow$ m exceeds the m $\rightarrow$ s flux in the jejunum and ileum. Thus, under the conditions of the Ussing chamber, the jejunum and ileum secrete Ca into the lumen in these segments.

These *in vitro* studies, however, may differ from what occurs physiologically. Since the tissue mounted in the Ussing chamber is in a nonphysiologic environment, it is difficult to extrapolate these data to project what happens *in vivo*. Secretion of Ca by the intestine might not occur *in vivo*. Under conditions of high Ca concentrations, *in situ* absorption studies show a similar magnitude of nonsaturable component throughout the intestine.[12,13] *In vitro,* the m $\rightarrow$ s flux is greater across the jejunum and ileum than across the duodenum. Other factors, then, may regulate paracellular Ca flux *in vivo*.

One factor that increases Ca flux is a complex of calcium:citrate:malate (CCM). Humans absorb Ca better from CCM than from Ca carbonate.[14] Increasing the citrate content of the CCM complex causes a dose-dependent increase in ^{45}Ca absorption in *in situ* loop experiments.[15] In studies using Ussing chambers, citrate increases paracellular transport of ^{45}Ca with net movement in the m $\rightarrow$ s direction. Citrate enhances the absorption of Ca to a greater extent in the ileum than in the duodenum.[15] Thus, citrate may enhance Ca absorption by increasing paracellular transport.

The paracellular movement of Ca through the tight junction is slower than predicted by simple diffusion, but hyperosmolar solutions can double or triple the rate of passive Ca flux. The increased rate of diffusion may occur because water moving into an area of hyperosmolarity expands tissues and widens the tight junctions. One theory to explain the increased paracellular transport of Ca is that of solvent drag.[16] As water moves through the tight junctions, Ca is brought along (see Figure 2).

B. TRANSEPITHELIAL CALCIUM MOVEMENT

The movement of Ca across intestinal epithelial cells requires three separate steps. Ca must (1) enter the cell across the mucosal membrane, (2) move across the cell through the cytoplasm, and (3) exit the cell at the serosal membrane.

1. Calcium Entry

Ca entry from the intestinal lumen across the brush-border membrane of the cell occurs down an electrochemical gradient. An electrical gradient of 40–70 mV exists with the interior of the cell

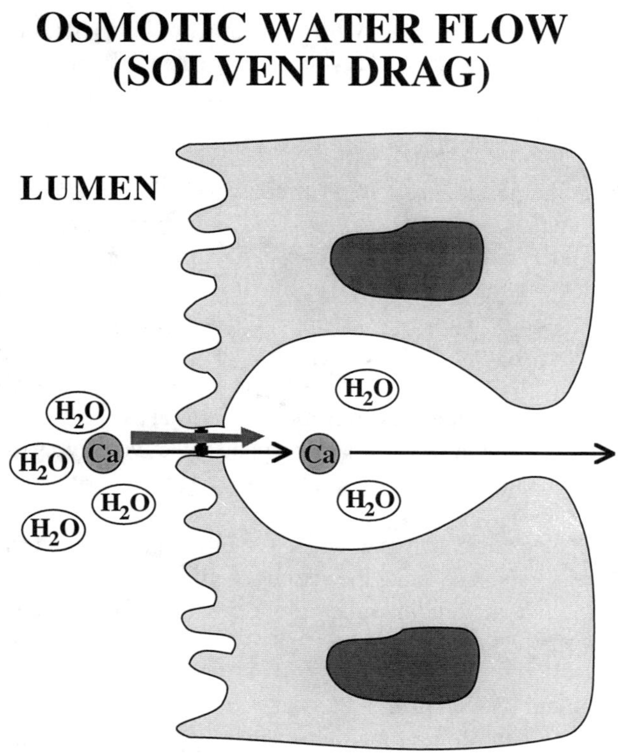

FIGURE 2. Working Model of Paracellular Movement of Calcium across the Rat Intestine. The net paracellular flux depends on the hydraulic conductivity of the tight junctions for calcium. This flux is controlled by the amount and direction of paracellular water flow. Movement of water from the lumen to the blood carries along calcium (solvent drag).

negative. The chemical gradient is about 10,000, with the intestinal luminal concentration of Ca in the millimolar range, and the intracellular free Ca concentration at 0.1–1 μM. Because Ca entry at the brush-border membrane is a saturable process, it has been ascribed to a Ca transporter or channel, although little direct evidence exists for either. Studies of Ca entry into cells have been performed on intact epithelia, isolated cells, and brush-border membrane vesicles (BBMV). The BBMV preparation has an outer layer of microvillar membrane with an entrapped vesicular space. The advantage of this preparation is the decreased interference from other tissue constituents when examining the Ca entry. BBMV prepared from vitamin D-deficient rats have greatly increased our understanding of Ca entry and the role of vitamin D in stimulating Ca movement across the brush border. Vesicles from vitamin D-deficient chicks showed a decreased initial rate of Ca uptake compared with vitamin D-repleted chicks. Ca uptake, measured for a longer period, did not differ in the amount of Ca entry due to treatment. These data suggest that vitamin D enhances the initial rate of entry, but does not affect the overall capacity for Ca entry.[7]

The vesicular uptake of Ca by BBMV is not dependent on energy. Using BBMV from rat intestine, the uptake of Ca can be broken down into two components: (1) Ca binding to the membrane and (2) transport into the vesicular space. The brush-border surface contains a small number of high-affinity anionic sites and a large number of low-affinity Ca-binding sites.[8] Although the specific proteins containing the binding sites have not been identified, the Kd for the high-affinity sites is 10^{-10} *M,* which is similar to other Ca-binding proteins such as calbindin (Ca-binding protein [CaBP]),[17] vitamin D-independent calmodulin,[18] and a calmodulin-binding protein.[19] One or more of these proteins might act to transport Ca from the lumen through the brush-border membrane into the cytoplasm. Calbindin-D is a likely candidate since it appears at the time Ca transport increases. Although binding proteins at the brush border have been identified, other aspects of the molecular mechanism for Ca entry across the brush border are not known or understood.

Vitamin D-stimulated Ca uptake by BBMV occurs within two hours of hormone administration,[20] which suggests that increased Ca entry does not require new protein synthesis.[21] It has been suggested that vitamin D-induced changes in membrane fluidity[22] may increase Ca uptake; however, this observation is unconfirmed. Vitamin D also increases alkaline phosphatase activity, and the possible interaction of calbindin-D with alkaline phosphatase on the brush-border surface has led investigators to examine the possible role of alkaline phosphatase in Ca entry. In rats, vitamin D deficiency decreases alkaline phosphatase activity,[23] and vitamin D injection increases brush-border alkaline phosphatase activity within 10 min, peaking at 45 min.[24] Since vitamin D also increases the low-affinity calcium-magnesium ATPase,[25] it was hypothesized that the two enzymes might act as a complex to stimulate Ca entry. However, several studies argue against a direct role for alkaline phosphatase in Ca transfer: vitamin D-stimulated Ca transport occurs before alkaline phosphatase activity increases;[26] alkaline phosphatase and Ca-ATPase activities appear at different times following vitamin D administration,[27] alkaline phosphatase and Ca-ATPase enzymes are separate molecular entities,[28] and neither inhibition of alkaline phosphatase activity by cyclohexamide[7,21] nor by theophylline[29] decreases Ca entry. These studies, therefore, suggest that alkaline phosphatase does not mediate Ca entry.

Our knowledge of the mechanisms though which Ca enters enterocytes is elementary. Although BBMV has allowed researchers to separate the actions of vitamin D from other tissue components, it remains difficult to separate the binding of Ca to the membrane from the transport of Ca across the brush-border membrane.

2. Intracellular Movement of Calcium

After Ca ions enter the cell, they must move across the cytoplasm and exit through the basolateral membrane. When large amounts of Ca enter the cell, one would expect Ca levels to increase. However, intracellular-free Ca levels remain stable within the nanomolar range. To prevent a large increase in cytosolic Ca, the calculated turnover of intracellular-free Ca must increase 25-fold.[30] Simple diffusion of Ca across the cell is two orders of magnitude slower than the experimentally measured movement of Ca across the cell.[31] To explain the enhanced transport, a Ca-binding protein was proposed by Wasserman[32] to ferry Ca across the cytosol. A Ca-binding protein (CaBP or calbindin), found in mammals and birds (9k Da and 28k Da, respectively), fulfills the requirements. The large amounts of CaBP can account for the measured transcellular transport rate. CaBP levels increase in response to vitamin D, which helps explain vitamin D-stimulated Ca absorption. Feher demonstrated *in vitro* that the addition of vitamin D-dependent CaBP to everted sac preparations significantly enhances Ca flux,[33] and that a linear relationship exists between Ca transported and CaBP content. Duodenal transport of Ca decreases to near zero when CaBP levels are undetectable.[34] Inhibition of mRNA transcription and protein synthesis abolishes the induction of CaBP and inhibits vitamin D-augmented Ca transport in the ileum.[35]

Of the other soluble Ca-binding proteins that facilitate intracellular transfer, only calmodulin approaches the millimolar cellular concentration of CaBP. Unlike CaBP, calmodulin levels do not increase with vitamin D treatment.[18] Calmodulin also differs from CaBP by its lower affinity for Ca. This difference in affinity may facilitate the transfer of Ca from calmodulin to other transporters. Thus, calmodulin may act to buffer intracellular Ca, and the transfer of Ca may utilize other carriers.[36] Mitochondria, Golgi complex, and endoplasmic reticula have been proposed as Ca carriers, but studies neither strongly support nor refute these organelles as Ca carriers.[37] Since CaBP is the only vitamin D-dependent Ca-binding protein identified so far, CaBP may be assigned as the main facilitator of intracellular Ca transfer.

In contrast, an endosomal-lysosomal vesicular pathway has been proposed to move Ca across the cytosolic space by carrier proteins. When Ca absorption is stimulated in the chick intestine, lysosomes of intestinal epithelial cells contain high levels of Ca[38] as demonstrated by biochemical, histological, and electron microprobe analyses. When vitamin D-depleted rats or chicks were repleted with vitamin D, electron-microscopic studies showed increased numbers of Ca-containing vesicles.[39] Vitamin D repletion increased the subcellular distribution of Ca in organelles, with the highest amounts found in lysosomes. Immunofluorescence studies of intestinal tissue sections show movement of endosomal-lysosmal vesicles to the basolateral membrane within 3 min following vitamin D administration.[37]

In double perfusion studies in which radiolabeled Ca is perfused in the duodenum of vitamin D-depleted animals, and the organ vasculature is perfused separately, addition of vitamin D to the vascular perfusate increases within minutes the amount of radiolabeled Ca transferred from the duodenum to the vasculature.[40] The rapid stimulation of Ca transport signifies a nongenomic effect of vitamin D because it is so much quicker than the genomic process involving transcription and protein synthesis of CaBP. This type of transport was named "transcaltachia" to describe movement of Ca ions across the epithelial cell in endocytic and lysosomal vesicles.

In the experiments on endosomal-lysosomal vesicular Ca transport (see Chapter 12), data were reported as a percentage of the values of the control group. The absolute amount of Ca transport is not shown, and it is therefore difficult to assess how much endosomal-lysosomal vesicular Ca transport contributes to overall transcellular Ca absorption.

3. Calcium Extrusion

In contrast to an electrochemical gradient that favors Ca entry, extrusion of Ca works against a gradient. The basolateral membranes of intestinal cells possess a Ca channel, an ATP-dependent Ca pump, a Na^+/Ca^{++} exchanger, and a Na^+/K^+ pump[41] (see Chapter 6). The ATP-dependent Ca uptake by basolateral membranes indicates the presence of an active component of transcellular Ca absorption. Extrusion has been attributed mostly to an ATP-dependent Ca pump. Although a Na^+/Ca^{++} exchanger exists in the basolateral membrane, it contributes little to Ca extrusion. The intestinal ATP-dependent Ca pump has been partially purified and resides specifically on the basolateral membrane of the epithelial cell. The location of the pump is further demonstrated by immunohistochemical studies showing antibody binding along the basolateral membrane.[42]

Administration of vitamin D increases both the rate of Ca uptake and the total amount of Ca accumulated by basolateral membrane vesicles (BLMV). Vitamin D treatment does not change the K_m of the pump, but it increases the V_{max} from 2.8 to 8.2 nmol/mg protein/min.[41] The vitamin D-augmented Ca transport could result from a synthesis of new Ca pumps, recruitment of existing Ca pumps in the cytosol, or direct activation of the Ca pump. Western blot analysis of homogenates from the intestinal mucosa by an antibody to an erythrocyte Ca pump showed that vitamin D treatment increased the number of Ca pumps in the membranes.[41] These results suggest that vitamin D stimulates the synthesis of new Ca pumps, although an enhanced recruitment of existing pre-formed pumps from intracellular stores also remains possible.

The activity of the Ca pump can be increased by calmodulin, CaBP, and other Ca-binding proteins. However, the increased rate of Ca uptake does not appear to be specific to proteins that bind Ca. Walters et al.[43] used basolateral membrane vesicles to show that EGTA (a Ca chelator) could increase Ca uptake. They theorized that Ca ions, complexed to EGTA or to proteins in the membrane or cytosol are more accessible to the pump.

In addition to Ca extrusion mediated by a vitamin D-stimulated Ca pump, a vitamin D-activated Ca channel on the basolateral membrane has been described.[44] The vitamin D-stimulated Ca uptake can be mimicked by Bay K8644, a Ca-channel agonist. Additionally, the vitamin D-stimulated uptake can be inhibited by the specific Ca-channel antagonist, nifedipine. Thus, vitamin D can augment Ca absorption at the basolateral membrane either by increasing the number of Ca pumps or by activating Ca channels. In contrast to the transfer of Ca by carrier proteins, the mechanism for Ca extrusion differs for transcaltachia. Endosomal-lysosomal vesicles transfer Ca to the extracellular environment by exocytosis at the basolateral membrane rather than by a Ca pump.

C. RATE-LIMITING STEP OF TRANSCELLULAR CALCIUM TRANSPORT

The rate-limiting step for movement of Ca from lumen into the blood may be one of the three defined steps for transcellular absorption: entry into the cell from the lumen, transport across the cytosolic space, or extrusion from the cell at the basolateral membrane. The activity of the

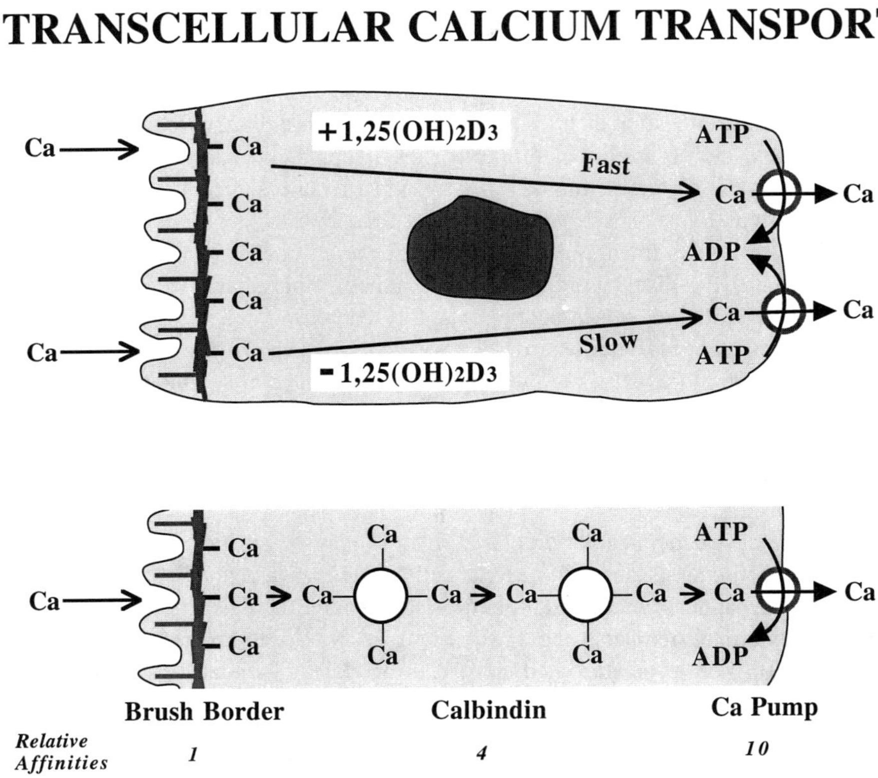

FIGURE 3. Transcellular Diffusional-Active Transport Model of Calcium Absorption. Calcium is initially bound to a brush border complex, then bound to calbindin, followed by binding to a ATP-dependent calcium pump on the basolateral membrane. There is an uphill gradient of binding affinity from the apical to the basal-lateral pole. In a vitamin D-sufficient state calcium diffusion increases from brush border to the basolateral membrane. (Adapted from Wasserman et al.[41])

basolateral membrane Ca pump is many-fold greater than necessary to accommodate active intestinal Ca transport.[31] Thus, extrusion of Ca from the cell is not the rate-limiting step. A speedy process of extrusion at the basolateral membrane ensures the maintenance of a low intracellular concentration (10^{-10} *M*) of Ca. If Ca exit were rate limiting, then the ionic concentration of intracellular Ca would rise following a meal.

The same reasoning can be applied to cytosolic transport. If transport were rate limiting, one would expect an increased intracellular ionic Ca concentration at the plasma membrane. A gradient could exist across the cytosolic space from millimolar concentrations to nanomolar concentrations at the basolateral membrane. Again, a gradient like this would result in increased intracellular ionic Ca concentrations. Some researchers have argued that the absence of an intracellular Ca gradient would not rule out transcellular transport as the rate-limiting step. Other organelles, which also can bind Ca, may regulate intracellular Ca concentrations (see Chapter 6). Because cytosolic Ca concentrations are low, if transcellular transport is not rate-limiting, the entry step is the remaining candidate for the rate-limiting step. Ca entry can be rate-limiting if the number of channels is small. Current understanding of Ca entry remains rudimentary, and further research is needed to clarify whether or not Ca entry at the brush-border membrane limits absorption.

Overall, the kinetics of Ca movement across the cell favors vectorial movement from intestinal lumen to blood. The affinity of CaBP to bind Ca exceeds the affinity of the brush border by a factor of four.[41] In turn, the basolateral Ca pump exceeds CaBP affinity for Ca by a factor of two. The vectorial movement and relative differences in affinities are illustrated in Figure 3. The uphill gradient of binding affinities from the entry at the brush-border membrane to extrustion at the basolateral Ca pump ensures movement of Ca across the cell and into the blood. Since vitamin D enhances movement of Ca at each of the three stages, the steps of Ca transport are coordinated.

During vitamin D deficiency, transcellular Ca absorption is slower than under conditions of vitamin D sufficiency, which decreases the quantity of Ca transferred to blood per unit time. In the vitamin D-repleted animal, vitamin D enhances Ca entry by 20–40%.

D. HUMAN STUDIES

Although *in vivo* human studies cannot pinpoint the particular route of absorption, they can still suggest what mechanisms are used. For example, the role of vitamin D for Ca absorption can be studied in patients with end-stage renal disease (ESRD), in which vitamin D would not be hydroxylated to 1,25-dihydroxyvitamin D ($1{,}25(OH)_2D$), the active form needed for biologic action. Figure 4 shows Ca absorption at different luminal Ca concentrations. Normal subjects show no difference in Ca absorption in the jejunum and ileum over a wide range of Ca concentrations. However, the pattern of absorption in the jejunum is curvilinear, and in the ileum the pattern is linear with no hint of saturation. The pattern in the ileum is consistent with passive absorption. ESRD patients have marked deficiencies in Ca absorption. In the jejunum Ca absorption is lower than normal, but still increases with higher luminal Ca concentrations. Between 5 and 20 m*M* Ca absorption is mainly mediated by passive mechanisms. Since the pattern of absorption among normal, ESRD + vitamin D, and ESRD patients is similar, vitamin D does not have a major influence on passive absorption in the jejunum. In contrast, the absorption of Ca by the ileum in ESRD patients is reduced and does not increase with higher concentrations of Ca.[45] Two possible explanations could explain the data. First, if higher Ca concentrations were administered to normal subjects and showed saturable absorption, then ileal absorption would be active. Although not demonstrated in this figure, other data suggest that the ileum can actively transport Ca because the normal ileum can absorb against a concentration gradient.[46] This would explain the increase in Ca absorption with administration of vitamin D. Second, both active and passive Ca absorption in the ileum may depend on vitamin D. However, in this case the active transport would be very small compared with the passive component so that a curvilinear (saturable) pattern is not detected.[46] Studies in animals provide evidence for and against vitamin D influences on passive absorption,[46] although not to the extent that would explain the ileal absorption of Ca in ESRD patients.

E. SUMMARY

Ca is absorbed from the intestine by two main routes, either through or between the cells. Movement through the cell involves cellular machinery and movement of Ca into, across, and extruded from the cell. Ca enters the cell across the brush-border membrane down a chemical gradient via a channel or carrier. Ca moves across the cell bound to a Ca-binding protein, whose biosynthesis is induced by vitamin D. A Ca-ATPase pump then extrudes Ca against a gradient. Another less likely manner of Ca absorption through the cell involves pinocytosis. Ca is engulfed into membrane vesicles and moves across the cell, then fuses with the plasma membrane and releases Ca into the extracellular space.

Movement of Ca between the cells (paracellular) is driven by chemical gradients. The amount of Ca absorbed paracellularly is also influenced by the structure of the tight junctions. Different factors in foods can alter the tight junctions, changing the rate of Ca absorption. Paracellular transport predominates in the ileum and accounts for the majority of Ca absorbed in the intestine. Thus, total Ca absorption is the sum of paracellular and transcellular routes. Larger amounts of Ca are absorbed paracellularly, but the mechanism for transcellular transport is better understood.

IV. TRADITIONAL METHODS TO MEASURE CALCIUM ABSORPTION

Many techniques exist for the measurement of Ca absorption. Use of a particular method depends on the subjects tested and the object of the investigation. Intestinal perfusion and balance studies are performed on animals and humans to measure the apparent absorption of Ca from a meal. Isolated

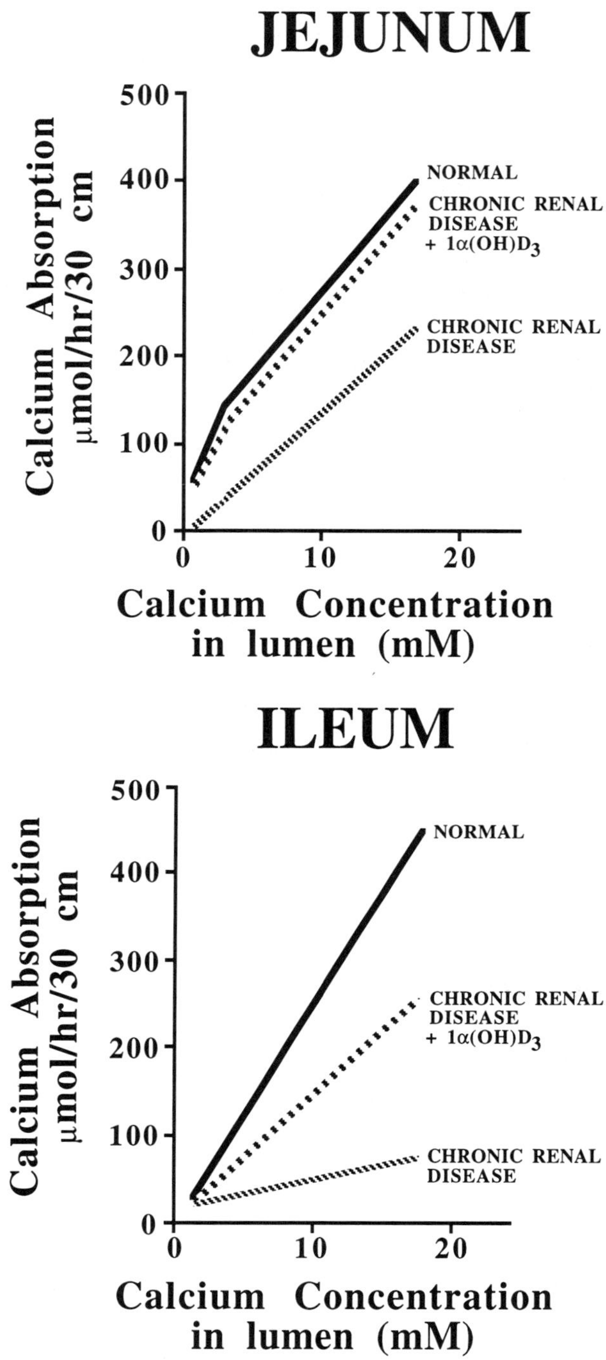

FIGURE 4. Schematic Diagram of Calcium Absorption Efficiencies at Different Luminal Calcium Concentrations in the Jejunum and Ileum. Groups studied are normal subjects and patients with end-stage renal disease with or without treatment with 1α-hydroxyvitamin D_3 (1α(OH)D_3). (Adapted from Sheikh et al.[46])

intestinal cells and organelles, *in situ* loops, and everted intestinal sacs are useful models to determine the mechanisms that mediate Ca absorption.

A. INTESTINAL BALANCE

The intestinal balance study represents a crude, overall method for determining Ca absorption. This method measures the amount of Ca ingested and the amount excreted. Output is subtracted from input to calculate net Ca absorption. The simplest method provides a known amount of Ca in food for the subject to ingest, followed by measuring Ca in the stool. A nonabsorbable marker (e.g., carmine red or chromium oxide) is typically given at the beginning of the study period, and collections are made until the second marker appears. Intervals for study are usually 6 days for humans. These studies measure net amounts of Ca absorbed by saturable and nonsaturable mechanisms. The intestinal balance method does not distinguish between the two processes. An increase in one pathway may disguise a decrease in the other pathway, thus not revealing what changes a treatment may impose.

Intestinal balance studies also cannot distinguish between nonabsorbed dietary Ca and secreted endogenous Ca that is not reabsorbed. Even if one assumes that endogenous Ca is absorbed at the same rate as exogenous Ca, the amounts of endogenous Ca secreted may differ over time or under diverse conditions. Thus, the amount of Ca in the stool does not accurately reflect true Ca absorption.

A true measure of Ca absorption accounts for the endogenous Ca in the stool and would provide a better estimate of the dietary Ca absorbed. To estimate the endogenous secretion of Ca, subjects ingest a marker to label their stools and simultaneously receive an intravenous injection of radioactive Ca to label the endogenous pool of Ca. Samples of plasma and stool are measured for radioactive Ca. The amount of radioactivity excreted into the stool is calculated as a function of the integral of plasma Ca-specific activity over the collection period. Thus, the radioactive marker in plasma gives an estimate of the total Ca pool, and the radioactivity in the stool represents the proportion of endogenous Ca secreted into the intestine.

Although double isotope studies should be used to estimate the amount of endogenous secretion, some studies have used single isotope methods[46] to measure true Ca absorption. There are problems with the use of single isotopes for measuring the true absorption of Ca. The primary reason is isotope equilibrium. The labeled ion from one side of the membrane is exchanged for an unlabeled ion on the other side. Equilibrium may exist for Ca, but not for the radiolabel over the short time frame of the study, and thus, net transfer is not measured. Another problem with isotopic equilibrium is the simple diffusion of label from one side to another through tight junctions. Again, one sees the transfer of tracer without measurement of net Ca movement. Because unidirectional fluxes of isotope are equated with mass movement of Ca, isotopic equilibration methods overestimate both the amount of Ca secreted into and that absorbed by the gut. The movement of the isotope may not be the same as the movement of Ca. This incorrect assumption leads to the erroneous calculation of the amount of Ca moved, which usually results in the overestimation of endogenous fecal Ca. The method for true absorption of Ca must be critically evaluated, and this is best done when the method is coupled with intestinal balance studies.

Although the balance method is limited by its inability to identify segments of the gastrointestinal tract that absorb or secrete Ca, it is useful as a method to collect data on human subjects. Other techniques have been developed for direct determination of Ca absorption in animal models or *in vitro*.

B. *IN SITU* LOOPS

The use of *in situ* loops provides a method to study absorption from different segments of the intestine. In anesthesized rats the segment studied is ligated and radiolabeled Ca of known specific activity is injected. Absorption over time is quantified by measuring the remaining radioactivity in the lumen. Figure 5[31] illustrates the absorption pattern of various Ca concentrations in rats. If one analyzes and presents the data as a Michaelis-Menten function, at concentrations below 50 mM Ca, transport has a maximum velocity (V_{max}) of 22 μmol/hr/loop and a K_m of 3.9 mM. At Ca concentrations above 50 mM, transport does not follow the theoretical curve modeled by the Michaelis-Menten equation, because Ca efflux exceeds predicted transport. In fact, a greater proportion of Ca transport uses a system that does not saturate at low concentrations. Thus, nonsaturable systems are also involved in Ca transport. This pattern can also be seen by examining the data in Figure 5 in another fashion. At a concentration of 200 mM, half of the Ca is absorbed in approximately 2 hr, in contrast to lower Ca concentrations (10 mM or less) where Ca is completely absorbed by this time.

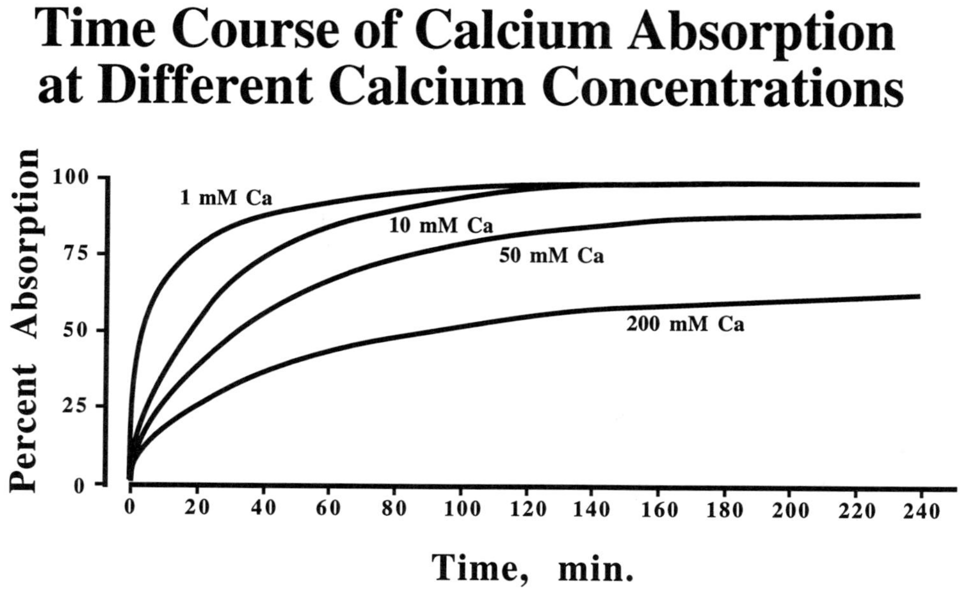

FIGURE 5. Time Course of Calcium Absorption by In Situ Duodenal Loops. Calcium absorption is dependent on both saturable and nonsaturable processes. When Ca is instilled into the lumen at increasing concentrations, the absorption of Ca is completed at lower concentrations much quicker than at higher concentrations. In the original experiment, absorption was calculated as the amount of ^{45}Ca lost at the indicated times. (Adapted from Bronner et al.[31])

If Ca absorption occurs entirely by simple diffusion (nonsaturable passive process), the fractional rate of Ca removal would be independent of Ca concentration, and the curves would be superimposable. As seen in Figure 5, however, the efficiency of Ca removal depends on the Ca concentration and, therefore, Ca transport also involves a saturable process. The *in situ* loop not only allows for study of absorption from different intestinal segments, but also allows for discrimination between saturable and nonsaturable Ca transport systems.

C. INTESTINAL PERFUSION

Since the study of saturable and nonsaturable Ca transport in humans using *in situ* loops is impractical, investigators have used an intestinal perfusion method. Ca solutions can be perfused into the whole, or specific segments of, intestine at a constant rate. With perfusion of low Ca concentrations, one can calculate the saturable components, V_{max} and K_m, in a manner similar to that for *in situ* loops. To separate the effects of treatment on saturable or nonsaturable Ca transport, concentrations of Ca should either be low enough for the saturable process to predominate, or high enough for the nonsaturable process to predominate.

D. EVERTED GUT SAC

The everted gut sac procedure is used to study active transport of Ca. One can evert the intestinal segment, ligate the ends, and bathe the sac both inside and outside in solutions containing the same concentration of buffer. Since the outside bathes in a volume much larger than the inside, an excess supply of Ca is available for transport. In oxygenated buffer, if the ratio of Ca from the inside (serosal) to the outside (mucosal) solution increases, the existence of active transport is demonstrated. Ca is concentrated on the serosal side against a moderate gradient in the duodenum, but not in the ileum. If nitrogen is substituted for oxygen, active transport ceases.

E. SUMMARY

Various methods can be used to study Ca absorption, depending on the type of mechanism one wants to examine. In humans, intestinal perfusion studies can indicate whether paracellular and/or transcellular routes exist for Ca transport but cannot determine the separate contribution of each. If one wants to separate transcellular from paracellular Ca movement, certain experimental conditions must be established.

Intestinal balance studies can be used for determining overall Ca absorption. In human balance studies the amount of Ca absorption measured is influenced by Ca secreted by the intestine, so the amount of endogenously secreted Ca must therefore be measured.

V. CALCIUM BIOAVAILABILITY

Mineral bioavailability from dietary sources is the percentage of available Ca that is absorbed and metabolically active. In practice, measurement of potential absorbability is difficult to achieve. Many physiological factors influence Ca absorption, in particular whether or not the subject is Ca deficient or repleted. Physiological factors can also influence Ca absorption. Many studies address mineral bioavailability, but these studies should be carefully examined in terms of the physical status of the animals or human subjects. Another confounding factor in studying Ca bioavailability is the fecal excretion of endogenous Ca. Endogenous fecal excretion of Ca (EFCa) is not affected by homeostatic regulation of body Ca. Thus, EFCa is not influenced by the physiological state of the organism. In contrast, the physiological state and diet directly affect urinary Ca excretion.[47,48] In general, bioavailability of Ca should be viewed as a relative rather than an absolute quantity.

Dairy products are the major source of Ca, supplying 60% of the Ca intake for adults and up to 75% for children. Vegetables, fruits, and grain products supply most of the rest, whereas meat, poultry, and fish supply only very small amounts. Many of these foods have molecular components that influence the bioavailability of Ca. In addition to these influences, most of the dietary Ca is complexed to components in food that must be degraded prior to absorption. The bioavailability of Ca depends on the solubility of Ca ions in the intestinal lumen. Insoluble Ca cannot be absorbed. Cow milk contains 40% of its Ca in solution and 60% is associated with casein. In a meal of steak, cheese, and French fries, 58% of the Ca is soluble and 42% insoluble.[46]

The combination of acid pH and the presence of CaBP in the duodenum and upper jejunum probably explains why the rate of Ca absorption is much greater from these segments than from the ileum, although the absolute amount of Ca absorbed is greatest in the ileum. After eating, the pH of the proximal jejunum increases to approximately 6 and beyond the mid portion of the small bowel to 7.6. Ca precipitates from solutions when the pH is greater than 6.1. Thus, the duodenum and jejunum absorb more dietary Ca per unit length than the ileum does. In addition, intestinal CaBP is found mainly in the duodenum with only relatively small amounts in the jejunum.

A. DIETARY COMPONENTS THAT AFFECT CALCIUM ABSORPTION

The following section reviews how several molecules in foods affect Ca absorption.

1. Lactose

Calcium ions in dairy products are readily absorbed and utilized. The enhancing effect of lactose on Ca absorption was demonstrated as early as 1926.[47] The mechanism for the effect of lactose on Ca absorption, however, has not been identified conclusively. Although studies show that lactose and Ca must be in the same segment of the intestine for lactose to exert its effect, lactose does not increase the *in vitro* solubility of Ca, suggesting that lactose does not act by increasing the luminal concentration of soluble Ca.[47] This finding, of course, does not rule out the possibility that lactose, present in the lumen under *in vivo* conditions, will increase Ca solubility.

Key findings from studies with lactose show that lactose increases the percentage of Ca absorption from an oral dose about two-fold, but the effect is not uniform for all intestinal segments. In the rat, lactose enhances absorption in the ileum by 320%, but only 42% in the duodenum and 31% in the jejunum.[49] Lactose enhances Ca absorption in vitamin D-deficient as well as vitamin D-replete animals. Reports of the effects of lactose on Ca absorption in humans vary, making conclusions difficult. Lactose at levels normally present in dairy products may not significantly affect Ca absorption by healthy adults consuming normal diets. In contrast, lactose improves the Ca absorption of human infants. Kobayashi[50] reported the effects of infant formula, lactose-free formula, and lactase-treated formula on the Ca balance of infants under 8 months of age. Ca absorption was 60% with the formula, 36% with lactose-free formula, and 72% with formula treated with lactase to hydrolyze lactose. These data suggest that lactose itself may not be important for enhanced absorption, but that the glucose and galactose released by lactose hydrolysis were effective in improving Ca absorption. A study using lactulose, a nonhydrolyzable sugar similar to lactose, also shows enhanced Ca absorption when lactulose is given with a meal. In contrast to the above findings, addition of the breakdown products (lactulose, galactose, and fructose) did not enhance Ca absorption.[51]

The question of whether or not lactose-intolerant humans absorb significantly lower amounts of Ca remains unsettled. Studies using radioactive ^{47}Ca given in milk and lactose-free milk to healthy adults show that absorption is greater from milk containing lactose. When the milk was fed to lactose-intolerant subjects, they absorbed Ca from lactose-free milk at rates similar to those of lactose-tolerant subjects.[52] The presence of lactose in milk actually reduces Ca absorption as judged by the postprandial appearance of ^{47}Ca in serum. However, one cannot assume that lactose intolerance impairs Ca balance. There is no increase in the amount of ^{47}Ca excreted in the feces, suggesting that ^{47}Ca may be absorbed at a later time period when it moves to lower segments of the intestine.[53] These Ca balance studies suggest that lactose intolerance has a negligible effect on Ca absorption.

2. Phytate

Calcium bioavailability is affected by the phytate content of several plant foods. Although increased intake of unrefined cereals or cereal brans reduces Ca absorption in the short term, long-term effects have not been systematically examined.[53] For many years it was thought that feeding whole wheat products to humans resulted in a negative Ca balance and that this was due to the phytate, which binds Ca and makes it unabsorbable.[53,54] Although calcium phytate per se is not absorbed, phytate is at least partially digested in the lower intestine, allowing Ca ions freed from the complex to be absorbed.

3. Fiber

Another plant component, diverse dietary fiber molecules, also influences Ca bioavailability. Evidence now exists that fiber itself impairs Ca absorption. Fiber in fruits and vegetables has little effect on mineral bioavailability,[55] but whole grain cereal fibers have a greater effect.[54] Thus, the soluble or gel-forming fibers in fruits and vegetables affect mineral absorption less than do insoluble fibers, which predominate in cereals, including cellulose, lignans, and some hemicelluloses.

4. Oxalates

Some vegetables, such as spinach and rhubarb, contain large amounts of oxalate, which binds Ca. Although these vegetables contain significant amounts of Ca, the presence of oxalate significantly reduces the bioavailability of Ca from these food items.[56,57] However, recent evidence suggests that oxalates alone cannot completely explain the poor absorption of Ca from spinach.[58] A study of the combination of milk and Ca oxalate ingestion in humans showed that oxalates did not interfere with absorption of Ca from milk.[59] The amounts of oxalate typically ingested are not sufficient to effectively lower the overall Ca absorption.

5. Fat

A diet high in fat will decrease the bioavailability of dietary Ca only in cases of fat malabsorption. Ca precipitates with fatty acids to form insoluble soaps. However, medium chain triglyceride:Ca complexes enhance Ca absorption.[60] These complexes can move through paracellular spaces, especially the tight junction, more easily than free Ca can.

B. DIETARY COMPONENTS THAT AFFECT URINARY CALCIUM EXCRETION

The bioavailability of Ca is dependent on both the absorption of Ca by the gut epithelial cells and by the retention of Ca by the body. The latter process is regulated primarily by the urinary excretion of Ca, which can be affected by dietary intakes of protein or phosphorus.

1. Protein

Calcium bioavailability is also affected by dietary protein. Usually protein does not affect Ca absorption,[61] but protein can enhance Ca absorption when the Ca intake is in the range of 800–1400 mg/day.[62]

In contrast, protein can markedly affect the renal handling of Ca. Increased dietary protein increases urinary Ca excretion.[63] For every gram of protein metabolized, there is an incremental loss of 1 mg of Ca in the urine. This loss is probably due to the excretion of sulfate resulting from the metabolism of sulfur-amino acids. Therefore, the loss of Ca in the urine is greater for meat protein than for dairy protein, whereas vegetable protein produces the smallest increase in urinary Ca excretion.

2. Phosphorus

Under normal dietary conditions P also does not affect Ca absorption.[64] In contrast to protein, increasing dietary phosphate (P) reduces urinary Ca excretion.[64] Protein and P affect the renal handling of Ca. Thus, foods high in protein that also have a large P content would have a less severe effect on the Ca balance. Since dairy products have high levels of protein, Ca, and P, increased dairy protein consumption may have a net positive effect on the Ca balance, even though dairy products have high levels of protein.[47]

C. SUMMARY

The bioavailability of Ca depends on the solubility of Ca ions in the gut lumen. Insoluble or bound Ca cannot be absorbed. When food is digested, acidification may release insoluble Ca, but digestion would also release P, oxalate, phytate, and fiber, which bind Ca. The luminal concentration of soluble Ca following a meal, which has been studied at various levels of the small intestine, falls as Ca travels from proximal to distal small intestine, due mainly to Ca precipitation.[65] Our understanding of how these food components affect the amount of Ca absorbed and of the various mechanisms responsible for Ca absorption needs to be fully evaluated in terms of the current dietary patterns of consumption. Knowledge of the interactions between factors that affect bioavailability and those that affect mechanisms of absorption would permit us to develop strategies that enable populations to avoid the risk of Ca deficiency.

VI. SUMMARY

Absorption of Ca from the intestine is dependent on a variety of factors. These factors may affect either transcellular (a multistep process of transferring Ca through the cell) or paracellular (between cells) absorption of Ca. Understanding of cellular events has increased over the past several years, and our knowledge of transcellular absorption of Ca far exceeds our knowledge of the mechanisms by which Ca moves paracellularly. Even less is known about how factors affecting *in vivo* Ca absorption act at the cellular level.

Molecules in foods alter bioavailability of Ca for absorption by acting on the solubility of Ca. If Ca is complexed to food components, the concentration of free, ionized Ca available for absorption in the intestinal lumen, i.e., the bioavailability, decreases. The most commonly used measurement of Ca bioavailability in humans is the balance technique. There are limits to these methods, in particular, the measurement of endogenously secreted Ca, which could alter the calculated amount of Ca absorbed. Radioisotopic studies can rectify this problem, but such studies are limited because of concerns over the use of radioactivity.

Understandings of Ca absorption and Ca bioavailability have improved, but as concern over osteoporosis increases, improved knowledge of the bioavailability of Ca from food and supplements is needed. Information on the bioavailability of Ca under diverse conditions should help individuals obtain the recommended daily intakes of Ca throughout the life cycle.

REFERENCES

1. **Birge, S. J., Peck, W. A., Berman, M. and Whedon, G. D.,** Study of calcium absorption in man: a kinetic analysis and physiologic model, *J. Clin. Invest.*, 48, 1705, 1969.
2. **Wensel, R. H., Rich, C., Brown, A. C. and Volwiler, W.,** Absorption of calcium measured by intubation and perfusion of the intact human small intestine, *J. Clin. Invest.*, 48, 1768, 1969.
3. **Krejs, G. J., Nicar, M. J., Zerwekh, J. E., Norman, D. A., Kane, M. G. and Pak, C. Y.,** Effect of 1,25-dihydroxyvitamin D_3 on calcium and magnesium absorption in the healthy human jejunum and ileum, *Am. J. Med.*, 75, 973, 1983.
4. **Heaney, R. P., Weaver, C. M. and Fitzsimmons, M. L.,** Influence of calcium load on absorption fraction, *J. Bone Miner. Res.*, 5, 1135, 1990.
5. **Allen, L. H. and Wood, R. J.,** Calcium and Phosphorus, in *Modern Nutrition in Health and Disease*, Shils, M. E., Olson, J. A., and Shike, M., eds., Lea & Febiger, Philadelphia, 1994.
6. **Heaney, R. P., Recker, R. R., Stegman, M. R. and Moy, A. J.,** Calcium absorption in women: relationships to calcium intake, estrogen status, and age, *J. Bone Miner. Res.*, 4, 469, 1989.
7. **Rasmussen, H., Fontaine, O., Max, E. E. and Goodman, D. B.,** The effect of 1-alpha-hydroxyvitamin D_3 administration on calcium transport in chick intestine brush border membrane vesicles, *J. Biol. Chem.*, 254, 2993, 1979.
8. **Miller, A. and Bronner, F.,** Calcium uptake in isolated brush-border vesicles from rat small intestine, *Biochem. J.*, 196, 391, 1981.
9. **Schedl, H. P. and Wilson, H. D.,** Calcium uptake by intestinal brush border membrane vesicles. Comparison with in vivo calcium transport, *J. Clin. Invest.*, 76, 1871, 1985.
10. **Nellans, H. N. and Kimberg, D. V.,** Cellular and paracellular calcium transport in rat ileum: effects of dietary calcium, *Am. J. Physiol*, 235, E726, 1978.
11. **Karbach, U.,** Segmental heterogeneity of cellular and paracellular calcium transport across the rat duodenum and jejunum, *Gastroenterology*, 100, 47, 1991.
12. **Zornitzer, A. E. and Bronner, F.,** In situ studies of calcium absorption in rats, *Am. J. Physiol.*, 220, 1261, 1971.
13. **Pansu, D., Bellaton, C. and Bronner, F.,** Effect of Ca intake on saturable and nonsaturable components of duodenal Ca transport, *Am. J. Physiol.*, 240, G32, 1981.
14. **Smith, K. T., Heaney, R. P., Flora, L. and Hinders, S. M.,** Calcium absorption from a new calcium delivery system (CCM), *Calcif. Tissue. Int.*, 41, 351, 1987.
15. **Louie, D., Zhong, Z. and Glover, W.,** Enhanced calcium absorption in the ileum and duodenum by calcium:citrate:malate, *Gastroenterology*, 104, A633, 1993.
16. **Karbach, U.,** Paracellular calcium transport across the small intestine, *J. Nutr.*, 122 (suppl. 3S), 672, 1992.
17. **Miller, A., Ueng, T. H. and Bronner, F.,** Isolation of a vitamin D-dependent, calcium-binding protein from brush borders of rat duodenal mucosa, *FEBS Lett.*, 103, 319, 1979.
18. **Bikle, D. D., Munson, S. and Chafouleas, J.,** Calmodulin may mediate 1,25-dihydroxyvitamin D-stimulated intestinal calcium transport, *FEBS Lett.*, 174, 30, 1984.
19. **Bikle, D. D. and Munson, S.,** The villus gradient of brush border membrane calmodulin and the calcium-independent calmodulin-binding protein parallels that of calcium-accumulating ability, *Endocrinology*, 118, 727, 1986.
20. **Bikle, D. D., Munson, S. and Zolock, D. T.,** Calcium flux across chick duodenal brush border membrane vesicles: regulation by 1,25-dihydroxyvitamin D, *Endocrinology*, 113, 2072, 1983.
21. **Bikle, D. D., Zolock, D. T., Morrissey, R. L. and Herman, R. H.,** Independence of 1,25-dihydroxyvitamin D_3-mediated calcium transport from de novo RNA and protein synthesis, *J. Biol. Chem.*, 253, 484, 1978.
22. **Matsumoto, T., Fontaine, O. and Rasmussen, H.,** Effect of 1,25-dihydroxyvitamin D_3 on phospholipid metabolism in chick duodenal mucosal cell. Relationship to its mechanism of action, *J. Biol. Chem.*, 256, 3354, 1981.
23. **Norman, A. W., Mircheff, A. K., Adams, T. H. and Spielvogel, A.,** Studies on the mechanism of action of calciferol. 3. Vitamin D-mediated increase of intestinal brush order alkaline phosphatase activity, *Biochim. Biophys. Acta*, 215, 348, 1970.
24. **Nasr, L., Monet, J. D. and Lucas, P. A.,** Rapid (10-minute) stimulation of rat duodenal alkaline phosphatase activity by 1,25-dihydroxyvitamin D_3, *Endocrinology*, 123, 1778, 1988.

25. **Haussler, M., Nagode, L. A. and Rasmussen, H.,** Induction of intestinal brush border alkaline phosphatase by vitamin D and identity with Ca-ATPase, *Nature*, 228, 1199, 1970.
26. **Bikle, D. D., Morrissey, R. L. and Zolock, D. T.,** The mechanism of action of vitamin D in the intestine, *Am. J. Clin. Nutr.*, 32, 2322, 1979.
27. **Lane, S. M. and Lawson, D. E.,** Differentiation of the changes in alkaline phosphatase from calcium ion-activated adenosine triphosphatase activities associated with increased calcium absorption in chick intestine, *Biochem. J.*, 174, 1067, 1978.
28. **Ghijsen, W. E., De Jong, M. D. and Van Os, C. H.,** Dissociation between Ca^{2+}-ATPase and alkaline phosphatase activities in plasma membranes of rat duodenum, *Biochim. Biophys. Acta*, 599, 538, 1980.
29. **Pansu, D., Bellaton, C., Roche, C. and Bronner, F.,** Theophylline inhibits transcellular Ca transport in intestine and Ca binding by CaBP, *Am. J. Physiol.*, 257, G935, 1989.
30. **Nellans, H. N. and Goldsmith, R. S.,** Transepithelial calcium transport by rat cecum: high-efficiency absorptive site, *Am. J. Physiol.*, 240, G424, 1981.
31. **Bronner, F., Pansu, D. and Stein, W. D.,** An analysis of intestinal calcium transport across the rat intestine, *Am. J. Physiol.*, 250, G561, 1986.
32. **Wasserman, R. H. and Taylor, A. N.,** Vitamin D_3-induced calcium-binding protein in chick intestinal mucosa, *Science*, 152, 791, 1966.
33. **Feher, J. J.,** Facilitated calcium diffusion by intestinal calcium-binding protein, *Am. J. Physiol.*, 244, C303, 1983.
34. **Roche, C., Bellaton, C., Pansu, D., Miller, A. and Bronner, F.,** Localization of vitamin D-dependent active Ca^{2+} transport in rat duodenum and relation to CaBP, *Am. J. Physiol.*, 251, G314, 1986.
35. **Tsai, H. C. and Norman, A. W.,** Studies on the mode of action of calciferol. VI. Effect of 1,25-dihydroxy-vitamin D_3 on RNA synthesis in the intestinal mucosa, *Biochem. Biophys. Res. Commun.*, 54, 622, 1973.
36. **Glenney, J. R., Jr. and Glenney, P.,** Comparison of Ca^{++}-regulated events in the intestinal brush border, *J. Cell Biol.*, 100, 754, 1985.
37. **Nemere, I.,** Vesicular calcium transport in chick intestine, *J. Nutr.*, 122, 657, 1992.
38. **Nemere, I., Leathers, V. and Norman, A. W.,** 1,25-dihydroxyvitamin D_3-mediated intestinal calcium transport. Biochemical identification of lysosomes containing calcium and calcium-binding protein (calbindin-D_{28K}), *J. Biol. Chem.*, 261, 16106, 1986.
39. **Sampson, H. W., Matthews, J. L., Martin, J. H. and Kunin, A. S.,** An electron microscopic localization of calcium in the small intestine of normal, rachitic, and vitamin-D-treated rats, *Calcif. Tissue Res.*, 5, 305, 1970.
40. **Nemere, I. and Norman, A. W.,** Transcaltachia, vesicular calcium transport, and microtubule-associated calbindin-D_{28K}: emerging views of 1,25-dihydroxyvitamin D_3-mediated intestinal calcium absorption, *Miner. Electrolyte Metab.*, 16, 109, 1990.
41. **Wasserman, R. H., Chandler, J. S., Meyer, S. A., Smith, C. A., Brindak, M. E., Fullmer, C. S., Penniston, J. T. and Kumar, R.,** Intestinal calcium transport and calcium extrusion processes at the basolateral membrane, *J. Nutr.*, 122 (suppl. 3S), 662, 1992.
42. **Borke, J. L., Caride, A., Verma, A. K., Penniston, J. T. and Kumar, R.,** Cellular and segmental distribution of $Ca^{2(+)}$-pump epitopes in rat intestine, *Pflugers Arch.*, 417, 120, 1990.
43. **Walters, J. R., Howard, A., Charpin, M. V., Gniecko, K. C., Brodin, P., Thulin, E. and Forsen, S.,** Stimulation of intestinal basolateral membrane calcium-pump activity by recombinant synthetic calbindin-D_{9K} and specific mutants, *Biochem. Biophys Res. Commun.*, 170, 603, 1990.
44. **De Boland, A. R., Nemere, I. and Norman, A. W.,** $Ca^{2(+)}$-channel agonist BAY K8644 mimics 1,25$(OH)_2$-vitamin D_3 rapid enhancement of Ca^{2+} transport in chick perfused duodenum, *Biochem. Biophys. Res. Commun.*, 166, 217, 1990.
45. **Vergne-Marini, P., Parker, T. F., Pak, C. Y., Hull, A. R., DeLuca, H. F. and Fordtran, J. S.,** Jejunal and ileal absorption in patients with chronic renal disease. Effect of 1-alpha-hydroxycholecalciferol, *J. Clin. Invest.*, 57, 861, 1976.
46. **Sheikh, M. S., Schiller, L. R. and Fordtran, J. S.,** In vivo intestinal absorption of calcium in humans, *Miner. Electrolyte Metab.*, 16, 130, 1990.
47. **Miller, D. D.,** Calcium in the diet: food sources, recommended intakes, and nutritional bioavailability, *Adv. Food Nutr. Res.*, 33, 103, 1989.
48. **Heaney, R. P., Recker, R. R. and Saville, P. D.,** Menopausal changes in calcium balance performance, *J. Lab. Clin. Med.*, 92, 953, 1978.
49. **Lengemann, F. W., Wasserman, R. H. and Comar, C. L.,** Studies on the enhancement of radiocalcium and radiostrontium absorption by lactose in the rat, *J. Nutr.*, 68, 443, 1959.
50. **Kobâyashi, A., Kawai, S., Obe, Y. and Nagashima, Y.,** Effects of dietary lactose and lactase preparation on the intestinal absorption of calcium and magnesium in normal infants, *Am. J. Clin. Nutr.*, 28, 681, 1975.
51. **Brommage, R., Binacua, C., Antille, S. and Carrié, A.-L.,** Intestinal calcium absorption in rats is stimulated by dietary lactulose and other resistant sugars, *J. Nutr.*, 123, 2186, 1993.
52. **Kocian, J., Skala, I. and Bakos, K.,** Calcium absorption from milk and lactose-free milk in healthy subjects and patients with lactose intolerance, *Digestion*, 9, 317, 1973.
53. **Allen, L. H.,** Calcium bioavailability and absorption: a review, *Am. J. Clin. Nutr.*, 35, 783, 1982.

54. **Weaver, C. M., Heaney, R. P., Martin, B. R. and Fitzsimmons, M. L.,** Isotopic exchange of ingested calcium between labeled sources. Evidence that ingested calcium does not form a common absorptive pool. Human calcium absorption from whole-wheat products, *J. Nutr.*, 121, 1769, 1991.
55. **Heaney, R. P.,** Nutritional factors in osteoporosis, *Annu. Rev. Nutr.*, 13, 287, 1993.
56. **Heaney, R. P., Weaver, C. M. and Recker, R. R.,** Calcium absorbability from spinach, *Am. J. Clin. Nutr.*, 47, 707, 1988.
57. **Heaney, R. P. and Weaver, C. M.,** Calcium absorption from kale, *Am. J. Clin. Nutr.*, 51, 656, 1990.
58. **Weaver, C. M. and Heaney, R. P.,** Isotopic exchange of ingested calcium between labeled sources. Evidence that ingested calcium does not form a common absorptive pool, *Calcif. Tissue. Int.*, 49, 244, 1991.
59. **Heaney, R. P. and Weaver, C. M.,** Oxalate: effect on calcium absorbability, *Am. J. Clin. Nutr.*, 50, 830, 1989.
60. **Sulkers, E. J., Lafeber, H. N., Degenhart, H. J., Lindemans, J. and Sauer, P. J.,** Comparison of two preterm formulas with or without addition of medium-chain triglycerides (MCTs). II: effects on mineral balance, *J. Pediatr. Gastroenterol. Nutr.*, 15, 42, 1992.
61. **Hegsted, M., Schuette, S. A., Zemel, M. B. and Linkswiler, H. M.,** Urinary calcium and calcium balance in young men as affected by level of protein and phosphorus intake, *J. Nutr.*, 111, 553, 1981.
62. **Linkswiler, H. M., Joyce, C. L. and Anand, C. R.,** Calcium retention of young adult males as affected by level of protein and of calcium intake, *Trans. N.Y. Acad. Sci.*, 36, 333, 1974.
63. **Linkswiler, H. M., Zemel, M. B., Hegsted, M. and Schuette, S.,** Protein-induced hypercalciuria, *Fed. Proc.*, 40, 2429, 1981.
64. **Spencer, H., Kramer, L., Osis, D. and Norris, C.,** Effect of phosphorus on the absorption of calcium and on the calcium balance in man, *J. Nutr.*, 108, 447, 1978.
65. **Fordtran, J. S. and Locklear, T. W.,** Ionic constituents and osmolality of gastric and small-intestinal fluids after eating, *Am. J. Dig. Dis.*, 11, 503, 1966.

Chapter 5

THE ROLE OF THE KIDNEY IN DIVALENT MINERAL NUTRITION

Charles P. McKay, M.D.

TABLE OF CONTENTS

0-8493-7845-1/95/$0.00+$.50

I. INTRODUCTION

The kidney, intestine, and bone are the three major effector organs that respond to changes in mineral nutrition and metabolism. These organs are regulated by the actions of parathyroid hormone (PTH), 1,25-dihydroxycholecalciferol ($1,25(OH)_2D$), and calcitonin (CT), which are secreted in response to changes in mineral homeostasis. In the intact organism, all of these organs and hormones respond in a coordinated fashion to nutritional stresses. This chapter overviews the mechanisms of normal renal handling of calcium (Ca) and phosphorus (P), as well as their control by the calciotropic hormones. The primary renal responses to nutritional changes in Ca and P are also reviewed.

II. NORMAL RENAL CALCIUM HANDLING

Excretion of Ca or any other substance by the kidneys is the result of glomerular filtration followed by the sum of the processes of tubular reabsorption and secretion. The amount of Ca filtered at the glomerulus (the filtered load) is determined by the glomerular filtration rate (GFR) and the plasma concentration of ultrafiltrable Ca. Ultrafiltrable Ca is that portion of Ca that is either ionized (Ca^{++}) or complexed to small molecular weight anions, but excludes protein-bound Ca.[1] With a normal glomerular filtration rate of 180 L/day and an ultrafilterable Ca of 58 mg/L, approximately 10.5 grams of Ca are filtered daily, of which only 2% is excreted. This daily Ca excretion of about 200 mg generally is equal to the amount absorbed by the intestine.

A. CALCIUM HANDLING BY DIFFERENT RENAL SEGMENTS

Tubular reabsorption of filtered Ca occurs in the proximal tubule, thick ascending limb of the loop of Henle, distal nephron and, collecting duct (see Figure 1). Approximately 70% of the filtered load of Ca is reabsorbed in the proximal tubule and 20% in the thick ascending limb through bulk reabsorption in association with Na^+ reabsorption.[2] The distal tubule actively reabsorbs 5–10% of the filtered Ca by a process regulated by PTH.

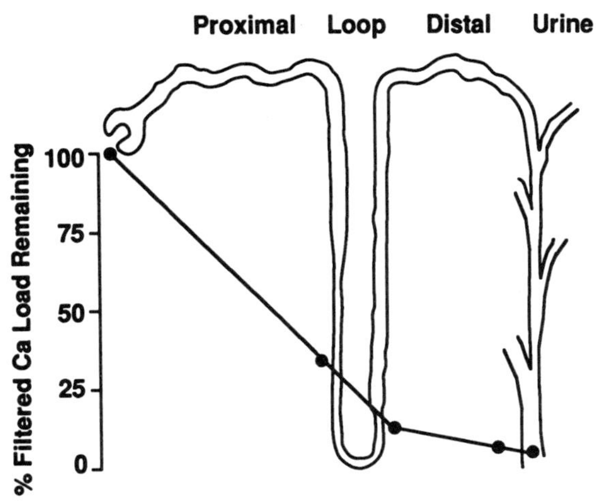

FIGURE 1. Model of Calcium Reabsorption along the Segments of the Mammalian Renal Tubule. (From Suki, W. N. and Rouse, D. in *The Kidney*, 4th ed., Brenner, B. M. and Rector, F. C., eds., Saunders, Philadelphia, 1991. With permission.)

Ca reabsorption in the proximal renal tubule is in parallel with Na^+ and water. Whereas in the superficial proximal convoluted tubule the concentration of Ca^{++} in the tubular fluid is the same as that of the glomerular filtrate (TF:GF = 1.0), later in the proximal tubule this ratio rises to 1.2. The mechanism for this increase relates to the paracellular passage of Ca^{++} following Na^+ and water by solvent drag across the tight junctions. As this segment of the proximal tubule becomes more restrictive to Ca than to Na^+ and water, molecular sieving results and Ca reabsorption lags behind Na^+ and water reabsorption. Another potential mechanism may be the increasing formation of Ca^{++} complexes with anions making Ca^{++} unavailable for reabsorption. In addition to this primary paracellular passive mechanism, controversy exists over the presence of an active transcellular component as well. Certain studies have suggested that up to one-third of the Ca^{++} reabsorption in the proximal tubule may be by active transport. Similar to the proximal convoluted tubule, the proximal straight tubule displays primarily a passive transcellular mechanism of Ca^{++} reabsorption. Again, at least some studies suggest an active mechanism as well.

The loop of Henle accounts for 20–25% of the Ca^{++} reabsorption with only a negligible portion of this occurring in either the descending or thin ascending portions of the loop.[3] In contrast, the thick ascending limb of the loop of Henle is a major site for Ca^{++} reabsorption. In the medullary portion of the thick ascending limb, the mechanism is a passive paracellular transport driven by the lumen-positive transepithelial potential difference in this segment. In addition to this voltage-driven mechanism, the cortical thick ascending limb displays active transport in some studies as well. In this segment, furosemide, which blocks the formation of the positive transepithelial potential difference, inhibits Ca^{++} reabsorption as well. Ca reabsorption is stimulated by CT in the medullary segment and by PTH in the cortical segment.

The distal convoluted tubule is responsible for only 5–10% of Ca^{++} reabsorption, but it is in this segment that the major regulation of Ca^{++} reabsorption occurs. This segment is also unique because of the dissociation of Ca^{++} reabsorption from Na^+ reabsorption. This dissociation can be demonstrated by administration of PTH or thiazide diuretics, or by phosphate (Pi) depletion. Along this segment the ratio TF:GF for Ca^{++} falls from 0.6 at the beginning to 0.3. More complete reabsorption is limited by the complexing of the tubular Ca^{++} to nonreabsorbable anions and not by any limit in the capacity of the active transcellular mechanism. The intraluminal voltage is negative, requiring the transport mechanism to work against both chemical and electrical gradients.

Ca enters the distal tubular epithelial through dihydropyridine-sensitive channels independent of any effect of Na^+. Calbindin-D_{28K}, the vitamin D-dependent Ca binding protein, has been localized to this segment. This suggests a possible role of this protein in transcellular movement to the basolateral surface, where exit from the cell occurs via Ca^{++}-ATPase and Na^+/Ca^{++} exchange transporters (see Figure 2). It is also in this segment that PTH exerts its control over Ca reabsorption. The mechanism for PTH regulation of Ca^{++} reabsorption is discussed next.

Finally, a small amount of Ca^{++} is reabsorbed by the collecting duct. However, PTH does not regulate Ca^{++} reabsorption in this segment.

B. REGULATION OF RENAL CALCIUM HANDLING

1. Control by PTH

A variety of hormonal and nonhormonal factors influence Ca^{++} reabsorption (see Table 1). Dietary changes in Ca and P affect renal Ca metabolism and will be covered in detail later. The primary hormonal control of Ca^{++} reabsorption is by PTH. A major mechanism by which PTH regulates extracellular Ca^{++} is through stimulation of renal Ca^{++} reabsorption. PTH not only stimulates distal renal tubular Ca^{++} reabsorption, but, through nonrenal mechanisms, it also increases serum Ca^{++} and the filtered load for Ca^{++}. In hyperparathyroidism, the increased filtered load may overwhelm the renal capacity to reabsorb Ca^{++} and result in hypercalciuria despite the enhanced Ca^{++} reabsorption (see Figure 3).

The *in vitro* effect of PTH is to activate adenylate cyclase in the proximal tubule, cortical thick ascending limb, distal tubule, and connecting tubule. Unlike the proximal tubule where PTH does

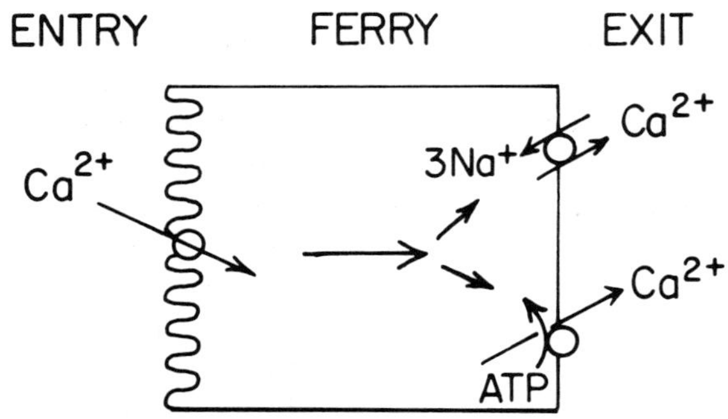

FIGURE 2. Cellular Mechanisms for the Transport of Calcium across the Renal Tubule. (From Yanagawa, N. and Lee, D. B. N. in *Disorders of Bone and Mineral Metabolism,* Coe, F. L. and Favus, M. J., eds., Raven Press, New York, 1992. With permission.)

TABLE 1
Factors Influencing Renal Tubular Calcium Reabsorption

Increase	Decrease
PTH	Phosphate depletion
Vitamin D	Volume expansion
Alkalosis	Acidosis
Thiazide diuretics	Loop diuretics
Calcium depletion	Hypercalcemia

not clearly enhance Ca^{++} reabsorption, the distal tubule and connecting tubule are the major sites for the regulation of Ca^{++} excretion. The exact site of action may be species specific. The mechanism is protein kinase A mediated and is independent of any effect on potential difference, Na^+, or water transport. The cellular mechanism is through an increase in the number of active Ca channels responsible for Ca entry. In addition, PTH also enhances Ca^{++} reabsorption in the cortical, but not in the medullary thick ascending limb by activating transcellular transport by a cyclic AMP (cAMP)-dependent mechanism. CT has been shown to activate Ca^{++} reabsorption in the medullary portion of the thick ascending limb, but the physiologic significance of this is not clear.

2. Control by Vitamin D

$1,25(OH)_2D$ has been reported to modulate Ca^{++} reabsorption but the exact effect is greatly dependent on the experimental conditions (see Figure 4). One potential mechanism for this effect is activation of reabsorption in the distal tubule by the stimulation of calbindin-D_{28K} formation. As with PTH, the extrarenal effects of vitamin D may result in an absolute increase in Ca^{++} excretion despite direct activation of Ca^{++} reabsorption.

3. Control by Other Hormones

Other hormones that display effects on Ca^{++} excretion include insulin, glucagon, growth hormone, thyroid hormone, glucocorticoids, mineralocorticoids, and estrogens. Insulin inhibits Ca^{++} reabsorption in the proximal renal tubule and results in increased Ca^{++} excretion. Glucagon increases both Na^+ and Ca^{++} excretion, probably by increasing the GFR. Chronic but not acute administration of growth hormone increases both Ca^{++} intestinal absorption and Ca^{++} excretion. Thyroid hormone and glucocorticoids also increase Ca^{++} excretion but through a mechanism involving enhanced bone resorption and increased filtered load of Ca^{++}. In contrast, estrogens inhibit bone resorption and Ca^{++}

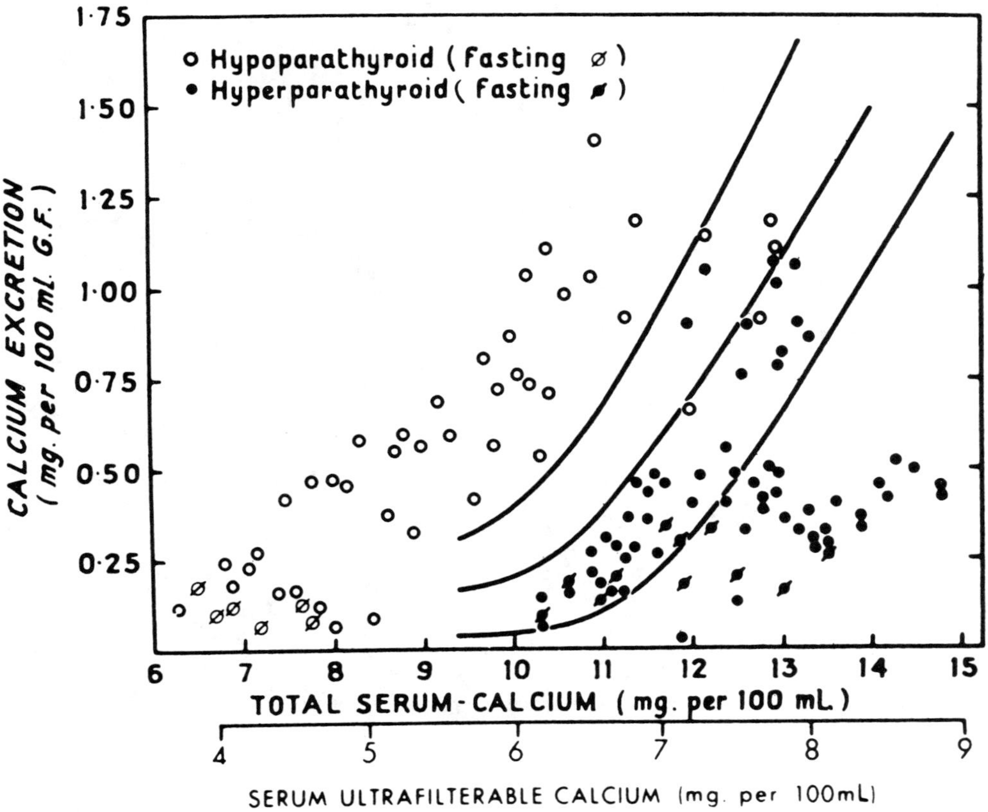

FIGURE 3. Effect of Parathyroid Hormone and Plasma Calcium on Urinary Calcium Excretion. (From Peacock, M., Robertson, W. G., and Nordin, B. E. C., Relationship between serum and urinary calcium with particular reference to parathyroid activity, *Lancet*, 1, 384, 1969. With permission.)

excretion. Mineralocorticoids, similar to Na^+ loading, also result in hypercalciuria. The mechanism for mineralocorticoid-induced hypercalciuria is an increase in the filtered load for Ca^{++} by an increase of the GFR.

4. Control by Extracellular Volume and Diuretics

Increasing the extracellular volume inhibits Ca^{++} reabsorption by decreasing that portion which is coupled to proximal Na^+ and water reabsorption. Diuretics also affect Ca^{++} excretion by mechanisms related to their site of action. Mannitol causes parallel increases in Ca^{++} and Na^+ excretion by its osmotic diuretic effect. Loop diuretics, e.g. furosemide, increase Ca^{++} excretion by inhibiting the potential difference-driven paracellular transport in the thick ascending limb. This results in a parallel increase in Na^+ and Ca^{++} excretion. Chronic administration of thiazide diuretics result in a decrease in Ca^{++} excretion. In addition to their hypovolemic effect, which enhances proximal reabsorption, these agents activate early distal tubular Ca^{++} reabsorption, possibly by enhancing basolateral Na^+/Ca^{++} exchange. The potassium-sparing diuretics also are hypocalciuric by enhancing Ca^{++} reabsorption at a site distal to the site of action of the thiazides. Finally, metabolic acidosis increases, and metabolic alkalosis decreases Ca^{++} excretion by direct effects on renal tubular Ca^{++} reabsorption.

In summary, renal Ca^{++} excretion results from filtration of the nonprotein-bound plasma Ca at the glomerulus followed by reabsorption of Ca^{++} by the proximal tubule, thick ascending limb, and distal tubule. The distal tubule is the site for regulation of Ca^{++} reabsorption by PTH.

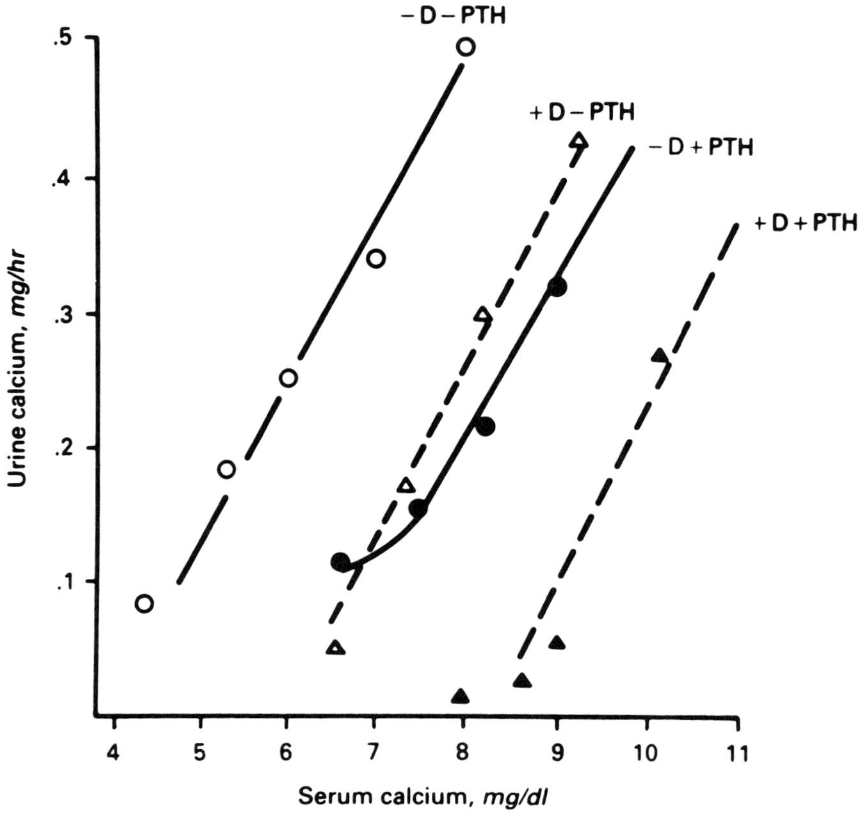

FIGURE 4. Role of Vitamin D and Parathyroid Hormone on the Relationship between Serum Calcium and Urinary Calcium Excretion. (From Yanagawa, N. and Lee, D. B. N. in *Disorders of Bone and Mineral Metabolism,* Coe, F. L. and Favus, M. J., eds., Raven Press, New York, 1992. With permission.)

III. NORMAL RENAL PHOSPHATE HANDLING

The filtered load of Pi, as with Ca, is the product of the GFR and the ultrafilterable Pi. In plasma, Pi exists in two forms: HPO_4^{2-} and $H_2PO_4^-$. At physiologic pH, the ratio of these two species is 4:1, respectively. Despite the fact that 15–20% of plasma Pi is protein bound, the filtered load of Pi equals the serum Pi × GFR because this partition is effectively nullified by the effect of the Gibbs-Donnan distribution of this anion and the correction for volume of the protein-free plasma water. Normally, about 20% of the filtered load of Pi is excreted, but this can vary greatly as a result of a number of factors. The most significant of these are the PTH level and Pi intake. Pi is reabsorbed by the renal tubule, but no evidence exists for secretion of this anion. This reabsorption displays saturation kinetics; that is, there exists a filtered load above which the transport capacity is reached, and all additional filtered Pi is excreted. This limit on transport capacity is known as the tubular maximum for Pi or T_mP. Normalizing the T_mP for the rate of glomerular filtration, T_mP/GFR, is the best index by which to assess renal Pi handling (see Figure 5).[4]

A. PHOSPHATE HANDLING BY DIFFERENT RENAL SEGMENTS

The proximal renal tubule is normally responsible for reabsorption of approximately 70% of the filtered Pi, which means that only minimal amounts of Pi are normally reabsorbed beyond the proximal tubule (see Figure 6).[5] The most avid reabsorption occurs in the first quarter of the proximal renal tubule. In this segment the ratio of the concentration of Pi in the tubular fluid to that of the glomerular filtrate (TF:GF) falls from 1.0 to 0.7. Tubular reabsorption in this segment, which

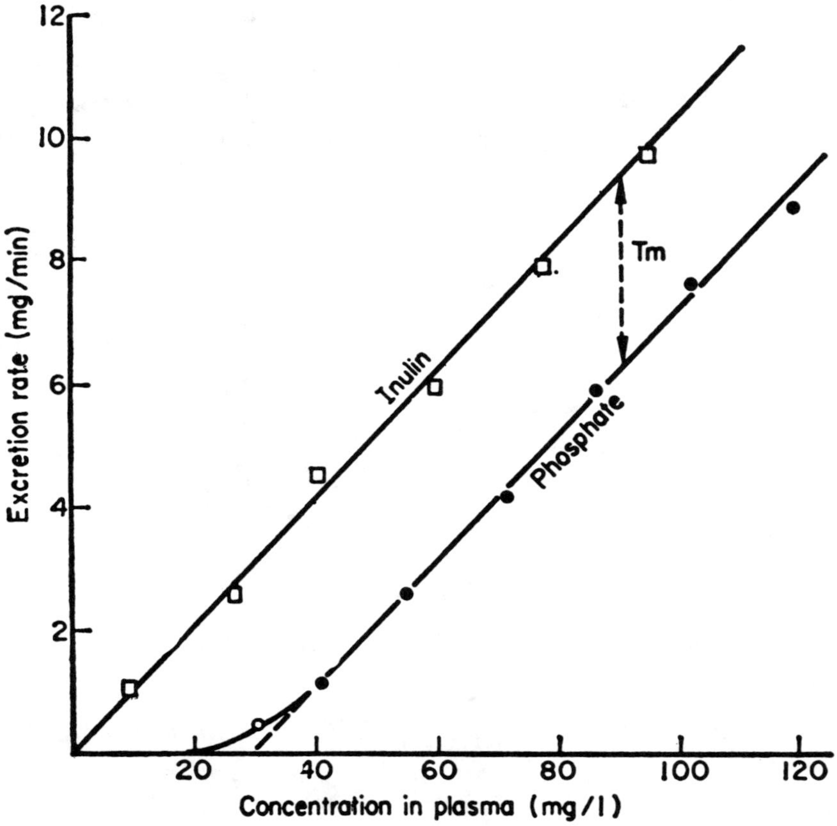

FIGURE 5. Relationship between the Filtered Load of Phosphate as Determined by Inulin Clearance and Urinary Phosphate Excretion Rate in a Normal Human. The x-intercept of the lower line is the T_mP/GFR or "theoretical renal phosphate threshold." (From Bijvoet, O. L. M., Relation of plasma phosphate concentration to renal tubular reabsorption of phosphate, *Clin. Sci.*, 37, 23, 1969. With permission.)

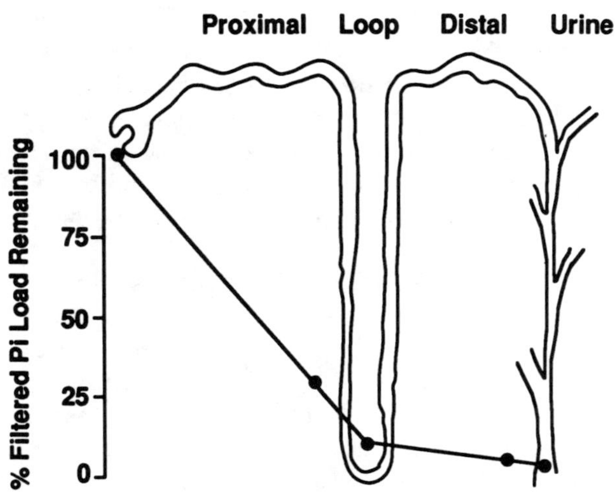

FIGURE 6. Model of Phosphate Reabsorption along the Segments of the Mammalian Renal Tubule. (From Suki, W. N. and Rouse, D. in *The Kidney*, 4th ed., Brenner, B. M. and Rector, F. C., eds., Saunders, Philadelphia, 1991. With permission.)

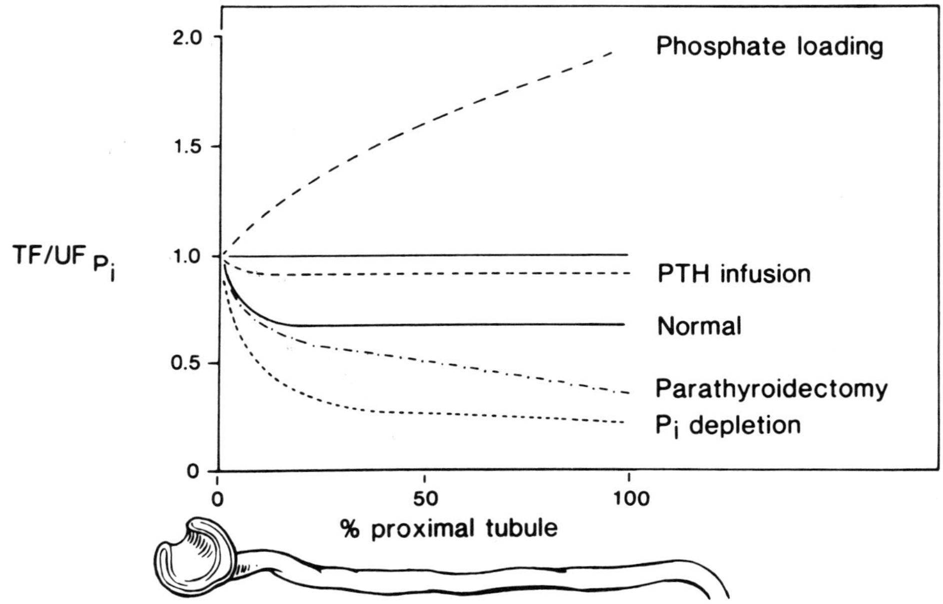

FIGURE 7. Effect of Parathyroid Hormone and Dietary Phosphate on Reabsorption of Phosphate along the Proximal Renal Tubule. TF/UF below 1 reflects net reabsorption. (From Knox, F. G. and Haramati, A., Renal regulation of phosphate excretion, in *The Kidney: Physiology and Pathology*, Seldin, D. W. and Giebisch, G., eds., Raven Press, New York, 1985. With permission.)

correlates to reabsorption of 40% of the filtered load, results from more avid reabsorption of Pi than either Na^+ or water (see Figure 7). Whereas little Pi reabsorption occurs in the remaining proximal convoluted and straight tubules in the presence of PTH, significant reabsorption occurs along the entire proximal tubule in its absence. There is little Pi reabsorption along the rest of the renal tubule until the distal tubule is reached, where up to 10% of filtered Pi is reabsorbed. Pi reabsorption in this segment is under strict control by PTH. In the collecting tubule, up to 3% of the filtered load of Pi is reabsorbed.

The percentage of Pi reabsorbed is dramatically altered in the presence of Pi deficiency (see later), which has differential effects on the two populations of nephrons that make up the kidney. The superficial nephrons often display qualitatively different functional properties than the deep or juxtamedullary nephrons do. In thyroparathyroidectomized rats on a normal Pi intake, the superficial nephrons reabsorb less of the filtered load than do the deep nephrons. Moreover, the superficial nephrons respond to low or high Pi intake by either halving or doubling their Pi reabsorption, respectively.

Transport of Pi across the renal tubular epithelium must first overcome the electrochemical gradient opposing the entry of Pi into cells.[6] This gradient is primarily determined by the 60–64 mV potential difference across the luminal membrane opposing Pi entry. Pi therefore requires active transport to enter the cell by an electroneutral Na^+-Pi cotransporter that is driven by the favorable Na^+ electrochemical gradient generated by the basolateral Na^+,K^+-ATPase (see Figure 8). This Na^+-Pi cotransport is modulated by intracellular and luminal pH, phosphorylation of the cotransporter by the protein kinases A and C, and ADP-ribosylation of the cotransporter. In contrast to the Na^+-dependent entry into the tubular cells, exit of Pi is most likely Na^+-independent and may involve an anion exchange mechanism.

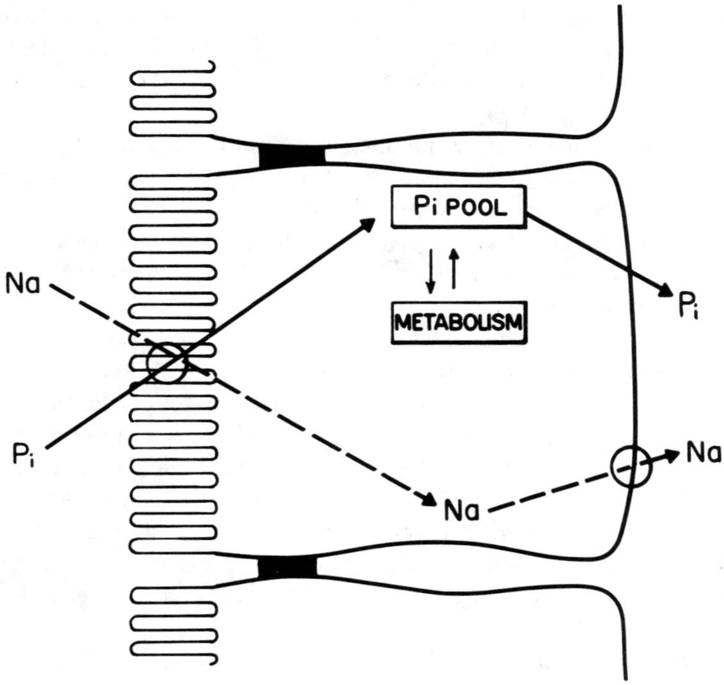

FIGURE 8. Cellular Mechanisms for the Transport of Phosphate across the Proximal Renal Tubule. (From Yanagawa, N. and Lee, D.B.N. in *Disorders of Bone and Mineral Metabolism,* Coe, F. L. and Favus, M. J., eds., Raven Press, New York, 1992. With permission.)

TABLE 2
Factors Influencing Renal Tubular Phosphate Reabsorption

Increase	Decrease
Phosphate depletion	PTH
Respiratory alkalosis	Respiratory acidosis
Hypercalcemia	Volume expansion
Growth hormone	Glucocorticoids
Insulin	Atrial natriuretic factor
	Fasting

B. REGULATION OF RENAL PHOSPHATE HANDLING

Many hormonal and nonhormonal factors modulate Pi transport (see Table 2). The most powerful regulator is the level of dietary Pi, which is discussed later in greater detail. Many of the modulators of Pi transport are discussed in regard to whether transport is activated by Pi depletion or inhibited by PTH.

1. Control by Acid-Base Status

Acid-base status significantly affects Pi transport. Respiratory acid-base changes have more pronounced effects on Pi excretion than metabolic acid-base changes do. Respiratory acid-base changes affect both the filtered load and the renal tubular handling of Pi. Respiratory acidosis increases plasma Pi and inhibits sodium-dependent Pi uptake in the proximal renal tubule, both of which increase Pi excretion. In contrast, respiratory alkalosis decreases plasma Pi and increases Pi reabsorption by the proximal straight tubule. Respiratory alkalosis also blunts the phosphaturic effect of PTH and dibutyryl cAMP on the straight, but not the convoluted, segment of the proximal tubule, possibly by activating the β_2-adrenoreceptors. In Pi-deprived rats, respiratory acidosis restores the phosphaturic effect of PTH.

Acute metabolic acidosis attenuates the phosphaturic effect of PTH but otherwise does not affect Pi reabsorption. Chronic metabolic acidosis also decreases reabsorption in the proximal renal tubule, but the effect is seen in normal and Pi-deprived states and may be dependent on activation of glucocorticoid secretion. Acute metabolic alkalosis can suppress Pi reabsorption but only with phosphate loading and maximal Pi reabsorption. Chronic metabolic alkalosis enhances Pi reabsorption by blocking glucocorticoid secretion.

2. Control by Extracellular Volume and Diuretics

Changes in the extracellular fluid volume also result in marked changes in Pi reabsorption. Volume expansion suppresses Pi reabsorption through the inhibition of transport in the proximal renal tubule, whereas Pi reabsorption is enhanced in volume depletion. Diuretics also affect Pi reabsorption through their relative inhibition of carbonic anhydrase. Inhibition of carbonic anhydrase reduces hydrogen secretion in the proximal renal tubule, which results in a reduction of Pi reabsorption. Therefore, acetazolamide has the greatest phosphaturic effect followed by thiazides and furosemide, both of which also have some abilty to inhibit carbonic anhydrase.

3. Control by Serum Calcium

Serum Ca^{++} suppresses Pi excretion by a variety of mechanisms. First, serum Ca^{++} decreases the filtered load of Pi by decreasing both ultrafiltrable Pi and the glomerular filtration rate by causing renal vasoconstriction. Secondly, serum Ca^{++} in at least some studies enhances Pi reabsorption in the proximal convoluted tubule. Thirdly, and probably most significantly, serum Ca^{++} suppresses PTH secretion. Decreasing the profound inhibitory effect of PTH on Pi reabsorption enhances the conservation of this anion.

4. Hormonal Control of Renal Phosphate Handling

Renal handling of Pi is affected by circulating concentrations of many hormones. Although PTH, vitamin D, and growth hormone are the most important regulators of renal Pi excretion, CT, thyroid hormones, insulin, and others also may have effects under some conditions.

a. Control by PTH

Of all the hormonal regulators of Pi excretion, PTH has the most significant effects. PTH plays a very fundamental role in the normal control of Pi excretion. At the cellular level, PTH binds to a basolateral membrane receptor and activates phospholipase C at low concentrations and adenylate cyclase at higher concentrations. These enzymes result in the phosphorylation of the Na^+-Pi cotransporter. Parathyroid hormone-related peptide (PTHrP) also has been shown to inhibit Pi transport, presumably by activating the same group of receptors.

PTH inhibits Pi reabsorption primarily in the proximal tubule, but Pi reabsorption is inhibited in the distal tubule as well. The cellular mechanism by which PTH inhibits Pi reabsorption may differ in the different segments. PTH inhibits Pi transport in the deeper nephrons more than in the superficial nephrons. This action of PTH is modulated by other factors that affect Pi transport. Acute Pi deprivation, respiratory alkalosis, and vitamin D block the ability of PTH to suppress Pi reabsorption through a mechanism localized to the proximal straight tubule.

b. Control by Vitamin D

Vitamin D also affects Pi excretion, but the relationship is less clear. Acutely, $1,25(OH)_2D$ activates Pi transport in the brush-border membrane of the proximal renal tubule. The mechanism for this effect has been shown to be associated with changes in the membrane lipids.[7] These effects can be obscured by other effects of vitamin D, which include increasing intestinal absorption of Ca and P and increasing serum Ca^{++}, as well as suppressing PTH secretion. Pi repletion from increased absorption would be expected to increase both the filtered load of Pi, as well as affecting its tubular transport. Changes in plasma Ca have direct effects on Pi handling and indirect effects through changes in PTH. Therefore, the role of $1,25(OH)_2D$ on controlling Pi excretion is complex.

c. *Control by Growth Hormone*

Growth hormone has significant effects on the control of Pi metabolism. Growing infants and adults with acromegaly have high serum Pi concentrations and relatively decreased Pi excretion. Growth hormone, either directly or through activation of insulin-like growth factor-1 (IGF-1) formation, stimulates Na^+-Pi cotransport in the proximal renal tubule. This effect is additive to the effect of Pi deprivation. Other effects of growth hormone in the kidney include activation of 1α-hydroxylase, which catalyzes the formation of $1,25(OH)_2D$. Other studies have shown that growth hormone is needed for stimulation of $1,25(OH)_2D$ formation by Pi deprivation. This effect may also be a direct effect of IGF-1 rather than growth hormone. Growth hormone, thus, has primary effects on Pi metabolism, as well as playing a role in the control of Pi metabolism during Pi depletion.

d. *Other Hormonal Control*

Other hormones have also been shown to modulate renal Pi excretion. CT induces hyperphosphaturia, probably as a result of directly blocking Pi reabsorption by the proximal tubule. Thyroxine and triidothyronine both directly stimulate reabsorption of Pi, which is additive to the effect of Pi depletion. Insulin also has a direct stimulatory effect on renal tubular Pi reabsorption and decreases Pi excretion, although the primary effect of insulin is to lower serum Pi by causing extrarenal redistribution into cells. Glucocorticoids demonstrate broad effects on mineral metabolism. In addition to their extrarenal effects, glucocorticoids inhibit Pi reabsorption by decreasing the membrane Na^+-Pi cotransporter as well as by activating the brush-border membrane Na^+-H^+ exchange resulting in luminal acidosis, which further inhibits Pi reabsorption. Atrial natriuretic factor also inhibits proximal tubule Pi reabsorption through inhibition of the Na^+-Pi cotransporter. Finally, catecholamines are hypophosphaturic as a result of hypophosphatemia secondary to redistribution into cells in addition to their activation of Pi reabsorption by modulating Na^+ reabsorption. β-adrenergic agents interact with the phosphaturic effect of PTH in a variety of physiologic situations. β-adrenergic antagonists restore the phosphaturic effect of PTH in respiratory alkalosis. In short term Pi depletion, β-adrenergic antagonists restore some of the phosphaturic effect of PTH, but neither these agents nor PTH are effective after long-term Pi depletion.

In summary, the majority of the reabsorption of the filtered Pi occurs in the proximal renal tubule. It is at this site that the regulation of Pi reabsorption by PTH and Pi depletion occurs. Other agents also affect Pi transport at the proximal tubule, but normally, the magnitude of their control is much less.

IV. DIETARY REGULATION OF RENAL CALCIUM HANDLING

In addition to hormonal regulation of renal Ca excretion, the nutritional state of an individual also may alter the handling of Ca by the kidney. In addition to a modest effect of Ca intake on Ca excretion, there are also effects of other nutrients, including vitamin D, sodium, and, especially, protein.

A. REGULATION BY DIETARY CALCIUM

In contrast to the profound effect of the state of Pi nutrition on its renal excretion (discussed later), only minimal changes in renal excretion of Ca occur when the Ca intake is altered. In humans, only 6%–8% of the change in dietary intake of Ca will be reflected in the urinary excretion (see Figure 9).[8,9] Most of the modulation of the ingested Ca load occurs by decreased intestinal absorption

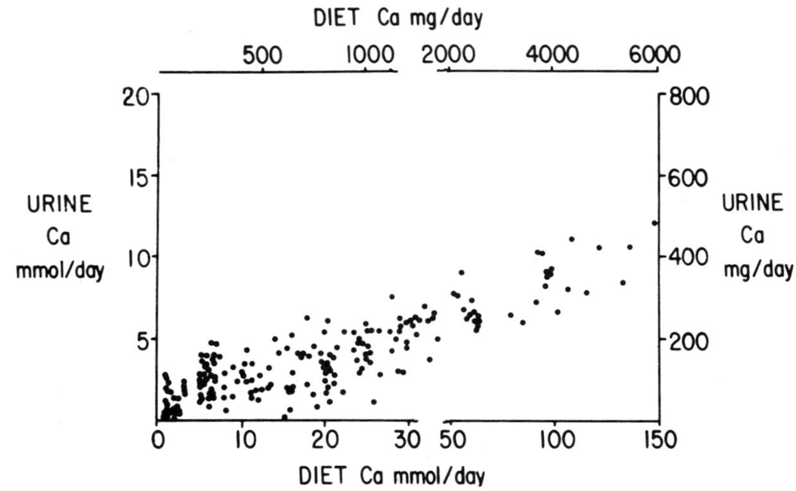

FIGURE 9. Effect of Dietary Calcium on Urinary Calcium Excretion in Normal Humans. (From Lemann, J., Adams, N. D. and Gray, R. W. in *New Engl. J. Med.*, 301, 536, 1979. With permission.)

mediated by the parathyroid-vitamin D axis. The small percentage of Ca that is absorbed is excreted by both an increase in filtered load and decreased distal tubular reabsorption as a result of the suppression of PTH secretion. In a study of young growing rats, Ca deprivation for a total of eight days led to a decrease in Ca excretion within 24 hours by increased Ca reabsorption.[10] Measurement of PTH and $1,25(OH)_2D$ at the eighth day showed increased levels of both. This study confirmed the renal conservation of Ca during states of deprivation, but it did not provide evidence for primary renal mechanisms. Hypercalcemia from infusing Ca, but not by feeding Ca, inhibits tubular reabsorption of Ca^{++} in both the proximal[11] and distal tubule.[12] The role of the suppression of PTH secretion by the high Ca^{++} in these studies was not clear.

B. REGULATION BY DIETARY PHOSPHATE

Pi depletion has clearly been shown to be associated with hypercalciuria in both man and animals.[13] The tubular segment responsible for the hypercalciuria is not clearly defined, but both proximal and distal renal tubular sites have been suggested.[14] Though proximal handling may be affected, it is likely that changes in the final urinary excretion of Ca reflect distal effects. Pi depletion in at least some studies caused inhibition of both Ca^{++} and Na^{+} reabsorption in the proximal tubule, whereas its effect in the distal renal tubule was specific for Ca^{++}. The exact role for either PTH or $1,25(OH)_2D$ as a mediator of this process has not been clearly established,[15] and some data suggest that Pi depletion may interfere with the action of PTH on the renal tubule.[16] Other studies of chronic Pi depletion have demonstrated suppressed distal renal tubular reabsorption of Ca^{++} that is resistant to correction by PTH.[17] Conversely, Pi loading has been associated with a decrease in Ca^{++} excretion and increased reabsorption of Ca^{++} in the distal tubule. Hyperphosphatemia likely causes transient hypocalcemia, which stimulates PTH secretion and results in increased Ca reabsorption by the distal tubule.[18]

C. EFFECT OF VITAMIN D DEFICIENCY

Vitamin D deficiency results in decreased intestinal Ca absorption and secondary hyperparathyroidism. Evidence exists for increased renal Ca excretion in vitamin D-deficient rats compared to vitamin D-replete rats with the same concentration of serum Ca (see Figure 4).[19] Thus, in vitamin D deficiency, a component of Ca wasting exists that is not correctable by PTH alone. The significance of this portion of the Ca transport is not clear.

D. EFFECT OF DIETARY PROTEIN AND CARBOHYDRATE

Dietary protein loading has also been shown to cause hypercalciuria.[20] Metabolism of animal protein as compared to that from other protein sources results in increased endogenous acid production, which inhibits Ca reabsorption. In addition, the increased urinary sulfate excretion as a result of metabolism of sulfur-containing amino acids may also have a direct hypercalciuric effect. Another potential mechanism is the stimulation by dietary protein of glucagon secretion, which then results in hypercalciuria.[21] In contrast to these findings, the ingestion of meat generally does not result in significant hypercalciuria, in part, due to the counteracting effect of the P contained in this source of protein.[22] Animal-protein intake has been shown, though, to be a risk factor for the formation of kidney stones.[23]

Carbohydrate loading, and in particular glucose, also can result in hypercalciuria.[24] Glucose inhibits Ca reabsorption partly by activating insulin secretion which is associated with hypercalciuria. Hypercalciuria, as a result of dietary protein or carbohydrate loading, may be increased in patients with stone disease.[25]

E. EFFECT OF DIETARY SODIUM

As would be assumed by the parallel reabsorption of sodium and Ca along several sites of the renal tubule, sodium intake, and thus excretion, will also directly influence Ca excretion.[26] This effect is seen with chronic sodium loading, but is not well demonstrated in studies of acute sodium loading using infusions of isotonic saline.[8] Studies in humans have shown an increase in urinary Ca excretion of approximately 0.6 mmol per 100 meq increase in urinary sodium.[8] This effect may be related to an increase in the filtered load of Ca.[27] The mechanism for the increased filtered load of Ca with increased dietary sodium in normal humans may result from enhanced PTH secretion and, hence, increased $1,25(OH)_2D$ formation and intestinal Ca absorption.[28] Again, renal stone patients may have an increased sensitivity to the hypercalciuric effect of sodium intake. In fact, a recent study has shown a correlation between sodium excretion and decreased bone mass in patients with absorptive hypercalciuria, suggesting a role for dietary sodium in the pathogenesis of hypercalciuria in this group of patients.[29]

In summary, variations in oral Ca intake result in only a limited change in Ca excretion due to regulation at the level of intestinal absorption. Other dietary influences such as decreased Pi intake, or increased intake of dietary acid, glucose, and sodium modulate renal Ca handling and result in increased Ca excretion.

V. DIETARY REGULATION OF RENAL PHOSPHATE HANDLING

Pi intake has direct effects on the kidney, as well as indirect effects mediated by hormonal changes related to Pi intake. The kidney is the major organ controlling Pi homeostasis, and therefore, the ability of the kidney to adapt to changes in Pi intake is very important.

A. REGULATION BY PHOSPHATE DEPLETION

Dietary factors, particularly Pi depletion, have significant effects on renal Pi handling.

1. Definition of Phosphate Depletion

Hypophosphatemia can be associated with normal total body Pi, or it can be associated with true Pi depletion.[30] Hypophosphatemia without total body deficiency can result from translocation from the extracellular to the intracellular compartment as a result of thermal burns, respiratory alkalosis, or as a consequence of Pi becoming trapped as phosphorylated intermediates of carbohydrate metabolism. In addition to these states of true hypophosphatemia, the kidney performs teleologically as if true hypophosphatemia existed during periods of increased need for Pi, e.g., growth, pregnancy, or lactation. Pi depletion can result from decreased dietary intake through enteral or parenteral

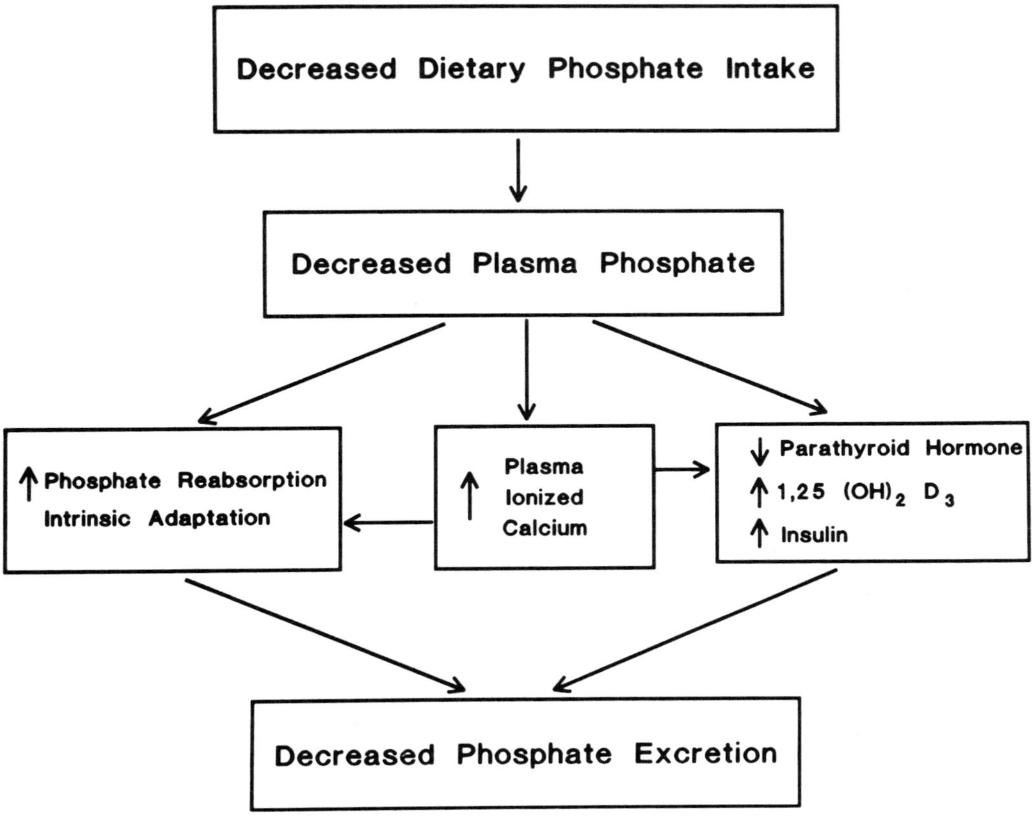

FIGURE 10. Mechanism of Decreased Phosphate Excretion with Phosphate Depletion. (From Berndt, T. J. and Knox, F. G. in *The Kidney: Physiology and Pathophysiology*, 2nd ed., Seldin, D. W. and Giebisch, G., eds., Raven Press, New York, 1992. With permission.)

routes, or it can result from decreased intestinal absorption, despite normal intake, due to the administration of Pi-binding antacids, malabsorption states, or in the presence of vitamin D deficiency.

2. Effect of Phosphate Depletion on Calciotropic Hormones

It has long been known that animals fed a low-Pi diet excrete a urine that is almost totally lacking in Pi.[31] Clearance studies demonstrated that Pi reabsorption at any level of plasma Pi was greater when the Pi intake was low.[32] Pi depletion can lead to hypercalcemia, which suppresses PTH secretion and, therefore, results in increased renal tubular reabsorption of Pi. Hypophosphatemia also increases formation of $1,25(OH)_2D$, which also enhances Pi reabsorption.[33] Finally, evidence of an increase in insulin secretion in response to Pi depletion has been reported.[34]

3. Direct Effect of Phosphate Depletion on the Renal Tubule

Despite the contribution of these potential mechanisms to enhance Pi reabsorption (see Figure 10), the most striking feature of Pi depletion is its ability to activate intrinsic renal tubular Pi reabsorption independent of these other factors.[35] This effect was first suggested by clearance studies demonstrating decreased Pi excretion with Pi depletion in animals, despite thyroparathyroidectomy or changes in plasma Ca. Also, not only is the mechanism by which Pi depletion decreases Pi excretion largely independent of effects of PTH, but Pi depletion blunts the ability of PTH[36] or cAMP[37] to enhance Pi excretion. The intrinsic ability of the renal tubule to respond to Pi depletion has now been well defined by studies with isolated renal tubules and cell culture studies.

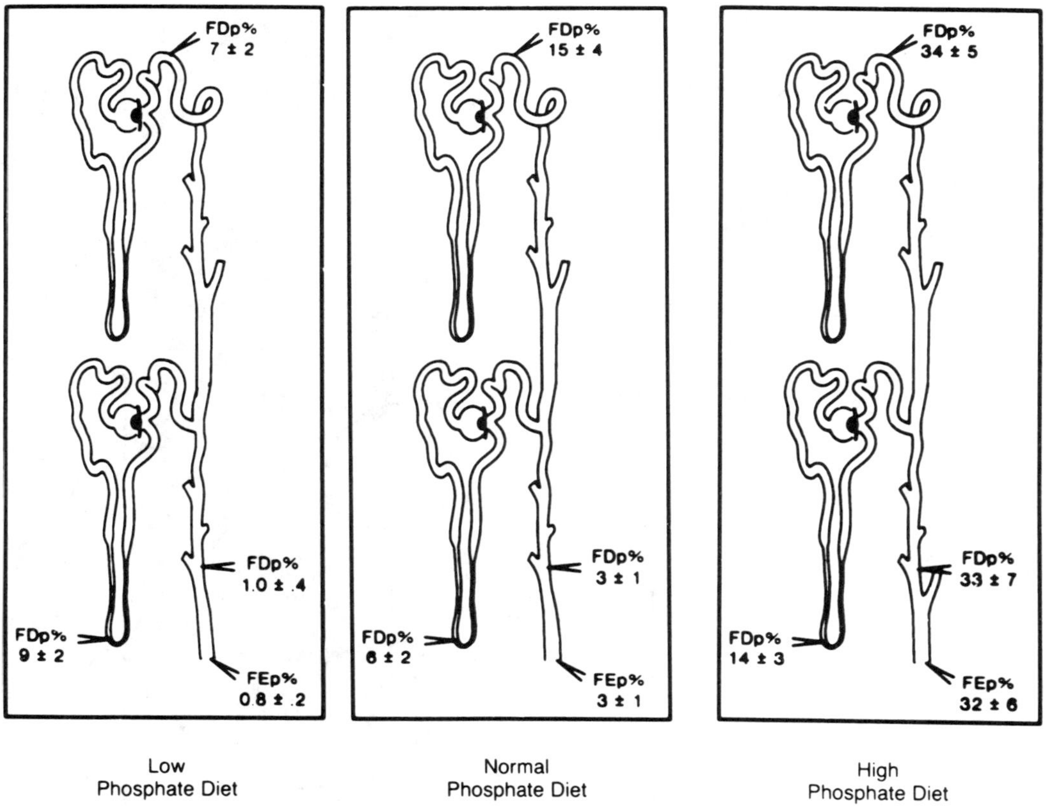

FIGURE 11. Role of Superficial and Deep Nephrons in the Renal Response to Dietary Phosphate Intake. (From Berndt, T. J. and Knox, F. G. in *The Kidney: Physiology and Pathophysiology*, 2nd ed., Seldin, D. W. and Giebisch, G., eds., Raven Press, New York, 1992. With permission.)

a. Segmental Renal Tubular Effects

Pi depletion enhances renal tubular handling of Pi to a greater extent than any other known condition. The primary site for adaptation to Pi depletion occurs in the proximal renal tubule,[38] but the effect is not limited to this segment.[39] In micropuncture studies it has been shown that the superficial nephrons can decrease their Pi excretion by half in response to Pi depletion (see Figure 11). In contrast to the deep nephrons though, the most dramatic characteristic of the superficial nephrons is to double the Pi excretion in response to a Pi load in the thyroparathyroidectomized rat.[40] In the thyroparathyroidectomized rat a more distal site of enhanced Pi reabsorption has been demonstrated as well. More recent microperfusion studies of the proximal convoluted tubule have shown that both the early and late portions of this segment respond to Pi depletion, although transport is relatively greater in the earlier portions of the proximal renal tubule (see Figure 12).[41] In addition to its inhibitory effects on the proximal convoluted tubule, Pi depletion also affects the proximal straight tubule, and it is at this site that the resistance to the phosphaturic effect of PTH is manifested.[42] At least in rabbits fed a low-Pi diet, the enhanced Pi transport in the proximal renal tubule is specific for Pi with no change in either sodium or glucose reabsorption. In hamsters time-course studies have demonstrated that the effect of low Pi is fairly rapid, occurring after only 2 to 4 hours of Pi depletion.[43]

b. Cell Culture Studies and Mechanisms

Studies with renal tubular cell lines in culture have further clarified the mechanisms by which Pi depletion enhances Pi reabsorption. Incubation of LLC-PK, MDCK, OK, and JTC-12.P3 renal cell

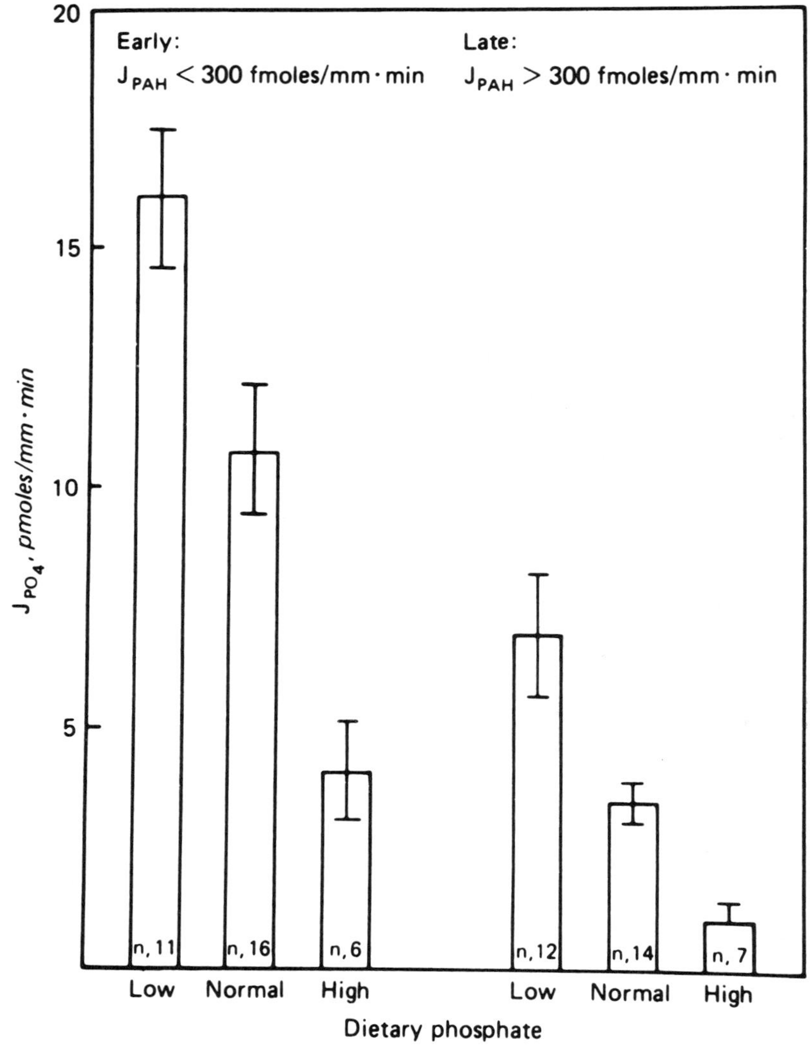

FIGURE 12. Effects of Dietary Phosphate on Renal Phosphate Transport along the Early and Late Proximal Convoluted Tubule. (From Brazy, P. C., et al., Comparative effects of dietary phosphate, unilateral nephrectomy, and parathyroid hormone on phosphate transport by the rabbit proximal tubule, *Kidney Int.*, 17, 788, 1980. With permission.)

lines in low-Pi media results in increased Na^+-Pi cotransport in each. The changes in Pi transport have been localized to the brush-border Na^+-Pi cotransporter by studies of membrane vesicles.[44] These changes occur within hours and are dependent on *de novo* protein synthesis. Recent studies have suggested that the mechanism involves control at a posttranscriptional, pretranslational step in protein synthesis. Characterization of the Na^+-Pi cotransport with Pi depletion demonstrates an increase in the V_{max} with no change in the K_m.[45] Studies in cultured cells have also suggested the presence of an even faster mechanism that is independent of protein synthesis.[46] Also, studies of the lipid composition of the brush-border membrane have shown changes with Pi depletion that would result in increased membrane fluidity.[47] A change in membrane fluidity could accelerate Pi transport by increasing the activity of the Na^+-Pi cotransport without necessarily increasing their number. A model has been proposed for the control of Pi transport wherein Pi depletion results in increased insertion of Na^+-Pi cotransporters either from preformed pools or by activating the synthesis of new transporters.[48] The signal transduction pathway by which Pi depletion activates Pi reabsorption is not known, but a role for decreased intracellular Pi has been suggested.[49]

B. EFFECT OF FASTING

In contrast to the effects of Pi depletion alone, fasting increases Pi excretion through the inhibition of tubular reabsorption.[50] In fact, fasting will reverse the increased tubular reabsorption to Pi depletion alone and allow a renal tubular response to PTH. Fasting suppresses the activation of Na^+-Pi cotransporters in membrane vesicles.[51] The signals by which fasting decreases Pi reabsorption are not totally known, but possible factors include acidosis[52] and enhanced glucagon secretion.[53]

C. REGULATION BY CALCIUM

Studies of the effect of serum Ca^{++} on Pi excretion have been performed using Ca infusions rather than changes in Ca^{++} intake. Changes in serum Ca^{++} affect Pi excretion, but the direction and magnitude are dependent on the experimental conditions. The presence of both PTH-independent and Ca^{++}-dependent mechanisms of Pi reabsorption has been described in X-linked hypophosphatemic rickets.[54] Though there is evidence for a primary effect of Ca^{++} on renal tubular Pi reabsorption,[55] it has not been consistently confirmed by other studies. Thus, the effect of changes of serum Ca^{++} on Pi excretion are mostly due to either PTH modulation of renal tubular handling of Pi or Ca^{++}-induced changes in the filtered load of Pi.

D. EFFECT OF VITAMIN D DEFICIENCY

As in studies of the effect of Ca^{++} on Pi excretion, it is difficult to separate the primary effects of vitamin D deficiency on renal P handling from the secondary effects induced by changes in PTH secretion, intestinal absorption, and bone resorption. Vitamin D deficiency in rats is associated with an increase in excretion of Pi, even when the secondary hyperparathyroidism is prevented.[56] Despite the evidence for a direct effect of vitamin D deficiency on the kidney, it is likely that the nonrenal effects of vitamin D deficiency predominate in the resulting changes in Pi excretion.

In summary, Pi depletion results in activation of Pi reabsorption by a direct tubular effect, as well as by extrarenal effects. Pi depletion results in marked enhancement of Pi reabsorption that may overide the effect of other modulators of renal Pi handling. Decreased Ca intake also will decrease Pi excretion, but through effects on PTH secretion or the filtered load of Pi.

VI. SUMMARY

The kidney plays a very key role in mineral homeostasis. By the modulation of the excretion of the 10.5 grams of Ca and the 6.5 grams of Pi that are filtered daily, the kidney is uniquely positioned to control the total body content of these minerals. The kidney also plays an endocrine role as the source of $1,25(OH)_2D$ formation. Control of Ca and Pi excretion is regulated by a number of hormonal and nonhormonal factors, the most important one being PTH. Normally the major response organ to changes in Ca intake is the intestine and not the kidney. In response to the challenge of dietary deprivation of Ca, the kidney does participate in maintaining the level of serum Ca, but in conjunction with the intestine and bone through stimulation by PTH and $1,25(OH)_2D$. In contrast, the kidney regulates Pi reabsorption in response to changes in Pi intake largely independent of the effect of PTH or other hormones. The ability of the kidney to respond intrinsically to changes in dietary Pi make it arguably the most important effector organ in Pi homeostasis.

REFERENCES

1. **Suki, W. N. and Rouse, D.,** Renal transport of calcium, magnesium, and phosphorus, in *The Kidney*, 4th ed., Brenner, B. M. and Rector, F. C., eds., Saunders, Philadelphia, 1991.
2. **Yanagawa, N. and Lee, D. B. N.,** Renal handling of calcium and phosphorus, in *Disorders of Mineral Metabolism,* Coe, F. L. and Favus, M. J., eds., Raven Press, New York, 1992.

3. **Costanzo, L. S. and Windhager, E. E.,** Renal regulation of calcium balance, in *The Kidney: Physiology and Pathophysiology*, 2nd ed., Seldin, D. W. and Giebisch, G., eds., Raven Press, New York, 1992.
4. **Bijvoet, O. L. M.,** Relation of plasma phosphate concentration to renal tubular reabsorption of phosphate, *Clin Sci.*, 37, 23, 1969.
5. **Bendt, T. J. and Knox, F. G.,** Renal regulation of phosphate excretion, in *The Kidney: Physiology and Pathophysiology*, 2nd ed., Seldin, D. W. and Giebisch, G., eds., Raven Press, New York, 1992.
6. **Murer, H. and Biber, J.,** Renal tubular phosphate transport, in *The Kidney: Physiology and Pathophysiology*, 2nd ed., Seldin, D.W. and Giebisch, G., eds., Raven Press, New York, 1992.
7. **Tsutsumi, M., Alvarez, U., Avioli, L. V. and Hruska, K. A.,** Effect of 1,25-dihydroxyvitamin D_3 on phospholipid composition of rat renal brush border membrane, *Am. J. Physiol.*, 249, F117, 1985.
8. **Lemann, J., Adams, N. D. and Gray, R. W.,** Urinary calcium excretion in human beings, *New Engl. J. Med.*, 301, 535, 1979.
9. **Lemann, J.,** Composition of the diet and calcium kidney stones, *New Engl. J., Med.*, 328, 880, 1993.
10. **Bourdeau, J. E., Bouillon, R., Zikos, D. and Langman, C. B.,** Renal responses to calcium deprivation in young rabbits, *Miner. Electrol. Metab.*, 14, 157, 1988.
11. **Edwards, B. R., Sutton, R. A. and Dirks, J. H.,** Effect of calcium infusion on renal tubular reabsorption in the dog, *Am. J. Physiol.*, 227, 13, 1974.
12. **Quamme, G. A.,** Effect of hypercalcemia on renal tubular handling of calcium and magnesium, *Can. J. Physiol. Pharmacol.*, 60, 1275, 1982.
13. **Coburn, J. W. and Massry, S. G.,** Changes in serum and urinary calcium during phosphate depletion: studies on mechanisms, *J. Clin. Invest.*, 49, 1073, 1970.
14. **Lau, K., Agus, Z. S., Goldberg, M. and Goldfarb, S.,** Renal tubular sites of altered calcium transport in phosphate-depleted rats, *J. Clin. Invest.*, 64, 1681, 1979.
15. **Dominguez, J. H., Gray, R. W., and Lemann, J.,** Dietary phosphate deprivation in women and men. Effects on mineral and acid balances, parathyroid hormone, and the metabolism of 25(OH) vitamin D, *J. Clin. Endocrinol. Metab.*, 43, 1065, 1976.
16. **Guruprakash, G. H., Babino, H., Duffy, W. B., Krothapalli, R. K., Senekjian, H. O., Eknoyan, G. and Suki, W. N.,** Microinjection study of renal calcium absorption in the phosphate-depleted rat, *Miner. Electrol. Metab.*, 11262, 1985.
17. **Goldfarb, S., Westby, G. R., Goldberg, M. and Agus, Z. A.,** Renal tubular effects of chronic phosphate depletion, *J. Clin. Invest.*, 59, 770, 1977.
18. **Wong, N. L. M., Quamme, G. A., Sutton, R. A. L. and Dirks, J. H.,** Effect of phosphate and calcium infusion on renal phosphate and calcium transport in the dog, *Renal Physiol.*, 8, 30, 1985.
19. **Kurokawa, K.,** Calcium-regulating hormones and the kidney, *Kidney Int.*, 32, 760, 1987.
20. **Goldfarb, S.,** Dietary factors in the pathogenesis and prophylaxis of calcium nephrolithiasis, *Kidney Int.*, 34, 544, 1988.
21. **Anderson, J. J. B., Thomsen, K. and Christiansen, C.,** High protein meals, insular hormones and urinary calcium excretion in human subjects, in *Osteoporosis 1987*, Christiansen, C., Johansen, J. S. and Riis, B. J., eds., Osteopress ApS, Denmark, 1987.
22. **Spencer, H., Kramer, L., Lesniak M., de Bartola, M., Norris, C. and Osis D.,** Calcium requirements in humans, *Clin. Orthop. Rel. Res.*, 184, 270, 1984.
23. **Curran, G. C., Willett, W. C., Rimm, E. B. and Stampfer, M. J.,** A prospective study of dietary calcium and other nutrients and the risk of symptomatic kidney stones, *New Engl. J. Med.*, 328, 833, 1993.
24. **Lemann, J., Lennon, E. J., Piering, W. F., Prien, E. L., Jr. and Ricanati, E. S.,** Evidence that glucose ingestion inhibits net renal tubular reabsorption of calcium and magnesium in man, *J. Lab Clin. Med.*, 75, 578, 1970.
25. **Wasserstein, A. G., Stolley, P. D., Soper, K. A., Goldfarb, S. and Agus, Z. S.,** Case-control study of risk factors for idiopathic calcium nephrolithiasis, *Miner. Electrol. Metab.*, 13, 85, 1987.
26. **Kleeman, C. R., Bohannan, J., Bernstein, D., Ling, S. and Maxwell, M. H.,** Effect of variation in sodium intake on calcium excretion in normal humans, *Proc. Soc. Exp. Biol. Med.*, 115, 29, 1964.
27. **McCarron, D. A., Rankin, L. I., Bennet, W. M., Krutzik, S., McClung, M. R. and Luft, F. C.,** Urinary calcium excretion at extremes of sodium intake in normal man, *Am. J. Nephrol.*, 1, 84, 1981.
28. **Breslau, N. A., McGuire, J. L., Zerwekh, J. E. and Pak, C. Y. C.,** The role of dietary sodium on renal excretion and intestinal absorption of calcium and on vitamin D metabolism, *J. Clin. Endocrinol. Metab.*, 55, 369, 1982.
29. **Pietschmann, P., Breslau, N. A. and Pak, C. Y. C.,** Reduced vertebral bone density in hypercalciuric nephrolithiasis, *J. Bone Min. Res.*, 7, 1383, 1992.
30. **Knochel, J. P.,** The clinical and physiological implications of phosphorus deficiency, in *The Kidney: Physiology and Pathophysiology*, 2nd ed., Seldin, D. W. and Giebisch, G., eds., Raven Press, New York, 1992.
31. **Crawford, J. D., Osborne, M. M., Talbot N. B., Terry M. L. and Morrill. M. F.,** The parathyroid glands and phosphorus homeostasis, *J. Clin. Invest.*, 29, 1448, 1950.
32. **Anderson, G. H. and Draper, H. H.,** Effect of dietary phosphate on calcium metabolism in intact and parathyroidectomized adult rats, *J. Nutr.*, 102, 1123, 1972.

33. **Gray, R. W. and Napoli J. L.,** Dietary phosphate deprivation increases 1,25-dihydroxyvitamin D_3 synthesis in rat kidney *in vitro, J. Biol. Chem.*, 258, 1152, 1983.
34. **Allon, M., Rodriguez, M. and Llach, F.,** Insulin in the acute renal adaptation to dietary phosphate restriction in the rat, *Kidney Int.*, 37, 14, 1990.
35. **Steele, T. H. and DeLuca, H. F.,** Influence of dietary phosphate in the parathyroidectomized rat, *J. Clin. Invest.*, 57, 867, 1976.
36. **Steele, T. H.,** Renal resistance to parathyroid hormone during phosphorus deprivation, *J. Clin. Invest.,* 58, 1461, 1976.
37. **Berndt, T. J., Onsgard, M. J. and Knox, F. G.,** Effect of cAMP analogue infusion on phosphate reabsorption in phosphate-deprived rats, *Am. J. Physiol.,* 255, F96, 1988.
38. **Wen, S.-F., Boynar J. W. and Stoll R. W.,** Effect of phosphate deprivation on renal phosphate transport in the dog, *Am. J. Physiol.*, 234, F199, 1978.
39. **Muhlbauer, R. C., Bonjour J.-P. and Fleisch H.,** Tubular localization of adaptation to dietary phosphate in rats, *Am. J. Physiol.,* 233, F342, 1977.
40. **Haramati, A., Haas, J. A. and Knox, F. G.,** Adaptation of deep and superficial nephrons to changes in dietary phosphate intake, *Am. J. Physiol.*, 244, F265, 1983.
41. **Brazy, P. C., McKeown, J. W., Harris, R. H. and Dennis, V. W.,** Comparative effects of dietary phosphate, unilateral nephrectomy, and parathyroid hormone on phosphate transport by the rabbit proximal tubule, *Kidney Int.*, 17, 788, 1980.
42. **Pastoriza-Monuz, E., Mishler, D. R. and Lechene, C.,** Effect of phosphate deprivation on phosphate reabsorption in the rat nephron: role of PTH, *Am. J. Physiol.*, 244, F140, 1983.
43. **Levine, B. S., Ho, K., Hodsman, A., Kurokawa, K. and Coburn, J. W.,** Early renal brush border membrane adaptation to dietary phosphorus, *Miner. Electrol. Metab.*, 10, 222, 1984.
44. **Caverzasio, J., Brown, C. D. A., Biber J., Bonjour, J.-P. and Murer, H.,** Adaptation of phosphate transport in phosphate-deprived LLC-PK_1 cells, *Am. J. Physiol.*, 248, F122, 1985.
45. **Cheng, L., Liang, C. T. and Sactor, B.,** Phosphate uptake by renal membrane vesicles of rabbits adapted to high and low phosphorus diets, *Am. J. Physiol.*, 245, F175, 1983.
46. **Biber, J. and Murer, H.,** Na^+-P_i cotransport in LLC-PK_1 cells: fast adaptive response to P_i deprivation, *Am. J. Physiol.,* 249, C430, 1985.
47. **Yusufi, A. N. K., Szczepanska-Konkel, M., Kempson, S. A., McAteer, J. A. and Dousa, T. P.,** Differential mechanisms of the increase in Na^+/P_i cotransport across the renal brush border membrane by thyroid hormone and by dietary phosphate deprivation, *Am. J. Physiol.*, 256, F852, 1989.
48. **Biber J.,** Cellular aspects of proximal tubular phosphate reabsorption, *Kidney Int.*, 36, 360, 1989.
49. **Barac-Nieto, M., Towd, T. L., Spitzer, A.,** Effect of P_i restriction on the relationship between the intracellular P_i and renal Na^+-P_i cotransport in growing guinea pigs, *Kidney Int.*, 37, 453, 1990.
50. **Beck, N., Webster, S. K. and Reineck, H. J.,** Effect of fasting on tubular phosphorus reabsorption, *Am. J., Physiol.*, 247, F241, 1979.
51. **Kempson, S. A., Shah, S. V., Werness, P. G., Berndt, T., Lee, P. H., Smith L. H., Knox, F. G. and Dousa, T. P.,** Renal brush border membrane adaptation to phosphorus deprivation: effects of fasting versus low-phosphorus diet, *Kidney Int.,* 18, 36, 1980.
52. **Kempson, S. A.,** Effect of metabolic acidosis on renal brush border membrane adaptation to low phosphorus diet, *Kidney Int.,* 22, 225, 1982.
53. **Saudek, C. D., Boulter, R. R. and Arky, R. A.,** The natriuretic effect of glucagon and its role in starvation. *J. Clin, Endocrinol. Metab.*, 36, 761, 1973.
54. **Glorieux, F. and Scriver, C. R.,** Loss of a parathyroid hormone-sensitive component of phosphate transport in X-linked hypophosphatemia, *Science*, 175, 997, 1972.
55. **Amiel, C., Kuntziger H., Coutte, S., Coureau, C. and Bergounioux, N.,** Evidence for a parathyroid hormone independent calcium modulation of phosphate transport along the nephron, *J. Clin. Invest.*, 57, 256, 1976.
56. **Kurnik, B. R. C., Huskey M. and Hruska K. A.,** 1,25-Dihydroxycholecalciferol stimulates renal phosphate transport by directly altering membrane phophatidylcholine composition, *Biochim. Biophys. Acta*, 917, 81, 1987.

Chapter 6

REGULATION OF CALCIUM METABOLISM IN CELLS

Brian Herman, Ph.D.

TABLE OF CONTENTS

I. INTRODUCTION

For many years, it has been recognized that the level of cytosolic free calcium (Ca_i^{2+}) is critical to proper cell functioning. Over a hundred years ago, Ca was found to be necessary for muscle contraction; based on research performed over the past 20 years, it is clear that alterations in Ca_i^{2+} are involved in a large number of biological functions (see Table 1). In this short review, we (1) examine mechanisms by which cells maintain tight control over Ca_i^{2+}, (2) show how Ca_i^{2+} is measured in cells, and (3) provide a few specific examples illustrating the importance of Ca_i^{2+} in normal cell function.

II. CALCIUM HOMEOSTASIS IN CELLS

All cells are exposed to a relatively high extracellular concentration of Ca (in the millimolar range). However, Ca_i^{2+} is kept at a very low level (ten to hundreds of nanomoles) inside of cells[1] (see Figure 1). Thus, a thousand- to ten thousand-fold gradient exists between intra- and extracellular Ca. Adding to this concentration gradient is the fact that the electrical potential difference between the inside and outside of the cell creates a driving force for Ca to enter cells. To maintain Ca_i^{2+} at nanomolar levels, cells maintain a low passive plasma membrane permeability to Ca, use ATP-dependent Ca extrusion mechanisms, sequester Ca in intracellular organelles, and utilize Ca-binding proteins (Figure 1).

0-8493-7845-1/95/$0.00+$.50

TABLE 1
Calcium-Regulated Biological Functions

Acetylcholine Release
Anaphase Initiation
Cell Differentiation
Egg Fertilization
Glycogen Synthesis
Interaction of Actin with Myosin
Neuronal Function
Stimulation of Cell Growth
Stimulation of Gene Expression

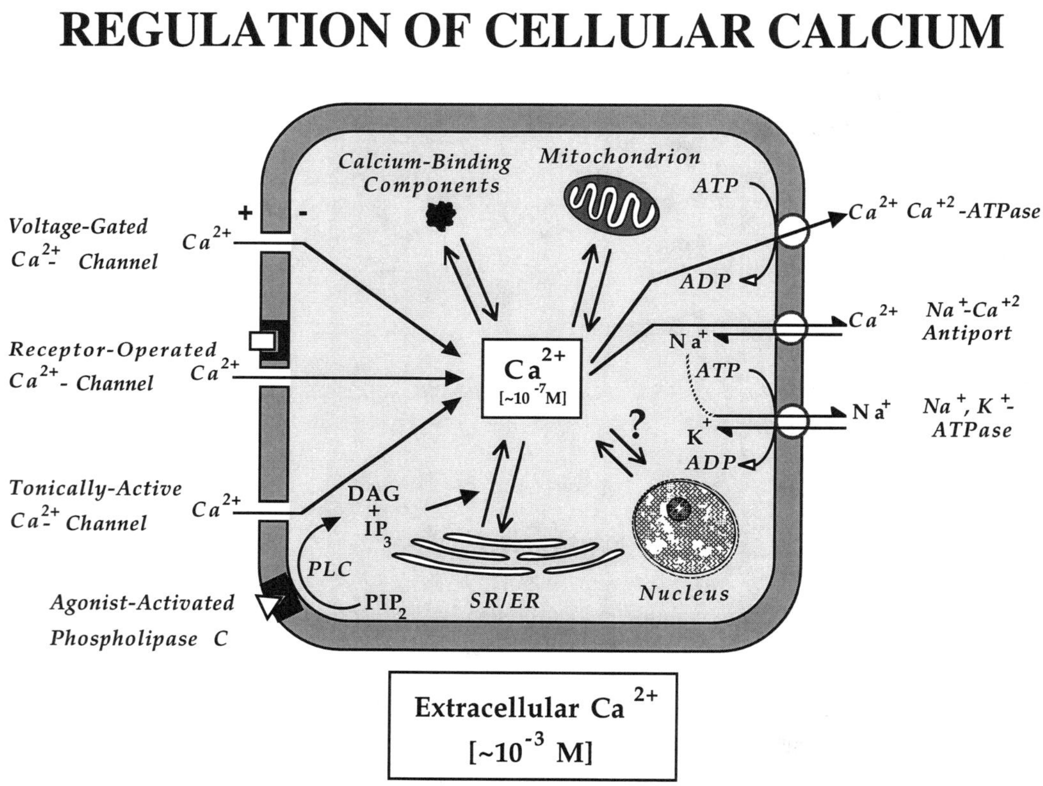

FIGURE 1. Regulation of Cellular Calcium. Calcium regulation at the plasma membrane involves a Ca^{2+}-translocating ATPase, a Na^+/Ca^{2+} exchanger, voltage-dependent and receptor-generated Ca^{2+} channels, and a transmembrane calcium leak. Intracellular modulation of cytosolic calcium can be attained through calcium binding proteins, release and resequestration of calcium in the sarcoplasmic/endoplasmic reticulum, and by calcium sequestration in the mitochondria. (Modified from References 3 and 51)

Ca is viewed as a ubiquitous second messenger that links cell surface activation events with subsequent biological activities. For this function, cells must be able to keep Ca_i^{2+} at a low concentration, yet also be able to vary Ca_i^{2+} rapidly and precisely in different cell compartments in keeping with the requirements of the functional cycle of cells. As noted previously, cells employ a number of mechanisms to accomplish this, with the result that Ca_i^{2+} is 10,000-fold less than extracellular Ca. The importance of this large gradient is that only a small increase in the permeability of the plasma membrane can lead to large increases in Ca_i^{2+}.

TABLE 2
Calcium Transport Proteins

	Protein	Binding Affinity	Transport Capacity
Plasma Membrane	Ca-Mg-ATPase	<0.5 μ*M*	0.5 nmol/mg/sec
	Na-Ca exchanger	1–20 μ*M*	20 nmol/mg/sec
SR/ER	Ca-ATPase	<0.5 μ*M*	70 nmol/mg/sec
Mitochondria	Uniporter	1–10 μ*M*	10 nmol/mg/sec
	Na-Ca exchanger	1–10 μ*M*	0.2–0.3 nmol/mg/sec

III. CALCIUM TRANSPORT PROTEINS

Ca transport proteins facilitate the repetitive movement of Ca into or out of cells and thus play a major role in the long-term maintenance of Ca levels between the intra- and extracellular environment. A large number of transporters have been identified, but no redundancy of action exists due to differences in kinetic properties of the different transporters which are necessary to satisfy the various functional demands of the cell. Ca transport proteins fall into two broad categories: those that facilitate Ca entry into cells (voltage-gated, receptor-operated, second-messenger operated, mechanically operated tonically active, and gap-junction channels),[2] and those that pump Ca out of cells (mainly the Ca^{2+}-Mg^{2+}-ATPase and Na^+/Ca^{2+} exchanger).[3]

A. PLASMA MEMBRANE

The Ca^{2+}-Mg^{2+}-ATPase of the plasma membrane is a high-affinity system for the fine regulation of Ca in the submicromolar range (see Table 2). The Ca^{2+}-Mg^{2+}-ATPase removes Ca from cells with high affinity (K_M for $Ca^{2+} < 0.5\ \mu M$) against a steep concentration gradient in exchange for two H^+ ions using the energy of ATP hydrolysis.[4] The Ca^{2+}-Mg^{2+}-ATPase is a 1000 amino acid multiple-pass membrane protein with some homology to the Na^+-K^+-ATPase.[5] Although it has a relatively high K_M, it has a low transport capacity (0.5 nmol/mg/sec). It is a P class ATPase (i.e. an aspartyl phosphate linkage is generated during ATP hydrolysis), which is vanadate sensitive and, in some tissues, is stimulated by calmodulin, which increases the V_{max} of the enzyme and decreases the K_M for Ca. The activity of this transporter can also be increased by cAMP-linked phosphorylation, acidic phospholipids, polyunsaturated fatty acids, and limited proteolysis.

The Na^+-Ca^{2+} exchanger is composed of subunits of 82, 70, and 33 kilodaltons (kDa).[6] It utilizes energy from the electrochemical gradients of other ions (i.e. Na^+) to move Ca. The Na^+-Ca^{2+} exchanger can move Ca either into or out of cells with the direction being dictated by the transmembrane Na^+ gradient, membrane potential, and Ca_i^{2+}. In resting muscle cells with a large negative membrane potential, the exchanger is poised towards Ca efflux; as the membrane potential becomes less positive, the exchanger can pump Ca into cells. Movement of Ca out of cells by this exchanger is electrogenic in that three Na^+ ions are transported in exchange for each Ca^{2+}. This exchanger has a high capacity (20 nmols of Ca/mg/sec) but low affinity for Ca^{2+} (K_M 1–20 μM). The K_M for Ca can be increased by kinase-linked phosphorylation; activation of this exchanger is largely responsible for the positive inotropic effect of digitalis in heart muscle.

Voltage-gated Ca channels (VGCC) are the most studied of the Ca entry pathways.[2] There are four types of VGCC now recognized, L, T, N, and P. Each of these four VGCC displays characteristic differences in terms of voltage dependence of activation, organ distribution, and pharmacologic sensitivities. However, common to all of these types of Ca channels is their depolarization-dependent activation and their selectivity for Ca over other ions.

The L-type VGCC is activated by a large depolarization of the membrane potential and inhibited by dihydropyridines (DHPs).[7] These VGCC are intimately involved in excitation-contraction coupling in cardiac and smooth muscle cells and excitation-secretion coupling in endocrine and some neuronal cells.[8] In cardiac muscle, the L-type channel resides in the T tubule and is activated by a depolarizing voltage change leading to the entry of extracellular Ca and subsequent release of intracellular stores of Ca from the sarcoplasmic reticulum (SR). Skeletal muscle L-type channels seem to differ from cardiac channels in that their activation is much slower and an influx of Ca through the channel is not required for contraction.[9] The activity of these channels can be modulated by catecholamines acting through cAMP-dependent protein phosphorylation or the GTP-binding protein G_s.

Using chimeric constructs of the cardiac and skeletal L-type VGCC, researchers have identified the sequences responsible for Ca release from the SR, voltage sensing, and DHP binding. As a class, the DHP-sensitive VGCC are composed of five subunits; α_1, α_2, β, γ, and δ.[9] The α_1 portion has a molecular weight of approximately 170 kDa, with four repeat units of homology, each containing 6 α-helical segments, all of which are thought to cross the plasma membrane. The α subunit of the DHP-sensitive VGCC contains the voltage-sensor, drug receptor, and multiple phosphorylation sites; expression of this subunit by itself has indicated that it is sufficient for some Ca channel function and possibly excitation-contraction coupling.[10] The α_2 subunit has a molecular weight of approximately 140 kDa and is covalently linked to the δ subunit via a disulphide linkage.[11] It is a hydrophilic protein distributed in a wide variety of tissues, and whereas it does not demonstrate channel activity on its own, when coexpressed with the α_1 subunit, it augments the activity of this subunit.[12] The β subunit is a peripheral membrane protein thought to be associated with the cytoplasmic surface of the plasma membrane.[13] It has a molecular weight of 58 kDa and may be a target for regulation by cAMP-dependent phosphorylation acting through linkages with the cytoskeleton. The γ subunit has also been cloned, and while its function is unknown, it has only been found in skeletal muscle and is thus thought to have a special function in excitation-contraction coupling in this tissue.[14]

The T-type VGCC is involved in pacemaker activity and repetitive firing in the heart and neurons.[15] These VGCC require only small depolarizations (at negative membrane potentials) to open and are rapidly inactivated in a voltage-dependent fashion. They are essentially resistant to DHP antagonists and can be blocked by Ni^{2+} and octanol. Interestingly, these VGCC are not found in adrenal chromaffin cells or sympathetic neurons.

N-type VGCC, like L-type VGCC, are activated by large depolarizations. However, they differ from L-type channels in that they are insensitive to DHP and are inhibited by ω-conotoxin. The unitary conductance of the N-type VGCC is much smaller than that of the L-type (1–20 pS vs 22–28 pS).[15,16] N-type VGCC are only found in neurons, with an exception being adrenal glomerulosa cells. Based on this distribution and the fact that ω-conotoxin blocks neurotransmitter release, N-type VGCC are thought to play a role in transmitter release.

P-type VGCC are also activated by large changes in membrane potentials but are not inhibited by DHP or ω-conotoxin.[17] Activity is inhibited by a low molecular weight toxin isolated from the funnel web spider. Like the N-type VGCC, P-type channels have been found to be involved in neurotransmitter release in brain and peripheral synapses.

Receptor-operated channels (ROC) open in direct response to ligand binding at the cell surface and allow the influx of Ca into cells in the absence of any intermediate messengers. These channels are often involved in rapid responses (i.e., synaptic transmission) and can be subclassified into two types based on their dependence on membrane potential. One type of ROC is the N-methyl-D-aspartate receptor (NMDAR), which opens in response to glutamate and whose activity is enhanced by depolarization.[18] This ROC is thought to be involved long-term potentiation.[19] The other type of ROC is not influenced by depolarization and is opened in response to extracellular ATP (ATPR).[20] Such ROC have been found in arterial smooth muscle cells.

Second messenger-operated Ca channels (SMOC) differ from ROC in that a second messenger, induced by ligand binding at the cell surface, regulates the opening of the channel.[21] These channels have been mostly studied in blood cells (neutrophils, platelets, T-lymphocytes, and mast cells). In some instances the second messenger has been identified (i.e. IP_3 in lymphocytes), but in other cases it is not known. It is also interesting that these SMOC demonstrate a voltage dependence opposite to that of the VGCC; SMOC Ca entry is enhanced by hyperpolarization and, as such, are strongly influenced by K^+ and Cl^- channels.[22]

Mechanically operated Ca channels (MOC) are activated by stretch and may serve a mechanosensor function.[23] These channels have been identified in endothelial cells, where they may be important in the regulation of vascular tone as well as in both skeletal and smooth muscle.

Tonically active Ca channels allow Ca to leak into cells.[24] Such activity has been found in smooth, cardiac, and skeletal muscle sarcolemma, and in conjunction with Ca efflux mechanisms of cells, it may help establish and regulate resting levels of Ca_i^{2+}.

Gap junctions provide a conduit for the movement of Ca from one cell to another.[25] The junctions are made up of subunits known as connexons and allow the passage of solutes between cells of less than 1500 molecular weight. The existence of such intercellular channels may facilitate information flow from one cell to another, leading to the coordination of activity of a group of cells or of tissue initiated as a localized response.

B. SARCOPLASMIC/ENDOPLASMIC RETICULUM

The major function of the sarcoplasmic/endoplasmic reticulum (SR/ER) membrane system is to provide a site for Ca storage that can be released rapidly and in a spatially controlled manner. Thus, these membrane systems require the ability to both sequester and release Ca. The Ca stored in these organelles is used for the most part to acutely alter Ca_i^{2+}.

Ca accumulation in the SR/ER utilizes a Ca^{2+}-ATPase active in high Mg^{2+} deriving energy from ATP hydrolysis.[26] This Ca^{2+}-ATPase has a molecular weight of 115 kDa and, is a high affinity (K_M <0.5 μM) P-type ATPase that transports two Ca ions into the SR/ER for every ATP hydrolyzed. Once in the lumen of the SR/ER, the Ca can bind to calsequestrin. This Ca^{2+}-ATPase is present in high amounts and thus can move large quantities of Ca (70 nmol/mg/sec in the SR). The activity of this ATPase can be modulated by acidic phospholipids and phospholamban, a protein phosphorylated by cAMP and calmodulin-dependent protein kinases.

Ca release from the SR/ER is thought to occur mainly through two distinct mechanisms involving different receptors. These two Ca-release proteins have been named the ryanodine receptor (based on the inhibition of Ca release from the SR/ER by the plant alkaloid ryanodine)[27] and the IP_3 receptor,[28] which binds IP_3, causing Ca release. It should be stated that whereas the ryanodine receptor has been localized to the interface between the SR and T tubules, the exact location of IP_3 receptors is still under debate.

The ryanodine receptor is a tetramer with a molecular weight of 1800 kDa in its functional state. It is responsible for Ca-induced Ca release (CICR) where sudden increases in Ca_i^{2+} can trigger further release of Ca.[29] A transient change in Ca_i^{2+} concentration appears required for activity, as prolonged increases in Ca_i^{2+} seem to inhibit CICR. CICR is operant in heart, smooth muscle, neurons, and adrenal chromaffin cells; the mechanism of activation is thought to be depolarization leading to the initial Ca release. Some data indicate that the ryanodine receptor shares characteristics with the nicotinic acetylcholine receptor, ligand-gated channels, and the *Shaker* K^+ channels.[2] The activity of purified ryanodine receptor can be inhibited by ruthenium red and procaine and stimulated by caffeine, Ca, and adenine nucleotides. Many researchers equate an effect of caffeine on Ca_i^{2+} with CICR; however, caffeine has other effects on cells; therefore, invoking CICR based on caffeine activity seems premature.

The IP_3 receptor releases Ca from internal nonmitochondrial stores in response to increases in IP_3 concentration. IP_3 is formed following ligand activated phospholipase C_γ (PLC_γ)-stimulated breakdown of phosphatidyl inositol-4,5-bisphosphate (PIP_2). Recent data also indicate a role for the G protein G_q in IP_3-mediated Ca release.[30] The actual localization of the IP_3 receptor is still a matter of debate. Data has been garnered to suggest that the IP_3 receptor is localized in the ER or an organelle termed the calciosome.[31] Whether the calciosome is a distinct organelle or just a specialized portion of the ER is yet to be determined. The IP_3 receptor is a tetramer of 260 kDa subunits and is negatively regulated by Ca_i^{2+} via the accessory Ca-binding protein calmedin[32] and by cAMP-dependent phosphorylation of the IP_3 receptor. Binding of IP_3 to its receptor can also be inhibited by heparin.

Whereas the ryanodine and IP_3 receptor are structurally and functionally distinct, interaction between the pools of Ca regulated by these receptors has been hypothesized to underlie the temporal and spatial alteration in Ca_i^{2+} seen in cells in response to ligand stimulation. The first model to explain Ca_i^{2+} changes elicited in cells in response to ligand suggests that an initial pulse of Ca_i^{2+} is released from an IP_3-sensitive store and that propagation of the Ca signal occurs through CICR.[33] In effect, changes in Ca_i^{2+} in this model would occur via diffusion of Ca across the cytoplasm releasing new stores of Ca as it diffuses. Whether the IP_3-sensitive and CICR pools of Ca are distinct or one in the same is not clear. The second model suggests that instead of Ca_i^{2+}, IP_3 acts as the diffusible messenger.[34] Ca, initially released from an IP_3-sensitive store, locally activates PLC, which is activated by Ca_i^{2+} and G_q. PLC_β produces more IP_3, which then diffuses across the cell releasing more Ca from IP_3-sensitive stores. Which of these models is correct (or at least the most feasible)? According to measurements of the velocity of the Ca spread and the diffusion of radiolabeled IP_3 and Ca in cells, IP_3 was found to diffuse at a rate nearly equivalent to the Ca spread, whereas the diffusion of Ca was approximately tenfold slower. In addition, the time required for the initiation of the Ca wave was consistent with the need to generate a second messenger (i.e., IP_3), and much slower than the time required for direct activation of a Ca channel. Thus, at present, the model where IP_3 serves as the diffusible messenger appears the more likely; however, both types of amplification may exist in cells where IP_3 could regulate long-distance Ca_i^{2+} changes, which could be locally amplified via CICR.

C. MITOCHONDRIA

The outer mitochondrial membrane is freely permeable to Ca and thus does not regulate mitochondrial Ca. Ca is transported into and out of the mitochondria across the inner mitochondrial membrane. An electrophoretic uniporter moves Ca into the matrix.[35] The uniporter is ruthenium red sensitive, inhibited by low levels of Ca_i^{2+} and high Mg_i^{2+}, has a K_M of 1–10 μM and transports 10 nmols/mg/sec. Efflux of Ca occurs via an electroneutral carrier protein that exchanges Ca^{2+} for 2 H^+ in nonexcitable cells and Ca^{2+} for 2 Na^+ in excitable tissue. Intramitochondrial pyridine nucleotides and membrane protein thiols may also modulate Ca fluxes.[36] In normal cells, resting mitochondrial Ca is relatively low, and thus mitochondria are not thought to serve as a storage site for Ca.[37] However, in certain disease states, mitochondria can accumulate a large amount of Ca and serve to buffer this ion at high capacity.

D. NUCLEAR MEMBRANE

Whether the nuclear membrane has specific Ca transporting proteins or channels is a topic of current investigation and debate. For many years, it was assumed that because of large nuclear pores, the nucleus was freely permeable to ions. However, the recent description of alterations in nuclear free Ca (Ca_n^{2+}) levels which are distinct from those of Ca_i^{2+} (in the same cell),[38] coupled with the ability of isolated nuclei to accumulate Ca in an ATP-dependent fashion[39] and release Ca after exposure to IP_3,[40] has suggested that the nucleus may not be freely permeable to Ca. Many characteristics of the purported nuclear membrane Ca^{2+}-ATPase are identical to those of the ER Ca^{2+}-ATPase, including inhibition by lanthanum and thapsigargin, and almost identical proteolytic cleavage patterns.[41] This ATPase can be modulated by calmodulin. A key question in these studies is whether purified nuclear membranes are contaminated by ER membranes. IP_3-mediated release of Ca followed by resequestration into a nuclear non-IP_3-sensitive compartment has also been demonstrated in isolated nuclei. These results tantalizingly suggest that the level of Ca in the nucleus may be as tightly controlled as that in the cytoplasm, and that nuclear specific changes in Ca may be one mechanism by which cell surface activation can be transduced into nuclear action.

TABLE 3
Calcium-Binding Proteins

Calcium-Binding Protein	Function
Annexins	Calcium channels
Calcineurin	Phosphatase
Calmodulin	Calcium-binding — alter enzyme activity
Calsequestrin	Calcium-binding — sequestration
Parvalbumin	Calcium-binding
Recoverin	Calcium sensor — inhibits phosphorylation of rhodopsin
Troponin C	Muscle contraction
Visinin	Calcium-binding in retinal cones

IV. CALCIUM-BINDING PROTEINS

Increases in Ca_i^{2+} are transduced into biological activity by binding to intracellular receptors (Table 3). Binding of Ca results in a conformational change in the protein that can either activate or inhibit other enzymatic activities or serve to buffer Ca. For example, Ca binding to troponin C induces a conformational change in the protein leading to muscle contraction. Ca calmodulin complexes in smooth muscle activate myosin light-chain kinase (MLCK) leading to contraction via phosphorylation of myosin light chain.

A large body of work exists describing molecular changes that occur in the Ca-binding proteins when they bind Ca and/or their substrates. Most of these proteins share a common structure, with the Ca-binding domain being a 29-residue helix-loop-helix EF hand structure.[42] Prototypical of this class of proteins is parvalbumin. This protein has repeated domains of 2 alpha helices oriented perpendicular to each other when Ca is bound. Whereas the Ca-binding domain of the different proteins is highly conserved, there is a wide range of affinities of these proteins for Ca. For example, the K_ds for parvalbumin is 10^{-9}, *M* whereas that of calmodulin is 10^{-5} *M*. The ability of parvalbumin to bind Ca is rather limited because the concentration of this protein is low in most cells. Calmodulin buffers to ~8 μ*M*, whereas troponin buffers between 6 and 80 μ*M* depending on the cell type. Calmodulin binds four molecules of Ca, is highly selective for Ca over Mg^{2+}, and makes up 1% of the total cell protein. It thus represents a significant Ca-binding protein in cells. Myosin, another Ca-binding protein, binds two Ca molecules/myosin molecule.

Ca-binding proteins also exist that lack an EF hand structure. These are the annexins,[43] the vision related proteins recoverin,[44] visinin,[45] and frequenin, as well as calcineurin.[46] Annexins were originally isolated as phospholipid- and Ca-binding proteins; they have since been shown to act like Ca channels. It is still unclear, however, how active these proteins are in terms of their Ca-binding or channel activities. Recoverin and its relatives are thought to be involved in sensing Ca_i^{2+} in rod outer segments and activating guanylate cyclase, which leads to the synthesis of cGMP and opens cationic channels in the rod outer segment membrane. This allows Ca to increase to 400 n*M*, which places the rods in their dark state. Recoverin is myristoleoylated, as is calcineurin, a phosphatase. Interestingly, recoverin and related proteins are activated by a decrease in Ca rather than an increase as seen in the other Ca-binding proteins.

V. MEASUREMENT OF CELLULAR CALCIUM

A variety of techniques have been developed to measure Ca_i^{2+} or Ca transport across biological membranes. These fall under the categories of electrical, radioactive, or microscopic techniques. To study Ca currents in cells and membranes, patch-clamp techniques can be employed.[2] In a patch clamp, a small patch of membrane is tightly attached to the end of a pipette so that current injected into the micropipette can only pass through the micropipette by passing through channels in the membrane covering its tip. This approach can be applied to the study of whole-cell Ca currents or single-channel Ca currents. Another technique for looking at Ca influx and efflux at the external surface of the plasma membrane of intact cells or organisms is that using a Ca-specific vibrating probe.[47] The probe electrode is placed next to the cell membrane and vibrates in one or two dimensions via piezo-electric elements at a certain frequency. This approach measures electrical or net charge currents generated by cells or organisms; because ions diffuse through the medium according to Fick's law, it is possible to map and measure patterns of specific ion flow across a system's surface by measuring the ion's orientation gradients near the surface. Radioactive measurements of Ca influx, efflux, and sequestration usually utilize $^{45}Ca^{2+}$ coupled with kinetic analysis and subcellular fractionation. This approach is rather complicated because very sophisticated mathematical models that require a fair number of assumptions need to be applied to the analysis of the data.

Microscopic techniques to measure Ca have been developed at both the electron and light microscopy level. Electron probe X-ray microanalysis[48] and ion imaging[49] are two electron microscopic techniques for measuring Ca content in cells and tissues. The principle behind x-ray microanalysis is that each ion in biological material, when bombarded with electrons, gives off specific energies that can be quantitated. Unfortunately, this technique requires that the material being studied must be frozen and can only measure total ion content. Thus it is not possible to measure dynamic events or free versus bound Ca using this approach. Ion microscopy can also be used to measure Ca and other ions in cells or tissue. Here, visual images of isotopic gradients in relation to cell morphology (with a spatial resolution of ~0.5 μm) can be generated. The technique, based on secondary ion mass spectrometry (SIMS), can distinguish between isotopes on the basis of their mass-to-charge ratio. For Ca, $^{40}Ca^{2+}$ and $^{44}Ca^{2+}$ are employed. As with electron probe x-ray microanalysis, the actual samples have to be cryogenically prepared, and thus dynamic or serial/temporal measurements in the same cell or tissue cannot be made.

At the light microscopic level, the availability of fluorescent probes sensitive to Ca has greatly enhanced our understanding of Ca metabolism in cells and tissues.[50] Some of the current Ca-sensitive probes include Fura-2, Fura-Red, Aequorin, Indo-1, Fluo-3, Ca Green, Crimson Orange, and Quin-2. Ca_i^{2+} can be quantitated using these probes by photometric or imaging approaches. The advantage of these probes is that they can be loaded into the cytoplasm (or other organelles) of living cells to provide a mechanism to study the quantitative 2- or 3-dimensional distribution of Ca during cell functioning.

VI. ROLE OF CALCIUM IN BIOLOGICAL EVENTS

To illustrate the importance of Ca_i^{2+} in biological events, three examples are described. Contraction of voluntary (skeletal) muscle is triggered by a signal from a nerve, which causes depolarization of the sarcolemma. Depolarization flows from the sarcolemma to the T-tubules that release stored Ca. The depolarization continues until it reaches the SR where more Ca is released; the Ca released from the T-tubules and the SR then bind to troponin C (4 Ca molecules/troponin molecule). The binding of Ca to troponin C releases the inhibition of actin binding to myosin by moving tropomyosin into the groove of the F-actin filament. The reaction is terminated by resequestration of Ca into the SR by a Ca^{2+}-ATPase.

In contrast to skeletal muscle, in smooth muscle cells, agonist binding to a receptor or depolarization of the plasma membrane causes an increase in Ca_i^{2+} by the influx of extracellular Ca as well as the release of Ca from IP_3-sensitive stores (calciosome). This Ca then complexes with calmodulin and activates MLCK. The activated MLCK phosphorylates myosin on serine 19 on each of the two 20,000 kDa myosin light chains, allowing them to interact with actin. Myosin light chain phosphatase dephosphorylates the myosin light chains, and Ca is both pumped out of the cell and resequestered into the calciosome.

Addition of growth factors to many cells results in a rapid, transient increase in Ca_i^{2+}. These increases can be either monophasic or oscillatory in nature. The mechanisms underlying the regulation of growth factor-induced alterations in Ca_i^{2+} encompass many of the mechanisms previously described in this chapter (e.g., ROC, VGCC, IP_3-sensitive stores, Ca^{2+}-Mg^{2+}-ATPase, etc.). Growth factor binding can also activate protein kinase C, which can stimulate Ca influx into cells. The fact that growth factor-induced changes in Ca_i^{2+} are important in mediating the activity of growth factors is demonstrated by the findings that inhibition of increases in Ca_i^{2+} caused by growth factor binding is necessary at various times for movement of cells from G_0 into G_1 and S phase. The recent introduction of "caged" physiological mediators, which can be loaded into single cells and released by photolysis using ultraviolet light, will provide the ability to further study the role of Ca, not only in growth factor action, but in other biological events as well.

VII. SUMMARY

Ca is an ubiquitous messenger involved in many cellular activities. Tight control of the concentration of Ca_i^{2+} is exerted to serve its role as a messenger but prevent unwanted detrimental effects in cells. The regulation of cellular Ca metabolism is under active study in the hope that new information will provide therapeutic targets for diseases where Ca metabolism has gone awry. Similarly, the search for cellular targets of Ca (i.e., Ca^{2+}-dependent genes, kinases, and biological activities) continues unabated. As Ca plays such a central role in cellular activity and homeostasis, the generation of new information regarding Ca function in cells will have fundamental importance in terms of our understanding of the biology of cells and tissues.

REFERENCES

1. **Cheung, J. Y., Bonventre, J. V., Malis, C. D. and Leaf, A.,** Calcium and ischemic injury, *N. Engl. J. Med.*, 314, 1670, 1983.
2. **Tsien, R. Y.,** Calcium channels, stores, and oscillations, *Annu. Rev. Cell Biol.*, 6, 715, 1990.
3. **Herman, B., Gores, G. J., Nieminen, A.-L., Kawanishi, T., Harman, A. and Lemasters, J. J.,** Calcium and pH in anoxic and toxic injury, *Crit. Rev. Toxicol.*, 21, 127, 1990.
4. **Grollman, E. F.,** Calcium signals in the liver, in *The Liver, Biology and Pathobiology*, Arais, I. A., Jacoby, W. B., and Popper, H., eds., Raven Press, New York, 1988.
5. **Carafoli, E.,** The Ca^{2+} pump of the plasma membrane, *J. Biol. Chem.*, 267, 2115, 1992.
6. **Blaustein, M. P.,** Effects of internal and external cations and of ATP on sodium-calcium and calcium-calcium exchange in squid axons, *Biophys. J.*, 20, 79, 1977.
7. **Tsien, R. W., Hess, P., McCleskey, E. W. and Rosenberg, R. L.,** Calcium channels: mechanisms of selectivity, permeation and block, *Annu. Rev. Biophys. Chem.*, 16, 265, 1987.
8. **Rane, S. G., Holz, G. G. and Dunlap, K.,** Dihydropyridine inhibition of neuronal calcium currents and substance P release, *Pflügers Arch.*, 409, 361, 1987.
9. **Tanabe, T., Mikami, A., Numa, S. and Beam, K. G.,** Cardiac-type excitation-contraction coupling in dysgenic skeletal muscle injected with cardiac dihydropyridine receptor cDNA, *Nature*, 344, 451, 1990.
10. **Tanabe, T., Beam, K. G., Powell, J. A. and Numa, S.,** Restoration of excitation-contraction coupling and slow calcium current in dysgenic muscle by dihydropyridine receptor complementary DNA, *Nature*, 336, 134, 1988.
11. **Takahashi, M. and Catterall, W. A.,** Identification of an alpha subunit of dihydropyridine-sensitive brain calcium channels, *Science*, 136, 88, 1987.
12. **Mikami, A., Imoto, K., Tanabe, T., Niidome, T., Mori, Y., Takeshima, H., Narumiya, S. and Numa, S.,** Primary structure and functional expression of the cardiac dihydropyridine-sensitive calcium channel, *Nature*, 340, 230, 1989.
13. **Ruth, P., Rohrkasten, A., Biel, M., Bosse, E., Regulla, S., Meyer, H. E., Flockerzi, V. and Hofmann, F.,** Primary structure of the β subunit of the DHP-sensitive calcium channel from skeletal muscle, *Science*, 245, 1115, 1989.
14. **Jay, S. D., Ellis, S. B., McCue, A. F., Williams, M. E., Vedvick, T. S., Harpold, M. M. and Campbell, K. P.,** Primary structure of the g-subunit of the DHP-sensitive calcium channel from skeletal muscle, *Science*, 248, 490, 1990.

15. **Tsien, R. W., Lipscombe, D., Madison, D. V., Bley, K. R. and Fox, A. P.,** Multiple types of neuronal calcium channels and their selective modulation, *Trends Neurosci.*, 11, 431, 1988.
16. **Hess, P.,** Calcium channels in vertebrate cells, *Annu. Rev. Neurosci.*, 13, 1337, 1990.
17. **Llinas, R., Sugimori, M., Lin, J. W. and Cherksey, B.,** Blocking and isolation of a calcium channel from neurons in mammals and cephalopods utilizing a toxin fraction (FTX) from funnel-web spider poison, *Proc. Natl. Acad. Sci. USA*, 86, 1689, 1989.
18. **Mayer, M. L. and Westbrook, G. L.,** The physiology of exitatory amino acids in the vertebrate central nervous system., *Prog. Neurobiol.* 28, 197, 1987.
19. **Collingridge, G. L. and Bliss, T. V. P.,** NMDA receptors — their role in long-term potentiation, *Trends Neurosci.*, 10, 298, 1987.
20. **Benham, C. D. and Tsien, R. W.,** A novel receptor-operated Ca^{2+}-permeable channel activated by ATP in smooth muscle, *Nature*, 328, 275, 1987.
21. **Meldolesi, J. and Pozzan, T.,** Pathways of Ca^{2+} influx at the plasma membrane: voltage-, receptor-, and second messenger-operated channels, *Exp. Cell Res.*, 171, 271, 1987.
22. **Penner, R., Matthews, G. and Neher, E.,** Regulation of calcium influx by second messengers in rat mast cells, *Nature*, 334, 499, 1988.
23. **Lansman, J. B., Hallam, T. J. and Rink, T. J.,** Single stretch-activated ion channels in vascular endothelial cells as mechanotransductors? *Nature*, 325, 8, 1987.
24. **Benham, C. D. and Tsien, R W.,** Calcium-permeable channels in vascular smooth muscle: voltage-gated, ligand-gated and receptor-operated channels, *Soc. Gen. Physiol. Symp.*, 42, 45, 1987.
25. **Cornell-Bell, A. H., Finkbeiner, S. M., Cooper, M. S. and Smith, S. J.,** Glutamate induces calcium waves in cultured astrocytes: long range glial signaling, *Science*, 247, 470, 1990.
26. **Pedersen, P. L. and Carafoli, E.,** Ion motive ATPases. I. Ubiquity, properties and significance to cell function, *TIBS*, 12, 146, 1987.
27. **Fleisher, S. and Inui, M.,** Biochemistry and biophysics of excitation-contraction coupling, *Annu. Rev. Biophys. Biophys. Chem.*, 18, 333, 1989.
28. **Berridge, M. J. and Irvine, R. F.,** Inositol phosphates and cell signalling, *Nature*, 341, 197, 1989.
29. **Fabiato, A.,** Calcium-induced release of calcium from the cardiac sarcoplasmic reticulum, *Am. J. Physiol.*, 245, C1, 1983.
30. **Smrcka, A. V., Hepler, J. R., Brown, K. O. and Sternweis, P. C.,** Regulation of polyphosphoinositide-specific phospholipase C activity by purified G_q, *Science*, 251, 804, 1991.
31. **Volpe, P., Krause, K.-H., Hashimoto, S., Zorzato, F., Pozzan, T., Meldolesi, J. and Lew, D. P.,** "Calciosome," a cytoplasmic organelle: the inositol 1,4,5-trisphosphate-sensitive Ca^{2+} store of nonmuscle cells? *Proc. Natl. Acad. Sci. USA*, 85, 1091, 1988.
32. **Danoff, S. K., Supattapone, S. and Snyder, S. H.,** Characterization of a membrane protein from brain mediating the inhibition of inositol 1,4,5-trisphosphate receptor binding by calcium, *Biochem. J.*, 254, 701, 1988.
33. **Berridge, M. J.,** Calcium oscillations, *J. Biol. Chem.*, 265, 9583, 1990.
34. **Meyer, T. and Stryer, L.,** Calcium spiking, *Annu. Rev. Biophys. Chem.*, 20, 153, 1991.
35. **Famulski, K. and Carafoli, E.,** Calcium transporting activity of membrane fractions isolated from the post-mitochondrial supernatant of rat liver, *Cell Calcium*, 3, 263, 1982.
36. **Akerman, K. E. O. and Nicholls, D. G.,** Physiological and bioenergetic aspects of mitochondrial calcium transport, *Rev. Physiol. Biochem. Pharmacol.*, 95, 149, 1983.
37. **Nieman, A.-L., Gores, G. J., Dawson, T. L., Herman, B. and Lemasters, J. J.,** Toxic injury from mercuric chloride in rat hepatocytes, *J. Biol. Chem.*, 265, 2399, 1990.
38. **Diliberto, P. A., Periasamy, A. and Herman, B.,** District Oscillations in Cytosolic and Nuclear Free Calcium in Single Intact Living Cells Demonstrated by Confocal Microscopy, in *Proc. Forty Ninth Annual Meeting Electron Microscopy Society of America*, 228, 1991.
39. **Nicotera, P., McConkey, D. J., Jones, D. P. and Orrenius, S.,** ATP stimulates Ca^{2+} uptake and increases the free Ca^{2+} concentration in isolated rat liver nuclei, *Proc. Natl. Acad. Sci. USA*, 86, 453, 1989.
40. **Nicotera, P., Orrenius, S., Nilsson, T. and Berggren, P.-O.,** An inositol 1,4,5-trisphosphate-sensitive Ca^{2+} pool in liver nuclei, *Proc. Natl. Acad. Sci. USA*, 87, 6858, 1990.
41. **Carafoli, E.,** The Ca^{2+} pump of the plasma membrane, *J. Biol. Chem.*, 267, 2115, 1992.
42. **Strynadka, N. C. J. and James, M. N. G.,** Crystal structures of the helix-loop-helix calcium-binding proteins, *Annu. Rev. Biochem.*, 58, 951, 1989.
43. **Huber, R., Berendes, R., and Burger, A., Schneider, M., Karshikov, A., Luecke, H., Roemisch, H. and Papues, E.,** Crystal and molecular structure of human annexin V after refinement. Implications for structure, membrane binding and ion channel formation of the annexin family of proteins, *J. Mol. Biol.*, 223, 683, 1992.
44. **Dizhoor, A. M., Ray, S., Kumar, S., Niemi, G., Spencer, M., Brolley, D., Walsh, K. A., Philipov, P. P., Hurley, J. B. and Stryer, L.,** Recoverin: a calcium sensitive activator of retinal rod guanylate cyclase, *Science*, 251, 915, 1991.
45. **Yamagata, K., Goto, K., Kuo, C.H., Kondo, H. and Miki, N.,** Visinin: a novel calcium-binding protein expressed in retinal cone cells, *Neuron*, 4, 469, 1990.

46. **Liu, J., Farmer, J. D., Jr., Lane, W. S., Friedman, J., Weissman, I. and Schreiber, S. L.,** Calcineurin is a common target of cyclophillin cyclosporin A and FKBP-FK506 complexes, *Cell,* 66, 807, 1991.
47. **Kühtreiber, W. M. and Jaffe, L. F.,** Detection of extracellular calcium gradients with a calcium-specific vibrating electrode, *J. Cell Biol.,* 110, 1565, 1990.
48. **Lefurgey, A., Ingram, P. and Mendel, L. J.,** Heterogeneity of calcium compartmentalization: electron probe analysis of renal tubules, *J. Membr. Biol.*, 94, 191, 1986.
49. **Chandra, S., Ausserer, W. A. and Morrison, G. H.,** Subcellular imaging of calcium exchange in cultured cells with ion microscopy, *J. Cell Sci.*, 102, 417, 1992.
50. **Tsien, R. Y.,** Fluorescent indicators of ion concentrations, *Methods Cell Biol.*, 30, 127, 1989.
51. **Wasserman, R. H.**, Cellular calcium: action of hormones, in *Calcium in Human Biology*, Nordin, B. E. C., ed., Springer-Verlag, London, 1988.

Section II.

HARD TISSUES: STRUCTURES AND FUNCTIONS

Although the term "hard tissues" includes both bones and teeth, the emphasis on the skeletal tissues, especially in Sections IV and V of this text, makes understanding the material presented in the chapter (Chapter 7) on skeletal tissues and mineralization essential prior to continuing on to other chapters. The mineralized phase of bone tissue is highlighted with illustrative examples of the structures of bone tissue and bone cells, and of the current methods used for the measurement of bone mass. The role of cytokines in regulating bone turnover is also covered. Dental tissues are reviewed in Chapter 8, which probes especially into the function of the tooth-forming cells. The chapter on collagen (Chapter 9) provides a chemical view of type I collagen as it underlies the structural organization of hard tissues. Detailed illustrations display current understandings of the complexity of this triple-helical protein. Changes in collagen that result from the diseases, osteogenesis imperfecta and osteoporosis, are also reviewed. Finally, Chapter 10 provides an overview of the biomarkers that are measured to assess the state of bone metabolism. These biochemical markers have been receiving increasing attention because of their use in interpreting the extent of bone turnover, either resorption or formation, under various conditions of health and disease.

The knowledge provided in this section on the components of hard tissue, both mineral and organic matrix, serves as the basis for understanding the actions of the calcium-regulating hormones on bone tissue, which are overviewed in section III. In addition, bone cytokines are introduced, and biochemical markers released during either bone formation or resorption are detailed. Both types of molecules will be covered further in later chapters of the book.

Chapter 7

SKELETAL TISSUES AND MINERALIZATION

Sanford C. Garner, Ph.D., John J. B. Anderson, Ph.D., and Wallace W. Ambrose, M.S.

TABLE OF CONTENTS

0-8493-7845-1/95/$0.00+$.50

I. INTRODUCTION

The skeleton performs a number of essential functions for the maintenance of life in vertebrates, some of which involve the obvious rigid structure provided by bone, and others that result from the dynamic organization of bone at the microscopic level. Bone provides both mechanical support for the body, including attachment for locomotor muscles, and protection for portions of soft tissue, such as brain, spinal cord, heart, and lungs. In addition, all blood cell formation or hematopoiesis takes place in the bone marrow. A less obvious function of bone is that it serves as a metabolic reservoir for calcium and other minerals. A constant exchange of calcium (Ca), phosphate (inorganic phosphorus or Pi), and other mineral elements occurs between bone mineral surfaces and extracellular fluid in bone tissue. This constant ebb and flow of Ca and Pi is the result primarily of the active exchange of these minerals that occurs at the interface of bone mineral surfaces with the extracellular fluid and, secondarily, of the remodeling processes within bone that renew bone microstructure throughout life.

Bone can be described at several levels. Bone may be considered first as a structural material; a mixture of organic matrix and inorganic (mineral) materials. Bone may also be viewed at the level of a mechanical device, with a characteristic resistance to bending, to compression, and to fracture. At a gross physical (organ) level, long bones such as the leg or arm bones may be separated into anatomical regions of epiphysis, metaphysis, and diaphysis. The total bone structure also consists of an arrangement of trabecular and cortical bone. Bone microstructure, i.e., the mixture of trabecular and cortical bone in different bones or in different portions of the same bone, may be equally, if not more, important than the absolute amount of bone mineral in determining strength and resistance to fracture. The structural analysis of bone is beyond the scope of this chapter, but the reader is referred to references 1–5 for additional information.

Bone may also be discussed at a microscopic or histological (tissue) level, because it consists of osteoblasts and osteoclasts that create and destroy bone, respectively. Bone as a metabolic entity serves as a storage reservoir for minerals, especially Ca and phosphorus (P), but also for other trace minerals. As a dynamic part of the body's response to the changing availability of these minerals, bone mineral is essential for maintaining Ca and Pi concentrations in the extracellular fluid compartment within limits acceptable for numerous functions essential to the continued well-being of the individual (see Chapter 3). Bone also undergoes extensive changes during growth and maintenance of skeletal tissues throughout the life cycle (for more information see Chapter 17).

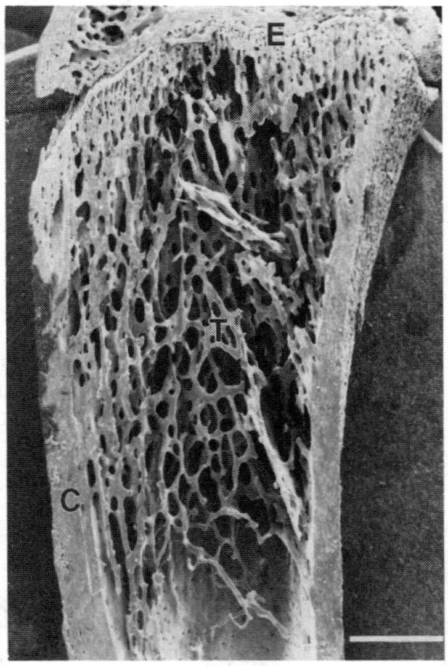

FIGURE 1. Compact and Cancellous Bone. The low-power (10×) scanning electron micrograph of a hemisectioned rat tibia illustrates the relationship between compact (C) and cancellous (trabecular) bone (T) in the long bones. The epiphyseal growth plate (E) is also evident. The bar indicates a 1 mm distance.

II. BONE AS AN ORGAN

Bone is considered a portion of the body's connective tissue, but together with teeth and cartilage, it shares the ability to add mineral to the underlying organic matrix of collagen and noncollagenous proteins, i.e., to become calcified. All bone consists of mineral (hydroxyapatite) deposited within an organic (collagen) matrix (see Chapter 9). The mineral alone is hard, rigid, and brittle and is effective mainly in resistance to compression. The collagen matrix, on the other hand, remains flexible and is mainly tension resistant, reducing fractures. In combination, the organic and inorganic components of bone produce a material that is one-third the weight but ten times as flexible and with approximately equal tensile strength as cast iron.[1]

A. STRUCTURE

Bone is organized into two types of structures that are intermixed within each bone. These structures are compact (cortical) bone, which forms the shafts of the long bones and the outer surface of almost all bones; and trabecular bone, also called cancellous or spongy bone, which fills the ends of the shafts of the long bones and forms most of the structure of the vertebrae (see Figure 1). Most of the volume occupied by compact bone consists of calcified matrix (80–90%), whereas only a small portion (15–25%) of trabecular bone volume is calcified.

B. GROSS ANATOMY

Anatomists separate bone into two types, the flat bones such as skull bones, scapula, mandible, and ilium and the long bones such as tibia, femur, and humerus. The long bones consist of 3 anatomic divisions, as illustrated in Figure 2. The inner surface of the bone is called the endosteum and the outer surface the periosteum. The shaft, or diaphysis, is a hollow cylinder of compact bone. The ends of the bone are known as the epiphyses and consist of a thin, cortical layer of compact bone surrounding a region of trabecular bone. The metaphysis is a tapering, transitional region between the epiphysis and the diaphysis containing both cortical and trabecular bone. The epiphysis and metaphysis are separated by a plate of hyaline cartilage called the epiphyseal growth plate (or physis). The growth plate is the site at which elongation of the long bones occurs by proliferation

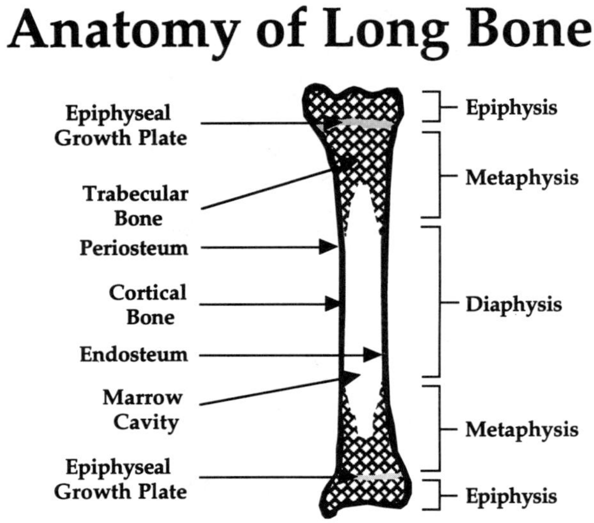

FIGURE 2. Anatomy of Long Bones. The long bones, i.e., the tibia, femur, humerus, and radius, are divided anatomically into three segments: the epiphyses, the metaphyses, and the diaphysis. The composition of cortical and trabecular bone varies as one moves from segment to segment.

of chondrocytes, cartilage-forming cells. Calcification of this cartilaginous area at puberty results in closure of the growth plate and cessation of longitudinal growth.[6,7,8]

III. BONE AS TISSUE

Bone tissue contains a number of different cell types that perform the functions necessary to build and maintain bone structure and carry out the homeostatic functions of bone. Thus, there are osteoblasts responsible for the formation of bone, cells derived from the osteoblasts that are present in mature bone, and osteoclasts capable of resorbing bone tissue during turnover of bone. In addition to the cellular components of bone tissue, the majority of bone tissue consists of hydroxyapatite crystals (see Section III.B.) deposited within a protein matrix that consists primarily of type I collagen. However, the other protein constituents of bone organic matrix are quite varied, and the role of many of these molecules remains to be discovered.

A. MICROSCOPIC ANATOMY (BONE CELLS)

Bone cells can be divided into two general types, bone-forming cells and bone-resorbing cells, which are derived from different osteoprogenitor cells. The bone-forming cells, or osteoblasts, are believed to give rise to related cell types with different functions in bone, e.g., the osteocyte and the resting osteoblast, or bone-lining cell. The osteoclast is the major cell responsible for bone resorption.

1. Bone-forming Cells (Osteoblasts)

The osteoblasts are derived from mesenchymal cells and are related to fibroblasts and the cells forming the walls of blood vessels (see Figure 3). Preosteoblasts are found in the tissue layers near bone-forming surfaces. They are elongated cells lacking the full ability of the mature osteoblasts to synthesize bone-matrix proteins, but they retain the ability to divide.

Osteoblasts are bone-forming cells that secrete collagen to form the osteoid or unmineralized bone matrix, and also regulate the processes that initiate mineralization. Osteoblasts are metabolically active cells and are characterized by an abundant rough endoplasmic reticulum and Golgi apparatus for synthesis and export of proteins (see Figure 4). These cells also express characteristic

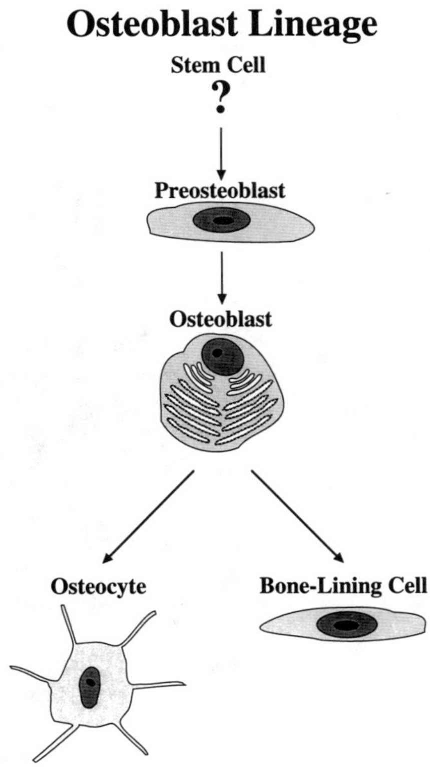

FIGURE 3. Osteoblast Lineage. The osteoblast is derived from the same stem-cell population that gives rise to mesenchymal cells, including fibroblasts; however the source of these stem cells has not been identified. Once the stem cell differentiates to the preosteoblast, the daughter cells of this line are committed to osteoblastic development. The fate of osteoblasts once bone has been formed is threefold: (1) They may undergo apoptosis, (2) remain on the surface of the bone as biosynthetically inactive bone-lining cells, or (3) completely enclose themselves in bone, forming an osteocyte.

membrane proteins, particularly the enzyme alkaline phosphatase (see Chapter 10), which has been proposed as a regulator of mineralization for many years, although its function remains undefined. Osteoblasts possess receptors for two of the major Ca- and bone-regulating hormones, parathyroid hormone (PTH) and 1,25-dihydroxyvitamin D (1,25$(OH)_2$D). It is generally accepted that the major effects of these hormones on maintenance of plasma Ca and on bone turnover are controlled via osteoblastic cells.

2. Osteoblast-Derived Cells of Mature Bone

Osteoblasts give rise to two cell types within bone that maintain some osteoblastic characteristics but no longer synthesize collagen for the formation of new bone.

a. Osteocytes

Osteocytes are bone cells that lie within small cavities, or lacunae, that are completely surrounded by bone (see Figure 4). They are osteoblasts that have surrounded themselves with matrix and remain connected with each other and with cells on the bone surface by thin processes that pass through thin tubular channels or canaliculi. The canaliculi provide a passageway for the diffusion of nutrients from extracellular fluid to these cells.

b. Bone-Lining Cells

Bone-lining cells are also called resting osteoblasts or surface osteocytes (see Figure 4). As the names imply, these cells are osteoblasts that are no longer actively forming bone but are not

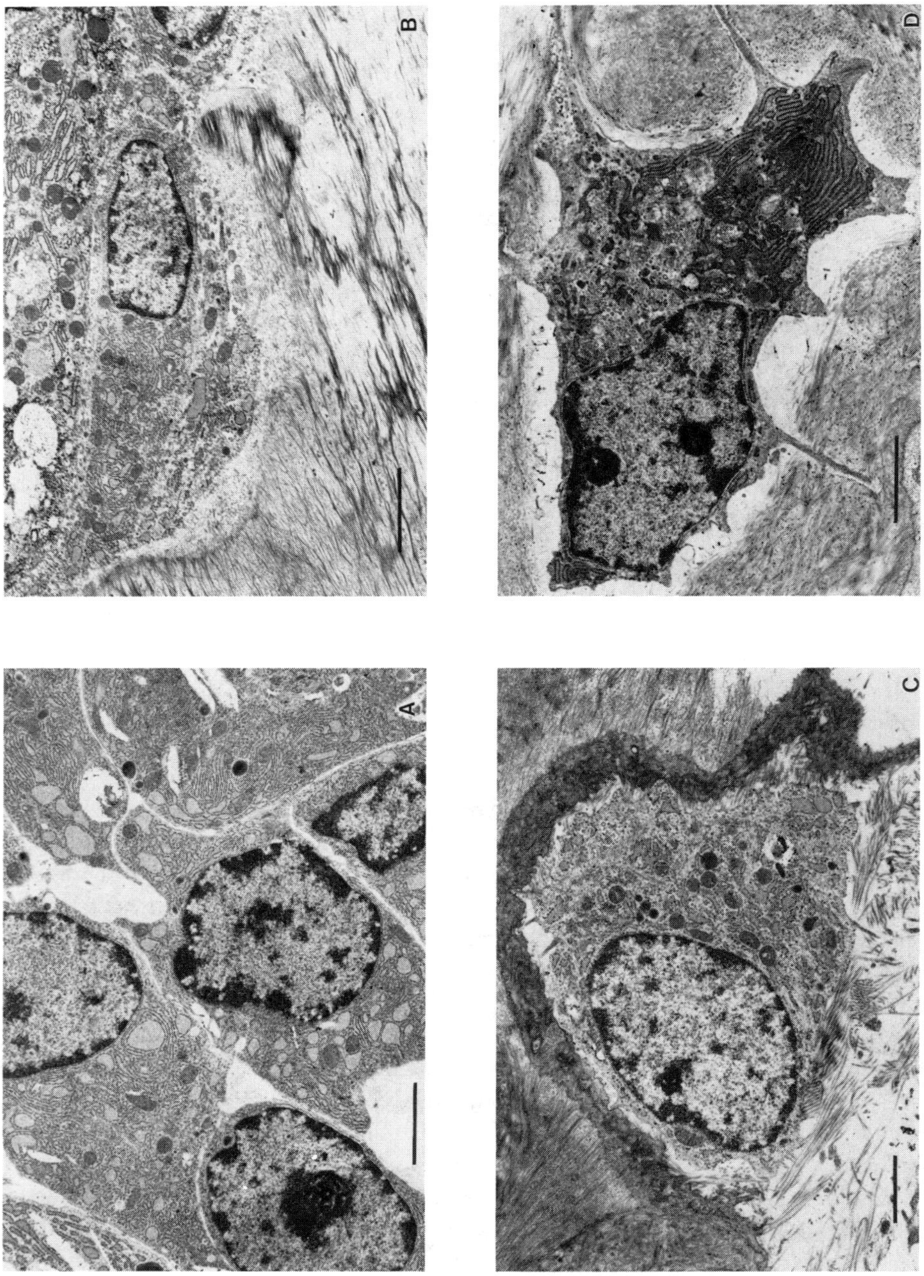

FIGURE 4. Bone Cells — Electron Micrographs. Cells of the osteoblast lineage are illustrated by the electron micrographs. (A) Osteoblastic cells. (B) Bone lining cells. (C) An osteoblast in an apparent transition phase to becoming an osteocyte. (D) An osteocyte completely surrounded by bone. The bar in each figure is equal to two microns (2 μm).

completely surrounded by bone. These lining cells are central to maintenance of blood Ca levels, perhaps by actively pumping Ca ions from the bone fluid compartment to the extracellular fluid compartment. Although it is likely that these cells represent another developmental stage of the osteoblast similar to the osteocyte, it has been suggested that these cells are formed directly from preosteoblasts, which they resemble histologically. It has been demonstrated that the bone-lining cells can be stimulated to differentiate into active osteoblasts.

3. Bone-Resorbing Cells (Osteoclasts)

Osteoclasts are multinucleated, giant cells that are capable of resorbing both bone mineral and matrix.[9] The osteoclasts are formed from cells of the monocyte-phagocyte lineage (see Figure 5). The cellular lineage of the osteoclast was defined in experiments with the disease osteopetrosis, a condition of dense bone growth without osteoclastic remodeling. Animal models with this disease either lack the mononuclear precursor cells or these cells fail to respond to the cytokines that signal cell proliferation and maturation. In either case, functional osteoclasts are not present in sufficient numbers to resorb substantial amounts of bone and, hence, bone turnover is significantly depressed in osteopetrosis.

The osteoclast resorbs bone in a region of attachment of the cell to the bone surface where the cell membrane is elaborately folded, resulting in the characteristic appearance of this area called the "ruffled border" (see Figure 6). Bone resorption involves the lowering of the pH in the region between the osteoclast and the bone surface through secretion of hydrogen ions (H^+), which are generated within the osteoclasts by carbonic anhydrase II (the same enzyme that is present in H^+-secreting cells of the stomach and kidney). The site of bone resorption is separated from the surrounding tissue by a ring of contractile proteins, the sealing zone or clear zone, which is formed by actin filaments anchored through integrins to the bone surface. Within this zone the bone surface is exposed to low pH and concentrated lysosomal enzyme activity, leading to the description of this region as a "secondary lysosome." However, as Blair et al.[9] have pointed out, the ability of the osteoclast to acidify the region of bone adjacent to the ruffled border vastly exceeds the transport of H^+ into cytoplasmic lysosomes.

B. CHEMICAL STRUCTURE

Although bone is organized into different structural components, at the molecular level all bone tissue shares a common composition. Bone consists of an inorganic or mineral phase composed primarily of hydroxyapatite crystals deposited within an organic phase of cross-linked collagen fibers. The mineral phase provides stiffness and resistance to compression, whereas the organic phase gives the bone strength and resistance to breaking. Together this composite structure has both rigidity and resistance to fractures. Hydroxyapatite has the chemical structure $Ca_{10}(PO_4)_6(OH)_2$ and makes up approximately 60–65% of bone by weight. Type I collagen fibers make up 90% of total bone proteins. When bone is first formed as part of a newly modeled bone or as part of the repair of a fracture, the collagen fibers are randomly oriented, and this bone is referred to as woven bone. However, as bone is remodeled during growth or as part of normal bone turnover, the collagen fibers are laid down in parallel arrays that are visible under polarized light as layers within the bone. Thus, this mature bone is referred to as lamellar bone.

C. COLLAGEN AND NONCOLLAGENOUS PROTEINS OF BONE MATRIX

As stated above, type I collagen makes up approximately 90% of bone matrix protein (see Chapter 9). The remaining 10% of total bone proteins consists of a mixture of proteins (Table 1) that are either synthesized by osteoblasts or are serum derived.[10] Whether the serum-derived proteins play a role in bone metabolism or whether they are simply trapped during the formation of bone matrix is not known. The remaining noncollagenous proteins of bone matrix are synthesized by

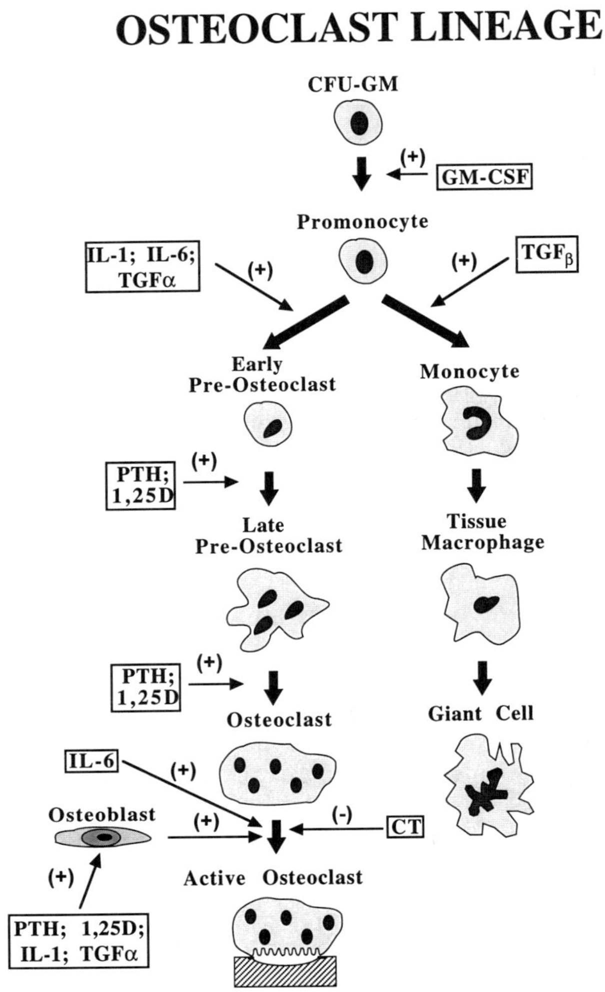

FIGURE 5. Osteoclast Lineage. Osteoclasts derive from a stem cell population (colony forming unit-granulocyte/macrophage or CFU-GM) that is capable of giving rise to osteoclasts or monocytes/macrophages. CFU-GM are stimulated by granulocyte-macrophage colony stimulating factor (GM-CSF) to differentiate into premonocytes. The premonocyte may commit to either the osteoclastic or monocytic pathway under the stimulus of local factors (cytokines), including interleukin-1 (IL-1), interleukin-6 (IL-6), and transforming growth factor-α (TGF_α) for the osteoclastic lineage, and transforming growth factor-β (TGF_β) for the monocytic lineage. Further development of the osteoclastic cell is stimulated by PTH and $1,25(OH)_2$-Vitamin D, which may act directly on the differentiating osteoclasts or may act through the osteoblast. Other cytokines, such as IL-1 and TGF_α, also stimulate resorptive activity through the osteoblast. The active osteoclast may also be regulated directly through stimulatory cytokines such as IL-6 and by inhibitory agents such as the circulating peptide, CT.[22-24]

osteoblasts and possibly other bone cells, and are likely to have functions as either structural or chemical signaling proteins. These proteins can be divided into the four general classes discussed next.

1. Cell-Attachment Proteins

Cell attachment is mediated by the family of proteins that constitute the integrins. Integrins are membrane-spanning proteins that recognize the amino acid sequence Arg-Gly-Asp (RGD) in extracellular proteins. Bone cells synthesize four proteins, fibronectin, thrombospondin, osteopontin, and bone sialoprotein [BSP], that are part of the extracellular matrix and serve as sites for cell attachment. Only BSP is confined primarily to bone, whereas the other proteins are found in many nonskeletal connective tissues.

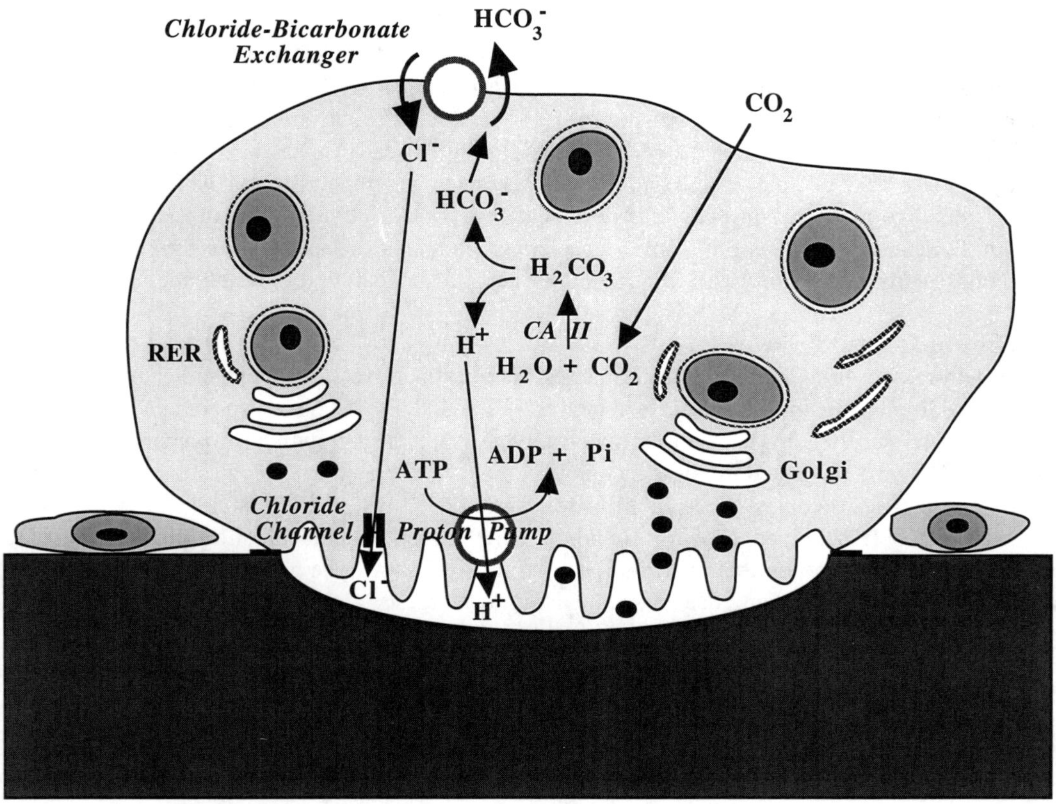

FIGURE 6. Osteoclast. The principal, and perhaps only, bone resorbing cell is the osteoclast. This multinucleated cell forms a "sealing zone" with the bone surface that allows a local area of bone to be exposed to low pH, which is produced by an active pumping of hydrogen ions into the resorption pit and a high concentration of proteolytic enzymes, which are released from lysosomes into the area of resorption.

TABLE 1
Noncollagenous Proteins of Bone Matrix

Noncollagen Protein of Bone Matrix	Possible Function
Thrombospondin	Cell attachment
Fibronectin	Cell attachment
Bone Sialoprotein (BSP)	Cell attachment
Osteopontin	Cell attachment
Proteoglycan I (Biglycan)	Unknown
Proteoglycan II (Decorin)	Unknown
Osteonectin	Calcium binding
Osteocalcin	Calcium binding
Matrix Gla-protein	Unknown
Insulin-like Growth Factor-1 (IGF-1)	Growth-related
Platelet-derived Growth Factor (PDGF)	Growth-related
Transforming Growth Factor-β (TGF-β)	Growth-related

2. Proteoglycans

Proteoglycans consist of a central core protein to which acidic polysaccharide side chains are attached. The side chains or glycosaminoglycans in bone are primarily chondroitin sulfate and heparin sulfate. The proteoglycans may facilitate osteoblast interaction with cell-attachment and other proteins, but their function remains unknown.

3. γ-Carboxylated (Gla) Proteins

The bone Gla-proteins contain γ-carboxylated glutamine residues that are the product of a vitamin K-dependent enzymatic process. The addition of the second carboxyl group to the side chain of the glutamine residue produces a binding site for Ca ions. Since Ca ions are essential cofactors in the function of γ-carboxylated proteins of the blood-clotting cascade, it has been suggested that the ability of these bone Gla-proteins to bind Ca may regulate bone mineralization. Osteocalcin (a bone Gla-protein) is found only in bone, where its synthesis by osteoblasts is regulated by $1,25(OH)_2$ vitamin D. The serum concentration of osteocalcin is often regarded as a marker for bone turnover. A second γ-carboxylated protein is matrix Gla-protein, which is found in both bone and cartilage.

4. Growth-Related Proteins

Growth-related proteins represent the largest number of different protein molecules found in bone. In addition to the insulin-like growth factors (IGF-1 and IGF-2), bone also contains $TGF_{\beta 1\text{-}5}$ and other proteins secreted by osteoblasts that stimulate osteoblast growth in a paracrine/autocrine manner.[11] One role suggested for these factors after they are liberated by osteoclastic action has been the recruitment of osteoblasts to areas of bone resorption.

Other osteoblast-derived proteins found in bone matrix include alkaline phosphatase and osteonectin, a glycoprotein that makes up approximately 2% of bone protein in developing bone. Alkaline phosphatase has long been associated with osteoblasts, and its synthesis and secretion by these cells is considered a marker of bone formation. The function of alkaline phosphatase in bone cell biology, however, must be considered unknown. Osteonectin is found in both proliferating bone and growing tissues, and its role in bone formation remains to be established.

IV. BONE FORMATION

All bone is formed by deposition of hydroxyapatite crystals within a collagen matrix. However, the process by which the collagen matrix is laid down differs according to the two major types of bone formation, intramembranous and endochondral (bone modeling on a cartilaginous structure).

A. INTRAMEMBRANOUS BONE FORMATION

The flat bones of the skull, the jaw, and the ribs are formed by intramembranous bone formation. In this process, mesenchymal cells differentiate directly into preosteoblasts and then into osteoblasts in areas of highly vascular embryonic connective tissue. The bone matrix synthesized by these cells is randomly oriented (or woven), and calcification is accomplished in irregular patches rather than in the orderly fashion seen in remodeling bone. Eventually this bone is remodeled to form lamellar bone.

B. ENDOCHONDRAL BONE FORMATION (BONE MODELING)

The long bones are formed *de novo* by calcification of a cartilaginous structure that serves as a model for the new bone. Cartilage is formed by chondroblasts, cells that are derived from prechondroblasts arising from the same mesenchymal cells that form osteoblasts. The chondrocytes secrete a collagen matrix, eventually enclosing themselves into lacunae. Because cartilage consists primarily of collagen fibers and is not rigid, chondrocytes can continue to enlarge and divide, expanding the lacunar spaces. Cartilage also expands at the periphery by appositional (circumferential) growth.

Cartilage is an avascular tissue, and the cells receive their nutrients by diffusion through the fluid surrounding the collagen fibers. Invasion of the cartilage by blood vessels initiates the process of mineralization of the organic matrix. As a result of the reduced diffusion of nutrients to the chondrocytes after mineralization, these cells begin to die. Not all chondrocytes are destroyed during initial calcification of the bone model, however. At each end of the bone, a layer of epiphyseal cartilage remains (see Figure 2), and this epiphyseal growth plate serves as the site of bone formation for elongation during growth. As chondrocytes proliferate, the oldest layers begin to calcify. This calcified cartilage is resorbed by osteoclasts, leaving calcified longitudinal septa. Osteoblasts form additional woven bone on these septa to form trabeculae of the primary spongiosa. As additional remodeling of these trabeculae takes place, lamellar bone replaces the woven bone, and secondary spongiosa is formed.

The epiphyseal cartilage calcifies after puberty as a result of increases at that time of estrogens in females and testosterone in males. Epiphyseal closure occurs at an earlier age in females resulting in earlier cessation of longitudinal growth. Delayed puberty, for almost any reason except undernutrition, results in elongation of the long bones and increased height in both females and males.

C. MINERALIZATION

Bone mineralization involves the formation of hydroxyapatite crystals within calcifying cartilage or newly laid down organic matrix (osteoid) in remodeling bone or new, woven bone. Two distinct mechanisms operate to deposit mineral in bone.[12-14] In lamellar bone formed during remodeling, mineral is deposited in association with the tightly spaced collagen fibrils and associated noncollagenous proteins. In the more open environment of randomly oriented collagen fibrils in cartilage and woven bone, mineralization is characterized by matrix vesicles that provide a site for hydroxyapatite crystal formation. These vesicles are formed by exocytosis from the plasma membrane of osteoblasts. Crystallization eventually produces a crystal larger than the original vesicle, and the vesicle is destroyed. Thus, the earliest bone formation either in endochondral bone formation, or in woven bone, proceeds by vesicle-driven mineralization. In the remodeling of mature bone, mineralization occurs directly within the collagen matrix without vesicle formation.

When bone matrix is first synthesized, it requires a period of time before mineralization can occur. It is not known whether this is due to the removal of inhibitors of crystal formation or to the formation of proteins that are necessary for the initiation of mineralization. Thus, sites of active bone formation are marked by a layer of unmineralized bone matrix, or osteoid, that is not yet calcified. The time required for calcification to begin, the osteoid maturation period, is approximately 10 days. Several inhibitors of bone mineralization have been identified, including pyrophosphate and phosphoproteins associated with calcified tissues.[13] The rate of mineralization appears to be related to the presence of these inhibitor molecules.

V. BONE RESORPTION

Bone resorption is defined as the removal of both bone mineral and organic matrix to produce a cavity in the bone structure, i.e., a resorption pit or Howship's lacuna. This process is carried out primarily by the osteoclast (Figures 6 and 7). Although resorption of the lacunar space around osteocytes has been described in a process called "osteocytic osteolysis," bone resorption results in distinctive changes in bone mineral and matrix that are not observed in osteocytic spaces.[15] The osteocyte may be capable of modifying the mineral phase at the surface of the osteocytic lacunae, but the organic matrix is not removed.[16]

Osteoclasts remove bone in a regulated fashion essential for both the remodeling process and for reconfiguring bone during the modeling process in endochondral bone formation. The major difference in osteoclastic regulation in these two processes is the time-dependent coupling of bone resorption with bone formation that is a characteristic of bone remodeling and the simultaneous, but physically separated, resorption and formation during modeling.

Once bone is dissolved beneath the osteoclast, the Ca and Pi ions and amino acids resulting from protein hydrolysis are removed from the resorption pit (Howship's lacunae) by these possible mechanisms: (1) translocation of individual components through the cytoplasm, (2) bulk transfer of these products via endocytotic vesicles, or (3) release of products when the osteoclast detaches along the sealing zone. The last mechanism is supported by microscopic evidence that osteoclasts are capable of moving along the surface of bone and forming multiple resorption pits. This suggests that the osteoclast is capable of continued bone resorption, but local factors may regulate the maximum size of a given resorption pit.

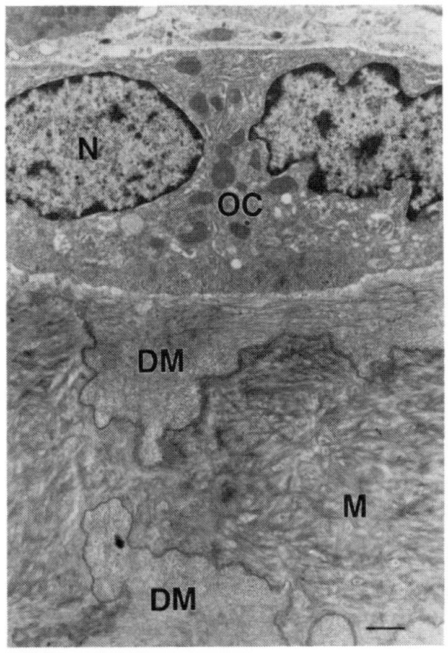

FIGURE 7. Osteoclast — Electron Micrograph. The osteoclast (OC) on the surface of rat trabecular bone contains two nuclei (N) in the area shown. It is adjacent to an area of demineralized (DM) bone and a larger mass of mineralized bone. The area of demineralized bone in the lower portion of the figure is due to another osteoclast. The bar is equal to one micron (1 μm).

Resorption of bone on the surface of either trabecular or compact bone results in excavation of shallow Howship's lacuna. However, in compact bone a group of osteoclasts may continue to resorb bone deep into the compact bone, forming a cylindrical opening through the bone; this cylindrical structure is known as an osteon or Haversian system. Osteoblasts will line the surface of this cylinder and lay down new bone in concentric rings until they have filled the excavation except for a central region through which blood vessels and nerves extend. This structure is also known as a Haversian system, or osteon (see Figure 8).

The activity of the osteoclasts is stimulated by PTH and vitamin D, whereas osteoclasts are inhibited by calcitonin (CT) and estrogens. Although recent reports of PTH receptors on avian osteoblasts have appeared,[17] binding of PTH to these receptors is associated with inhibition of osteoclastic activity rather than with stimulation. Thus, the regulation of osteoclastic activity by these hormones is believed to be mediated by cytokines secreted by the osteoblasts.[18] Osteoblasts are responsive to both PTH and vitamin D and are believed to produce factors with osteoclast resorption-stimulating activity (ORSA) that are either secreted into the surrounding extracellular fluid or are bound to the cell membrane of the osteoblast (or extracellular matrix) and affect the osteoclasts in direct contact with the cell.[19]

VI. BONE REMODELING

During growth, bones must be constantly reshaped to maintain their optimal shape for support. As elongation occurs, the protuberance of the epiphysis must be reduced by osteoclastic resorption, as this volume is filled first by the metaphyseal region and eventually by the cylindrical diaphysis (see Figure 9). In growing bone, bone resorption and formation take place in separate regions of the bone with formation exceeding resorption, so that gains in bone mass occur as part of early-life skeletal development.

In mature bone, osteoblastic bone formation occurs only at sites of osteoclastic activity, and ideally results in replacement of the exact quantity of bone removed by resorption (see Figure 10). When bone formation fails to keep pace with bone resorption, a net decrease in bone mass results; osteoporosis is marked by such a discrepancy between removal of bone and its replacement.

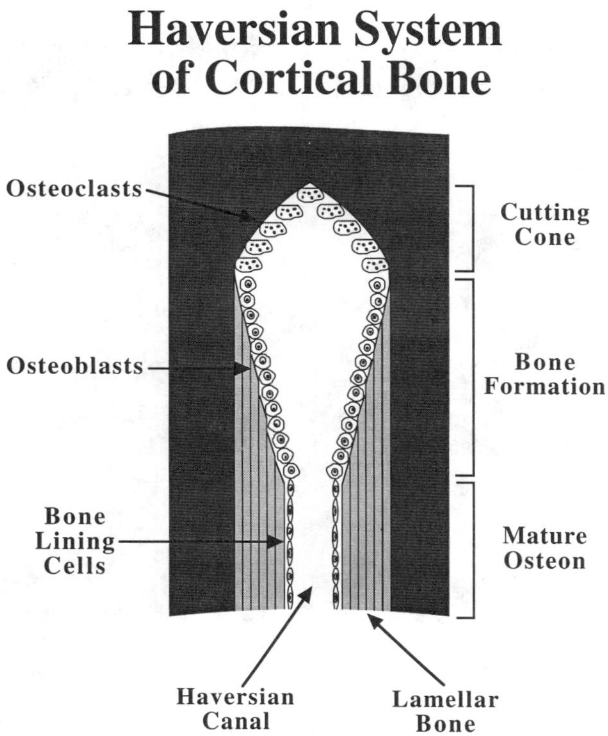

FIGURE 8. Haversian Systems. The Haversian systems (osteons) of compact bone are formed when a "cutting cone" of several osteoclasts excavates an area of bone. At the reversal zone between the cutting cone and area of bone formation, osteoblasts move in and begin replacing the bone with concentric layers of lamellar bone. An opening is left through the center of the Haversian canal through which blood vessels and nerves pass.

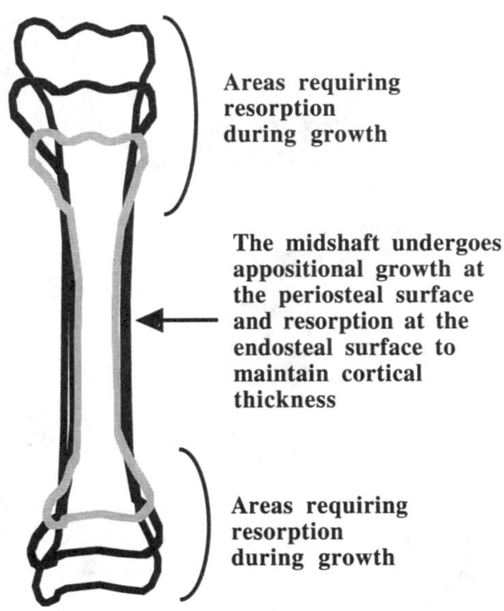

FIGURE 9. Reshaping of a Long Bone During Growth (Modeling). During growth, the bones must be reshaped to maintain the bone model. The outer aspect of the epiphysis is resorbed as the bone length increases at the epiphyseal plate. The midshaft undergoes both resorption on the endosteal surface and growth on the periosteal surface to maintain a similar cortical thickness as the diameter of the bone increases. The process of modeling is distinct from that of remodeling (see Figure 10), in which the resorption of bone and its subsequent formation are tightly coupled at individual sites.

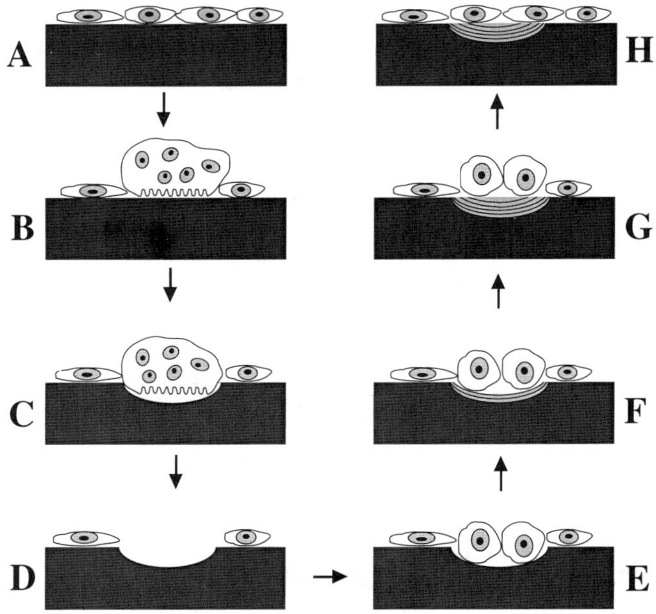

FIGURE 10. Coupling of Remodeling in Howship's Lacunae. Remodeling of bone is a multistep process beginning with (A) activation at an area of bone surface covered by bone-lining cells. (B) Osteoclast(s) are recruited to this site and (C) excavate a resorption pit (Howship's Lacuna). During the (D) reversal phase, the osteoclast moves away from the resorption pit and (E) osteoblasts move in and (F) begin replacing the resorbed bone with new layers of bone. (G) Once this process is complete and the bone tissue has been completely restored (H), the osteoblasts are replaced by quiescent bone-lining cells again. (Adapted from Talmage et al.[36])

A. THE BONE MULTICELLULAR UNIT (BMU) AND BONE REMODELING

The concept of bone remodeling was advanced by Frost.[20] He later introduced the concept of the bone multicellular unit (BMU) for the multicellular sequence of changes in bone that resulted in renewal of bone matrix and mineral in distinct units.

As the organic matrix ages, it becomes brittle and weak and undergoes microfractures. Bone remodeling replaces it with new matrix. This process of remodeling of mature bone consists of a predictable and ordered sequence of bone resorption followed by bone formation, and it can be divided into the following 3 stages:

Activation of osteoclasts
Resorption by osteoclasts
Formation by osteoblasts

The periods of resorption and formation are also separated by a period sometimes called the "reversal phase," as osteoclasts are replaced by osteoblasts at the resorption site.

B. REGULATION OF BONE REMODELING

The processes of bone remodeling also are involved in the response of bone to strain, such as repeated exercise, that results in greater bone mass and in stronger bone, and remodeling is essential for the healing of bone fractures. Bone remodeling may occur in either a random fashion, intersecting the site of microfracture damage by chance, or by a regulated process that favors remodeling in areas of damaged bone.[21] The latter possibility has been proposed by several investigators, but evidence for directed remodeling is difficult to obtain experimentally.

That osteoclasts are specifically recruited to an area to initiate remodeling may be argued, but once that process has begun, it is clear that the process by which osteoblasts replace the bone removed from the bone surface is closely regulated.

The regulation of bone remodeling requires interactions between bone-resorbing and bone-forming cells. Experiments with isolated osteoblasts and osteoclasts have demonstrated that osteoclasts alone are not responsive to stimulation; however, when co-cultured with osteoblasts, the addition of PTH or $1,25(OH)_2D$ can promote bone resorption by osteoclasts. In addition, exposing osteoclasts to medium conditioned by osteoblasts stimulated by PTH or $1,25(OH)_2D$ has a similar stimulatory effect on bone resorption. Therefore, osteoblasts must synthesize a factor that promotes bone resorption by the osteoclast. Numerous proteins are present in bone along with collagen. Several of these are large glycoprotein molecules that likely serve primarily a structural function. Many soluble proteins, however, are also incorporated into mineralized bone at the time of matrix formation. As discussed earlier (see the section on noncollagenous proteins of bone matrix), protein growth factors secreted by osteoblasts or adsorbed from plasma are almost always present in mature bone. Liberation of these factors during bone resorption may serve as signals for the recruitment of osteoblasts to resorption sites.

The local factors secreted by osteoblasts and other cells of the bone marrow or stromal cells are proteins known collectively as cytokines.[22-24] Cytokines may either stimulate osteoclastic bone resorption or inhibit resorption and stimulate bone formation. Factors in the local environment of bone that stimulate osteoclastic bone resorption include interleukin-1 (IL-1), transforming growth factors-α (TGF-α), tumor necrosis factor-α (TNF-α), and interleukin-6 (IL-6). Bone resorption is inhibited by transforming growth factor-β (TGF-β), γ-interferon, and interleukin-4 (IL-4). Since these agents are secreted by cells of the lymphocyte and macrophage lineages, bone marrow is a rich source for these peptides.

The existence of these multiple factors has been established; however, the physiologic role of one or more of these peptides in the local regulation of bone remodeling has not been proven. This represents an exciting area of research in attempting to modulate bone remodeling. The possibility that these or other local factors may stimulate bone formation by osteoblasts suggests the possiblity of therapies that could increase bone formation even in those who have lost bone due to osteoporosis.

The investigation of the role of cytokines in bone remodeling and in the regulation of bone cell metabolism will be greatly accelerated in the near future by the development of specific animal models with selected deletion or overexpression of specific cytokines and/or their receptors. In many cases, researchers may be able to specifically target these mutations to cells of bone, or they may mutate the genes for these proteins in all cells.

VII. EFFECT OF EXERCISE (STRAIN) ON BONE

Considerable evidence supports a role for mechanical loading (strain) or gravitational force in maintaining bone mass.[25] Individuals confined to long term bed rest or those who have participated in space flights lose bone. However, the role of exercise in the accumulation of peak bone mass, and particularly in preventing the loss of bone associated with the menopause and with aging, remains controversial.[26,27] Although extensive loss of bone can be observed in a relatively short period of time with inactivity or weightlessness,[28,29] the gain in bone mass with exercise is much smaller. Comparison of bone mineral content and bone density in young women suggests that increased physical activity may offset, at least in part, an inadequate dietary Ca intake.[30] (see Chapter 19 for additional information on this topic.)

VIII. AGING AND OSTEOPOROSIS

Aging is generally associated with a net loss of bone tissue at all skeletal sites. The bone appears normal, and excessive osteoclasts cannot be found, but too little bone, or osteopenia, exists. Such bone is more susceptible to fracture, especially the trabecular bone tissue. Osteoporotic fractures occur most commonly to the vertebrae, distal radius and ulna (wrist), proximal femur (hip), or humerus (upper arm). Osteoporosis and related dietary issues are discussed in greater detail in chapters 17, 20, and 21.

IX. ASSESSMENT OF BONE MASS AND BONE TURNOVER

There is a great need for accurate methods of assessing bone mass and bone turnover either for diagnosis in subjects believed to be at risk for bone loss or for assessment of treatment modalities in those who have already lost bone. Although the most accurate information on bone quality and bone remodeling activity at a particular site can be obtained by bone histomorphometry, the invasive nature of this procedure limits its usefulness in the diagnosis and treatment of bone disorders. Although X-rays can be used to provide some information about gross changes in bone structure, the need to measure much smaller changes in bone mineral content (BMC) or bone mineral density (BMD) has led to the development and refinement of instruments that can be used to noninvasively determine bone quality in a particular area with continually improving accuracy and reproducibility. Several general types of these instruments are discussed later.

Although BMC and/or BMD can be measured with accuracy and reproducibility approaching 1–2%, this provides information only on the current status of the bone, not on changes in bone formation and resorption that can be related to treatment. Some of the molecules present in blood and/or urine are discussed later as possible markers for the dynamic processes occurring within bone.

A. BONE HISTOMORPHOMETRY

The most accurate estimates of bone mass are obtained by direct sampling of the bone, e.g., transiliac bone biopsy, followed by biochemical and histological analyses. Because of the invasive nature of this procedure, which requires removal of a cylindrical core of bone through the iliac crest, it is not in routine use. However, as a research tool, this procedure can provide valuable information about the rates of bone formation and turnover when bone is labeled *in vivo* with tetracycline, fluorescein, or other fluorescent markers of bone mineralization. Together with well-established staining techniques for bone, these fluorescent compounds can be used to measure the actual bone turnover rate during the period of study and define the status of the population of bone cells in the region examined.

B. *IN VIVO* MEASUREMENTS OF BONE MINERAL CONTENT AND DENSITY

The need to assess BMC and/or BMD in large numbers of individuals has prompted the development of several noninvasive methods that give quantitative results, as opposed to qualitative estimates from standard X-rays. The ideal for a useful method of measuring bone density is a technique that is both accurate (i.e., that provides an estimate of bone mass or density that is very close to the true value) and precise (i.e., that is able to reproducibly measure the same site in the skeleton). Because of the relatively slow rate of change in bone mass during most of the life cycle, precision in the range of 1–2% is necessary to measure meaningful changes in bone mass or density, even when studies extend over a year or more.

1. Radiographic Absorptiometry (RA)

This method uses X-rays of the hand bones to assess bone mass, but the method quantifies the density and, hence, it is called photodensitometry. The quantitation by this method rests on the use of a computer-controlled calculation of the bone density based on the X-ray intensity (black, white, and gray shadings), but only the hand bones (middle phalanges) can be used. Very little interference occurs because of soft-tissue attenuation at these sites. Accuracy with this technique is fairly good (6%), but precision is much better (2%). However, RA is not generally useful because the site of measurement is limited to the hand bones, and information is commonly needed on other parts of the appendicular skeleton or on the axial skeleton.

2. Single-Photon Absorptiometry (SPA) and Single-Energy X-Radiographic Absorptiometry (SPX)

SPA and SPX measurements are limited to single peripheral bones that have relatively little soft-tissue, e.g., forearm (radius and ulna), feet, hands, and lower shin. A monoenergetic photon (gamma) source is used (SPA), such as ^{125}I, and this source has to be replaced periodically, depending on the half-life of the specific radionuclide. A similar monoenergetic X-ray source (SPX) is also available now for conducting similar studies. These instruments are portable and, therefore, suitable for field investigations.

3. Dual-Photon Absorptiometry (DPA) and Dual-Energy X-Radiographic Absorptiometry (DEXA)

DPA and DEXA are essentially identical techniques, and only the source of the photons (radionuclide vs. X-ray generator) differs.[31] These instruments are typically found in radiology departments of hospitals where radiation safety is carefully monitored. With either of these methods the radiation dosages to subjects is very low, e.g., the amount received by a person flying at 40,000 feet from New York to Denver.

The basic principle of DEXA is that it utilizes two monoenergetic X-rays (gamma photons) that are generated by an X-ray machine and then focused on a target tissue site for a short period of time. A machine-driven tracking system allows the source to move across (laterally) different sites of interest or the entire body from head to toes. One of the X-rays is harder and the other is soft. The harder X-ray is stopped to a large extent by the skeletal (mineralized) tissue, whereas most of the soft X-rays are stopped by the soft tissue, including fat. The algorithm uses the weight, height, sex, and age of the individual, along with the X-ray attenuation data for calculating BMC or BMD, fat mass, and lean mass (LBM), exclusive of bone, i.e., a three-compartment model of body composition.

The major advantages of DEXA are its ease of utilization, relative independence of special operator skills and training, and precision (reproducibility) of measurement. Disadvantages include high cost of the equipment (over $100,000), requirement of a trained technician, uncertainty of the algorithm for calculating fat and lean compartments, and uncertainty of measurement accuracy of these compartments. The DEXA measurement of bone mineral content and density are generally accepted as being quite accurate (~5%) and precise (2–4%). One other potential disadvantage of this method that is somewhat problematic is its two-dimensional mode (as opposed to 3-D computed tomography), which is clearly a problem for obese subjects but not necessarily for those with body fat measurements of 20–40%.

Babies, small infants, and even pregnant women can be measured with the DEXA technique because of the low radiation doses, but of course an experimental study measuring the bone mass of pregnant women would be almost impossible to do.

The method of choice for many researchers has become DEXA. The reason for this preference lies in the instrument's capability of generating computerized readouts with little effort required by the investigator. The catch, however, is that the algorithms used by the manufacturers are based on the typical body composition values of relatively healthy young adults.

a. Bone

Measurements of BMC and BMD using DEXA are considered very accurate (3–4%) for normal-weight or thin individuals, but not for heavily muscled and obese subjects because of the greater attenuation by increased mass from soft tissues. Precision, however, remains good (2%) for all subjects. Measurements of both the axial skeleton and the appendicular skeleton can be made with this method. In addition, total body measurements from head to toe (or neck to toe) can be made. A special arm attachment (device) permits separated measurement of the radius and ulna. These measurements can be done quite rapidly (fast mode) or more slowly.

b. Fat

For the reasons just discussed, the normalized data set used by DEXA for comparison does not apply to very obese individuals (>50% body mass) or to sick patients who have lost much of their lean tissue, who may also be dehydrated, or who may have shifts of water (fluid) from blood to extravascular fluid compartments. The potential pitfalls of using DEXA have not so dampened the enthusiasm of investigators that they are discarding this method; to the contrary, they are trying different ways to improve the method for evaluating body fat under conditions of excessive obesity.

4. Quantitative Computed Tomography (QCT)

This is the only method considered here that obtains three-dimensional bone data, i.e., true volumetric bone density. The technique, however, is only used routinely for estimating vertebral bone density, especially of the lumbar region of the spine. Also, it only measures trabecular bone, and it is considered by many investigators to overestimate vertebral bone loss. A major disadvantage of this method is the high radiation exposure (~100–300 mrem per study versus 1–2 mrem per study for DEXA). A comparison of single measurements using QCT and DEXA cannot be made, but multiple measurement trends can be used for comparison.

5. Summary

The best experimental use of these bone-densitometric machines is for prospective investigations of BMC and BMD in the same individuals using the same machines and operators in order to limit errors, such as positioning and operator differences. DEXA has become the method of choice for experimental studies because of its wide availability, high precision, and ease of use, despite some disadvantages. Furthermore, the low radiation dose of DEXA machines makes them quite safe.

C. BONE MARKERS IN BLOOD AND URINE

The importance of balanced bone resorption and formation in the maintenance of bone health has resulted in continued efforts by researchers and clinicians to find molecules in urine or plasma that reflect bone resorption and/or formation.[32] These markers of bone turnover are likely to change over short time periods, e.g., hours or days, as opposed to the months or years required for the changes in bone mass or density (described earlier). Thus, these methods can be used to follow therapeutic intervention in metabolic bone diseases such as osteoporosis (see Chapter 10 for more detailed information on the markers of bone turnover in current use or under development).

1. Markers Of Bone Formation

Alkaline phosphatase is an enzyme that is characteristic of osteoblasts, and an increase in blood alkaline phosphatase may reflect increased bone formation; however, the synthesis of alkaline phosphatase isozymes in the liver, GI tract, and other tissues make measurement and interpretation of changes in alkaline phosphatase difficult.

Osteocalcin, also known as bone Gla-protein (BGP), is one of the proteins that make up bone matrix along with collagen, although its function is not known. Synthesis of this protein is dependent on vitamin K. Like collagen and alkaline phosphatase, osteocalcin is synthesized by the osteoblasts, and its blood levels may reflect the level of bone formation.

2. Markers of Bone Resorption

Hydroxyproline is a modified amino acid unique to collagen and measurable in both blood and urine. When collagen is degraded during bone resorption, the hydroxyproline residues are released from the protein and are not reused. Therefore, the amount of hydroxyproline in the blood and/or urine reflects the level of osteoclastic bone resorption, assuming no alteration in turnover of other body collagen.

Osteoclasts synthesize a tartrate-resistant acid phosphatase (TRAP) that may be measured in blood. Changes in serum concentrations of TRAP may be reflective of bone resorption by osteoclasts.

Mature collagen contains cross-links between adjacent protein molecules. These pyridinoline and deoxypyridinilone cross-links can be measured in urine and in some cases in serum, and they are indicative of the resorption of collagen molecules because the cross-links are not hydrolyzed before excretion. However, collagen molecules other than bone collagen contain significant amounts of pyridinoline cross-links.

3. Summary

Bone markers, although useful for estimating changes in turnover, have not yet been shown to be as accurate as would be desirable. Because this area of understanding is being actively investigated, better use of these markers should emerge in the future.

X. NUTRIENT REQUIREMENTS FOR BONE FORMATION AND MAINTENANCE

Bone formation and maintenance require many nutrients in addition to Ca and P.[33,34] An adequate intake of protein and energy is the first requirement for bone formation because the collagen matrix must be laid down before mineralization can occur. Formation and growth of bone obviously require an ample supply of Ca and P to adequately mineralize the organic matrix. This supply of minerals must be provided from the mother's body during pregnancy and during early life in breast-fed infants. During the remainder of life, these minerals must be obtained from foods, especially dairy products, but including dark green leafy vegetables and other foods.

Several vitamins are also essential for normal bone growth. A deficiency of vitamin D results in defects in mineralization and decreased linear growth. In children this condition is known as rickets, whereas in adults it is more commonly called osteomalacia. This defect in mineralization is associated with hypocalcemia and/or hypophosphatemia, which are secondary to decreased efficiency of absorption of both minerals from the gut (see Chapter 12).

Vitamin A deficiency decreases in bone resorption, collagen synthesis, and mineral accretion. In the absence of vitamin A, osteoclastic lysosomes do not release their contents as readily, and there is a failure of bone resorption. Although collagen synthesis is also decreased, the net effect is an increase in bone formation. Mellanby[35] demonstrated that continued vitamin A deficiency in puppies produced nervous lesions as nerve compression resulted from overgrowth of bones of the skull and spinal column.

Vitamin C deficiency impairs bone formation through decreased synthesis of collagen; this results from failure of proline and lysine hydroxylation after incorporation into the collagen molecule, a step in which vitamin C is a cofactor. Iron and oxygen are also required for this reaction. These hydroxylation reactions are essential for establishing the helical structure of collagen and forming of cross-links between collagen molecules that stabilize bone matrix (see Chapter 9).

Vitamin K deficiency results in undercarboxylation of glutamate residues and impaired collagen synthesis. Vitamin K is required for synthesis of proteins containing γ-carboxyglutamate. Bone contains several of these proteins, the most abundant of which is osteocalcin (see Table 1). A role for osteocalcin in bone mineralization has been proposed, but its function remains under investigation.

Both hypervitaminosis A and D stimulate bone resorption, which results in weaker bones.

Several mineral deficiencies, such as those of magnesium, zinc, and iron, may also contribute to inadequate bone formation and accumulation of bone mass.

XI. SUMMARY

As an organ, bone can be described by its anatomic location, shape, and function. The organization of bone into cortical and trabecular microstructure is essential for the supportive and metabolic functions provided by the skeleton. At the tissue level, bone contains several different types of cells that are responsible for bone formation (osteoblasts) and bone resorption (osteoclasts) during growth and maintenance of the skeleton.

Although bone appears externally to be an unchanging structure, its microenvironment is remarkably dynamic. Not only does bone undergo microscopic remodeling processes that are constantly replacing small packets of bone throughout the skeleton, but at the chemical level, bone is constantly exchanging Ca and Pi with extracellular fluid (ECF), and ultimately with the plasma.

The regulation of Ca homeostasis is complex, involving interactions with kidney and gut and with hormonal factors, especially PTH and vitamin D. The control of bone turnover is even more complex as circulating hormones known to affect bone include PTH, vitamin D, calcitonin, and estrogen. The roles of local bone factors, e.g., cytokines, growth factors, and noncollagenous matrix proteins, in the regulation of bone formation and remodeling are only now beginning to be elucidated.

Once the bone matures and the individual attains peak bone mass, a phenomenon that may occur at different ages for different parts of the skeleton (see Chapter 17), the maintenance of bone health is dependent on the balance between bone resorption and formation. When formation fails to replace the same amount of bone removed by osteoclastic resorption, bone mass decreases. In late life, the resulting low bone mass or osteopenia is eventually evidenced as osteoporosis when fractures occur. Current research suggests that physical activity and adequate nutrition during periods of bone accretion and bone maintenance contribute to attaining optimal peak bone mass, as well as to minimizing the rate of loss with aging in older individuals.

REFERENCES

1. **Albright, J. A. and Skinner, H. C. W.,** Bone: structural organization and remodeling dynamics, in *The Scientific Basis of Orthopaedics*, Albright, J. A. and Brand, R. A., Eds., Appleton & Lange, Norwalk, Connecticut, 1987.
2. **Currey, J.,** *The Mechanical Adaptations of Bones*, Princeton University Press, Princeton, NJ, 1984.
3. **Evans, F. G.,** *Mechanical Properties of Bone*, Charles C. Thomas, Springfield, IL, 1973.
4. **Mammone, J. F. and Hudson, S. M.,** Micromechanics of bone strength and failure, *J. Biomechanics*, 26, 439, 1993.
5. **Lanyon, L. E.,** Control of bone architecture by functional load bearing, *J. Bone Min. Res.*, 7 (suppl 2), S369, 1992.
6. **Jee, W. S. S.,** The skeletal tissues, in *Cell and Tissue Biology: A Textbook of Histology*, Weiss, L., ed., Urban & Schwarzenberg, Baltimore, 1988.
7. **Cormack, D. H.,** Bone, in *Ham's Histology*, Cormack, D. H., ed., J.B. Lippincott Company, London, 1987.
8. **Fawcett, D. W.,** Bone, in *Bloom and Fawcett: A Textbook of Histology*, Fawcett, D. W., ed., Chapman & Hall, New York, 1994.
9. **Blair, H. C., Schlesinger, P. H., Ross, F. P. and Teitelbaum, S. L.,** Recent advances toward understanding osteoclast physiology, *Clin. Orthop. Rel. Res.*, 294, 7, 1993.
10. **Termine, J. D.,** Non-collagen proteins in bone, in *Cell and Molecular Biology of Vertebrate Hard Tissues (Ciba Foundation Symposium 136)*, Wiley, Chichester, 1988.
11. **Hauschka, P. V., Chen, T. L. and Mavrakos, A. E.,** Polypeptide growth factors in bone matrix, in *Cell and Molecular Biology of Vertebrate Hard Tissues (Ciba Foundation Symposium 136)*, Wiley, Chichester, 1988.
12. **Bonucci, E.,** The locus of initial calcification in cartilage and bone, *Clin. Orthop. Rel. Res.*, 78, 108, 1971.
13. **Termine, J. D., Eanes, E. D. and Conn, K. M.,** Phosphoprotein modulation of apatite crystallization, *Calcif. Tissue Int.*, 31, 247, 1980.
14. **Skinner, H. C. W.,** Bone: mineralization, in *The Scientific Basis of Orthopaedics*, Albright, J. A. and Brand, R. A., eds., Appleton & Lange, Norwalk, Connecticut, 1987.
15. **Boyde, A.,** Evidence against osteocytic osteolysis, in *Bone histomorphometry, Metab. Bone Dis. Rel. Res. (suppl)*, Societe Nouvelle de Publications Medicals et Dentairs, Paris, 1981.
16. **Lanyon, L. E.,** Osteocytes, strain detection, bone modeling and remodeling, *Calcif. Tissue Int.*, 53 (suppl 1), S102, 1993.
17. **Agarwala, N. and Gay, C. V.,** Specific binding of parathyroid hormone to living osteoclasts, *J. Bone Min. Res.*, 7, 531, 1992.
18. **McSheehy, P. M. J. and Chambers, T. J.,** Osteoblastic cells mediate osteoclastic responsiveness to parathyroid hormone, *Endocrinology*, 118, 824, 1986.
19. **Fuller, K., Gallagher, A. C. and Chambers, T. J.,** Osteoclast resorption-stimulating activity is associated with the osteoblast cell surface and/or the extracellular matrix, *Biochem. Biophys. Res. Commun.*, 181, 67, 1991.
20. **Frost, H. M.,** *Bone Remodelling Dynamics*, Charles C. Thomas, Springfield, Illinois, 1963.
21. **Burr, D. B.,** Remodeling and the repair of fatigue damage, *Calcif. Tissue Int.*, 53 (suppl 1), S75, 1993.
22. **Chambers, T. J.,** The regulation of osteoclastic development and function, in *Cell and Molecular Biology of Vertebrate Hard Tissues, (Ciba Foundation Symposium 136)*, Wiley, Chichester, 1988.
23. **Mundy, G. R.,** Cytokines and local factors which affect osteoclast function, *Int. J. Cell Cloning*, 12, 215, 1992.
24. **Roodman, G. D.,** Role of cytokines in the regulation of bone resorption, *Calcif. Tissue Int.*, 53 (suppl 1), S94, 1993.

25. **Rubin, C. T. and Lanyon, L. E.,** Regulation of bone formation by applied dynamic loads, *J. Bone Jt. Surg.*, 66-A, 397, 1984.
26. **Drinkwater, B. L.,** Exercise in the prevention of osteoporosis, *Osteoporosis Int.*, 3 (suppl 1), S169, 1993.
27. **Block, J. E., Smith, R., Black, D. and Genant, H. K.,** Does exercise prevent osteoporosis?, *J. Am. Med. Assoc.*, 257, 3115, 1987.
28. **Donaldson, C. L., Hulley, S. B., Vogel, J. M., Hattner, R. S., Boyers, J. H. and McMillan, D. E.,** Effect of prolonged bed rest on bone mineral, *Metabolism*, 19, 1071, 1970.
29. **Vogel, J. M., Whittle, W. M., Smith, M. C. and Rambaut, P. C.,** Bone mineral measurement, experiment M078, in *Biomedical Results from Skylab*, Administration, National Aeronautics and Space Administration, GPO, Washington, DC, 1977.
30. **Metz, J. A., Anderson, J. J. B. and Gallagher, P. N., Jr.,** Intakes of calcium, phosphorus, and protein, and physical-activity level are related to radial bone mass in young adult women, *Am. J. Clin. Nutr.*, 58, 537, 1993.
31. **Wahner, H. W. and Fogelman, I.,** *The Evaluation of Osteoporosis: Dual Energy X-Ray Absorptiomety in Clinical Practice*, Martin Dunitz, Ltd., London, 1994.
32. **Delmas, P. D.,** Biochemical markers of bone turnover I: theoretical considerations and clinical use in osteoporosis, *Am. J. Med.*, 95 (suppl 5A), 11, 1993.
33. **Simmons, D. J., ed.,** *Nutrition and Bone Development*, Oxford University Press, New York, 1990.
34. **Guggenheim, K. Y., Wolinsky, I. and Ornoy, A.,** Nutrition and bone formation, in *Handbook of Nutritional Requirements in a Functional Context. Vol. I. Development and Conditions of Physiologic Stress*, Recheigl, M., Jr., ed., CRC Press, Boca Raton, FL, 1981.
35. **Mellanby, E.,** Nutrition in relation to bone growth and the nervous system, *Proc. R. Soc.*, B132, 28, 1944–5.
36. **Talmage, R. V., Grubb, S. A. and VanderWiel, C. J.,** Physiologic processes in bone, in *The Musculoskeletal System: Basic Processes and Disorders*, Wilson, F. C., ed., 2nd ed., 1983.

Chapter 8

DENTAL TISSUES

James W. Bawden, D.D.S., Ph.D., John J. B. Anderson, Ph.D., and Sanford C. Garner, Ph.D.

TABLE OF CONTENTS

I. INTRODUCTION

The teeth make up the other major class of calcified connective tissue. Unlike bone, the structure of the teeth is established during formation, and no physiologic remodeling of the tissues occurs during the remainder of life. Although bone and two of the dental tissues, dentin and cementum, share in common a mixed structure of collagen-based organic matrix and hydroxyapatite inorganic material, the arrangement of these two components is quite different in teeth.

The teeth begin their formation in the first few months of fetal life and development of successive teeth can continue through the teenage years. Development of the primary dentition is typically completed by about three years of age. These teeth are lost when the secondary dentition begins to erupt in the oral cavity. Cells derived from the oral epithelium are responsible for the development of enamel, and cells differentiated from the mesenchymal pulpal tissues form the dentin. An exquisite sequence of cell-to-cell and matrix-to-cell inductions leads to the deposition and mineralization of these highly refined biomineralized tissues. Keep in mind that the fully formed mineralized phases of teeth remain essentially inert, i.e., without cellular influences, after eruption. Therefore, the adequate provision of nutrients for tooth development must occur during a relatively narrow window of time. The enamel, and eventually the dentin and pulp, may be damaged by

0-8493-7845-1/95/$0.00+$.50

environmental conditions through the caries (tooth decay) process after eruption. However, under healthy conditions, the dentin and pulp are protected from systemic influences experienced by most other tissues and cell types. None of the dental (tooth) tissues is involved in the classical homeostatic-feedback mechanisms required to sustain systemic physiologic conditions.

This chapter covers in short sections the structure of the mature tooth and some of the early embryologic stages of tooth development. The primary focus of this chapter is placed on the transfer of calcium ions into the developing tissues that become mineralized, namely the dentin, enamel, and cementum. Finally, brief overviews are provided of the nutritional supply required for optimal tooth development and of the role of dietary fluoride in the maintenance of the enamel surfaces of erupted teeth and in caries prevention. Details of the oral epithelium and the periodontal tissues are not covered.

II. STRUCTURE OF TEETH

The adult human or secondary dentition consists of 32 permanent teeth, whereas the primary dentition comprises only 20 teeth. Each tooth, regardless of its external shape, consists of a crown and either single or multiple roots. By definition, the anatomical crown is covered by the enamel, the most highly calcified tissue of the body. The remainder of the crown is composed of the dentin, another calcified tissue that encompasses the central chamber filled with the unmineralized tissue of the tooth, the pulp. The dentin and pulp also constitute the tissues of the root. However, the outer surface of the root is covered by another calcified tissue called cementum. The enamel and cementum meet around the neck of the tooth, approximately at the gum line, and form the cemento-enamel junction. In younger people, this junction is not normally seen on the portion of the tooth exposed to the oral cavity because the epithelial tissue, the gingiva (gums), covering the alveolar process (jaw bone) extends for a short distance onto the crown. In older people, or younger people with periodontal disease that results in recession of the gum, parts of the root as well as the anatomical crown may be exposed in the oral cavity. Whatever portion of the tooth is actually seen in the mouth is called the clinical crown.

The basic structure of a mature, fully mineralized, erupted molar tooth consists of the following tissue components (see Figure 1): enamel, dentin, cementum, pulp, and periodontal ligament. As erupted teeth age, enamel occasionally may be worn away and reduced in thickness to a significant degree. However, this most highly mineralized of all mammalian mineralized tissues, is remarkably resistant to wear under normal conditions. Other changes in tooth surfaces with aging often occur because of infections in the periodontal tissues, caries formation, and the removal or malfunction of salivary glands, which normally secrete fluids that bathe the tooth surfaces with proteins and minerals that are protective to the tissue surfaces. No gender differences exist in tooth structure, but females typically have teeth somewhat smaller than those of males.

Whereas enamel is derived from epithelial tissues, dentin is a mesenchyme-derived tissue. The formative cells, the odontoblasts, are differentiated from the pulpal connective tissue. The odontoblasts remain on the surface of the dentin after the primary stage of dentin formation is complete, and their cellular processes extend deep into the dentin to provide continuing, but indirect, contact with the extracellular fluids. Cementum is also derived from cells in connective tissue, apparently from cells located in the periodontal ligament.

III. DEVELOPMENT OF TEETH

Two major processes make up the normal development sequence of tooth formation, namely, morphodifferentiation and cytodifferentiation. Each of these processes is briefly described, and then descriptions of the functional delivery of calcium and other mineral ions to the calcified tissues via specific cells provide the focus of the rest of this section.

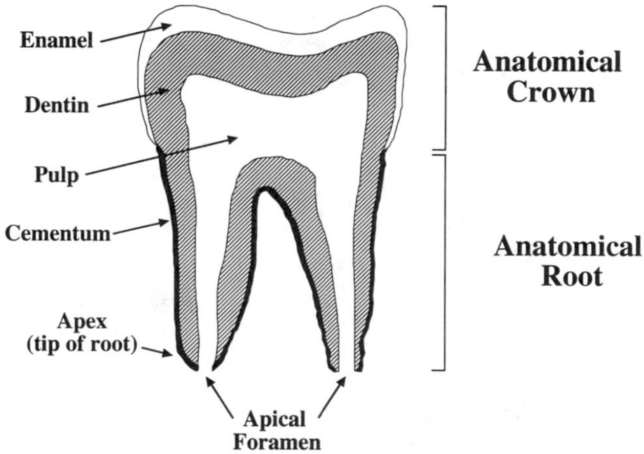

FIGURE 1. Anatomical Structure of a Mature (Erupted) Molar Tooth. The anatomical crown and the anatomical root of each tooth are covered by calcified tissues, the enamel and the cementum, respectively. Both the crown and the root consist primarily of a layer of calcified tissue, the dentin (shaded areas of diagram), and the pulp, which contains the only living cells of the mature tooth. The blood supply, nerves, and lymphatics enter and exit the tooth through the apical foramina.

A. MORPHODIFFERENTIATION

Each developing tooth of either primary or secondary dentition passes through the same developmental series, i.e., bud stage, cap stage, and bell stage.[1] The initiation of each tooth is in the horseshoe-shaped extension of the oral epithelium that gives rise to local cell growth to form balls of epithelial cells or buds, 10 in the upper jaw and 10 in the lower jaw for the primary dentition, and 16 in each jaw for the secondary dentition. The development of individual teeth through the cap stage is marked by development of the enamel organ, a specialized cellular structure that is responsible for the critical inductions leading to tooth formation. The final development of the tooth takes place during the bell stage in which the epithelial component, or enamel organ, forms the outer layer of the tooth, and the mesenchymal component forms both the dentin and the dental pulp.

B. CYTODIFFERENTIATION

Cytodifferentiation during tooth development is well defined and involves a tightly integrated series of inductions (see Figure 2).[2,3] The epithelial cells of the presumptive enamel organ induce the adjacent cells of the pulpal mesenchyme to differentiate into odontoblasts, which begin to secrete the predentin matrix. Soon after dentin matrix deposition begins, the epithelial cells of the enamel organ adjacent to the predentin differentiate to assume the general morphologic characteristics of ameloblasts. Immediately after that, dentin mineralization begins, followed quickly by the beginning of enamel matrix deposition by the ameloblasts. Enamel matrix deposition and mineralization is a highly refined, intricate process that is incompletely understood. Dentin formation is also a complex and only partially understood process. When development has been completed, the remaining mesenchymal tissues form the central portion of the tooth through which the blood supply and innervation are provided.

1. Odontoblasts and Dentin Formation

The dentin layer surrounds the pulp and underlies the enamel of the crown and the cementum of the root. The chemical composition of the dentin is 20% organic (mainly collagen), 10% water, and 70% inorganic, (mostly hydroxyapatite).

The odontoblasts retreat from the adjacent preameloblasts, laying down the dentin matrix, which remains unmineralized until a defined thickness is achieved (see Figure 2). Then, mineralization commences and follows the pulpal direction of matrix deposition. The odontoblasts leave behind

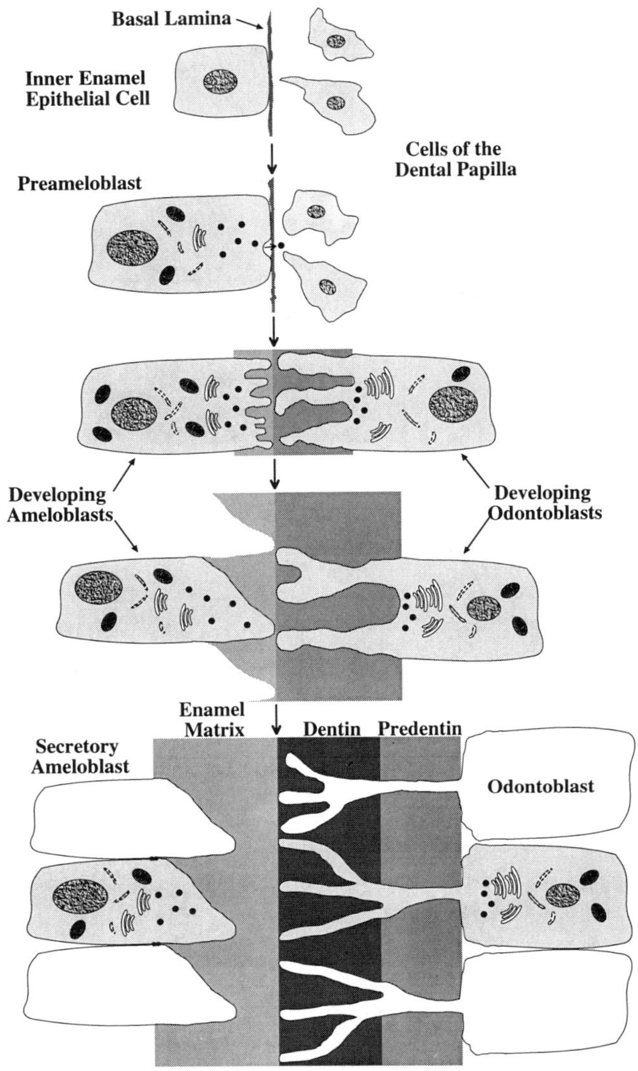

FIGURE 2. Cytodifferentiation of Odontoblasts and Ameloblasts. The inner epithelial cells of the enamel organ are separated from the mesenchymal cells of the dental papilla by a basal lamina. The preameloblasts secrete soluble factors that stimulate development of the odontoblasts. Contact between the dentin matrix and the preameloblasts is necessary for further differentiation and maturation into secretory ameloblasts. Both odontoblasts and ameloblasts are then committed to their final differentiation sequence, which results in the formation of unmineralized enamel and predentin, respectively. The odontoblast cell bodies withdraw from the enamel:dentin interface, but cell processes maintain contact between the cell body and the interface. The transfer of the large numbers of Ca ions required for calcification of the enamel matrix and predentin is regulated by ameloblasts and odontoblasts, respectively. (Adapted from References 1 and 9)

cellular extensions that penetrate the dentin to, or nearly to, its junction with enamel. After the prescribed thickness of dentin is laid down, matrix secretion and mineralization cease. However, odontoblasts continue to cover the surface of dentin, and they can be stimulated to deposit additional, protective dentin in response to advancing dental caries or other insults detrimental to normal physiology of the pulp.

2. Ameloblasts and Calcium Transport during Enamel Formation

The enamel is formed by a layer specialized of cells, the ameloblasts (see Figure 2), that synthesize a specialized organic matrix consisting of two classes of glycoproteins, the amelogenins and the enamelins. In contrast to the other mineralized tissues, enamel matrix is collagen free.

Whereas the organic matrices of bone and dentin require time for maturation before initiation of mineralization, the enamel matrix forms small hydroxyapatite crystals almost immediately after it is laid down. These crystals enlarge slowly until the entire thickness of the enamel is deposited. Upon completion of the secretory stage, the ameloblasts undergo marked, cyclic morphologic alterations to exercise control over the events that lead to the cleavage and removal of almost all of the matrix proteins and to rapid mineralization of the tissue. This process ultimately results in a structure that is the most highly calcified tissue in the body. Mature enamel is approximately 97% mineral by weight. The mineral is in the form of closely packed hydroxyapatite (calcium phosphate dihydrate) crystals arranged in rod-like structures that run perpendicular to the enamel surface and extend from the surface of the crown to the dentin-enamel junction.

Adequate amounts of calcium exist in the extracellular fluid to support crystal growth in the developing tooth, i.e., the Ca:P product is supersaturated in ECF relative to hydroxyapatite. The initial mineral phase in mammals is octacalcium phosphate, which hydrolyzes to a hydroxyapatite-like material.[4-6] Evidence exists that tight intercellular junctions between adjacent ameloblasts prevent direct access of ECF Ca to the surface of the mineralizing enamel. For example, lanthanum, which has a similar ionic radius to that of Ca, cannot penetrate the intercellular junctions of either secretory ameloblasts or maturation stage ameloblasts.[7,8] The mechanisms by which Ca moves downhill from a high concentration in the ECF to a lower concentration in the enamel fluid most likely requires transcellular transport because of the "tight" intercellular connections in the enamel organ.

A transcellular transport system for Ca ions must exist to move Ca ions from ECF (proximal membrane) to the enamel fluid (distal membrane) without producing a significant rise in intracellular Ca (see Chapter 6). Several mechanisms have been proposed for this Ca transfer:[9] (1) Ca could be packaged into vesicles that fuse with the distal cell membrane and release Ca into the enamel fluid; (2) Ca entering the cell at the proximal cell membrane could immediately be bound to a Ca-binding protein (CaBP) and transferred to the distal membrane for extrusion from the cell; (3) the cytosolic free Ca ion concentration across the cell from proximal to distal membrane could form a gradient to favor movement from ECF to enamel fluid; and (4) Ca ions may be transferred along the inner surface of the plasma membrane by membrane fluidity with various molecules of phosphatidyl serine acting as carriers. Although little evidence exists for the vesicular or membrane-bound transfer of Ca across the ameloblast cell layer, the transfer mechanisms of Ca bound to CaBP and transcellular diffusion appear to play a role in Ca transport.

The Ca-translocating mechanisms of the secretory and maturation phases of ameloblasts may differ because of variation in the morphology and function of these cells. The transport of Ca through the secretory ameloblasts is relatively limited, and the diffusion of Ca ions through the cytoplasm without a critical increase in cytoplasmic Ca concentration may be sufficient to account for the net transfer of Ca. During the maturation stage, however, the Ca flux to the enamel fluid is greatly increased to support rapid mineralization. The amount of Ca required for the mineralization of enamel is too great to be transported by transcellular diffusion without raising the intracellular Ca concentration. A likely explanation for the transport of Ca across the maturation stage cells adjacent to the rapidly mineralizing enamel is by binding Ca to a 9 kDa CaBP, which is present in higher concentrations in maturation stage ameloblasts but is not as abundant in the secretory ameloblasts. The formation of a Ca-CaBP complex at the proximal membrane and the release of Ca from the complex at the distal membrane with extrusion across the membrane could explain the transcellular movement of Ca without a corresponding increase in the cytoplasmic-free Ca concentration.

Thus, current evidence supports transcellular Ca transport by either diffusion (secretory ameloblasts) or CaBP-mediated transfer (maturation stage ameloblasts). During transcellular transport, Ca must enter the cell at the proximal membrane and exit the cell at the distal membrane. The secretory ameloblasts appear to contain Ca-ATPase-associated Ca pumps along the entire cell membrane. The direction of Ca transport at the proximal (ECF to cytoplasm) and distal cell membranes (cytoplasm to enamel fluid) may be explained by differences in the extracellular concentration of Ca^{2+} adjacent to the respective membranes. The [Ca^{2+}] in the ECF, which is in contact with the proximal membrane, is approximately 1 m*M*. In the enamel fluid, adjacent to the distal membrane, the [Ca^{2+}] is approximately 10 μ*M*. The export of Ca^{2+} at the proximal surfaces would be less than the Ca influx driven by the large transmembrane gradient. At the distal membrane, however, the gradient is much less, due to the lower Ca concentration in the enamel fluid. At that surface the Ca transported by the Ca-ATPase exceeds the Ca entering the cytoplasm down the concentration gradient from the ECF.

The cellular mechanisms responsible for the transcellular transport of Ca, though not fully explained, must move significant amounts of Ca ions in the maturation stage without a net increase in intracellular Ca, which would inhibit essential cell functions. In summary, the mature ameloblasts serve as amazing Ca-transport vehicles that enable the developing enamel surfaces to accumulate optimal quantities of Ca, phosphate, and other components of this mineral rich tissue.

3. Cementoblasts and Cementum Formation

The layer of calcified tissue covering the roots of teeth is the cementum, which is formed by a specialized connective tissue cell type, the cementoblast. Although it is clear that a protein matrix is deposited and subsequently mineralized, the details of cementum formation are poorly understood.

4. Fibroblasts and Pulp Formation

The soft tissue within the tooth, or pulp, consists of blood vessels, nerves, lymphatics, and fibroblasts. The pulp arises from the mesenchymal (fibroblastic) cells of the inner part of the dental papilla.

IV. NUTRIENT REQUIREMENTS DURING TOOTH FORMATION

The effective delivery of oxygen and nutrients is critical to tooth development and to the continuing health of the pulp after tooth development has been completed.

A. CALCIUM AND PHOSPHORUS

Adequate amounts of Ca ions (and phosphate ions) are essential for the development of enamel, dentin, and cementum. Because the diet almost always provides more than enough phosphorus, Ca is the most likely nutrient to be deficient during dental development. The delivery of adequate amounts of Ca to the dental tissues during development is essentially dependent on the maintenance of normal Ca concentrations in the extracellular fluids (plasma). Since the homeostatic mechanisms controlling the extracellular Ca ion concentration are highly efficient, only the most severe forms of Ca deprivation can result in hypomineralization of the dental tissues. The dental tissues do not, however, participate in the systemic Ca homeostatic mechanisms that result in Ca withdrawal from bone. Genetic defects, transient oxygen deprivation, or deficiencies of nutrients in addition to Ca may result in the formation of abnormal enamel, dentin, or cementum.[10,11]

B. OTHER NUTRIENTS

Trace elements other than fluorides appear to have insignificant effects on tooth development unless the integrity of the enamel organ is compromised during the formative process. Essentially, this statement can be made for water-soluble and fat-soluble vitamins.

V. SPECIAL ROLE OF FLUORIDE IN CARIES PREVENTION

Dental decay (caries) results from bacterial acid production on the tooth surfaces, most commonly the enamel. Bacterial colonies (or plaque) form in greater numbers on the surfaces of individuals with rich western-type diets, especially sugars that stick to the teeth for extended times. When sugar-rich foods were no longer available to Norwegian children during World War II, the rate of caries formation declined dramatically.[12] It has long been known that the pH of the oral cavity decreases well below 7.0 following the ingestion of certain types of foods, especially short carbohydrates, such as dextrins, and disaccharides. The retentive sugars, such as those found in toffees and similar candies, have been shown in the Vipeholm, Sweden, study to be particularly cariogenic.[13] On the other hand, foods, such as fruits, vegetables, and relatively unprocessed cereals and other plant sources help protect against caries. Phosphates, which are used as additives in many foods, also help prevent caries.[14] The major advance in preventing tooth caries, however, has come from the widespread use of fluoride products.

Fluorides are believed to prevent caries by three primary mechanisms: (1) reduction of enamel solubility, (2) enhancement of enamel remineralization, and, (3) reduction in acid production by cariogenic bacteria. The relative clinical importance of these mechanisms is a matter of controversy. However, enhancement of remineralization is generally agreed to be the most critical mechanism.

Fluorides may be administered systemically, primarily in drinking water or as fluoride supplements (drops and tablets). Their effect is both pre-eruptive and posteruptive. The balance between these components is a point of discussion at this time. Fluorides may be applied to the surfaces of the teeth (topical) in a variety of vehicles, concentrations, and frequencies. The use of a properly selected agent in the correct manner can be highly effective in the prevention of caries.[15-17]

The recommended concentration of fluoride in drinking water is approximately 1 ppm, depending on climate. Excessive concentrations consumed during the time of enamel formation can result in discoloration and malformation of enamel (fluorosis). Although fluoridated toothpastes are effective caries-preventive agents, over-ingestion of such toothpastes by small children can lead to fluorosis. Parental supervision of tooth brushing at an early age is urged.[18]

Fluoride accumulates in bone with age.[19] The effects of fluoride on bone fragility, especially in postmenopausal women, is a controversial issue. Current data suggest that fluoride ingestion at the optimal level is protective, but that ingestion of excessive amounts may lead to increased fragility.

VI. CONCLUDING REMARKS

The normal development of teeth, both *in utero* and during childhood, depends primarily on the proper function of homeostatic mechanisms and the availability of an adequate nutrient supply.[20] With rare exceptions, malformations in the dental tissues occur secondary to abnormal hormonal control, especially with respect to vitamin D and parathyroid hormone, excessive fluoride intake, and genetic defects.

After the teeth erupt, diet becomes important in caries prevention. Frequent exposure to sucrose and other cariogenic nutrients can result in rampant, destructive caries.

REFERENCES

1. **Moss-Salentijn, L. and Hendricks-Klyvert, M.,** *Dental and Oral Tissues: An Introduction*, 3rd ed., Lea & Febiger, Philadelphia, 1990.
2. **Warshawsky, H. and Smith, C. E.,** Morphological classification of rat incisor ameloblasts, *Anat. Rec.*, 179, 423, 1974.
3. **Josephson, K., Fejerskov, O., Baelum, V. and Weile, V.,** The effect of a single dose of 1-hydroxyethylidene-1,1-bisphosphonate (HEBP) on presecretory ameloblast differentiation in rat incisors, *J. Biol. Buccale*, 18, 321, 1990.
4. **Brown, W. E., Smith, J. P., Lehr, J. R. and Frazier, A. W.,** Crystallographic and chemical reactions between octacalcium phosphate and hydroxyapatite, *Nature*, 196, 1050, 1962.
5. **Brown, W. E., Crow, L. C., Siew, C. and Gruninger, S.,** Acidic calcium phosphate precursors in formation in enamel mineral, in *Tooth Enamel IV*, Fearnhead, R. W. and Suga, S., eds., Elsevier Science Publishers, Amsterdam, 1984.
6. **Brown, W. E., Eidelman, N. and Tomazic, B.,** Octacalcium phosphate as a precursor in biomineral formation, *Adv. Dent. Res.*, 1, 306, 1987.
7. **Takano, Y. and Crenshaw, M. A.,** The penetration of intravascularly perfused lanthanum into the ameloblast layer of developing rat molar teeth, *Arch. Oral Biol.*, 25, 505, 1981.

8. **Josephsen, K.,** Lanthanum tracer study on permeability of ameloblast junctional complexes in maturation zone of cat incisor enamel organ, in *Tooth Enamel IV*, Fearnhead, R. W. and Suga, S., eds., Elsevier Science Publishers, Amsterdam, 1984.
9. **Bawden, J.,** Calcium transport during mineralization, *Anat. Record*, 224, 226, 1989.
10. **Enwonwu, C. O.,** Influence of socio-economic conditions on dental development in Nigerian children, *Arch. Oral. Biol.*, 18, 95, 1973.
11. **Sweeney, E. A., Saffir, A. J. and Leon, R.,** Linear hypoplasia of deciduous incisor teeth in malnourished children, *Am. J. Clin. Nutr.*, 24, 29, 1971.
12. **Toverud, G.,** The influence of war and post-war conditions on the teeth of Norwegian schoolchildren, I, *Millbank Memorial Fund Q.*, 34, 354, 1956.
13. **Gustafsson, B. E., Quensel, C. E., Lanke, L. S., Lundquist, C., Grahnen, H., Bonow, B. E. and Krasse, B.,** The Vipeholm dental caries study: the effect of different levels of carbohydrate intake on caries activity in 436 individuals observed for five years, *Acta Odont. Scand.*, 11, 232, 1954.
14. **Bowen, W. H.,** The cariostatic effect of calcium glycerophosphate in monkeys, *Caries Res.*, 6, 43, 1972.
15. **Murray, J. J., Rugg-Gunn, A. J. and Jenkins, G. N.,** *Fluorides in Caries Prevention*, 3rd ed., Wright, Oxford, 1991.
16. **Newbrun, E.,** *Cariology*, 3rd ed., Quintessence Books, Chicago, 1989.
17. **Rugg-Gunn, A.J.,** *Nutrition and Dental Health*, Oxford Medical Publications, Oxford, 1993.
18. **Bawden, J. W., ed.,** Workshop Report (Fluorides), *J. Dent. Res.*, 71, 1218, 1992.
19. **Eble, D. M., Deaton, T. G., Wilson, F. C., Jr. and Bawden, J. W.,** Fluoride concentrations in human and rat bone, *J. Public Health Dentistry*, 52, 288, 1992.
20. **Coumoulos, H. and Mellanby, M.,** Dental conditions of 5 year old children in institutions and private schools compared with LCC schools, *Br. Med. J.*, i, 751, 1947.

Chapter 9

COLLAGEN : THE MAJOR MATRIX MOLECULE IN MINERALIZED TISSUES

Mitsuo Yamauchi, D.D.S., Ph.D.

TABLE OF CONTENTS

I. INTRODUCTION

Bone is regarded as a composite tissue made up of basically two phases, an organic and an inorganic one. The inorganic phase of bovine cortical bone, composed of calcium and inorganic orthophosphate, represents approximately 75%, the organic phase 25%.[1] The predominant constituent of the bone organic matrix is fibrillar type I collagen (90% of the total matrix), and the noncollagenous components constitute the remainder. There is some evidence that trace amounts of

0-8493-7845-1/95/$0.00+$.50

type V are present in bone.[2] However, the predominant organic component of bone and dentin is type I collagen. The two phases (mineral and type I collagen fibrils) are arranged in the tissue in a highly ordered fashion, and structurally, they are closely associated with each other. This specific structural arrangement seems to be critical for the mechanical properties of bone (see review by Glimcher).[3] Due to this well-organized architectural arrangement between mineral crystals and type I collagen fibrils, bone tissue is mechanically very durable against external forces, such as tension and compression, and much stronger than either component would be alone.

In this chapter, the basic biochemical nature and characteristics of type I collagen in the mineralized tissues and its potential roles in the process of mineralization are described.

II. COLLAGEN FAMILY

Collagen is the most abundant protein in the mammal, accounting for about 30% of total proteins. This major structural protein is present in the extracellular space in essentially all connective tissues of the body. The unique feature of collagen is the presence of highly repetitive sequences of amino acids $[\text{Gly (glycine)-X-Y}]_n$ (often X is proline and Y hydroxyproline). This repetitive sequence allows three polypeptide chains (called α chains) to fold into a unique triple-helical structure. Every third amino acid is situated in the center of the triple helix in a very restricted space that can hold only glycine (Gly), the smallest amino acid. Therefore, the occurrence of Gly as the third amino acid is crucial for the collagen triple-helical structure. Each chain is twisted in the form of a left-handed helix, and then the three helical chains are intertwined with one another in a higher order ropelike right-handed triple helix structure (see Figure 2).

A. COLLAGEN CLASSIFICATION

Since collagen has been recognized as a family of structurally related proteins, a number of genetically distinct collagen types have been identified. At present, at least nineteen collagen types and more than 30 unique α chains, have been identified.[4] Each type has a characteristic tissue distribution and apparently a unique biological function. The discoveries of these new types of collagen during the last twenty years have caused some confusion in the definition of collagen. The advent of sophisticated protein chemistry techniques and molecular biology has been responsible for the early definitions based on the morphological features to the ones more related to the amino acid sequence, the protein structure, and the functions.[5] The general definition of a collagen molecule now is that it is a structural protein that contains one or more domains of a triple helix comprised of three polypeptides and assembled into an aggregate in the extracellular space.

These different types of collagen could be classified into three groups ; (1) fibril-forming, (2) fibril-associated (FACITs) and (3) nonfibrillar collagens.

Collagen Family
1. Fibril-forming : Types I, II, III, V, XI
2. FACIT (Fibril Associated Collagen with Interrupted Triple Helices): Types IX, XII, XIV?, XIX?
3. Others: Types IV, VI, VII, VIII, X, XIII —.

B. FIBRIL-FORMING COLLAGENS

All collagens that belong to the first group form fibrils in the various tissues, and they appear as a characteristic cross striation with repeating axial periods (called D periods) of about 67 nm in electron micrographs. The rod-shaped collagen molecules are packed in parallel and are staggered longitudinally with respect to one another by some multiple of the fibril axial repeat distance of about 67 nm.[6] This molecular packing arrangement creates alternate zones of high and low packing density along the direction of the fibril axis, overlap, and gap (hole) zones, respectively (see Figure 1).

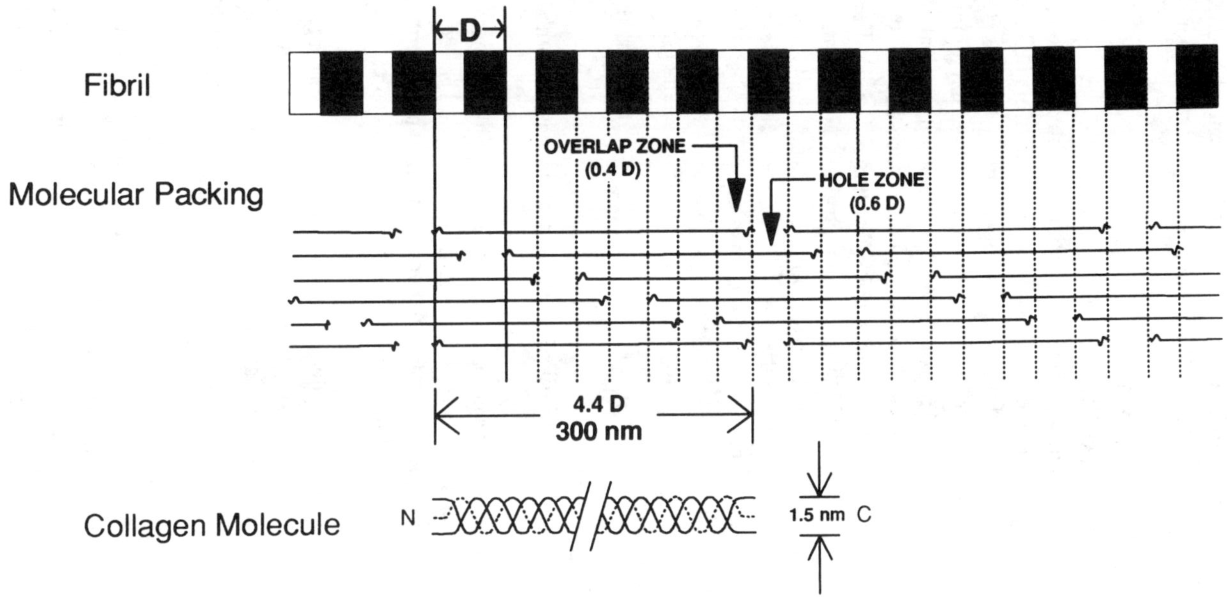

FIGURE 1. Two Dimensional Diagram of a Type I Collagen Fibril. The individual collagen molecules represented by lines are packed in parallel and staggered with respect to one another by 65-67 nm (called D period). This arrangement creates alternate regions of high (overlap) and low (gap or hole) packing density along the direction of fibrillar axis.

Although the overall striation pattern of these fibrils is similar in many connective tissues, detailed analyses using X-ray diffraction and electron microscopy have shown small but distinct differences in the D-period among different tissues. For instance, the D-period of skin and cornea fibrils is significantly shorter than that of tendon fibrils.[7,8] By identifying the structure, the quantity, and the molecular locus of the trifunctional intermolecular cross-link, histidinohydroxylysinonorleucine (HHL) (see later discussion), in the skin type I fibril, we and others have demonstrated that the molecular packing modality of skin is different from that of ligament and bone.[9-13] The specific molecular packing of skin and corneal fibrils likely generates the shorter D-period.

C. FIBRIL-ASSOCIATED COLLAGENS

Another group of collagens, types IX, XII, and XIV (possibly XIX), do not form fibrils themselves but appear to be closely associated with the fibrils. All these molecules contain more than one collagenous (triple helical) domain separated by noncollagenous (nontriple helical) domains.[14] The structure of these molecules can be divided into three main functional regions. One region serves for the interaction and adhesion of these molecules with the fibrils. A second region serves as a rigid arm that projects out of the fibril, and a third region serves for interaction with other matrix elements or with cells.[5] For instance, type IX collagen, the best characterized FACIT collagen, has three collagenous domains (COL 1-3) and four noncollagenous domains (NC 1-4). The NC 1 domain is present at the carboxy terminus and the NC4 at the amino terminus. NC2 connects COL 1 and 2, and NC3 connects COL 2 and 3. COL 1 and 2 appear to interact with the type II collagen fibrils, and COL 3 serves as the arm projecting out of the fibrils. It has been clearly demonstrated that the COL 2 domain of type IX is covalently cross-linked to nontriple helical domains of type II collagen.[15-17] A similar relationship may exist between types XII, XIV and type I fibrils. Thus, this group of collagens potentially functions as regulators of the fibril diameter and/or as bridges between fibrils and other components.

D. NONFIBRILLAR COLLAGENS

In addition to the fibril-forming and the fibril-associated collagens, a number of nonfibrillar collagens have been identified.

Type IV collagen, for example, is the principal collagenous component of basement membrane. This collagen, with other matrix components such as laminin, entactin, and perlecan, forms complex sheets underneath the basal lamina. This sheet-like network may provide a supporting framework with relatively large openings suitable for selective filtration of molecules through a basement membrane.

Type VI collagen is a heterotrimeric molecule with a short triple helix (100 nm) and two nontriple helical globular domains. These molecules are present in the extracellular space as oligomers that incorporate into microfibrils with a beaded appearance of 100 nm periodicity.[18] The type VI collagen microfibril may function as a connecting element between different fibrils, basement membrane, and cells.

Type VII contains a long discontinuous triple helical region (about 400 nm) with a large noncollagenous domain at the carboxyterminal end of the molecule. This collagen assembles into antiparallel dimers that overlap by 60 nm. The dimers then laterally aggregate, forming the principal component of anchoring fibrils that connects the epithelium to the dermis. A number of studies have indicated that inherited dystrophic epidermolysis bullosa, a disease with defects in anchoring fibrils, results from defects in the type VII collagen gene.

Type X collagen has a very restricted tissue distribution, which is in the zone of hypertrophic cartilage. The molecule is about half the size of the fibrillar collagens (138 nm vs. 300 nm), and it is composed of a small amino-terminal nonhelical domain, a triple helical domain, and a large carboxy-terminal nonhelical domain. It appears that type X collagen exists as fine filamentous mats surrounding hypertrophic chondrocytes or in association with the heterotypic (II-IX-XI) collagen fibrils in cartilage. Due to its highly restricted distribution at the interface between cartilage and

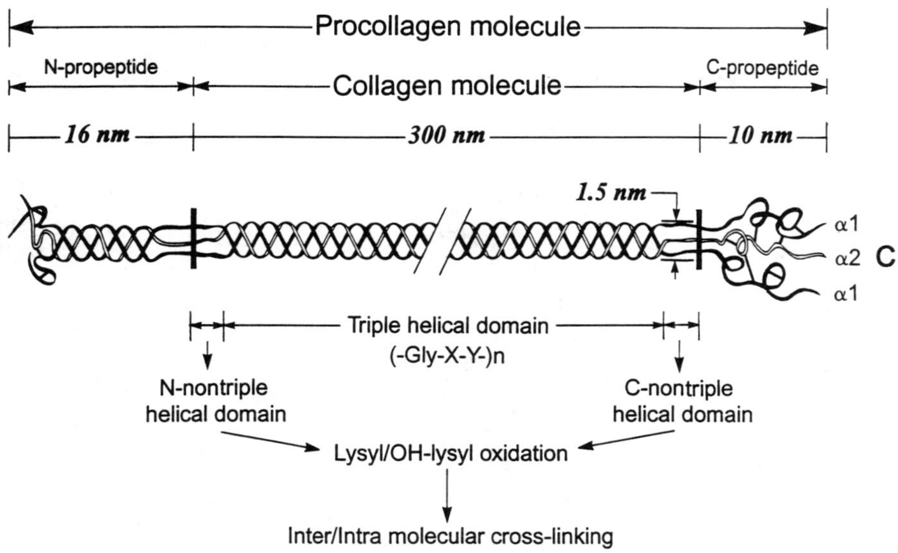

FIGURE 2. The Type I Procollagen Molecule Structure and Its Various Domains. After the C- and N-propeptide extensions are cleaved off during the extracellular processing, the collagen molecule has three domains: N-nontriple helical, triple helical, and C-nontriple helical domains. The central rodlike triple helical domain represents more than 95% of the molecule. Both C- and N-terminal nontriple helical domains contain Lysyl/OH-lysyl residues which can be converted to aldehyde (oxidative deamination) leading to cross-linking.

bone, the potential role of type X collagen in cartilagenous mineralization has been proposed. Immunohistochemical studies using antibodies against type X collagen showed the strongest reactivity at the mineralization boundary.[19]

Several studies have indicated an association of type X collagen to the matrix vesicles (MVs) that have been suggested by some investigators to play a critical role in the initiation of mineralization.[20-21] A recent study showed that the uptake of Ca^{2+} by MVs was markedly reduced when the MV-associated collagens II and X were removed from the MVs[22], indicating the binding of types II and X to MVs might play a role in cartilage mineralization. In addition, it has been reported that transgenic mice with a dominant negative mutation in type X collagen develop compression of hypertrophic growth plate cartilage and a decrease in newly formed bone, although mineralization itself is normal.[23] Some other data, however, have indicated that type X collagen has no effects on mineralization[24] or that it has rather an inhibitory effect on mineralization.[25] Possibly type X collagen provides the structural support in hypertrophic cartilage matrices by forming a pericellular polymeric lattice.[26]

The detailed structures and potential functions of these and other collagens have been provided in several excellent reviews and books.[5,27-30]

Of all these collagens, fibrillar type I collagen is by far the most abundant genetic product in the body. This type of collagen essentially represents the major extracellular matrix component in most tissues and organs.

III. TYPE I COLLAGEN

The type I collagen molecule is a heterotrimer composed of two α1 chains and one α2 chain, $[\alpha 1(I)_2\alpha 2(I)]$. This molecule consists of three domains: the NH_2-terminal nontriple helical, the triple helical, and the COOH-terminal nontriple helical domains. The single (uninterrupted) triple helical domain represents more than 95% of the molecule. The molecule is secreted by the cell as its precursor form, procollagen. The collagen molecule is generated outside the cell by enzymatic cleavages at both the C- and the N-terminal ends of the procollagen molecule (see Figure 2).

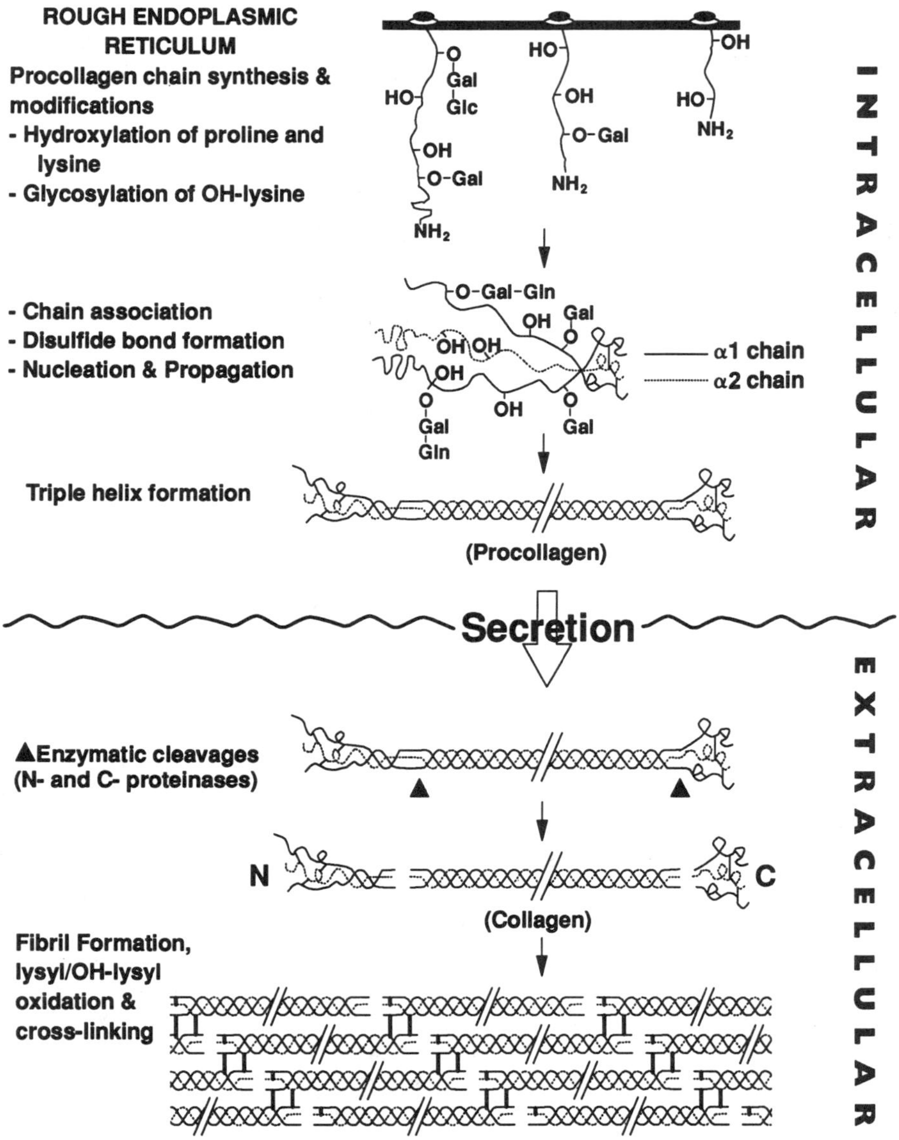

FIGURE 3. Sequential Events in the Biosynthesis of Type I Collagen. The individual proα chains are synthesized on the ribosomes of the rough endoplasmic reticulum and subjected to a number of co- and post-translational modifications. After hydroxylations of the specific prolyl and lysyl residues and glycosylations of the specific hydroxylysyl residues, the proα chains are associated, and the triple helix is formed from the C-terminal portion of the molecule by nucleated growth. The newly formed procollagen molecules are packed into the secretory vesicles and tranported to the extracellular space for further modifications. Both C- and N-propeptides of the procollagen molecules are cleaved off by specific enzymes to form the collagen molecules. The fully processed collagen molecules then self-assemble in a specific staggered manner to form fibrils. The molecules in the fibril are then stabilized by extensive intermolecular cross-linking.

A. BIOSYNTHESIS

The biosynthesis of type I collagen is a complicated, multistep process.[31] Translation of the mRNAs of pre-procollagen chains is initiated with the synthesis of signal peptide extensions, and the newly synthesized polypeptides acquire a number of co- and posttranslational modifications. These modifications that take place intra- and extracellularly require the act of at least 10 different enzymes, and many of them are unique to collagens and other proteins containing collagenous sequences (see Figure 3).

B. INTRACELLULAR MODIFICATION

The important intracellular modifications of procollagen polypeptide (proα) chains include hydroxylation of specific lysyl and prolyl residues and the glycosylation of specific hydroxylysine residues. Prolyl (Pro) residues at the N-terminal side of glycine (-Pro-Gly) are hydroxylated to form hydroxyproline (Hyp) catalyzed by prolyl hydroxylases (prolyl-4- and prolyl-3-hydroxylases). In a similar manner some of the lysyl (Lys) residues in -Lys-Gly sequences are hydroxylated to form hydroxylysine (Hyl) catalyzed by lysyl hydroxylase. All three enzymes appear to be inactive against a triple helical structure; therefore, these modifications must occur before the formation of the triple helix. Hydroxyproline is important for stabilization of the triple helical structure of the collagen molecule. Hydroxylysine is for directing certain cross-linking pathways, and it also is the glycosylation site of the molecule. Two types of O-linked glycosylation (galactosyl- and glucosyl-galactosyl-) are known to occur on the specific hydroxylysine residues present in triple-helical domains. These glycosylations are catalyzed by hydroxylysyl galactosyl transferase and galactosyl hydroxylysyl glucosyl transferase, respectively. The role of glycosylation of hydroxylysine residues is still not well understood; however, the presence of these bulky groups within the molecule could sterically hinder the lateral packing of collagen molecules.[32] The less dense packing of type II collagen fibrils could be due to the high degree of glycosylation of the molecules. Glycosylation of hydroxylysine residues also could influence cross-linking maturation.[9,33] The N-linked glycosylation of an asparagyl residue in the C-propeptide also occurs. Two proα1(I) chains and one proα2(I) chain are then intertwined through the COOH-terminal propeptides. This association allows a nucleus of triple helix formation. Once the nucleus of triple helix forms, it rapidly propagates in a zipper-like fashion from the C- to the N-terminus of the protein.[34] Finally, formed procollagen molecules are packaged in saccules, transformed into secretory granules, and secreted to extracellular space, passing through the Golgi complex.

C. EXTRACELLULAR PROCESSING

Outside the cell, the procollagen molecule is further processed by cleavages of both the N- and C-terminal propeptide extensions to form a collagen molecule. The cleavages take place by the action of two distinctive proteinases, procollagen N-proteinase and procollagen C-proteinase. These propeptide extensions in the tissue have been proposed to play a role in fibrillogenesis.[35] The processed collagen molecules then spontaneously self-aggregate through clusters of charge and hydrophobicity of the triple helical portion of the molecule to form a fibril.

Type I collagen molecules appear to be packed together into fibrils in a very specific manner in which the molecules are longitudinally staggered with respect to one another by specific multiples of 67 nm and have specific lateral orientations with respect to one another.[6]

Although type I collagen, a product of two single genes (α1 and α2), is the most ubiquitous protein in the body's various connective tissues, the chemistry varies from tissue to tissue because of posttranslational modifications. As briefly described above, the modality of molecular packing as well as the cross-linking chemistry of type I collagen (see below) are tissue-specific, and this specificity seems to be important for the physiological functions of each tissue.

IV. TYPE I COLLAGEN IN MINERALIZED TISSUES

The fibrillar type I collagen has a number of essential roles in the mineralization of bone. Type I collagen, first of all, defines compartments within the tissue that become impregnated with mineral. It then provides a periodic, three-dimensional template for the orderly deposition and packing of the bone mineral crystals. The final result of the presence of type I collagen is the formation of a rigid, space-filling biomaterial that is very strong for its weight and much stronger than either component would be alone. Type I collagen may also serve as a stable substrate for the polyanionic matrix components in the tissue that facilitate the initiation of mineralization.

The collagen in the mineralized tissues is present in the form of axially periodic fibrils consisting of type I collagen molecules. It has been well documented that, at least in vertebrate systems, fibrillar collagen and mineral crystals are closely associated to each other.[36-37] When Hodge and Petruska proposed the D-staggered model of the collagen fibril,[6] they suggested that the gap (hole) zones created between the ends of the molecules could be the sites of mineral deposition in bone. In fact, electron micrographs of mineralized tissues have shown that the initial mineral crystal deposition occurs preferentially at the gap zones corresponding to the axial repeat of the collagen fibrils.[38-40] In addition, data from a number of recent reports indicate that the initial crystals are plate-shaped, that they are mainly located within the collagen fibrils (preferentially in the gap zones), and that they are oriented in parallel to each other and to the long axis of the collagen fibrils.[41-43]

The size and growth, as well as the orientation of the initial crystals, suggest that they are accommodated by channels or grooves in the collagen fibril formed by contiguous adjacent gaps. This arrangement is consistent with the molecular packing model proposed previously.[44,45] It has also been reported that during collagen mineralization, changes take place in the shape of the collagen fibrils[46,47] and in the geometry of the molecular organization within a fibril.[45,48,49] All these studies indicate that the bone collagen fibril itself has a structure providing an organized space and a stable template for the orderly deposition of mineral crystals within the fibrils. Later it properly distorts encasing a large mass of minerals. What is the molecular basis of this dynamic nature of collagen fibrils that seems to be important for the proper mineralization? Are there any differences in type I collagen fibrils between nonmineralized and mineralized tissues?

Although bone (and dentin) type I collagen has essentially the same chemical composition, molecular structure, and chain composition as those of soft connective tissues, its physicochemical properties differ significantly from other type I collagens. Bone collagen, for example, has different mechanical properties, has the ability to renature after thermal denaturation, is highly insoluble, and fails to swell in mild acid.[3] Because all the type I collagens possess essentially the same primary structure, these distinct physicochemical differences are most likely derived from the differences in the posttranslational modifications of bone collagen. Indeed, for instance, rat bone type I collagen contains 15 residues of hydroxylysines/1,000 amino acids, whereas rat skin type I collagen contains only 5 residues/1,000. Also, dentin collagen contains two to three times as much hydroxylysine than that of skin.[50-51] However, the most distinct feature of type I collagen in mineralized tissues can be seen in its cross-linking chemistry and molecular packing structure.

V. CROSS-LINKING OF COLLAGEN

The process of cross-linking of collagen is crucial in order for the connective tissues to function properly. The intermolecular cross-linking provides the fibrillar matrices with various mechanical properties such as tensile strength and viscoelasticity.[52] Collagen cross-linking has been extensively reviewed by several authors during the last decade.[53-56] In this section, therefore, only the basic mechanisms of cross-linking of type I collagen, the characteristics of cross-linking of mineralized tissue collagens, and the potential roles of these in mineralization are described.

A. BASIC MECHANISMS OF CROSS-LINKING

All the known cross-links of type I collagen (proven by the isolation and characterization of the cross-linked peptides) are condensation products between the prosthetic groups of juxtaposed specific peptidyl residues of lysine (Lys), hydroxylysine (Hyl), and histidine (His). The process of cross-linking is initiated by the enzymatic oxidative deamination by lysyl oxidase of ε-amino groups on specific peptidyl Lys and Hyl to aldehyde (see Figure 4). These are located at both the carboxy- and the amino-terminal nontriple helical domains of a molecule (hereafter referred to as C-domain and N-domain, respectively), the 16^C residues are on the C-domains and the 9^N residues are on the N-domains of the two $\alpha 1$ chains, and the residue 5^N is on the N-domain of the single $\alpha 2$ chain in the molecule.[57] Therefore, there are five residues (two at the C-domain and three at the N-domain) that are potentially converted to aldehyde. The aldehydes formed are 5-amino-5-carboxypentanal

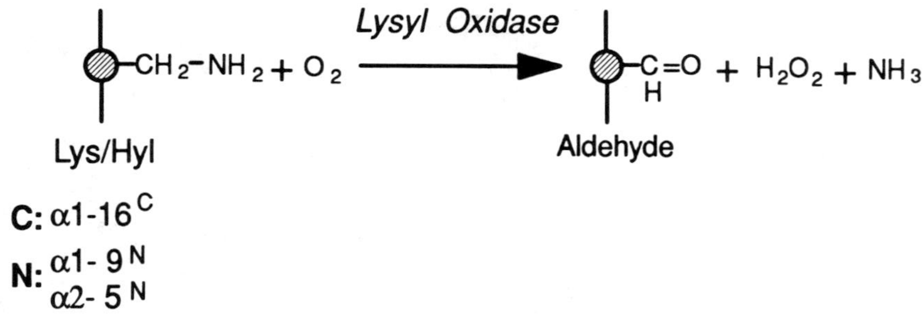

FIGURE 4. Formation of Aldehyde of Specific Peptidyl Lysyl and Hydroxylysyl Residues through the Action of Lysyl Oxidase. These residues are located at the 16th position in the C-nontriple helical domain of α1 chains, the 9th and 5th in the N-nontriple helical domains of α1 and α2 chains, respectively.

(Lys^{ald} , α-amino adipic acid-δ-semialdehyde, allysine) and 2-hydroxy-5-amino-5-carboxypentanal (Hyl^{ald}, δ-hydroxy-α-amino adipic acid-δ-semialdehyde, hydroxyallysine), respectively.

Lysyl oxidase (EC 1.4.3.13) is a copper-dependent amine oxidase that requires molecular oxygen and a carbonyl cofactor. Although the latter compound is not precisely identified, some data suggest a role for pyrroloquinoline quinone (methoxatin, PQQ) in the function of this enzyme.[58] The early studies have indicated that this enzyme binds to and is highly reactive to the fibrils but not against the collagen molecules in solution or α chains.[59] Our recent studies, however, indicate that, at least in some tissues, most if not all Lys/Hyl at the C-nontriple helical domains of all collagen molecules in the type I fibrils are converted to aldehyde.[9,11,60,61] This implies that the oxidative deamination reaction of Lys/Hyl has to take place during fibrillogenesis, probably at a very early stage. Irreversible inhibition of the lysyl oxidase by lathyrogens such as β-aminopropionitrile and D-penicillamine at high doses causes connective tissue fragility and rupture because of the lack of cross-linking.[52] This classical example of inhibition of a biochemical pathway clearly indicates the biological relevance of collagen cross-linking.

The aldehydes formed (Lys^{ald} and Hyl^{ald}) then undergo a series of condensation reactions to form complex intra- and inter molecular cross-links in the fibril. The iminium divalent intermolecular cross-links seem to be the first to form (see Figure 5) and then mature into more complex multivalent cross-links.[55]

The patterns of cross-linking, including the pathways, the concentration of the individual cross-links, and their molecular distributions, vary from tissue to tissue.[54-55] These patterns seem to be tissue specific and are probably related to the tissue's physiological functions but not to the particular types of collagen. Even within the same tissue, the cross-linking to some extent varies depending on sites within the tissue.[62] The tissue specificity of cross-linking could be due to various factors. Because cross-link condensation reactions, except for the initial oxidation step, are spontaneous, turnover rate is an important factor in regulating cross-link maturation. Periodontal ligament collagen, for instance, has little mature stable cross-links, likely due to its high rate of turnover.[9] The lack of the stable cross-links, in turn, makes the periodontal ligament collagen degrade more readily. The degree of hydroxylation of Lys is also a factor in regulating the pathway.[64] The degree of Hyl glycosylation can possibly influence cross-link maturation.[9,33] The modality of molecular packing is undoubtedly a key factor for the cross-link patterning because it determines the microenvironment for the reaction of the specific amino acid residues. For instance, a fraction of molecules in skin collagen fibrils are packed almost in register, which allows the fibril to form a particular trifunctional cross-link in a mature animal.[10,12,13] The packing in ligament, tendon, and bone appears to be different.[9,65,66] The diagram in Figure 6 represents the major cross-linking pathway in nonmineralized tissues.

There are two types of pathways that derive from Lys^{ald}. One leads to the formation of dehydro-histidinohydroxymerodesmosine (deH-HHMD) via aldol. Another leads to the formation of histidino-hydroxylysinonorleucine (HHL)[10, 67] via the iminium cross-link, dehydro-hydroxylysinonorleucine

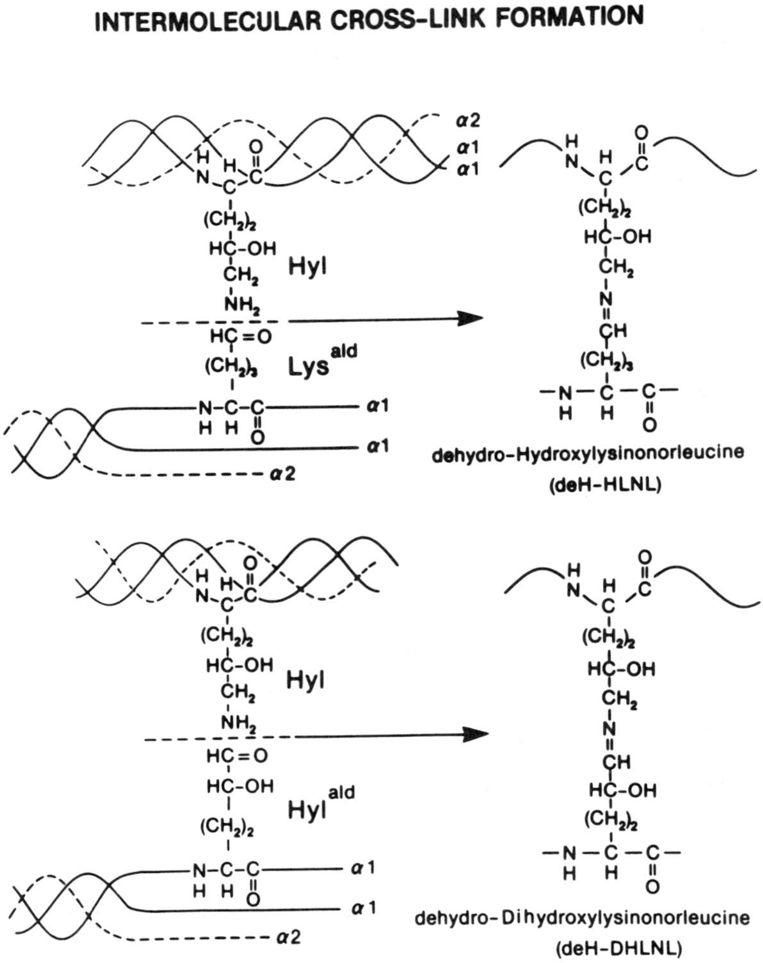

FIGURE 5. Formation of Bifunctional Intermolecular Cross-Links.

(deH-HLNL). The former mainly occurs in the N-domain of the collagen molecule in soft connective tissues such as ligament, tendon, skin, and cornea.[68-69] The latter occurs in the C-domain of the molecule in skin[10,12,33] and cornea (Yamauchi, unpublished data).

The pathway that derives from Hyl^{ald} is predominant in skeletal tissues such as bone, cartilage, tendon, and dentin. Pyridinoline[70,71] is probably the maturational cross-link in this pathway (see Figure 7).[54] In mineralized tissues such as bone and dentin, the major Hyl^{ald} and its cross-linking pathway is located at the C-domain of the molecule.[11,60,61,67,72] Recently, it has been shown that mineralizing collagens have a distinct cross-linking chemistry and 3-dimensional structure that correlate well with their function in the process of mineralization.[9,11,13,60,61,66]

B. BONE COLLAGEN CROSS-LINKING AND ITS POTENTIAL ROLE IN MINERALIZATION

The intermolecular cross-linking of bone collagen is intimately related to the the way collagen molecules are arranged in a fibril. Cross-linking is initiated with the conversion of the specific peptidyl Hyl, mainly at the C- domain of the collagen molecules soon after the molecule is synthesized. These aldehydes are located at the boundaries of the "hole" zones and react with the juxtaposed Hyl on neighboring molecules to form bifunctional cross-links (dehydro-dihydroxylysinonorleucine, deH-DHLNL (see Figure 5) prior to mineralization.[11,60,61] These cross-links are capable of tautomerizing between an iminium and a keto form. When two such cross-links

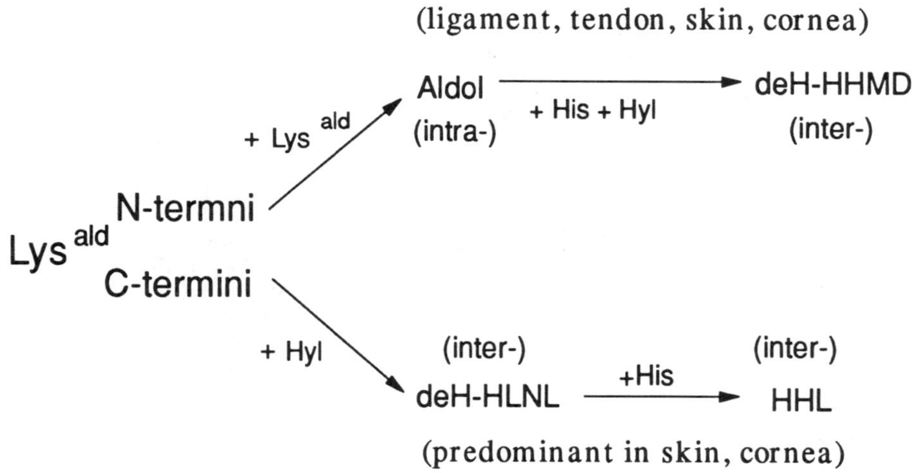

FIGURE 6. Lys^{ald}-Derived Pathways. These are the major cross-linking pathways in nonmineralized tissues.

are able to contact each other, they can condense to form a complex cross-link, pyridinoline.[55,73] Whether pyridinoline ties three collagen molecules or only two molecules is not certain at present. The latter imposes fewer constraints on the arrangements of fibrils than does the former. As a minor form, the lysyl analog of pyridinoline (deoxypyridinoline or lysylpyridinoline) is present in some tissues. It comprises two Hyls and one Lys and appears to be present mainly in mineralized tissues.[54,66] The ratio of pyridinoline to deoxypyridinoline cross-links in human bone is 3 or 4 to 1 and they appear to reach the maximum concentration by 10–15 years of age and remain in the same range throughout adult life.[74]

It has been found that the cross-linking between the C-domain aldehyde and the Hyl on an adjacent molecule is stereospecific in nature, favoring the Hyl on α1 chains over an α2 chain.[11] By using a computer simulation model (Monte Carlo method) Katz et al. found that such specificity was due to the stereospecific packing of the bone collagen molecules themselves.[13] The results of this bifurcating cross-linking pattern in a stereospecific manner is to connect groups of the molecules laterally in a sheet-like structure. These laterally-connected molecules become the mechanical element of a bone collagen fibril. Such cross-linking also laterally connects adjacent "hole" regions into zones having plate-like shapes, with overall dimensions similar to those determined on isolated bone mineral crystals.[41] Moreover, the connectivity established by the initial lateral cross-linking appears to decrease by dissociation of the iminium bond of the deH-DHLNL cross-link when collagen is mineralized. This is possibly due to the deformation of collagen fibrils brought about by the growth of mineral crystals within the fibrils. This occurs in dentin,[60] mineralizing turkey tendon,[66] and bone.[61] These findings indicate that collagen cross-linking and fibrillar structures are dynamic during mineralization, regulating the size, shape, and location of mineral crystals within the fibrils and are in agreement with X-ray diffraction and NMR studies (see Figure 8).

The state of the N-domain seems to be another unique structural feature of mineralizing collagens. Our indirect data suggest that this portion of the molecule does not participate in cross-linking reactions as much as the C-domain does. As collagen mineralization appears to begin at the N-domain ends of the hole zones,[75] an epitaxial role for the N-domain ends in bone is possible.

Histidinoalanine and lysinoalanine are two nonreducible cross-linking amino acids isolated from calcified tissue matrices.[76,77] These cross-links were originally thought to be derived from mineralized tissue collagen; however, more recent studies by Kuboki and his co-workers indicate that these cross-links are rather associated with phosphoproteins.[78-79] Whether these cross-links tie phosphoproteins to collagen fibrils is still not known.

In addition to the lysyl oxidase-mediated cross-links described above, sugar-derived (nonenzymatically glycosylated or glycated) cross-links have been reported to occur in extracellular

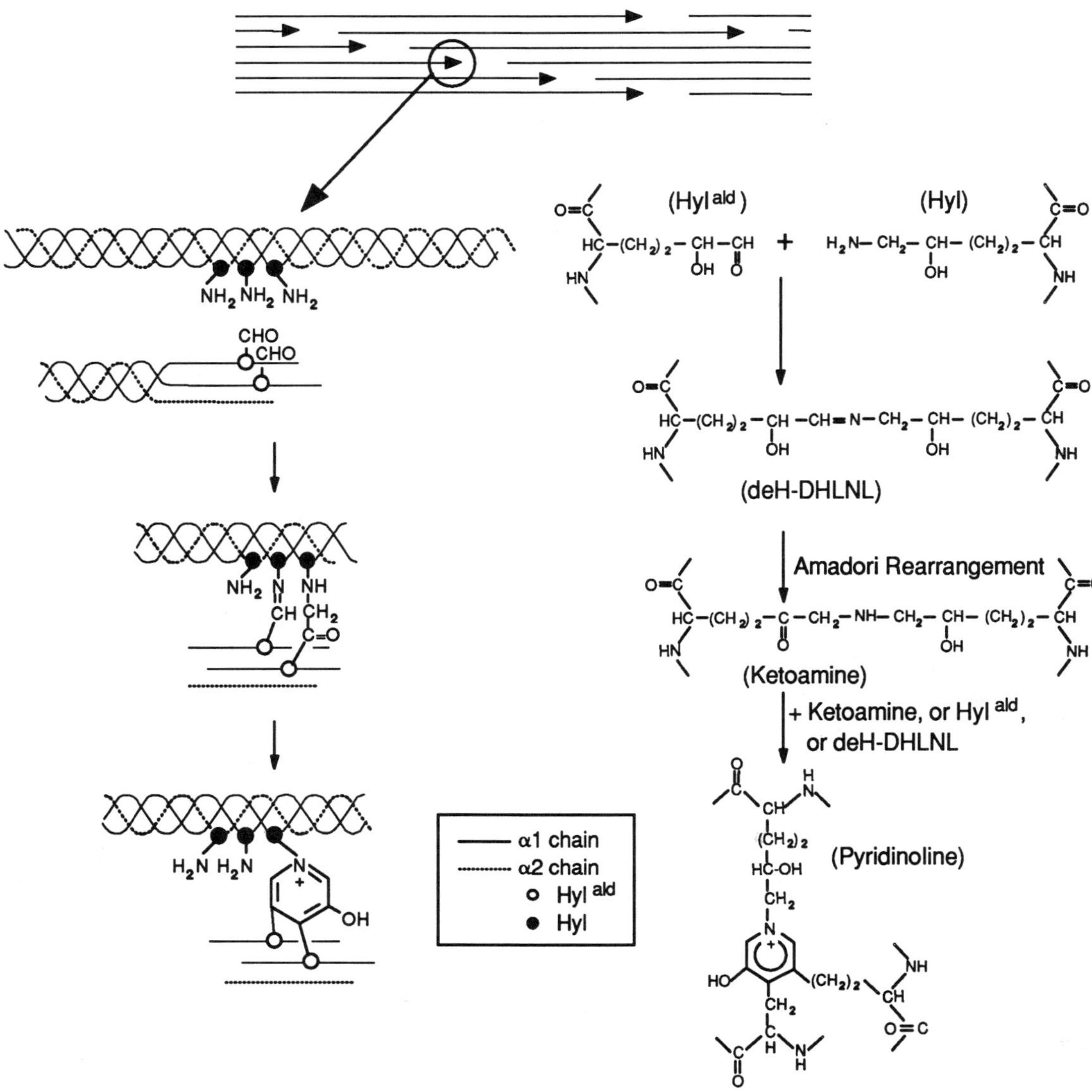

FIGURE 7. The Major Cross-Linking Pathway in Mineralized Tissue Collagen. In the top panel, each horizontal line represents a collagen molecule with an arrow being the C-termini of the molecule. On the left the schematic diagram of cross-linking pathway at the C-nontriple helical domain is shown. On the right, the detailed chemistry corresponding to the left side diagram is shown. Note that the direction of the molecules on the right panel does not correspond to that of the left. The mechanism for the formation of pyridinoline is not completely clear at present. The feasible mechanism would be the condensation between a ketoamine and an iminium cross-link.[55] Several data have indicated that not all deH-DHLNL cross-links mature into pyridinoline.

matrix proteins including collagen, and these are thought to be related to aging and diabetes.[80,81] Recently, the preferential glycation sites of type I collagen have been determined by analyzing the various peptide fragments generated by CNBr and trypsin treatments.[82] The occurrence and significance of these types of cross-links in mineralized tissue collagens are yet to be determined.

VI. BONE DISORDERS AND COLLAGEN

Two major bone disorders involving collagen alterations, namely osteogenesis imperfecta and osteopororis, are briefly reviewed in the following sections.

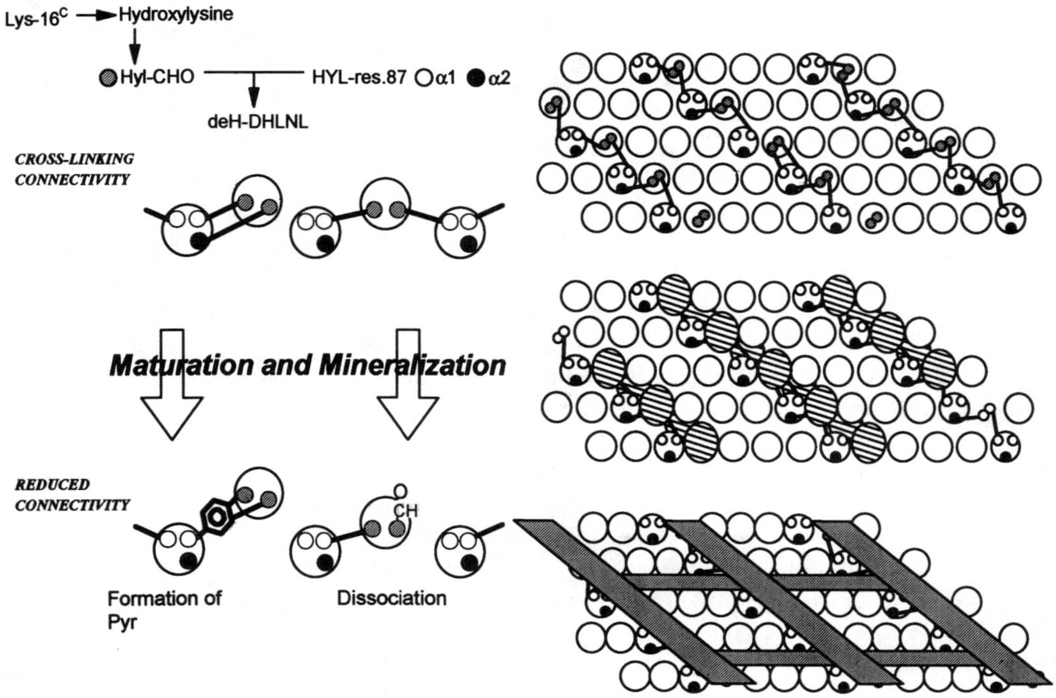

FIGURE 8. Cross sectional illustration of the COOH-Terminal Cross-Linking Connectivity and Mineralization. On the left, the type I collagen molecules are represented as large circles with the position of 87-Hyl in α1 chains indicated by small open circles, 87-Hyl in α2 chains by small closed circles, and the two α1 chain 16^C-Hyl^{ald} residues by small shaded circles. Before mineralization, the bifunctional cross-link, deH-DHLNL is formed between α1 chain 16^C-Hyl^{ald} and 87-Hyl in α1 chain or α2 chain on staggered adjacent molecules. The ratio of cross-links involving 87-Hyl from α1 chains to those involving α2 chains (about 3 to 1) strongly indicates the fixed angular orientation of the molecules. As a result, the collagen molecules are laterally connected to one another forming a sheet (see the top panel on the right) providing the young nonmineralized fibrils with a stable template. Such a template may facilitate the orderly precipitation of mineral at the early stage of mineralization (see the middle panel on the right.) Then some of the bifunctional cross-links mature into a trifunctional cross-link, pyridinoline, as a result of maturation, but, some dissociate back to the their reactant state, Hyl^{ald} and Hyl, as a result of mineralization (see the text). This proper distortion as a result of reduction of cross-link connectivity may allow the fibrils to encase the large quantity of mineral crystals mass (see the bottom panel on the right). (Modified from References 45 and 60)

A. OSTEOGENESIS IMPERFECTA

Osteogenesis imperfecta (OI) is characterized by "a brittleness of bone" that is apparent early in life. The disease is heterogenous and classified into several phenotypes. A number of biochemical and genetic studies have demonstrated that almost all cases of OI are due to mutations in type I collagen.[4] The mutations include partial gene deletion, partial gene duplications, and RNA splicing mutations, but the most common mutations so far are single-base substitutions that convert a codon for Gly to a codon for another amino acid within the major triple helical domain of proα1 or proα2 chains.[83] As has been described above, the triple helical domain of the molecule (>95% of the molecule) contains a large number of repetitive tripeptide units (338 triplets), Gly-X-Y. The occurrence of Gly as every third amino acid is essential for triple helical formation (see earlier). A single mutation that causes the conversion of Gly to an amino acid with a bulkier side chain, therefore, can cause deleterious effects on the chain folding leading to an impediment to the triple helical conformation. These Gly substitutions can generate procollagen molecules with incorrect structures, which cause their degradation as they are slowly secreted in a process referred to as "procollagen suicide".[84] In some cases a triple helix is formed, but there are subtle changes in the conformation of the protein such as a flexible kink within the triple helical domain.[85] The collagen containing such a kink drastically disrupts the proper fibril formation. Other mutated collagens are incorporated into fibrils, but the fibrils are weaker than normal.[84]

In bone, the fibrils that contain mutated molecules may not generate the proper structure of molecular packing that is important for proper cross-linking and mineralization (see earlier). In that case, the deposition and growth of mineral crystals within the fibrils could be impaired, leading to poorly organized mineralization. In fact, calcifying tendon of OI mice (oim/oim) contains collagen fibrils that are disorganized and do not appear to have a continuous channel generated by connected hole zones. Mineral crystals are larger and irregular when compared to those of normal animals, indicating that their size and growth are not well controlled.[86] These data also indicate the importance of an organized molecular packing structure of collagen fibrils for proper mineralization. The domain-specific interaction of collagen fibrils with other macromolecules such as phosphoproteins and/or proteoglycans could also be disrupted by the incorporation of mutated molecules into the fibrils. In the past alterations were reported in cross-linking in bone collagen in OI patients, although these analyses were limited to reducible cross-links.[87,88] Further studies are necessary to understand the molecular mechanisms of the bone brittleness induced by these mutations.

B. OSTEOPOROSIS

It is often difficult to distinguish the mild type of OI from osteoporosis. Similar mutations in the type I collagen gene (Gly → Ser, Gly → Cys) have recently been reported in some patients with osteoporosis[89,90] indicating a phenotypic overlap between OI and osteoporosis. Most patients with osteoporosis due to the mutations in type I collagen reported so far have not only osteoporosis but also other abnormalities. Other types of mutation such as substitutions of the X or Y position of the triplets (Gly-X-Y) may not cause OI but may cause milder diseases such as osteoporosis.[4] This type of mutation could again alter the fibrillar packing structure leading to alteration of mineralization. Cross-link alterations in monkey bone collagen from disuse osteoporosis[91] and also in human osteoporosis[92] have been reported.

Other bone disease states also have shown cross-link changes such as those that occur in vitamin D deficiency,[93-95] osteogenic osteoblastoma,[95,96] and osteopetrosis.[97] These data indicate that collagen cross-linking is altered under various pathological conditions of bone that could, in turn, possibly have deleterious effects on the mineralization process resulting in impaired mechanical properties of bone.

VII. INTERACTION BETWEEN COLLAGEN AND ACIDIC MACROMOLECULES IN MINERALIZED TISSUES

Although it has been demonstrated that collagen fibrils provide sites for mineralization, the initiation of mineralization (nucleation) is likely regulated by many other factors, i.e. macromolecules that can associate with the collagen fibrils, and at the same time, interact with Ca^{2+}. Such components can enhance Ca^{2+} concentration near the collagen fibrils and then initiate the nucleation of the apatite crystals. There are several phosphoproteins identified in bone and dentin, e.g., osteopontin (OPN), bone sialoprotein (BSP), bone acidic glycoprotein-75 (BAG-75), and dentin phosphophyryns (dPPs).[98,99] Of these, the dPP seems to offer interesting characteristics that can be related in many ways to the mineralization process of dentin.[100,101] It has been shown that (1) the dPPs are deposited directly at the mineralization front of dentin,[102,103] (2) the protein possesses a very unusual composition that makes it extremely acidic, and (3) it interacts with collagen fibrils.[104] More recently it has been shown that the dPP specifically binds to the locus of the e-band of the collagen fibril, a region near the hole (gap) zone of the fibril.[105] Since the dPP associated with collagen fibrils still retains the Ca^{2+}-binding property, the dPP secreted onto the surfaces of collagen fibrils in the dentin mineralization front could initiate the nucleation of apatite crystals around the gap zone of collagen fibrils.[101] Previous studies have also indicated that such an interaction between phosphophoryn and the stable polymer (i.e., collagen fibril) is critical for inducing mineralization from metastable solutions that do not spontaneously precipitate.[106,107] Whether this type of interaction between the collagen fibril and an anionic protein takes place in bone, and if so, which protein is involved in this process, remain to be investigated.

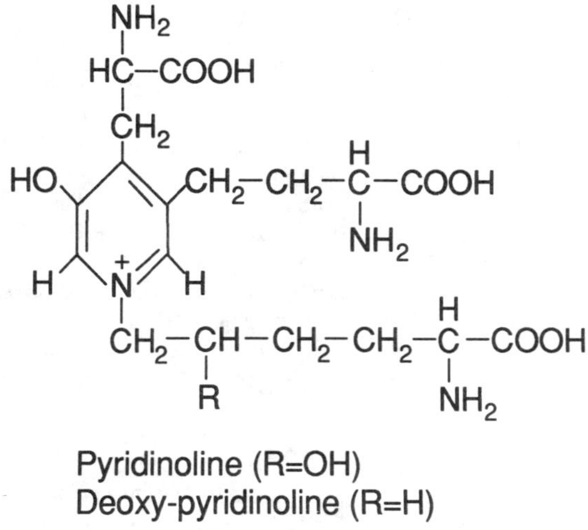

FIGURE 9. Structure of Pyridinoline and Deoxypyridinoline.

VIII. COLLAGEN CROSS-LINKS AS BIOMARKERS OF BONE RESORPTION

Recently there has been considerable interest in measurements of urinary pyridinoline and deoxypyridinoline (see Figure 9) as indices of bone resorption.[108,109] (also see Chapter 10)

Although pyridinoline is present in various connective tissues other than bone (cartilage, ligament, tendon, dentin, etc.), the urinary excretion from these tissues is much lower than that from bone because of their slow turnover in contrast to bone, which is a dynamic tissue undergoing remodeling throughout life. The measurement of urinary excretion seems to have many advantages over the conventional measurements due to its specificity and sensitivity, and both cross-links are promising markers for the assessment of bone resorption in various bone metabolic diseases.[110] Development of specific antibodies that recognize these cross-links and surrounding peptides will further improve the tissue specificity and sensitivity.

IX. SUMMARY

Fibrillar collagen makes up about 90% of the organic matrices of bone and dentin. Unlike other connective tissues, the collagen composition in bone and dentin is remarkably simple, consisting almost exclusively of type I. Although this ubiquitous protein is the product of two single genes (one for α1 chain and the other for α2 chain), the posttranslational chemistry varies from tissue to tissue. Recent studies have indicated that the type I collagen fibril structure in mineralized tissues may facilitate the proper mineralization, and intermolecular cross-linking appears to play a role in this process. The further elucidation of this dynamic nature of fibrillar structure is important in order to understand the fundamental mechanism(s) of mineralization.

This chapter focused on the structure of type I collagen in mineralized tissues and its relation to mineralization. A number of important subjects of mineralized tissue collagen such as regulation of synthesis, degradation, and assembly have not been detailed in this chapter. In order to understand the biological role of collagen in mineralized tissues, extensive studies including molecular genetics, protein chemistry, and metabolic studies will be needed.

ACKNOWLEDGMENT

This work was supported by NIH grant DE10489 and NASA grant NAGW-3946. The author thanks Ms. G.S. Chandler for her help in the preparation of this chapter.

REFERENCES

1. **Herring, G.M.,** The organic matrix of bone, in *The Biochemistry and Physiology of Bone,* vol 1, G.H. Bourne, ed., Academic Press, New York, 1972.
2. **Niyibizi, C. and Eyre, D. R.,** Identification of the cartilage α1 (XI) chain in type V collagen from bovine bone, *FEBS Lett.*, 242, 314, 1989.
3. **Glimcher, M. J.,** Composition, structure, and organization of bone and other mineralized tissues and the mechanism of calcification, in *Handbook of Physiology: vol 7 Endocrinology,* Greep, R.O. and Astwood, E.B., eds., American Physiological Society, Washington D.C., 1976.
4. **Kivirikko, K. I.,** Collagens and their abnormalities in a wide spectrum of diseases, *Annals of Medicine,* 25,113, 1993.
5. **van der Rest, M. and Garrone, R.,** Collagen family of proteins, *FASEB J.*, 5, 2814, 1991.
6. **Hodge, A. J. and Petruska, J. A.,** Recent studies with the electron microscope on ordered aggregates of the tropocollagen macromolecule, in *Aspects of Protein Structure,* Ramachandran, G. N., ed., New York, Academic Press, 1963.
7. **Brodsky, B., Eikenberry, E. F., and Cassidy, K.,** An unusual collagen periodicity in skin, *Biochem. Biophys. Acta,* 621, 162, 1980.
8. **Marchini, M., Morocutti, M., Ruggeri, A., Koch, M. H. J., Bigi, A. and Roveri, N.,** Differences in the fibril structure of corneal and tendon collagen. An electron microscopy and X-ray diffraction investigation, *Conn. Tissue Res.*, 15, 269, 1986.
9. **Yamauchi, M., Katz, E. P. and Mechanic, G. L.,** Intermolecular cross-linking and stereospecific molecular packing in type I collagen fibrils of the periodontal ligament, *Biochemistry,* 25, 4907, 1986.
10. **Yamauchi, M., London, R. E., Guenat, C., Hashimoto, F. and Mechanic, G.L.,** Structure and formation of a stable histidine-based trifunctional cross-link in skin collagen, *J. Biol. Chem.*, 262, 11428, 1987.
11. **Yamauchi, M., Katz, E. P., Otsubo, K., Teraoka, K. and Mechanic, G.L.,** Cross-linking and stereo-specific structure of collagen in mineralized and nonmineralized skeletal tissues, *Conn. Tissue Res.*, 21, 159, 1989.
12. **Mechanic, G. L., Katz, E. P., Henmi, M., Noyes, C. and Yamauchi, M.,** Locus of a histidine-based, stable trifunctional, helix to helix collagen cross-link: stereospecific collagen structure of type I skin fibrils, *Biochemistry,* 26, 3500, 1987.
13. **Katz, E. P. and David, C.,** Unique side-chain conformation encoding for chirality and azimuthal orientation in the molecular packing of skin collagen, *J. Mol. Biol.*, 228, 963, 1992.
14. **Shaw, L. M. and Olsen, B. R.,** FACIT collagens: diverse molecular bridges in extracellular matrices, *TIBS,* 16, 191, 1991.
15. **Eyre, D. R., Apone, S. and Wu, J. J.,** Collagen type IX: evidence for covalent linkages to type II collagen in cartilage, *FEBS Lett.*, 220, 337, 1987.
16. **van der Rest, M. and Mayne, R.,** Type IX collagen proteoglycan from cartilage is covalently cross-linked to type II collagen, *J. Biol. Chem.*, 262, 1615, 1988.
17. **Wu, J. J., Woods, P. E. and Eyre, D. R.,** Identification of cross-linking sites in bovine cartilage type IX collagen reveals an antiparallel type II-type IX molecular relationship and type IX to type IX bonding, *J. Biol. Chem.*, 267, 23007, 1992.
18. **Timpl, R. and Engel, J.,** Type VI collagen, in *Structure and Function of Collagen Types,* Mayne, R. and Burgeson, R. E., eds., Academic Press, Orlando, Florida, 1987.
19. **Schmid, T. M., Popp, R. G. and Linsenmayer, T. F.,** Hypertrophic cartilage matrix: Type X collagen, supramolecular assembly and calcification, *Ann. N.Y. Acad. Sci.*, 580, 64, 1990.
20. **Bonuci, E.,** Fine structure of early cartilage calcification, *J. Ultrastruct. Res.*, 20, 33, 1967.
21. **Anderson, H. C.,** Vesicles associated with calcification in the matrix of epiphyseal cartilage, *J. Cell Biol.*, 41, 59, 1969.
22. **Kirsch, T. and Wuthier, R. E.,** Stimulation of calcification of growth plate cartilage matrix vesicles by binding to type II and X collagens, *J. Biol. Chem.*, 269, 11462, 1994.
23. **Jacenko, O., LuValle, P. A. and Olsen, B. R.,** Spondylometaphyseal dysplasia in mice carrying a dominant negative mutation in a matrix protein specific for cartilage-to-bone transition, *Nature,* 365, 56, 1993.
24. **Boskey, A. L., Maresca, M. and Appel, J.,**The effects of noncollagenous matrix proteins on hydroxyapatite formation and proliferation in a collagen gel system, *Conn. Tis. Res.*, 21, 171, 1989.
25. **Poole, A. R. and Pidoux, I.,** Immunoelectron microscope studies of type X collagen in endochondral ossification, *J. Cell Biol.*, 190, 2547, 1989.
26. **Kwan, A. P. L., Cummings, C. E., Chapman, J. A. and Grant, M. E.,** Macromolecular organization of chicken type X collagen in vitro, *J. Cell Biol.*, 114, 594, 1991.
27. **Mayne, R. and Burgeson, R. E., eds.,** *Structure and Function of Collagen Types,* Academic Press, Orlando, Florida, 1987.
28. **van der Rest, M. and Bruckner, P.,** Collagen: diversity at the molecular and supramolecular levels. *Cur. Opi. Struct. Biol.*, 3, 430, 1993.
29. **Burgeson, R. E. and Nimni, M.,** Collagen structure and distribution, *Clin. Orthopaed. Rel. Res.*, 282, 250, 1992.

30. **Yurchenco, P. D., Birk, D. E. and Mecham, R. P., eds.,** *Extracellular Matrix Assembly and Structure*, Academic Press, San Diego, California, 1994.
31. **Olsen, B. R.,** Collagen Biosynthesis, in *Cell Biology of Extracellular Matrix*, 2nd ed., Hay, E. D., ed., Plenum Press, New York, 1991.
32. **Ibrahim, J. and Harding, J. J.,** Pinpointing the sites of hydroxylysine glycosides in peptide α1-CB7 of bovine corneal collagen, and their possible role in determining fibril diameter and thus transparency, *Biochim. Biophys. Acta*, 992, 9, 1989.
33. **Yamauchi, M., Noyes, C., Kuboki, Y. and Mechanic, G. L.,** Collagen structural microheterogeneity and a possible role for glycosylated hydroxylysine in type I collagen, *Proc. Natl. Acad. Sci. USA*, 79, 7684, 1982.
34. **Engel, J. and Prockop, D. J.,** The zipper-like folding of collagen triple helices and the effects of mutations that disrupt the zipper, *Ann. Rev. Biophys. Biophys. Chem.*, 20, 137, 1991.
35. **Fleischmajor, R., Perlish, J. S. and Olsen, B. R.,** Amino and carboxyl propeptides in bone collagen fibrils during embryogenesis, *Cell Tissue Res.*, 247, 105, 1987.
36. **Landis, W. J. and Christoffersen, J. A.,** Contribution with review to the description of mineralization of bone and other calcified tissues in vivo, *Anat. Rec.*, 230, 435, 1991.
37. **Glimcher, M. J.,** On the form and function of bone: from molecules to organs, in *The Chemistry and Biology of Mineralized Tissues*, Veis, A., ed., Elsevier Science Publishers, Amsterdam, 1981.
38. **Robinson, R. A. and Watson, M. L.,** Collagen-crystal relationships in bone as seen in the electron microscope, *Anat. Rec.*, 114, 383, 1952.
39. **Glimcher, M. J.,** Specificity of the molecular structure organic matrices in mineralization, in *Calcification in Biological Systems*, Sognnaes, R. F., ed., Washington DC., *Am. Assoc. Advanc. Sci.*, 1960.
40. **Nylen, M. J., Scott, D. B. and Mosley, V. M.,** Mineralization of turkey leg tendon, in *Calcification in Biological Systems*, Sognnaes, R. F., ed., Washington DC, Am. Assc. Adv. *Sci.*, 1960.
41. **Weiner, S. and Traub, W.,** Organization of hydroxyapatite crystals within collagen fibrils, *FEBS Lett.*, 206, 262, 1986.
42. **Traub, W., Arad, T. and Weiner, S.,** Three-dimensional ordered distribution of crystals in turkey tendon collagen fibers, *Proc. Natl. Acad. Sci. USA*, 86, 9822, 1989.
43. **Landis, W. J., Song, M. J., Leith, A., McEwen, L. and McEwen, B.F.,** Mineral and organic matrix interaction in normally calcifying tendon visualized in three dimensions by high-voltage electron microscopic tomography and graphic image reconstruction, *J. Struc. Biol.*, 110, 39, 1993.
44. **Katz, E. P. and Li, S. T.,** The intermolecular space of reconstituted collagen fibrils, *J. Mol. Biol.*, 73, 351, 1973.
45. **Katz, E. P., Wachtel, E., Yamauchi, M. and Mechanic, G. L.,** The structure of mineralized collagen fibrils, *Conn. Tis. Res.*, 21, 149, 1989.
46. **Lee, D. D. and Glimcher, M. J.,** The three-dimensional spacial relationship between the collagen fibrils and the inorganic calcium-phosphate crystals of pickeral and herring fish bone, *Conn. Tis. Res.*, 21, 247, 1989.
47. **Landis, W. J., Moradian-Oldak, J. and Weiner, S.,** Topographic imaging of mineral and collagen in the calcifying turkey tendon, *Conn. Tis. Res.*, 25, 181, 1991.
48. **Bonar, L. C., Lees, S. and Mook, H. A.,** Neutron diffraction studies of collagen in fully mineralized bone, *J. Mol. Biol.*, 181, 265, 1985.
49. **Bigi, A., Ripamonti, A., Koch, M. H. J. and Roveri, N.,** Calcified turkey leg tendon as structural model for bone mineralization, *Int. J. Biol. Macromol.*, 10, 282, 1988.
50. **Stoltz, M., Furthmayr, H. and Timpl, R.,** Increased lysine hydroxylation of rat bone and tendon collagen and localization of the additional residues, *Biochem. Biophys. Acta*, 310, 461, 1973.
51. **Butler, W. T.,** Dentin collagen, chemical structure and role in mineralization, in *Dentin and Dentinogenesis, vol II*, Linde, A., ed., CRC Press, Boca Raton, FL, 1984.
52. **Nimni, M. E. and Harkness, R. D.,** Molecular structure and function of collagen, in *Collagen. vol I*, CRC Press, Boca Raton, Florida, 1988.
53. **Robins, S. P.,** Analysis of the cross-linking components in collagen and elastin, *Methods Biochem. Anal.*, 28, 329, 1982.
54. **Eyre, D. R., Paz, M. A. and Gallop, P. M.,** Cross-linking in collagen and elastin, *Ann. Rev. Biochem.*, 537, 717, 1984.
55. **Yamauchi, M. and Mechanic, G. L.,** Cross-linking of collagen, in *Collagen, vol I*, CRC Press, Boca Raton, Florida, 1988.
56. **Reiser, K., McCormick, R. J. and Rucker, R. B.,** Enzymatic and nonenzymatic cross-linking of collagen and elastin, *FASEB J.*, 6, 2439, 1992.
57. **Tanzer, M. L.,** Cross-linking, in *Biochemistry of Collagen*, Ramachandran G. N. and Reddi, A. H., eds, Plenum, New York, 1976.
58. **Kagan, H. M. and Trackman, P. C.,** Properties and function of lysyl oxidase, *Am. J. Respir. Cell Mol. Biol.*, 5, 206, 1991.
59. **Siegel, R. C.,** Lysyl oxidase, *Int. Rev. Connect. Tissue Res.*, 8, 73, 1979.
60. **Yamauchi, M., Chandler, G. and Katz, E. P.,** Collagen cross-linking and mineralization, in *The Chemistry and Biology of Mineralized Tissues*, Slavkin, H. and Price, P., eds., Elsevier Science Publishers, Amsterdam, Netherlands, 1992.

61. **Otsubo, K., Katz, E. P., Mechanic, G. L., and Yamauchi, M.,** The cross-linking connectivity in bone collagen fibrils: the COOH-terminal locus of free aldehyde, *Biochemistry*, 31, 396, 1992.
62. **Yamauchi, M., Prisayanh, P., Haque, Z. and Woodley, D. T.,** Collagen cross-linking in sun-exposed and unexposed sites of aged human skin, *J. Invest. Dermatol.*, 97, 938, 1991.
63. **Tanner, J. H., Yamauchi, M. and Simpson, D. M.,** Collagen cross-linking in bovine gingiva, *Archs. Oral Biol.*, 36, 111, 1991.
64. **Eyre, D. R. and Glimcher, M. J.,** Reducible cross-links in hydroxylysine-deficient collagens of a heritable disorder of connective tissue, *Proc. Natl. Acad. Sci. USA*, 69, 2594, 1972.
65. **Nakamura, Y.,** Structure of type I collagen dimers, *Int. J. Macromol.*, 9, 281, 1987.
66. **Yamauchi, M. and Katz, E. P.,** The post-translational chemistry and molecular packing of mineralizing tendon collagens, *Conn. Tis. Res.*, 29, 81, 1993.
67. **Yamauchi, M., Woodley, D. T. and Mechanic, G. L.,** Aging and cross-linking of skin collagen, *Biochem. Biophys. Res. Commun.*, 152, 893, 1988.
68. **Kang, A. H., Faris, B. and Franzblau, C.,** Intramolecular cross-link of chick skin collagen, *Biochem. Biophys. Res. Commun.*, 36, 345, 1969.
69. **Tanzer, M. L., Housley, T., Berube, L., Fairweather, R., Franzblau, C. and Gallop, P. M.,** Structure of two histidine-containing cross-links from collagen, *J. Biol. Chem.*, 248, 393, 1973.
70. **Fujimoto, D.,** Isolation and characterization of a fluorescent material in bovine achilles tendon collagen, *Biochem. Biophys. Res. Commun.*, 76, 1124, 1977.
71. **Fujimoto, D., Moriguchi, T., Ishida, T. and Hayashi, H.,** The structure of pyridinoline, a collagen cross-link, *Biochem. Biophys. Res. Commun.*, 84, 52, 1978.
72. **Kuboki, Y., Tsuzaki, M., Sasaki, S., Liu, C. F. and Mechanic, G. L.,** Location of the intermolecular cross-links in bovine dentin collagen: solubilization with trypsin of cross-link peptides containing dihydroxylysinonorleucine and pyridinoline, *Biochem. Biophys. Res. Comm.*, 102, 119, 1981.
73. **Eyre, D. R. and Oguchi, H.,** The hydroxypyridinium cross-links of skeletal collagen: their measurement, properties and a proposed pathway of formation, *Biochem. Biophys. Res. Commun.*, 92, 404, 1980.
74. **Eyre, D. R., Dickson, I. R. and van Ness, K.,** Collagen cross-linking in human bone and articular cartilage, *Biochem. J.*, 252, 495, 1988.
75. **Berthet-Colominas, C., Miller, A. and White, S. W.,** Structural study of the calcifying collagen in turkey leg tendons, *J. Mol. Biol.*, 134, 431, 1979.
76. **Fujimoto, D., Hirama, M. and Iwashita, T.,** Histidinoalanine, a new crosslinking amino acid, in calcified tissue collagen, *Biochem. Biophys. Res. Commun.*, 104, 1102, 1982.
77. **Fujimoto, D., Hirama, M. and Iwashita, T.,** Occurrence of lysinoalanine in calcified tissue collagen, *Biochem. Biophys. Res. Commun.*, 103, 1378, 1982.
78. **Kuboki, Y., Fujisawa, R., Tsuzaki, M., Liu, C. F. and Sasaki, S.,** Presence of lysinoalanine and histidinoalanine in bovine dentin phosphoprotein, *Calcif. Tis. Int.*, 36, 126, 1984.
79. **Kuboki, Y., Takita, H., Fujisawa, R., Yamaguchi, H., Yamada, H., Tazaki, M., Ohnuma, Y., Mizuno, M. and Tsuzaki, M.,** Histidinoalanine-containing phosphoprotein in bone, *Calcif. Tis. Int.*, 48, 196, 1991.
80. **Monnier, V. M., Sell, D. R., Nagaraj, R. H., Miyata, S., Grandhee, S., Odetti, P. and Ibrahim, S. A.,** Maillard reaction-mediated molecular damage to extracellular matrix and other tissue proteins in diabetes, aging, and uremia, *Diabetes*, 41, 36, 1992.
81. **Reiser, K.,** Nonenzymatic glycation of collagen in aging and diabetes, *Proc. Soc. Exp. Biol. Med.*, 196, 17, 1991.
82. **Reiser, K. M., Amigable, M. A. and Last, J. A.,** Nonenzymatic glycation of type I collagen, *J. Biol. Chem.*, 267, 24207, 1992.
83. **Byers, P. H.,** Brittle bones-fragile molecules: disorders of collagen gene structure and expression, *Trends Genet.*, 6, 293, 1990.
84. **Prockop, D. J.,** Mutations that alter the primary structure of type I collagen, *J. Biol. Chem.*, 265, 5349, 1990.
85. **Vogel, B. E., Doelz, R., Kadler, K. E., Hojima, Y., Engel, J. and Prockop, D. J.,** A substitution of cysteine for glycine 748 of the $\alpha 1$ chain produces a kink at this site in the procollagen I molecule and an altered N-proteinase cleavage site over 225 nm away, *J. Biol. Chem.*, 263, 19249, 1988.
86. **Landis, W. J., Hodgens, K., Mello, C., Snowise, M., Feuerbach, R. J., Arena, J., Berkery, D. and McEwen, B. F.,** Insight into a biological basis for the strength of calcified tissue: three-dimensional ultrastructural studies of a brittle bone model by high voltage electron microscopic tomography and graphic image reconstruction, *Trans. Orthopaed. Res. Soc.*, 19, 16, 1994.
87. **Mechanic, G. L. and Bullough, P.,** The qualitative and quantitative cross-link structure of human normal and osteogenesis imperfecta bone collagens, in *Physical Chemistry and Crystallography of Apatites of Biological Interest*, C.N.R.S., Paris, 1974.
88. **Fujii, K. and Tanzer, M. L.,** Osteogenesis imperfecta: Biochemical studies of bone collagen, *Clin. Ortho. Rel. Res.*, 124, 271, 1977.

89. **Spotila, L. D., Constantinou, C. D., Sereda, L., Ganguly, A., Riggs, B. L. and Prockop, D.J.,** Mutation in the gene for type I procollagen (COL 1A2) in a woman with postmenopausal osteoporosis: evidence for phenotypic and genotypic overlap with mild osteogenesis imperfecta, *Proc. Natl. Acad. Sci. USA.*, 88, 5423, 1991.
90. **Shapiro, J. R., Stover, M. L., Burn, V. E., McKinstry, M. B., Burshell, A. L., Chipman, S. D. and Rowe, D. W.,** An osteopenic nonfracture syndrome with features of mild osteogenesis imperfecta associated with the substitution of a cysteine for glysine at triple helix position 43 in the Wproa1(I) chain of type I collagen, *J. Clin. Invest.*, 89, 567, 1992.
91. **Yamauchi, M., Young, D. R., Chandler, G. S. and Mechanic, G. L.,** Cross-linking and new bone collagen synthesis in immobilized and recovering primate osteoporosis, *Bone*, 9, 415, 1988.
92. **Bailey, A. J., Wotton, S. F., Sims, T. J. and Thompson, P.W.,** Post-translational modifications in the collagen of human osteoporotic femoral head, *Biochem. Biophys. Res. Comm.*, 185, 801, 1992.
93. **Mechanic, G. L., Toverud, S. U. and Ramp, W. K.,** Quantitative changes of bone collagen crosslinks and precursors in vitamin D deficiency, *Biochem. Biophys. Res. Commun.*, 47, 760, 1972.
94. **Mechanic, G. L., Toverud, S. U., Ramp, W. K. and Gonnerman, W. A.,** The effect of vitamin D on the structural cross-links and maturation of chick bone collagen, *Biochim. Biophys. Acta*, 393, 419, 1975.
95. **Yamauchi, M., Banes, A. J., Kuboki, Y. and Mechanic, G. L.,** A comparative study of the distribution of the stable cross-link, pyridinoline, in bone collagens from normal, osteoblastoma, and vitamin D-deficient chicks, *Biochem. Biophys. Res. Commun.*, 102, 59, 1981.
96. **Banes, A. J., Bernstein, P. H., Smith, R. E. and Mechanic, G. L.,** Collagen biochemistry of osteo-petrotic bone I: changes in bone collagen cross-links in virus induced avian osteopetrosis, *Biochem. Biophys. Res. Commun.*, 81, 1390, 1978.
97. **Dziedzic-Goclawska, A., Wojtowicz, A., Moutier, R., Marks, S. C. and Yamauchi, M.,** An increase in pyridinoline cross-links in bone of osteopetrotic rats, *Calcif. Tis. Int.*, 52, 58, 1993.
98. **Heinegard, D. and Oldberg, A.,** Structure and biology of cartilage and bone matrix noncollagenous macromolecules, *FASEB J.*, 3, 2042, 1989.
99. **Glimcher, M. J.,** The possible role of collagen fibrils and collagen-phosphoprotein complexes in the calcification of bone in vitro and in vivo, *Biomaterials*, 89, 7, 1990.
100. **Veis, A., Sabsay, B. and Wu, C. B.,** Phosphophoryns as mediators of mineralization, in Surface Reactive Peptides and Polymers, Steven Sikes, C. and Wheeler, A. P., eds., American Chemical Society, Washington, DC, 1991.
101. **Veis, A.,** Mineral-matrix interactions in bone and dentin, *J. Bone Min. Res.*, 8, S493, 1993.
102. **Weinstock, M. and Leblond, C. P.,** Radioautographic visualization of the deposition of a phospho-protein at the mineralization front in the dentin of the rat incisor, *J. Cell Biol.*, 56, 838, 1973.
103. **Maier, G. D., Lechner, J. H. and Veis, A.,** The dynamics of formation of a collagen-phosphophoryn conjugate in relation to the passage of the mineralization front in rat incisor dentin, *J. Biol. Chem.*, 258, 1450, 1983.
104. **Stetler-Stevenson, W. G. and Veis, A.,** Type I collagen shows a specific binding affinity for bovine dentin phosphophoryn, *Calcif. Tis. Int.*, 38, 135, 1986.
105. **Traub, W., Jodaikin, A., Arad, T. and Veis, A.,** Dentin phosphophoryn binding to collagen fibrils, *Matrix*, 12, 197, 1992.
106. **Lucci, A., Crenshaw, M. A. and Linde, A.,** Induction and inhibition of hydroxyapatite formation by rat dentine phosphoprotein in vitro, *Arch. Oral Biol.*, 33, 685, 1988.
107. **Crenshaw, M. A.,** Mineral induction by matrix from mineralized biological tissues, *Mat. Res. Soc. Symp. Proc.*, 218, 185, 1991.
108. **Delmas, P. D.,** Biochemical markers of bone turnover, *J. Bone Min. Res.*, 8, S549, 1993.
109. **Eyre, D.,** Editorial: new biomarkers of bone resorption, *J. Clin. Endocrin. Metab.*, 74, 470A, 1992.
110. **Robins, S. P., Black, D., Paterson, C. R., Reid, D. M., Duncan, A. and Seibel, M. J.,** Evaluation of urinary hydroxypyridinium cross-link measurements as resorption markers in metabolic bone diseases, *Eur. J. Clin. Invest.*, 21, 310, 1991.

Chapter 10

SERUM AND URINE MARKERS OF BONE TURNOVER

Gayle E. Lester, Ph.D.

TABLE OF CONTENTS

I. INTRODUCTION

An acute need exists for minimally invasive, sensitive means to determine rates of bone turnover in general, but especially in metabolic bone diseases such as osteoporosis where other conventional markers of calcium metabolism are relatively unaltered. Appropriate biochemical markers should reflect the formation or breakdown of factors specific to bone matrix or the activity of the bone cells, either osteoblasts or osteoclasts, that are responsible for bone remodeling. Numerous assay methods are available to monitor these cellular and matrix factors. Some assays have been available for many years, e.g., urinary hydroxyproline and serum alkaline phosphatase, whereas others are very new. Of the newer markers there are several that have not been well explored or validated by comparison with other indices. None to date has been shown to be unique for the diagnosis of metabolic bone disease, but some markers are more closely associated with certain diseases than others.

The current "Gold Standard" against which biochemical marker levels are compared is the histomorphometric interpretation of iliac crest specimens obtained from bone biopsy. Marker sensitivity, specificity, and relationship to resorption or formation are usually based on data obtained from both the clinical history and the histologic assessment of biopsy specimens.[1,2] Although histomorphometry is considered the standard, it is an invasive technique subject to the variability associated with biopsy site and mode of analysis;[1] thus, it is not an appropriate means for assessment of skeletal changes over short time intervals.

0-8493-7845-1/95/$0.00+$.50

TABLE 1
Biochemical Markers Related to Bone Turnover

Bone Formation	Bone Resorption
Alkaline phosphatase, total or skeletal isoenzyme, plasma	Hydroxyproline, urinary
Osteocalcin, plasma	Tartrate-resistant acid phosphatase, plasma
Procollagen I extension peptides, plasma	Hydroxylysine, urinary
	Pyridinoline/deoxypyridinoline, urinary

In assessment of biochemical marker suitability, the ability to detect the marker and sensitivity of the assay are two important issues. The influence of diurnal rhythms on marker levels must be predictable, and the marker should not be influenced by changes in dietary patterns.[2] It is also important to understand how the marker is cleared from the body and the influence of declining renal and hepatic function on the circulating and excreted levels. The assay used should be sufficiently sensitive to reflect subtle changes in the biochemical marker associated with clinical treatments and changes in disease status. Here, too, the specificity of the assay becomes very important in that interfering substances may mask actual changes in the biochemical marker of interest.

To some extent, marker proteins can be delineated as to whether they predominantly reflect changes in bone resorption or formation (Table 1). The appealing aspect of a serum or urine marker is the relatively short time frame over which it could be followed to monitor therapeutic treatments.[1,2] In contrast, bone density measurements and bone biopsy require a minimum of 6 months between determinations due to either the lack of sensitivity of the method or the invasive nature of the procedure. In this brief chapter, markers are addressed as shown in Table 1, according to their reflection of bone formation or resorption. Discussion will focus on the newer, more sensitive markers and the application of these markers to diagnosis and monitoring of metabolic bone diseases.

II. BONE FORMATION MARKERS

Markers for bone formation are most likely to be molecules that are synthesized by the bone-forming cells, the osteoblasts. The three markers discussed here are all synthesized by osteoblasts; however, the degree to which their appearance in plasma reflects the actual formation of bone remains unresolved.

A. TOTAL AND SKELETAL ALKALINE PHOSPHATASE

Skeletal alkaline phosphatase is an enzyme synthesized and released into the circulation by the osteoblast during bone formation and mineralization. Although it is a bone-specific isoenzyme, it is structurally very similar to the liver and kidney alkaline phosphatase isoenzyme, being a product of the same gene subjected to posttranslational modifications. The skeletal enzyme is a tetrameric glycoprotein localized in the plasma membrane of the osteoblast.[1] Because these isoenzymes are structurally similar, most common methods detect total serum alkaline phosphatase and not the bone-specific isoenzyme. Although half or less of circulating levels are derived from bone, elevated levels of total enzyme can be detected in pathologies associated with increased bone turnover.[2] However, moderate changes in total serum alkaline phosphatase are ambiguous and may very likely result from alterations in the hepatic isoenzyme. Recently, monoclonal antibodies have been produced against the purified skeletal enzyme, and highly specific and sensitive immunoradiometric assays are now available.[3] The serum levels of bone-specific alkaline phosphatase compare well to levels of total enzyme but are not influenced by diseases of the liver or kidney. Because there is no cross-reactivity with the hepatic isoenzyme, this new assay should be useful for monitoring subtle changes in osteoblastic activity associated with aging, menopause, and metabolic bone diseases.

B. OSTEOCALCIN (BONE GLA-PROTEIN, BGP)

Osteocalcin is a 49 amino acid, noncollagen protein that is specifically found in bone and dentin. It is a unique protein in that it contains 3 residues of glutamic acid that undergo posttranslational, vitamin K-dependent carboxylations. Its precise function is unknown; however, it is synthesized by the osteoblast and released into the circulation or incorporated into bone matrix. Despite a short elimination half-life, circulating forms of osteocalcin can be detected by a variety of radioimmunoassay methods.[4-6] Although well accepted as a marker of bone formation, two major problems exist: (1) there are wide differences observed in osteocalcin levels with available assay methods[7,8] and (2) intact osteocalcin and fragments are released from bone matrix during bone resorption.[9] The variability in normal levels is no doubt due to the use of polyclonal antibodies generated against different epitopes of the osteocalcin molecule in the assay methodologies. Recently, the circulating forms of osteocalcin have been characterized by Garnero and co-workers,[10] and these investigators have developed a panel of monoclonal antibodies with which to quantify the contribution of each of these fragments. They report that four major fragments of osteocalcin are found in plasma in addition to the intact molecule. The relative contribution of these fragments is similar in various diseases, and this indicates that these epitopes are due to specific, enzyme-driven cleavages[10] and not a result of increased bone resorption. The presence of these fragments might also explain some of the variability in normal circulating levels detected by the various radioimmunoassays based on polyclonal antibodies.

The application of monoclonal antibody technology to measurement of this serum factor will impart increased sensitivity and specificity to assays. Based on the assays available, osteocalcin levels have been shown to be increased with skeletal growth at puberty and various diseases associated with increased bone turnover, such as hyperparathyroidism, hyperthyroidism, and Paget's disease and to be decreased with glucocorticoid treatment and in diseases such as hypothyroidism and hypoparathyroidism. In a normal individual, where bone resorption and formation are coupled, osteocalcin is considered to be an adequate marker of bone turnover; in diseases where bone resorption and formation are uncoupled, serum osteocalcin is considered to be a reliable marker of bone turnover and formation.

Recently, it has been reported that a cohort of elderly women with elevated circulating levels of under carboxylated osteocalcin had a 5-fold relative risk of hip fracture.[11] Although the functional significance of increases in the under carboxylated form of osteocalcin is not known, this is a very exciting observation. It is the first report of the association of a serum marker with bone fragility. Application of this analysis (under carboxylated osteocalcin) to serum samples from other pathologies will be helpful in elucidating the usefulness of this potential marker.

C. PROCOLLAGEN I EXTENSION PEPTIDES

The markers just described are the most widely used to monitor bone formation; however, there are conditions in which circulating levels of these markers appear to be dissociated.[12] Although osteocalcin is one protein specific to bone, it represents only 1% of the total protein synthesized by the osteoblast. In contrast, type I collagen represents 90% of the protein synthesized by osteoblasts and thus should provide a sensitive index of bone formation. New assays have been developed based on the detection of the carboxy-terminal and amino-terminal segments of type I procollagen (PICP and PINP). As described in the chapter on collagens, these propeptides are cleaved from the precursor molecule, procollagen, in a 1:1 molar ratio to newly synthesized collagen (see Figure 3 in Chapter 9). These peptides are not incorporated into the matrix but are released into the extracellular fluid and found in the serum. Of these two peptides, PICP circulates as a 100 kDa glycoprotein in the serum, whereas PINP circulates as both a 64–70 kDa globular protein and various fragments.

Commercial assays are available for both of these peptides and have yielded information as to the usefulness of these peptides as markers of bone formation. The serum levels of PINP are

100-fold those of PICP with antibodies currently available. This implies that either these peptides are preferentially released from the bone or are cleared differently from the plasma. Perhaps related to these differences, there is a poor relationship between the serum levels of these two metabolites in normal and disease states. At present, there does not appear to be a consensus on the usefulness of these assays in monitoring bone formation or turnover.[12,13] PICP appears to be the more promising since levels of this peptide correlate better with osteocalcin and skeletal alkaline phosphatase levels. The correlation with bone formation rates obtained from histomorphometric analysis of bone biopsy samples has been reported to be both good[14] and poor.[12] Further studies are needed to assess the usefulness of measurement of these extension peptides in the clinical setting.

III. BONE RESORPTION MARKERS

Bone resorption is a result of osteoclastic activity that dissolves bone mineral and enzymatically digests collagen and other bone matrix proteins. Thus, markers for bone resorption include (1) proteins that are relatively specific to osteoclasts, such as tartrate-resistant acid phosphatase (TRAP) and (2) modified amino acids that are released by breakdown of collagen molecules. These modified amino acids include both hydroxylated proline and lysine as well as pyridinium crosslinks that are present in mature matrix.

A. HYDROXYPROLINE

Urinary hydroxyproline has long been known to be an inexpensive marker of bone resorption; however, it is a nonspecific index in that it reflects breakdown of total collagen from all tissues. Since half of collagen in the body is present in bone and the turnover rate of bone exceeds that of all soft tissues, urinary hydroxyproline excretion has served as a somewhat useful marker of increased bone resorption. Hydroxyproline is released into the circulation during the breakdown of collagen; breakdown products include peptide-bound hydroxyproline and free amino acid. The free amino acids are degraded in the liver, and only the peptide-bound form (approximately 10%) is found in the urine. In addition, ingestion of dietary proteins, such as gelatin, will result in increased hydroxyproline in the urine. Thus hydroxyproline is, in fact, a relatively insensitive, albeit convenient, marker of bone resorption. Measurement of this amino acid is by a colorimetric assay of hydrolyzed urine and thus gives an index of total, urinary hydroxyproline. Although levels are elevated in diseases of high bone turnover, such as Paget's disease, there is poor correlation of urinary hydroxyproline levels with bone resorption as determined by histomorphometric techniques on bone biopsy specimens.[15] This relative lack of sensitivity has led to the search for improved markers of bone resorption.

B. TARTRATE-RESISTANT ACID PHOSPHATASE

Tartrate-resistant acid phosphatase (TRAP) refers to a plasma isoenzyme that originates in part from the osteoclast.[16] TRAP is a lysosomal enzyme and is part of a family of isoenzymes that circulate in the blood. Plasma levels of TRAP increase in various metabolic bone diseases associated with increased bone turnover, but it may not be any more sensitive or specific than hydroxyproline.[17] Recently, there have been new assays developed for TRAP based on specific monoclonal antibodies against the bone isoenzyme.[18] These improved assays may show TRAP to be a more useful marker of osteoclastic activity than did previous assays.[19]

C. HYDROXYLYSINE GLYCOSIDES

Like hydroxyproline, hydroxylysine is an amino acid unique to collagen and collagen-like proteins. Although much less abundant than hydroxyproline, urinary levels of this amino acid could serve as a potential marker of collagen breakdown. Unlike hydroxyproline, hydroxylysine is released from collagen as either galactosyl-hydroxylysine (GHYL) or glucosyl-galactosyl-hydroxylysine (GGHYL). The ratio of these products is tissue dependent and thus, analysis of this ratio can be used to impart tissue specificity to the analysis.[20] Initial studies have shown increased levels of urinary GHYL with aging.[21] Unfortunately, the analysis of GHYL and GGHYL requires separation and quantitation by high-performance liquid chromatography (HPLC) and thus is not applicable as a routine clinical assay. Further evaluation of these markers is warranted as well as development of specific assays against the differentially glycosylated hydroxylysines.

D. PYRIDINOLINE AND DEOXYPYRIDINOLINE

Pyridinoline (hydroxylysylpyridinoline, Pyr) and deoxypydininoline (lysylpyridinoline, Dpyr) are nonreducible pyridinium crosslinks found in mature collagen. These crosslinks are thought to stabilize the collagen chains within the mature matrix (See Chapter 9) and are not present in procollagen molecules secreted by osteoblasts during matrix synthesis. They are found in bone and cartilage and to a lesser extent in other connective tissues except skin.[22] The ratio of Pyr to Dpyr in bone differs from that in cartilage and is similar to the ratio of these peptides in urine (4:1).[23] Thus, it is assumed that these peptides are released from bone matrix during degradation associated with bone resorption. These fluorescent peptides are not further metabolized in the body or reutilized during collagen synthesis and are found in the circulation and excreted into the urine unchanged. There is no contribution to these levels from food sources.[24] Approximately 30% of the Pyr/Dpyr is excreted as free cross-link, and 70% is excreted as a larger peptide-bound form.[25]

The amounts of Pyr/Dpyr excreted can be measured with fluorimetry following reverse-phase HPLC separation of hydrolyzed urine samples. The value of these peptides as an index of bone resorption has been proven with HPLC analysis of urine specimens from individuals with various pathological conditions. Levels of these peptides increase with the onset of menopause and can be reduced with hormone replacement therapy.[26,27] Cross-link levels correlate well, especially Dpyr, with bone turnover as measured by histomorphometric analysis of bone biopsy specimens[15] and with urinary hydroxyproline levels. Urinary levels of these metabolites are elevated in patients with tumor-associated hypercalcemia[28] and Paget's disease.[29] Excretion of these cross-links follows a circadian rhythm[30] similar to that observed with osteocalcin; this probably reflects a reported nocturnal increase in bone turnover.[31]

Although the pyridinoline cross-links appear to be appropriate markers for bone resorption, the technical difficulty of the HPLC assay has resulted in a search for more convenient means to measure these markers. Recently, immunoassays have been developed against either free pyridinoline or one of the two cross-linking domains (C-domain or N-domain, see Chapter 9).[32-34] Although there have not been many studies carried out using these assays, preliminary reports indicate that several of them are promising. Specifically, assays have been developed against the following: (1) free pyridinoline and free deoxypyridinoline,[32] (2) cross-linked N-telopeptides of type I collagen,[33] and (3) cross-linked C-telopeptides from type I collagen.[34]

For all assays developed, there are good correlations between increased urinary levels of the specific epitope and increased bone turnover as assessed by histomorphometric analysis of bone biopsy.[13,28,35] Difficulties arise when evaluating the sensitivity and specificity of these various assay methods in detecting changes in bone turnover as a result of clinical treatments[36,37] and in distinguishing "fast" bone losers.[38] Since most of these assays have only been commercially available for a short time, much work remains to be done to fully characterize the usefulness of each assay. The designation of urinary Pyr and Dpyr as the preferred markers for assessment of bone resorption has held up despite differences in the methods by which these are determined.

IV. USEFULNESS OF AND INTERRELATIONSHIP BETWEEN MARKERS

It is clear that no one marker will be completely diagnostic for any particular metabolic state of bone or any specific disease. Many markers appear to have a role to play in the diagnosis and

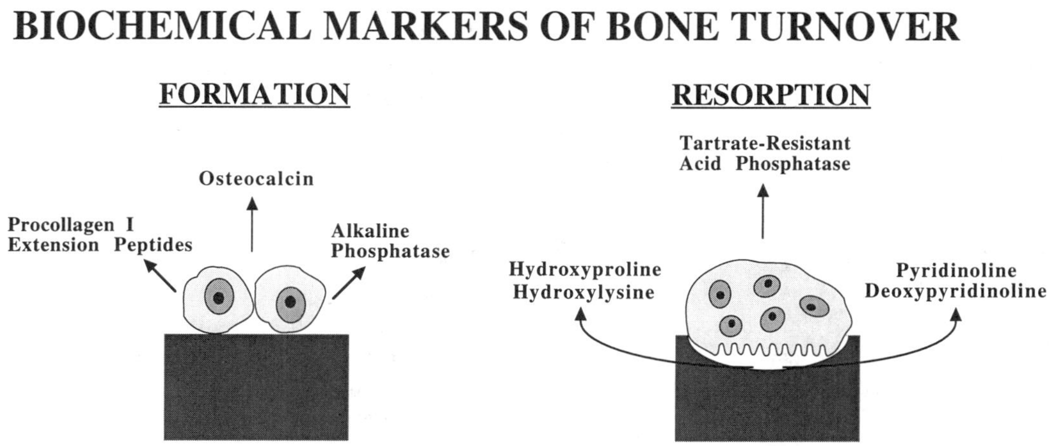

FIGURE 1. Sources of Biochemical Markers of Bone Formation and Resorption. Several markers of bone formation are released by osteoblasts, including procollagen I extension peptides, osteocalcin, and alkaline phosphatase. Possible markers for bone resorption are tartrate-resistant acid phosphatase and products of collagen degradation, such as the amino acids, hydroxyproline and hydroxylysine, and the collagen cross-links pyridinoline and deoxypyridinoline.

monitoring of changes in bone turnover. It is well known that bone turnover is increased in normal women after the fourth decade and further increased with the onset of menopause. Markers of bone formation and resorption are elevated during these periods and generally return to premenopausal levels with hormone replacement therapy.

Circulating osteocalcin has been proposed to be a very sensitive marker for bone formation. Several unresolved questions remain, however, about the metabolic and renal clearance of this protein. In addition, the relationship between incorporation of newly synthesized osteocalcin into matrix vs. its release into the circulation has not been well described. Furthermore, the significance of undercarboxylated osteocalcin in the circulation, and the significance of the various osteocalcin fragments found in serum need to be explored further. It is possible that new assays with improved specificity for skeletal alkaline phosphatase or measurement of the procollagen peptides might provide a better index of bone formation.

The degradative nature of bone resorption has added to the difficulty of finding accurate and sensitive markers. Analysis of the pyridinoline cross-links has been shown to provide a relatively accurate index of bone resorption. The newer assay methods need to be validated further, and many questions remain as to the precise relationship of these cross-links and peptide fragments to different disease states. Some investigators have used a panel of markers to predict rate of bone loss successfully.[29] Prediction of such a rate of loss has important clinical implications because patients with "high" bone turnover appear to respond differently to therapeutic interventions than those with "low" bone turnover.

V. SUMMARY

At present, although there are numerous markers available (Figure 1), no ideal marker or combination of markers for bone turnover has been identified. It appears that it will be necessary to combine several markers of formation with several markers of resorption in order to obtain a sensitive and specific assessment of bone loss.[39,40] A combination of the markers in conjunction with measurements of bone mineral density would be of most benefit in assessment of skeletal status. It has been proposed that the rate of bone loss may be a very significant factor in determination of bone quality.[41] Determination of bone loss rate in combination with bone density may improve our ability to predict fracture risk in individuals.

REFERENCES

1. **Delmas, P. D.,** Biochemical markers of bone turnover for the clinical investigation of osteoporosis, *Osteoporosis Int.*, Suppl 1, S81, 1993.
2. **Delmas, P. D.,** Biochemical markers of bone turnover I: theoretical considerations and clinical use in osteoporosis, *Am. J. Med.*, 95 (suppl 5A), 11S, 1993.
3. **Garnero, P. and Delmas, P. D.,** Assessment of the serum levels of bone alkaline phosphatase with a new immunoradiometric assay in patients with metabolic bone disease, *J. Clin. Endocrinol. Metab.*, 77, 1046, 1993.
4. **Price, P. A., Parthemore, J. G. and Deftos, L. J.,** New Biochemical marker for bone metabolism, *J. Clin. Invest.*, 66, 878, 1980.
5. **Lian, J. B. and Gundberg. C. M.,** Osteocalcin: biochemical considerations and clinical applications, *Clin. Orthop. Rel. Res.*, 226, 267, 1988.
6. **Delmas, P. D., Stenner, D., Wahner, H. W., Mann, K. G. and Riggs, B. L.,** Serum bone gla-protein increases with aging in normal women: implications for the mechanism of age-related bone loss, *J. Clin. Invest.*, 71, 1316, 1983.
7. **Tracy, R. P., Andrianorivo, A., Riggs, B. L. and Mann, K. G.,** Comparison of monoclonal and polyclonal antibody-based immunosassays for osteocalcin, *J. Bone Miner. Res.*, 5, 451, 1990.
8. **Taylor, A. K., Linkart, S., Mohan, S., Christenson, R. A., Singer, F. R. and Baylink, D.,** Multiple osteocalcin fragments in human urine and serum as detected by a midmolecule osteocalcin radioimmunoassay, *J. Clin. Endocrinol. Metab.*, 70, 467, 1990.
9. **Gundberg, C. and Weinstein, R. S.,** Multiple immunoreactive forms of osteocalcin in uremic serum, *J. Clin. Invest.*, 77, 1762, 1986.
10. **Garnero, P., Grimaus, M., Demiaux, B., Preaudat, C., Seguin, P. and Delmas, P. D.,** Measurement of serum osteocalcin with a human-specific two-site immunoradiometric assay, *J. Bone Miner. Res.*, 12, 1389, 1992.
11. **Szulc, P., Chapuy, M. C., Meunier, P. J. and Delmas, P. D.,** Serum undercarboxylated osteocalcin is a marker of the risk of hip fracture in elderly women, *J. Clin. Invest.*, 91, 1769, 1993.
12. **Ebeling, P. R., Peterson, J. M. and Riggs, B. L.,** Utility of type I procollagen propeptide assays for assessing abnormalities in metabolic bone diseases, *J. Bone Miner. Res.*, 7, 1243, 1992.
13. **Charles, P., Mosekilde, L., Risteli, L., Risteli, J. and Eriksen, E. F.,** Assessment of bone remodeling using biochemical indicators of type I collagen synthesis and degradation: relation to calcium kinetics, *Bone Miner.*, 24, 81, 1994.
14. **Eriksen, E. F., Charles, P., Melsen, F., Mosekilde, L., Risteli, L. and Risteli, J.,** Serum markers of type I collagen formation and degradation in metabolic bone disease: correlation with bone histomorphometry, *J. Bone Miner. Res.*, 8, 127, 1993.
15. **Delmas, P. D., Schlemmer, A., Gineyts, E., Riis, B. J. and Christiansen, C.,** Urinary excretion of pyridinoline crosslinks correlates with bone turnover measured on iliac crest biopsy in patients with vertebral osteoporosis, *J. Bone Miner. Res.*, 6, 639, 1991.
16. **Minkin, C.,** Bone acid phosphatase: tartrate-resistant acid phosphatase as a marker of osteoclast function, *Calcif. Tissue. Int.*, 34, 285, 1992.
17. **Delmas, P. D.,** Biochemical markers of bone turnover for the clinical assessment of metabolic disease, *Endocrinol. Metab. Clin. North. Am.*, 19, 1, 1990.
18. **Kraenzlin, M., Lau, K. H. W. and Liang, L.,** Development of an immunoassay for human serum osteoclastic tartrate-resistant acid phosphatase, *J. Clin. Endocrinol. Metab.*, 71, 442, 1990.
19. **Stepan, J. J., Silinkova-Malkova, E. and Havrenek, T.,** Relationship of plasma tartrate-resistant acid phosphatase to the bone isoenzyme of serum alkaline phosphatase in hyperparathyroidism, *Clin. Chim. Acta*, 133, 189, 1983.
20. **Grazioli, V., Casari, E., Murone, M. and Bonini, P. A.,** High-performance liquid chromatographic method for measuring hydroxylysine glycosides and their ratio in urine as a possible marker of human bone collagen breakdown, *J. Chromatography*, 615, 50, 1993.
21. **Moro, L., Mucelli, R. S. P., Gazzarrini, C., Modricky, C., Marotti, F. and de Bernard, B.,** Urinary β-1-galactosyl-O-hydroxylysine (GH) as a marker of collagen turnover of bone, *Calcif. Tissue. Int.*, 42, 87, 1988.
22. **Eyre, D. R.,** Collagen crosslinking amino acids, *Methods Enzymol.*, 144, 115, 1987.
23. **Eyre, D. R., Koob, T. J. and Van Ness, K. P.,** Quantitation of hydroxypyridinium crosslinks in collagen by high performance liquid chromatography, *Anal. Biochem.*, 137, 380, 1984.
24. **Colwell, A., Russell, R. G. G. and Eastell, R.,** Factors affecting the assay of urinary 3-hydroxy pyridinium crosslinks of collagen as markers of bone resorption, *Euro. J. Clin. Invest.*, 23, 341, 1993.
25. **Eyre, D. R.,** New biomarkers of bone resorption, *J. Clin. Endocrinol. Metab.*, 74, 470A, 1992.
26. **Hassager, C., Risteli, J., Risteli, L., Jensen, S. B. and Christiansen, C.,** Diurnal variation in serum markers of type I collagen synthesis and degradation in healthy premenopausal women, *J. Bone Miner. Res.*, 7, 1307, 1992.

27. **Seibel, M. J., Cosman, F., Shen, V., Gordon, S., Dempster, S. W., Ratcliffe, A. and Lindsay, R.,** Urinary hydroxypyridinium crosslinks of collagen as markers of bone resorption and estrogen efficacy in postmenopausal osteoporosis, *J. Bone Miner. Res.*, 7, 881, 1993.
28. **Body, J. J. and Delmas, P. D.,** Urinary pyridinium crosslinks as markers of bone resorption in tumor-associated hypercalcemia, *J. Clin. Endocrinol. Metab.*, 74, 471, 1992.
29. **Ubelhart, D., Gineyts, E. C., Chapuy, M. C. and Delmas, P. D.,** Urinary excretion of pyridinium crosslinks: a new marker of bone resorption in metabolic bone disease, *Bone Miner.*, 8, 87, 1990.
30. **Schlemmer, A., Hassager, C., Jensen, S. B. and Christiansen, C.,** Marked diurnal variation in urinary excretion of pyridinium crosslinks in premenopausal women, *J. Clin. Endocrinol. Metab.*, 74, 476, 1992.
31. **Eastell, R., Calvo, M. S., Burritt, M. R., Offord, K. P., Russell, R. G. G. and Riggs, B. L.,** Abnormalities in circadian patterns of bone resorption and renal calcium conservation in type I osteoporosis, *J. Clin. Endocrinol. Metab.*, 74, 487, 1992.
32. **Seyedin, S. M., Kung, V. T., Daniloff, Y. N., Hesley, R. P., Gomez, B., Nielsen, L. A., Rosen, H. N. and Zuk, R. F.,** Immunoassay for urinary pyridinoline: the new marker of bone resorption, *J. Bone Miner. Res.*, 5, 635, 1993.
33. **Hanson, D. A., Weis, M. A., Bollen, A. M., Maslan, A. L., Singer, F. R. and Eyre, D. R.,** A specific immunoassay for monitoring human bone resorption: quantitation of type I collagen cross-linked N-telopeptides in urine, *J. Bone Miner. Res.*, 7, 1251, 1993.
34. **Risteli, J., Elomaa, I., Niemi, S., Novamo, A. and Risteli, L.,** Radioimmunoassay for the pyridinoline cross-linked carboxy-terminal telopeptide of type I collagen: a new serum marker of bone collagen degradation, *Clin. Chem.*, 39, 635, 1993.
35. **Rosen, H. N., Dresner-Pollak, R., Moses, A. C., Rosenblatt, M., Zeind, A.J., Clemens, J. D. and Greenspan, A. L.,** Specificity of urinary excretion of cross-linked N-telopeptides of type I collagen as a marker of bone turnover, *Calcif. Tissue Int.*, 54, 26, 1994.
36. **Filipponi, P., Pedetti, M., Beghe, F., Giovagnini, B., Miam, M. and Cristallini, S.,** Effects of two different bisphosphonates on Paget's disease of bone: ICTP assessed, *Bone*, 15, 261, 1994.
37. **Hassager, C., Colwell, A., Assiri, A. M. A., Eastell, R., Russell, R. G. G. and Christiansen, C.,** Effect of menopause and hormone replacement therapy on urinary excretion of pyridinium crosslinks: a longitudinal and cross-sectional study, *Clin. Endocrinol.*, 37, 45, 1992.
38. **Fledelius, C., Riis, B. J., Overgaard, K. and Christiansen, C.,** The diagnostic validity of urinary free pyridinolines to identify women at risk of osteoporosis, *Calcif. Tissue Int.*, 54, 3811, 1994.
39. **Bettica, P., Moro, L., Robins, S. P., Taylor, A. K., Talbot, J., Singer, F. R. and Baylink, D. J.,** Bone resorption markers galactosyl hydroxylysine, pyridinium crosslinks, and hydroxyproline compared, *Clin. Chem.*, 38, 2313, 1992.
40. **Charles, P., Hasling, C., Risteli, L., Risteli, J., Mosekilde, L. and Eriksen, E. F.,** Assessment of bone formation by biochemical markers in metabolic bone disease: separation between osteoblastic activity at the cell and tissue level, *Calcif. Tissue Int.*, 51, 1405, 1992.
41. **Riis, B. J.,** Biochemical markers of bone turnover II: diagnosis, prophylaxis, and treatment of osteoporosis, *Am. J. Med.*, 95 (suppl 5A), 17S, 1993.

Section III.

HORMONAL REGULATION OF CALCIUM AND PHOSPHORUS

The calcium-regulating hormones, which are the focus of this section, not only act in bone to maintain homeostasis of blood calcium (Ca) and phosphorus (P), but they also act on the gut and kidneys. The integrated actions of these hormones, then, permit the organism to function well as a result of the constancy of Ca (and P) in the "milieu interieur" of Claude Bernard. Parathyroid hormone (PTH) is reviewed first in Chapter 11. The "classical" functions of this hormone are outlined, and new information on the control of PTH secretion by the parathyroid glands is given. The role of vitamin D, its biotransformation, and its physiologic significance under diverse physiological conditions is covered in Chapter 12. In addition, information about problems of inadequate or excessive intakes of this vitamin is provided. The functions, both real and putative, of calcitonin (CT), the third Ca-regulating hormone, are reviewed in Chapter 13. This most recently discovered of the three critical hormones involved in Ca homeostasis remains an enigma, because humankind can survive well without it, at least after the first year or so of life. The last hormones covered in this section, the steroids, both estrogens and corticosteroids (Chapter 14), are included, not because they are Ca-regulating per se, but because they have such powerful effects on skeletal tissues, either good or bad. Estrogens secreted by females (but probably not by males in sufficient amounts) exert powerful conserving effects on bone tissue, even though bone cells have many fewer estrogen receptors than cells of the reproductive organs. Corticosteroids have, on the other hand, adverse effects on bone that lead, in cases of excessive adrenal production or chronic therapy, to significant reductions in bone mass and the functions of several organs.

This section provides the information on hormones that act on bone, gut, and renal tissues and thereby greatly affect both the availability and the amounts of Ca ions in extracellular fluids.

Chapter 11

PARATHYROID HORMONE

Sanford C. Garner, Ph.D.

TABLE OF CONTENTS

0-8493-7845-1/95/$0.00+$.50

I. INTRODUCTION

The concentration of ionized plasma calcium (Ca^{++}) is the physiologic regulator of parathyroid hormone (PTH) secretion and is in turn tightly regulated by this peptide hormone. Plasma calcium (Ca) is maintained within very tight limits for an individual, typically within 2 to 3% of the mean value over time. However, in the absence of PTH, the physico-chemical equilibrium between free Ca in the blood and calcium phosphate crystals in the bone will result in a decrease of plasma Ca to 30–40% below its normal concentration (total) of approximately 10 mg/dL (2.5 m*M*). The fall of blood Ca in the absence of PTH results in abnormal nerve function and involuntary muscle contractions known as tetany. If this condition is not reversed by restoring Ca to the normal range, death will ensue. Thus, the parathyroid glands are essential for the maintenance of life in most mammalian species because of their role in regulating the blood concentrations of Ca and inorganic phosphorus (Pi).

PTH prevents the fall in Ca by increasing the movement of Ca ions from bone fluid to plasma and from urinary filtrate back into plasma, thus conserving the Ca that would be lost in the urine. In addition, PTH indirectly increases intestinal absorption of Ca by promoting formation of $1,25(OH)_2D$, the active metabolite of vitamin D.

This chapter summarizes all aspects of parathyroid physiology, from biosynthesis of PTH to regulation of its secretion and metabolism to its major functions in bone and kidney. In addition, the clinical disorders of PTH secretion are discussed, and the variations in parathyroid function across the lifecycle are briefly reviewed. The literature relating to PTH is quite large, and only a small portion of it is represented here. A thorough treatment of our current knowledge of PTH and the parathyroid has been published recently and provides information in greater depth on all aspects of parathyroid function, particularly clinically related changes in PTH secretion.[1]

II. PARATHYROID GLAND ANATOMY AND HISTOLOGY

In humans, the parathyroid glands are four small, compact bodies that generally are embedded beneath the capsule of the thyroid or, rarely, within the thyroid mass itself (Figure 1). The number and location varies slightly among species. The parathyroid cells arise embryologically from the neuroectoderm; thus, if migration into the thyroid tissue is not complete, ectopic parathyroid glands may be found in adults. Parathyroid tissue is found in all mammals, birds, and amphibians, but not in fish. However, a hypercalcemic factor in the fish pituitary, which may be the evolutionary precursor of PTH, has also been reported.

The parathyroid gland contains two major types of cells in humans. These are the chief cells that secrete PTH and the oxyphil cells that are mitochondria-rich but do not appear to be able to synthesize PTH. Although a conversion of chief cells to oxyphil cells likely occurs over time, particularly as individuals age, the regulation of this transition is not understood. Parathyroid glands also contain increasing numbers of fat cells with age.

III. PTH GENE AND REGULATION OF TRANSCRIPTION

A single copy of the gene for PTH exists in the human genome, and it is located on the short arm of chromosome 11. There are two introns inserted between three exons (Figure 2) that code for the

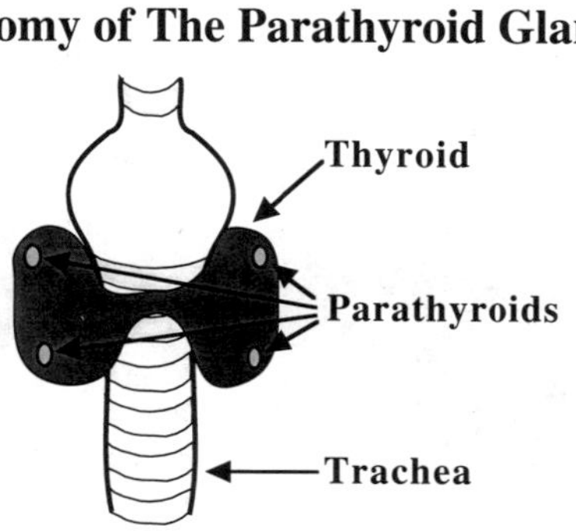

FIGURE 1. Anatomy of the Parathyroid Gland. The parathyroid gland normally consists of 4 small, separate lobes of tissue embedded in the surface of the thyroid gland. Although shown here on the front of the thyroid, the parathyroids are variable in location and are often found behind the thyroid. In addition, the usual number of 4 lobes may vary from 3 to 5 or even more in some individuals. Ectopic locations of the parathyroid are also common, with many individuals having one or more lobes distant from the thyroid.

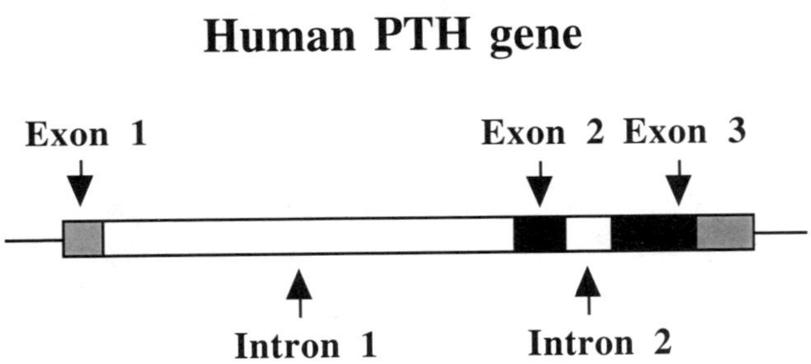

FIGURE 2. Human PTH Gene Structure. The gene for human PTH contains 3 exons that are transcribed to PTH mRNA; these 3 regions are separated by 2 introns containing 3400 and 103 base pairs, respectively. Exon 1 consists of a sequence of either 100 or 129 base pairs, depending on the initiation site for mRNA synthesis, and forms a 3′-untranslated region of PTH mRNA. Exon 2 contains a nucleotide sequence coding for most of the "prepro" sequence for PTH. Exon 3 contains the remainder of the "pro" sequence and the nucleotides coding for PTH_{1-84} (black area). The remainder of Exon 3 (gray area) codes for a 3′-untranslated portion of the PTH mRNA.[2,3]

complete PTH molecule.[2,3] Regulatory sequences in the upstream regions of the gene that are likely to control transcription of the PTH gene have been reported to include consensus sequences for cAMP- and vitamin D-response elements. In addition, a number of investigators have demonstrated that Ca concentration, vitamin D, and glucocorticoids can regulate the amount of messenger RNA for PTH in the parathyroid cell.

IV. SYNTHESIS AND SECRETION OF PARATHYROID HORMONE

Relatively small amounts of PTH are stored in parathyroid chief cells. Therefore, most of the PTH secreted in response to hypocalcemia is newly synthesized as a rapid response to the demand for PTH. PTH is synthesized as a 115 amino acid precursor molecule (preproPTH) containing two regions at the amino terminus that are removed during processing to the mature, biologically active molecule consisting of 84 amino acids.[4] As the preproPTH molecule is synthesized on ribosomes attached to the RER, it is transported into the cisternal space of the RER, where the leader or "pre" sequence of 25 amino acids is removed by proteolytic enzymes (Figure 3). ProPTH is transported from RER to the Golgi complex, where the "pro" sequence of 6 amino acids is removed to produce biologically active PTH_{1-84}. From the Golgi, PTH is packaged into secretory vesicles, from which secretion occurs by exocytosis.

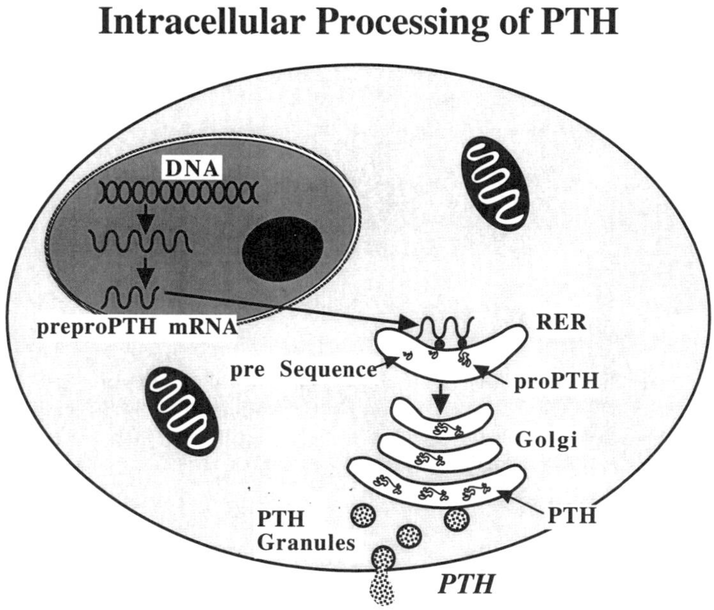

FIGURE 3. Intracellular Processing of PTH. The mRNA for preproPTH is produced by splicing of the sequence transcribed from the PTH gene. This mRNA is translated by ribosomes, which transfer the protein product into the cisternae of the rough endoplasmic reticulum, a process controlled by the "pre"- sequence of preproPTH. Cleavage of the "pre"-sequence occurs rapidly and the proPTH product is formed within the RER. As this product moves into the connecting Golgi apparatus, the "pro"-sequence is cleaved and $PTH_{1\text{-}84}$ is packaged into secretory granules together with PSP-I (chromogranin) for possible secretion.

Once PTH is packaged into secretory vesicles, it may experience one of three fates: (1) secretion, (2) storage, or (3) intracellular degradation (Figure 4). PTH secreted in response to decreased extracellular Ca comes mainly from newly synthesized hormone stores with the conventional (or "old") storage granules perhaps serving as an emergency supply of PTH. The latter class of granules is released preferentially by noncalcium secretagogues that increase intracellular cAMP.

A second major protein, parathyroid secretory protein-I (PSP-I), is synthesized and secreted by the parathyroid gland. This glycoprotein of molecular weight 72,000 or 64,000 is identical to the chromogranins, acidic glycoproteins present in storage vesicles for catecholamines in adrenal medullary cells. However, the functional significance of PSP-I in the parathyroid gland is unknown. Although the secretion of PSP-I is regulated by the same factors that control PTH secretion, expression of the gene for PSP-I is regulated somewhat differently.

The synthesis of PTH is relatively insensitive to factors, such as hypocalcemia, that control PTH secretion. An elevated extracellular Ca concentration rapidly suppresses PTH secretion by 80% or more, whereas it decreases the biosynthesis of the prohormone by only 15%.[5] Therefore, intracellular degradation of PTH serves as an important control point for PTH secretion as the need for more PTH secretion is met by a reduction in degradation. When parathyroid cells are exposed *in vitro* to high Ca over 48–72 hrs, PTH mRNA levels may be suppressed by approximately 50%.

A. CALCIUM CONTROL OF PTH SECRETION

The concept of the inverse relationship between the extracellular Ca concentration and the secretion of PTH is a well-established one as demonstrated in the 1940s by infusion of decalcified blood through the thyroparathyroid of the dog, which led to an increase in serum Ca in the peripheral circulation. The conclusion drawn from this response was that low blood Ca was a direct stimulus for the parathyroid gland to produce more hormone.

Additional evidence for a direct effect of Ca on PTH secretion was provided by Raisz et al.[6] using the *in vitro* incubation of rat parathyroid glands and an *in vitro* PTH bioassay. Low Ca in the medium

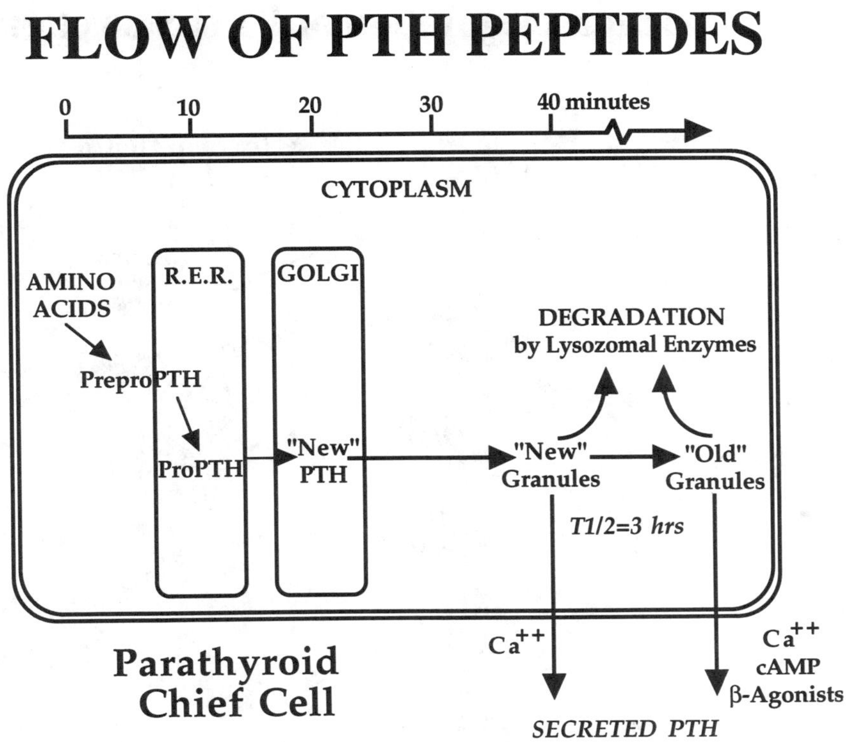

FIGURE 4. Flow of PTH Peptides. The processing of preproPTH to PTH is completed in approximately 20 minutes. However, once packaged into secretory granules, the maturation of granules appears to result in two pools of releasable PTH, a "new" population that is released preferentially by hypocalcemia and an "older" population that is released by both hypocalcemia and intracellular cAMP stimulated by β-adrenergic agonists or other hormonal stimuli. (Modified from Reference 49 with permission)

stimulated, and high Ca inhibited, amino acid uptake, nucleic acid and protein synthesis, hormonal secretion, and protein release by parathyroid tissue.

The availability of the newly developed radioimmunoassay for PTH in the late 1960s led to more direct demonstrations of the release of PTH from the isolated parathyroid gland; however, this assay technique also provided evidence for the presence in the circulation of fragments of PTH that lack biological activity (see Metabolism of PTH later). An inverse relationship between the serum Ca concentration and PTH release *in vivo* was demonstrated in several animal models, confirming the conclusion that Ca is the primary determinant of PTH secretion.

B. COUPLING OF EXTRACELLULAR CALCIUM AND PTH SECRETION

The stimulatory effect of low Ca on PTH secretion is nearly unique among endocrine cells. With the exception of renin secretion by juxtaglomerular cells of the kidney, other endocrine cells respond to an increase in extracellular Ca with an increase in secretion. Experiments with permeabilized parathyroid cells have demonstrated that increasing intracellular Ca in the millimolar range can stimulate secretion of PTH. This experimental finding, together with additional evidence provided by the demonstration that impermeant ions, such as lanthanum, and polyvalent cations, such as neomycin, can inhibit secretion of PTH despite being confined to the exterior of the cell, led to the proposal of a membrane receptor for Ca that mediates the response of the parathyroid cell to low extracellular Ca.

Recently, Brown and co-workers have reported the cloning of a protein with characteristics of a Ca sensor from a cDNA library derived from bovine parathyroid cell messenger RNA.[7] The protein derived from this cDNA has a predicted topological structure that is similar to the seven membrane-spanning domains of the G-protein-coupled superfamily of receptors. The receptor responds to

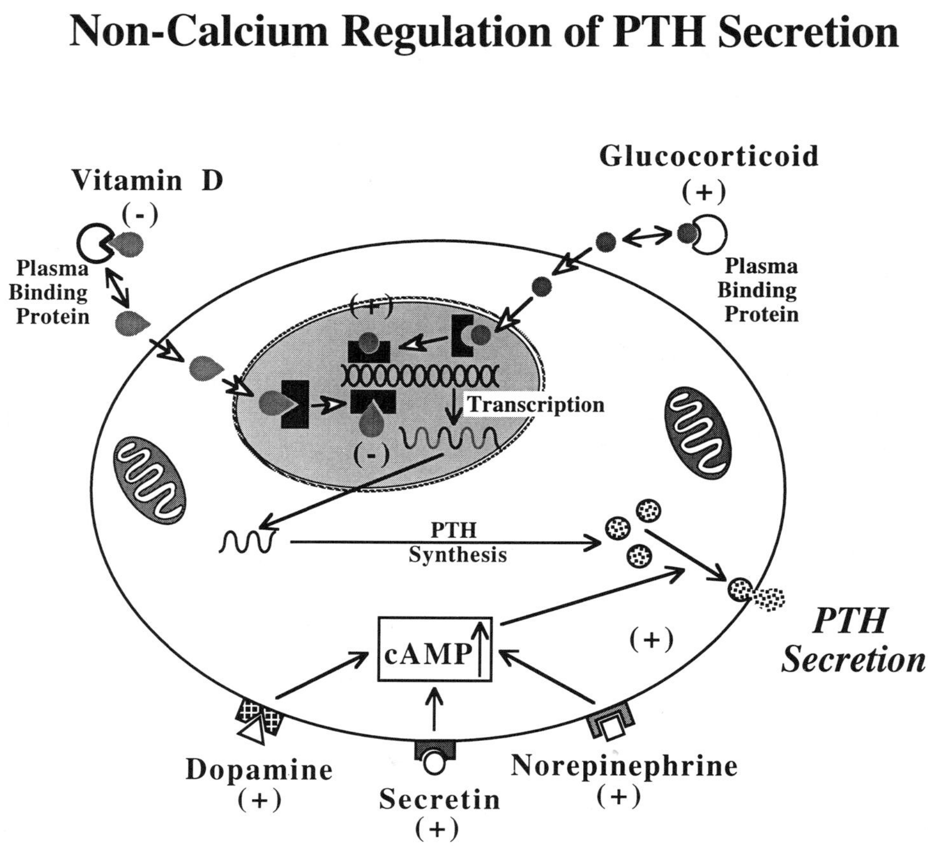

FIGURE 5. Noncalcium Regulation of PTH Secretion. Calcium is accepted as the primary regulator of PTH secretion; however, experimental evidence points to potential modulation of PTH secretion by either peptide hormones, such as norepinephrine, secretin, or dopamine that act through cAMP formation, or steroid hormones, such as vitamin D and glucocorticoids, e.g., cortisol, that regulate transcription of PTH mRNA. Vitamin D has been used clinically to control PTH secretion during parathyroid hyperplasia secondary to renal failure.

extracellular Ca and other polyvalent cations with an increase in intracellular phosphatidylinositol turnover. Using the bovine Ca receptor cDNA, studies have identified a similar nucleotide sequence in human parathyroid adenoma cells. Thus, the transducing mechanism for hypocalcemic stimulation of PTH secretion has begun to be elucidated.

The relationship between the decrease of extracellular Ca and the subsequent increase in secretion of bioactive PTH from parathyroid cells is well accepted; however, the intracellular second messenger system or systems through which activation of the cell-surface Ca receptor elicits an increase in PTH secretion is an area of active investigation. Several intracellular molecules have been proposed as second messengers, including intracellular Ca^{++}, cAMP, inositol phosphates, and diacylglycerol. Agents that increase intracellular cAMP in parathyroid cells, including β-adrenergic catecholamines, dopamine, secretin, and prostaglandin E_2, can stimulate PTH secretion (Figure 5). However, changes in cAMP do not correlate well with responses of parathyroid cells to physiologic changes in extracellular Ca^{++}. In addition, the pool of PTH granules released in response to cAMP appears to differ from the pool that is released in response to hypocalcemia (Figure 4). Similarly, the intracellular Ca^{++} concentration of parathyroid cells varies with extracellular Ca^{++}, but this alone is not adequate to explain the coupling of hypocalcemia and secretion. Brown et al.[8] have proposed that activation of protein kinase C stimulates PTH secretion. In their proposed model, increased phospholipid turnover as a result of decreased extracellular Ca^{++} would increase intracellular diacylglycerol levels, which in turn would activate protein kinase C. However, both diacylglycerol and inositol phosphate (IP_3) increase in parathyroid cells in the presence of elevated extracellular Ca^{++}, presumably through activation of phospholipase C.[9] Thus, the intracellular effectors for PTH secretion in response to decreased extracellular Ca^{++} are not yet identified. The recently described membrane Ca^{++} sensor and several second-messenger systems, possibly including intracellular Ca^{++}, cAMP, phospholipase C-generated messengers, protein kinase C, and possible inhibitors of protein kinase C from the sphingomyelin pathway, may form a complex regulatory system for the secretion of PTH.

C. NONCALCIUM SECRETAGOGUES FOR PTH

Despite the acceptance of hypocalcemia as the primary stimulus for PTH secretion, a role for other secretagogues continues to be investigated (Figure 5). Several circulating factors have been demonstrated to stimulate PTH secretion either *in vitro* or *in vivo,* and these putative modulators of PTH secretion have been reviewed elsewhere.[10,11] Stimulation of PTH secretion, probably through increased intracellular cAMP, has been reported for the peptide hormone, secretin, and for the neurotransmitters, β-adrenergic catecholamines and dopamine. In addition, steroid or steroid-like hormones have been shown to be either stimulatory, in the case of glucocorticoids, or inhibitory, in the case of $1,25(OH)_2$-vitamin D. Although considerable evidence exists that at least some of these agents are consistently effective in increasing or suppressing the secretion of PTH, either *in vitro* or *in vivo,* none of these agents has been demonstrated to have a normal physiologic function in modulating PTH secretion.

D. SIGMOIDAL RELATIONSHIP BETWEEN PTH AND CALCIUM

Sherwood et al.[12] postulated a linear relationship between extracellular Ca and PTH secretion. However, subsequent research has revealed a sigmoidal relationship between these two parameters. Mayer and Hurst[13] measured PTH secretion in calves by radioimmunoassay (RIA) of parathyroid venous blood over a range of plasma Ca obtained by intravenous infusion of Ca or EDTA solutions. They found that a plot of PTH vs. plasma Ca produced a sigmoidal relationship with a maximum secretion of PTH that was maintained at plasma Ca less than 7.5 mg/dL and a minimum secretion that could not be reduced further at plasma Ca greater than 10.5 mg/dL. A consistent finding has been that an irreducible level of PTH secretion with approximately 10–20% residual secretion persists no matter how high the Ca level is raised.

1. Theoretical Treatment of Set Point

The sigmoidal relationship between PTH secretion and extracellular Ca concentration can be modeled mathematically (see Figure 6). Brown[14] and others have calculated theoretical curves for *in vitro* secretion of PTH from dispersed human parathyroid cells in response to changing Ca. By comparing secretion from parathyroid cells over a range of Ca concentrations either *in vitro* or *in vivo,* one can compare the difference in response after adjusting the PTH concentrations to a maximum secretion rate determined at low Ca. In this way the effect of a change in the set point for secretion has been demonstrated to affect PTH levels *in vivo*. Differences in the set point have been demonstrated for pathological parathyroid tissue and for parathyroid tissue in young mammals.

2. Alteration of Set Point in Parathyroid Adenoma and Hyperplasia

When Ca control of secretion of PTH from parathyroid adenomas was first examined *in vitro* and *in vivo,* the suggestion was made that secretion from many adenomas was autonomous of control by Ca. However, subsequently Brown et al.[15,16] reported that the set point for normal human parathyroid cells was 1.0 m*M* whereas, for a majority of adenomas, the set point exceeded this value. Most adenomatous and hyperplastic parathyroid tissues have been responsive to inhibition of PTH secretion by hypercalcemia, but extraordinarily high levels of Ca may be required to demonstrate the inhibition of secretion.

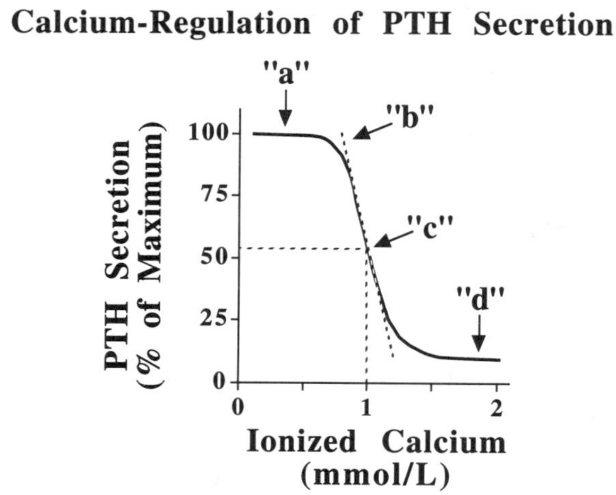

FIGURE 6. PTH Set Point. PTH secretion is characterized by suppressiblity by increasing extracellular ionized calcium concentrations. Due to the phenomena of maximum secretion rate and a minimum, nonsuppressible rate of secretion characteristic of parathyroid chief cells, the relationship between PTH secretion and ionized calcium concentration can be described by a sigmoidal curve defined by the following equation:

$$\text{PTH secretion} = ((a-d)/(1 + (x/c)^b)) + d$$

where a = maximum PTH release, b = slope of the curve at the set point, c = set point (Ca^{++} concentration causing half-maximal inhibition of secretion), and d = minimum PTH release.

V. METABOLISM OF PTH

In addition to the degradation of PTH that takes place within the parathyroid gland and is a major regulatory process in the control of PTH secretion, extensive metabolism of PTH occurs in peripheral tissues. The half-life for intact PTH molecules in plasma is less than 5 minutes. The Kuppfer cells of the liver are responsible for cleavage of the intact PTH molecule between residues 33–34 and 36–37. The kidney is responsible for clearance of the intact molecule and fragments by receptor-mediated uptake and glomerular filtration, respectively.[17] The carboxyterminal fragments accumulate in the blood at much higher concentrations than the intact PTH molecule does because of a much longer half-life in plasma. When renal function is impaired, the carboxyterminal fragments may reach extraordinarily high concentrations, even when the biologically active, intact PTH concentration is within normal limits.

Experiments with ^{125}I-labeled PTH injected into rats[18] have demonstrated the kinetics of PTH metabolism. A rapid (3 min) initial disappearance curve is followed by a slower (48 min) component. Similar results have been obtained by an assay of serum from patients undergoing surgery for the removal of parathyroid adenoma.

VI. PTH STRUCTURE AND FUNCTION

Parathyroid hormone consists of a single chain of 84 amino acids (Figure 7) in all species for which the structure has been determined, i.e., bovine, human, porcine, and rat. Tregear et al.[19] demonstrated that a peptide with the sequence of amino acids 1-27 of PTH had some bioactivity, but the amount of activity increased with addition of amino acids 28 and 29. Both the 1-34 and 1-84 sequences have full activity in most assay systems, although some exceptions have been proposed. Removal of the first amino acid from the N-terminus of PTH reduces bioactivity, and removal of amino acids 1 and 2 produces a molecule with antagonistic properties in some *in vitro* assay systems.

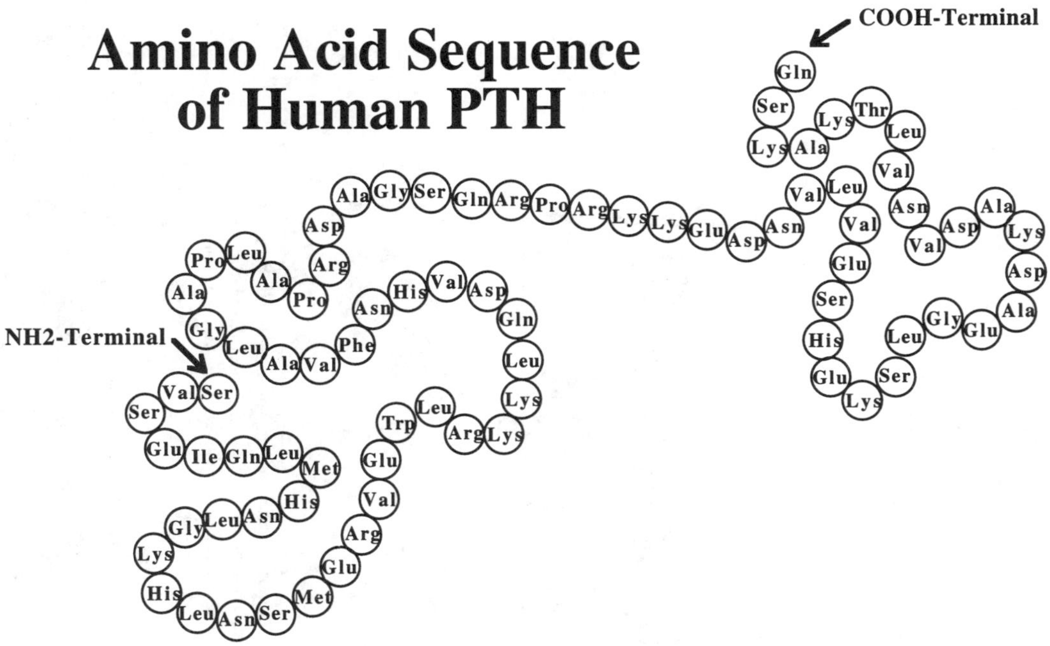

FIGURE 7. Secondary and Tertiary Structure of Human PTH. The arrangement of the amino acids of PTH into a tertiary structure with two cores of hydrophobic amino acids is based on the tertiary structural model proposed by Zull and Lev.[50]

Despite the finding that $PTH_{1\text{-}34}$ is equipotent with $PTH_{1\text{-}84}$ in most assay systems, the possibility still remains that the 2 forms of the hormone may have different functions in some systems. Doses of $PTH_{1\text{-}34}$ and $PTH_{1\text{-}84}$ that were equipotent for the stimulation of Pi excretion differed in their effect on the renal tubular reabsorption of Ca.[20] $PTH_{1\text{-}84}$ at the dose tested did not increase net Ca excretion, whereas an equimolar dose of $PTH_{1\text{-}34}$ did increase it. The conclusion was that $PTH_{1\text{-}84}$, but not $PTH_{1\text{-}34}$, increases the distal renal tubular reabsorption of Ca and thus enhances conservation of this cation.

The studies by Goltzman et al.[21] of the multiple molecular forms of bioactive PTH using gel filtration of sera from individuals with primary hyperparathyroidism and with secondary hyperparathyroidism due to renal insufficiency suggest that the bioactive PTH in primary hyperparathyroidism is $PTH_{1\text{-}84}$ with little or no $PTH_{1\text{-}34}$ present. However, in the patients with renal failure there were significant amounts of $PTH_{1\text{-}34}$ in the plasma. The source of this bioactive fragment was not determined, but its direct secretion by the parathyroid gland was ruled out.

A. PTH RECEPTORS

The PTH receptor has been reported to be a 585 amino acid protein[22] that belongs to the class of receptors that have seven transmembrane domains and that activate adenylate cyclase and phospholipase C through stimulatory G proteins (see Figure 8). This receptor binds both $PTH_{1\text{-}34}$ and parathyroid hormone-related peptide (PTHrP) and is believed to be responsible for the effects of both peptides to stimulate movement of Ca ions from bone or kidney into blood. Although the major calcemic effects of PTH are likely to be mediated through the PTH/PTHrP receptor molecule that binds the amino-terminal region of the hormone, some investigators have proposed a second receptor specific for the carboxyl-terminal portion of PTH.[23-25] Although the existence of this second receptor for PTH has not been confirmed experimentally, its existence could explain apparent discrepancies in the effects of $PTH_{1\text{-}34}$ and $PTH_{1\text{-}84}$ in some assays.

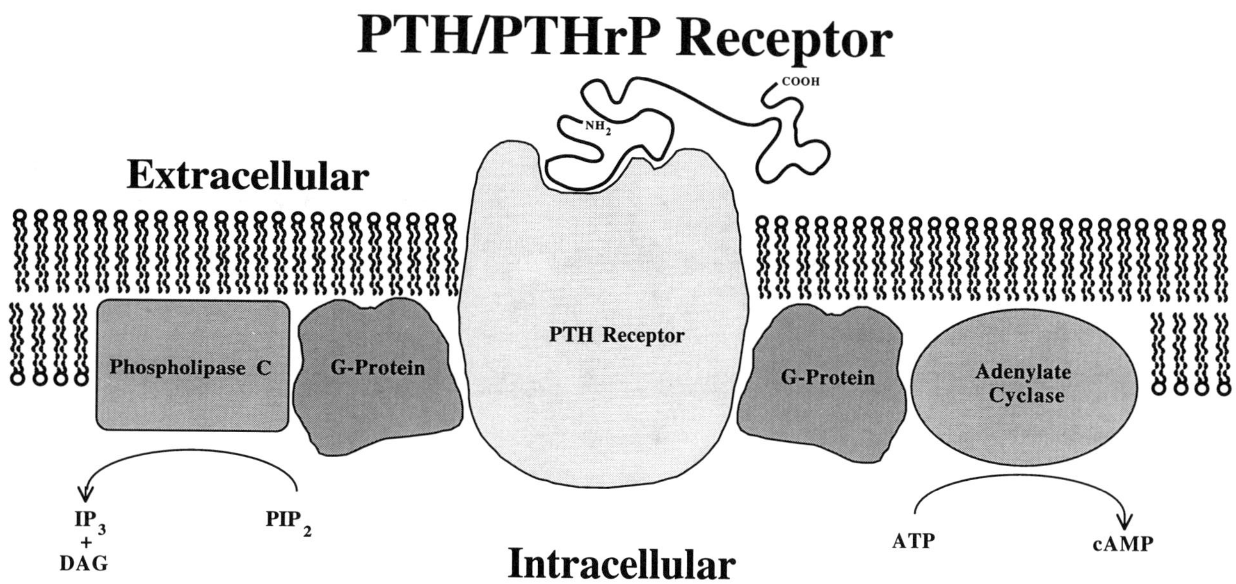

FIGURE 8. PTH Receptor and Intracellular Second Messengers. PTH and PTHrP share a common receptor in bone and kidney. The receptor recognizes the amino-terminal portion of the PTH molecule, and binding of PTH results in activation of adenylate cyclase and phospholipase C through a stimulatory G-protein. The increase in intracellular cyclic adenosine monophosphate (cAMP), diacylglycerol (DAG), and inositol trisphosphate (IP_3) mediates the effects of PTH on the target cells.

B. BIOLOGICAL EFFECTS OF PTH

PTH has 5 major biological effects: (1) mobilization of Ca from bone, (2) bone formation, (3) increased renal Pi excretion, (4) renal Ca retention, and (5) increased formation of $1,25(OH)_2D$. Therefore, the administration of large amounts of PTH produces several characteristic, easily measured responses. Within minutes both serum Ca and serum phosphorus (P) increase, and the urinary excretion of Ca decreases, whereas that of Pi increases. In addition, an increase in urinary cAMP can be detected. Over the longer term net loss of bone mineral and matrix follows and soft-tissue calcification may also occur. The resorption of bone leading to the degradation of collagen results in an increase in serum and urinary hydroxyproline. These effects are also seen in individuals with hyperparathyroidism. Although these effects of grossly elevated serum PTH are related to physiological responses to PTH, they may not accurately reflect the relative importance of these responses in the normal individual.

1. Effects of PTH on Bone

Mobilization of Ca from bone by physiologic concentrations of PTH involves the osteoblastic cells, and is probably mediated primarily by the bone-lining cells. Stimulation of osteoclasts by prostaglandin E results in increased bone resorption, but not in increased plasma Ca. Additional information on the regulation of extracellular Ca concentration by PTH has been obtained from isotopic studies that indicate that PTH increases the availability of Ca and P in the bone fluid compartment. Although the mechanism by which bone cells respond to PTH with movement of Ca from bone to blood is not known, Talmage et al.[26] concluded that osteoclasts are not involved in the short-term regulation of plasma Ca.

The first response to an injection of PTH is a small reduction in serum Ca that appears to be due to the increased permeability of bone cell membranes. This hypocalcemic response is followed by the efflux of Ca from bone fluid into the serum. Bone cells (primarily the osteoblasts) also respond to PTH with an increase in adenyl cyclase and phospholipase C activity. Increased intracellular Ca, cAMP, diacylglycerol (DAG), and inositol phosphate (IP_3) (DAG and IP_3 are products of phospholipase C activity) have been reported to serve as second messengers for the effects of PTH on bone cells.

If the dose of PTH is high enough, osteoclastic activity will be stimulated and bone resorption will result. Although PTH increases osteoclastic activity, receptors for PTH have only recently been reported to exist on the osteoclast.[27] Binding of PTH to these receptors has been reported to inhibit rather than stimulate osteoclastic activity. Therefore, the current hypothesis is that osteoblasts stimulate osteoclastic activity by either releasing soluble factors or by expressing a membrane-bound osteoclast stimulator. The catabolic effect of PTH on bone is an important one when serum PTH is increased well above normal circulating levels. The erosion of bone that accompanies hyperparathyroidism was an early indicator of this clinical condition. Physiologically, the stimulation of osteoclastic bone resorption by PTH may be important during periods of increased demand for Ca such as those of pregnancy and lactation.

Despite the emphasis given to the resorptive effects of high doses of PTH, the hormone also has an anabolic effect on bone. The PTH stimulation of bone formation probably occurs via direct stimulation of osteoblastic activity. The separation of anabolic and catabolic effects of PTH on bone depends, at least in part, on the mode of administration; intermittent administration of PTH by injection produces significant increases in bone mass in animal studies, whereas similar doses of PTH administered by continuous infusion do not.[28] Due to its ability to increase bone mass rather than only to decrease the rate of loss as most other anti-osteoporotic agents do, PTH as a possible treatment for osteoporosis is under investigation.

2. Effects of PTH on the Kidney

PTH reduces reabsorption of sodium, Ca, Pi, and bicarbonate in the proximal renal tubule. Most of the sodium is reabsorbed distally. PTH increases Ca reabsorption in the distal portion of the tubule and produces a net retention of Ca, contributing to the hypercalcemic effect of PTH. The anions, however, are not reabsorbed and an increased phosphaturia results. The urinary loss exceeds the increase in efflux of P from bone, and the net effect is a fall in serum P after PTH injection. Resorption of bone results in an efflux of Ca, P, and bicarbonate into plasma; the effect of PTH on the kidney is to promote excretion of the anions while conserving the Ca.

PTH also stimulates activity of the 1-hydroxylase that converts 25(OH)D to $1,25(OH)_2D$ in kidney cells. The $1,25(OH)_2D$ stimulates the intestinal absorption of Ca by increasing synthesis of Ca-binding proteins in intestinal absorptive cells.

3. Nonclassical Effects of PTH

Effects of PTH on targets other than bone or kidney have been reported. These effects have included abnormal electroencephalogram (EEG), inhibition of erythropoiesis, inhibition of platelet aggregation, chronotropic and inotropic effects on myocardium, and alterations in carbohydrate and lipid metabolism.[29] Vasodilatory effects of PTH have also been investigated. PTH has been shown by several investigators to produce a decreased arterial pressure in rats, dogs, and other species. PTH also has a direct effect to relax smooth muscle *in vitro.*

Although some of the these effects have been postulated to be responsible for some of the pathological manifestations of uremia due to secondary hyperparathyroidism, there is no evidence that PTH exerts important effects at physiological concentrations on any tissue besides bone and kidney. The effects of PTH on other functions were obtained with concentrations that were 1000–10,000 times normal circulating levels.

VII. PTH ASSAYS

The goal of PTH assays has historically been to increase the sensitivity of the assay sufficiently to measure the very small amount of PTH present in normal sera, approximately 10 pg/mL. However, this task has been made more difficult by the heterogeneous nature of circulating fragments of PTH. The types of assay methods for PTH fall into several categories: (1) *in vivo* bioassays, (2) *in vitro* bioassays, and (3) *in vitro* immunoassays. The *in vivo* bioassays may be further subdivided by the response to PTH that is measured and the species in which it is assayed. PTH bioassays may measure a change in serum Ca or altered urinary Pi excretion, for example. The *in vitro* bioassays for PTH fit into three subtypes based on the nature of the response measured: (1) release of Ca from whole rat or mouse bones, (2) synthesis of cAMP by bone or kidney cells, and (3) stimulation of glucose-6-phosphate dehydrogenase activity in kidney or bone cells. The basic types of the *in vitro* immunoassay are the radioimmunoassay (RIA), the immunoradiometric assay (IRMA), and the immunochemiluminometric assay (ICMA).

The first reliable technique for assaying PTH was developed by Collip in the 1920s using an increase in serum Ca concentration in the intact dog after infusion of parathyroid extracts.[30] Munson in the 1950s developed a method for the assay of PTH in parathyroidectomized (PTX) rats in which the injection of PTH prevented the initial fall in serum Ca that would normally follow PTX.[31] Other *in vivo* assays of this period used the hypercalcemic response of intact rats or chicks or the phosphaturic response of mice or rats to injection of PTH.

The most sensitive assay for PTH yet developed is the cytochemical bioassay of Chayen and co-workers as described by Chambers, et al.[32] This assay is based on an increase in the activity of glucose-6-phosphate dehydrogenase in distal tubule cells of guinea-pig kidneys in response to incubation with PTH. Although this assay is extremely sensitive and is able to measure PTH concentrations in the femtogram/mL range, it is also exceedingly time consuming and is used mainly for limited research applications. Other *in vitro* bioassays based on the stimulation of cAMP synthesis by renal membranes or by intact osteoblast-like cells derived from osteosarcoma have also shown promise of being sensitive enough to measure normal circulating levels of PTH, but these bioassays have not been widely used.

In the 1960s the technique of radioimmunoassay was developed and refined by Berson, Yalow, and co-workers.[33] PTH was one of the first hormones for which they developed an RIA, and at first it appeared that this method would reliably measure serum PTH. However, the existence of multiple forms of PTH or fragments of PTH in the circulation[34] have complicated the use of the RIA for clinical measurements of PTH. Not all of the circulating forms of PTH are biologically active.[35] Thus, although there was often good correlation between the levels of PTH measured by these RIAs and those measured by a bioassay, there was some question as to how reliably the values reflected the parathyroid status of an individual.

Today, the most commonly used clinical assay for PTH involves the use of two antibodies to different portions of the intact PTH molecule to provide a sensitive assay that measures only the biologically active molecule. In these assays, the first antibody, which is usually directed against the C-terminal portion of the molecule, is immobilized to a large polystyrene bead or to the surface of the assay tube to extract intact PTH and C-terminal fragments from the sample (Figure 9). The second antibody, which is usually directed against the N-terminal portion of the PTH molecule, is labeled with ^{125}Iodine (IRMA) or a chemiluminescent molecule (ICMA) to allow detection of the bound antibody. Because of the requirement for the complete PTH structure to form the antibody-antigen-antibody "sandwich," these assays are believed to recognize only the intact, biologically active molecule.[36]

VIII. CLINICAL DISORDERS INVOLVING PTH

Clinical disorders of parathyroid function include several types of both under- and over-activity of PTH, i.e., hypo- and hyperparathyroidism.

A. HYPOPARATHYROIDISM

Hypoparathyroidism may result from either decreased secretion or decreased peripheral action of PTH. The most direct consequences of hypoparathyroidism are hypocalcemia and hyperphosphatemia. The clinical manifestations of hypoparathyroidism are primarily a result of the hypocalcemia. Reduced plasma-ionized Ca causes increased neuromuscular excitability, which may result in tetany (uncontrollable muscular twitching) when the Ca drops to a low enough level. Four steps in the biological action of PTH at which defects could occur that would result in clinical manifestations of hypoparathyroidism are the following: (1) insufficient PTH secretion, (2) secretion of inactive PTH, (3) presence in plasma of a PTH antagonist, or (4) defect at the target cell involving the PTH receptor or intracellular second messengers.

Insufficient PTH secretion may result from a number of causes; these include (1) injury to the parathyroid during thyroid surgery, (2) hypomagnesemia, (3) suppression following hypercalcemia, and (4) cancer chemotherapy with doxorubicin or cytosine arabinoside. Deficient PTH secretion for which no discernible cause is found, i.e., "idiopathic" hypoparathyroidism, is rare. The suggestion has been made that autoimmunity may be responsible for some cases.

Hypoparathyroidism caused by a defect in PTH synthesis or processing that would result in the secretion of inactive PTH is a theoretical explanation for this condition. A few cases have been presented that may fall into this category, but this mechanism has not been confirmed.

B. PSEUDOHYPOPARATHYROIDISM

Pseudohypoparathyroidism (PHP) is characterized by a resistance to parathyroid hormone rather than by a lack of the hormone. The underlying defect explaining the resistance to PTH in PHP might be at any of several steps in the biological response to PTH, for example, (1) a circulating antagonist of PTH (2) abnormal PTH receptors or (3) an abnormal adenylate cyclase component other than the receptor, e.g., the guanine nucleotide binding protein, cAMP-dependent protein kinase, or kinase substrate. Evidence suggests that the last condition exists in many individuals with pseudohypoparathyroidism because the red blood cell guanine nucleotide binding protein is decreased.

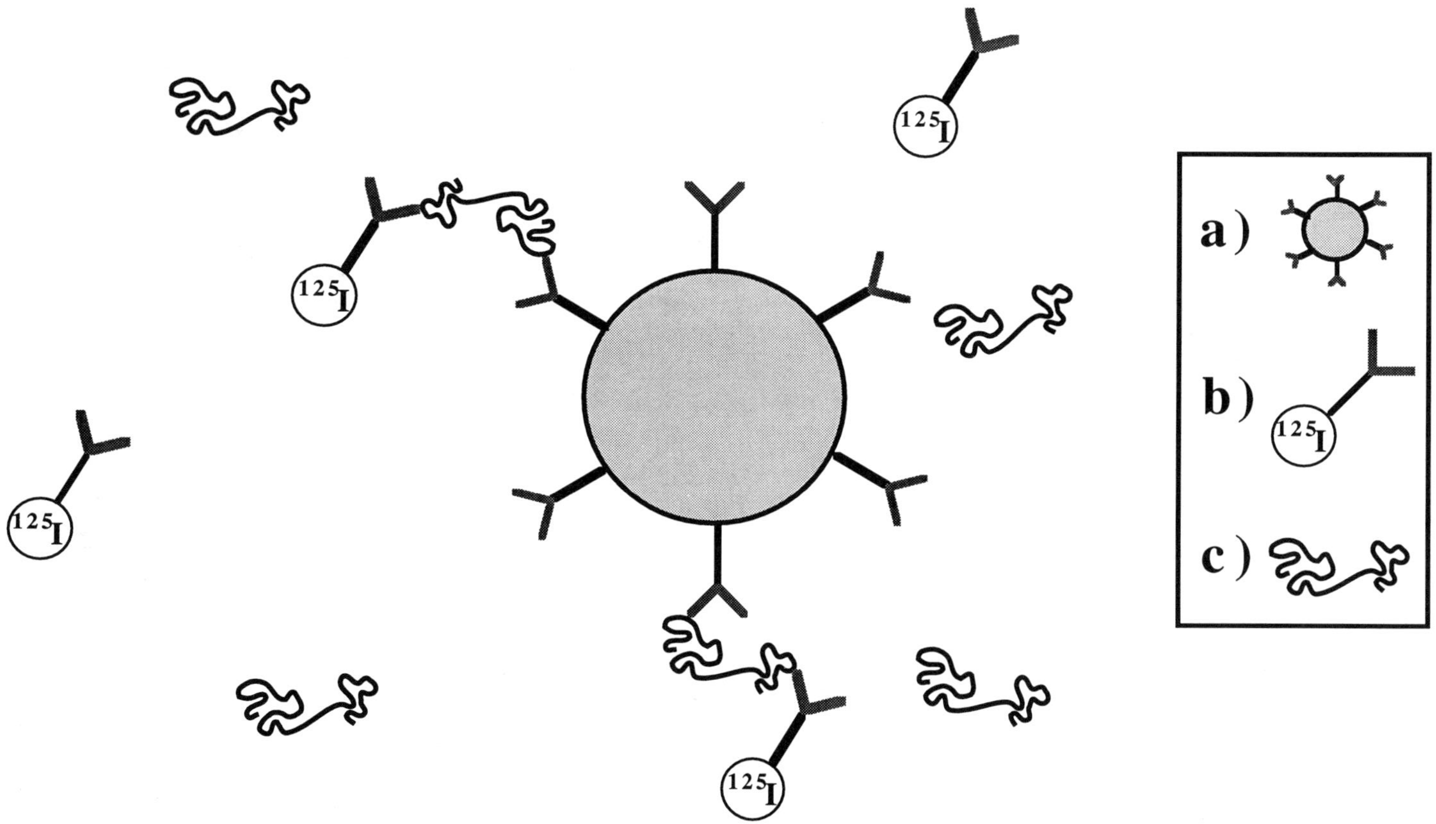

FIGURE 9. PTH Immunoradiometric Assay (IRMA). The immunoradiometric assay for PTH uses two antibodies, directed against two different segments of the amino acid sequence to measure the intact PTH_{1-84} molecule. The first antibody in this example (a) has selectivity for the carboxyl-terminal region of PTH and is covalently bound to a large polystyrene bead to “capture” the PTH molecules containing this part of the structure. The second antibody (b) is directed against the amino-terminal portion of PTH and is radiolabeled with ^{125}I for detection of the complex. Only molecules that contain both carboxyl- and amino-terminal portions of the molecule (c) are able to form the antibody-PTH-antibody “sandwich” necessary for retention of ^{125}I on the bead after extensive washing. The immunochemiluminometric assay (ICMA) is directly analogous to the IRMA, but the system for detecting the antibody-PTH-antibody complex is a luminescent molecule rather than a radionuclide.

However, the underlying defect in pseudohypoparathyroidism may also involve other defects in receptors or adenylate cyclase activity.

C. HYPERPARATHYROIDISM

Hyperparathyroidism may be classified as primary, secondary, or tertiary and involves the excessive secretion of PTH.

1. Primary Hyperparathyroidism

Primary hyperparathyroidism may be due to either hyperplasia of otherwise normal parathyroid cells or to an adenoma of the parathyroid gland. Adenomas have been postulated to develop from hyperplastic parathyroid glands. However, Arnold et al.[37] reported that adenomas were of clonal origin. The polyclonal nature of hyperplastic glands indicates that a fundamental difference exists among these types of hyperparathyroidism.

2. Secondary Hyperparathyroidism

Secondary hyperparathyroidism occurs when PTH is secreted in response to a tendency toward hypocalcemia. The hypocalcemia may result from renal insufficiency, intestinal malabsorption, and osteomalacia or rickets due to vitamin D deficiency among other causes. Immunoassayable serum PTH reaches extremely high levels in chronic renal failure due in part to decreased clearance of PTH fragments. However, biologically active PTH is also increased in later stages of the disease.

Hyperphosphatemia, decreased 1-hydroxylation of 25-hydroxyvitamin D, reduced intestinal absorption of Ca, and peripheral resistance to PTH may all contribute to PTH hypersecretion in renal failure. Renal retention of phosphate and the resulting rise in serum phosphate leads to hypocalcemia due in part to complexing of serum Ca by phosphate, resulting in a fall in serum-ionized Ca. The hyperphosphatemia also inhibits renal production of $1,25(OH)_2D_3$, which aggravates the hypocalcemia by reducing the intestinal absorption of Ca. Skeletal resistance to PTH also contributes to hypocalcemia, but the mechanisms for this resistance are not clear.

3. Tertiary Hyperparathyroidism

Tertiary hyperparathyroidism is the name given to secondary hyperparathyroidism that results in hyperplasia of the parathyroid similar to primary hyperparathyroidism.

D. HYPERCALCEMIA OF MALIGNANCY

Hypercalcemia of malignancy (HHM) may result from metastases of tumors to bone that produce bone resorption. However, increased bone resorption may also occur due to malignancies that do not have metastases on bone. In a few cases of hypercalcemia of malignancy, ectopic production of PTH by tumor cells has been demonstrated by assay of PTH secretion by the tumor *in vivo* and *in vitro*. In most cases, however, RIA of sera from patients with hypercalcemia associated with malignancy shows normal or suppressed levels of PTH.

In these cases of HHM serum immunoreactive PTH is normal; however, many individuals have a "PTH-like" substance that is not recognized by RIAs for PTH but do have activity in bioassays for PTH based on either renal or bone responses to PTH. This factor, which is larger than PTH, has been isolated and its sequence determined. Because it has effects on plasma calcium similar to those of PTH, this factor is most commonly called parathyroid hormone-related protein (PTHrP). PTHrP is synthesized as either a 139, 141, or 173 amino acid protein, depending on the splicing of the mRNA. The first 13 amino acids at the amino terminal portion of the PTHrP molecule have 70% homology with PTH, explaining, in part, the ability of this molecule to bind to the PTH receptor. PTHrP is made by a number of normal cells, including the lactating mammary gland, where expression of the PTHrP mRNA is regulated by prolactin. In addition PTHrP is synthesized in vascular smooth muscle and in smooth muscle of the gastrointestinal tract. Because PTHrP concentrations in plasma are below the limit of detection of current assays, it has been proposed that PTHrP is an autocrine/paracrine factor, which acts primarily on the cells that produce it or on nearby cells in the same tissue.

IX. PTH THROUGH THE LIFE CYCLE

The concentrations of PTH and ionized Ca may vary over the life cycle. Although marked changes occur at birth in both Ca and PTH, changes throughout the remainder of life are relatively small in comparison to the range of normal values. Because of the difficulty in assaying the biologically active PTH molecule before the development of the two-site immunoassays, the early reports of changes in serum PTH with age or during pregnancy and lactation must be interpreted cautiously.

A. PTH IN INFANCY, CHILDHOOD, AND ADOLESCENCE

Large amounts of calcium are transferred daily from mother to fetus via the placenta, resulting in higher blood calcium in the fetus relative to the mother. Samples of cord blood collected at birth demonstrate suppression of PTH, which increases markedly after birth as Ca decreases.[38] No evidence exists for neonatal hypoparathyroidism because the decrease in plasma Ca that occurs at birth elicits an increase in PTH secretion. Although few data are available for children from studies that have used the newer, more sensitive immunoassays for PTH, earlier reports do not suggest great differences during childhood in serum PTH concentrations or in the relationship between Ca concentrations and suppression of PTH secretion. Similarly, comprehensive cross-sectional or longitudinal studies of biologically active PTH in adolescence are not available. However, the studies that are in the literature suggest that adolescents have concentrations of immunoreactive PTH and ionized Ca similar to those of adults.

B. PTH IN ADULTS

Although serum-ionized Ca is tightly controlled for an individual and varies only moderately for normal adults (the mean value for serum ionized Ca is 1.25 mmol/L with ±5% variation), the serum immunoreactive PTH in adults varies over a fairly wide range between individuals. One major reference laboratory reports a range of 10 to 65 pg/mL for the 95% confidence interval for intact PTH. Adults below the age of 65 years do not differ in serum-ionized Ca or PTH concentrations, and most investigators have failed to find a significant difference between males and females. However, in a study performed in Denmark, a seasonal variation in serum PTH with higher levels in the winter was reported.[39]

Plasma PTH also varies for an individual over 24 hr. This circadian rhythm in PTH secretion results in a nocturnal increase in plasma PTH.[40] This pattern of changing PTH secretion during the day appears to be linked to changes in plasma-ionized Ca in most individuals, but there may be some involvement of adrenergic hormones.[41]

C. PTH DURING THE MENSTRUAL CYCLE

The most recent study on PTH concentrations during the menstrual cycle did not find any change throughout the cycle.[42] However, an earlier report found a rise in PTH at, or around, ovulation.[43]

D. PTH WITH AGING

Serum PTH has been reported by some investigators to be constant with advancing age, at least to age 65.[39] However, others found a gradual, significant increase of serum PTH with age in both normal men and women.[44] Even in individuals between 80 and 90 years of age, most serum PTH values lie within the range of 10 to 65 pg/mL described above.

E. PTH DURING PREGNANCY AND LACTATION

Pregnancy and lactation place additional stress on the mineral metabolism of the mother for maintenance of normal Ca concentration while she is providing mineral to the developing fetus and neonate, respectively, and a role for increased PTH secretion has been proposed. For many years there were reports in the literature on increased PTH during pregnancy, leading to a concept termed "physiological hyperparathyroidism of pregnancy." However, since the development of the sensitive 2-site immunoradiometric assays for PTH, Davis et al.[45] have reported on a group of 81 healthy women in their first pregnancy that their mean serum PTH was significantly lower than in a group of nonpregnant women with normal menstrual cycles. They confirmed this tendency by bioassay of serum PTH in a smaller number of pregnant and nonpregnant women.[45] Although the role of PTH in pregnancy and lactation does not appear to require major changes in circulating concentrations, there is clear evidence for significant changes in serum PTH in several animal species during pregnancy and/or lactation. The possibility exists that a modest change in serum PTH in humans is obscured by the variability of the hormone between individuals and by variations in diet or lifestyle that cannot be controlled in human studies.[46] In a study of lactational intensity effects, Greer et al.[47] found that PTH was significantly greater in women nursing twins compared to those nursing a single infant.

X. EFFECTS OF NUTRITIONAL MODIFICATION ON PTH SECRETION

Dietary intakes of Ca, P, and vitamin D within normal limits of variation do not appear to affect plasma PTH concentrations.[39] However, ingestion of a diet with high P combined with low Ca for 28 days has been demonstrated to increase circulating PTH.[48] Since this diet is representative of the typical intakes of Ca and P by many American teenagers and young adults, especially females, the possibility that chronically elevated PTH may impair the achievement of peak bone mass during these years has serious implications for long-term bone health.

XI. SUMMARY

There is a critical relationship between plasma-ionized Ca and PTH secretion; the negative feedback loop between these two circulating substances provides for very precise maintenance of plasma-ionized Ca. If it were not for the Ca-mobilizing effects of PTH on bone and kidney, there would be a rapid loss of Ca from the blood, resulting in life-threatening hypocalcemia. PTH also stimulates the maximum efficiency of Ca absorption by the small intestine when dietary Ca intakes are low. This effect is mediated through the kidney cells that hydroxylate 25-OH vitamin D to form 1,25$(OH)_2$-vitamin D.

Although several conditions of over- or undersecretion of PTH exist in human pathology, the relationship between PTH and Ca remains fairly constant throughout life for most of the population. Extremely high consumption of phosphates, coupled with inadequate dietary Ca, may produce a nutritional hyperparathyroidism by which the body's homeostatic mechanisms act to restore a normal plasma Ca concentration. Unfortunately, the long-term effects of this response to an improper diet are a loss of bone mass as the chronic stimulation of PTH secretion increases osteoclastic resorption of bone.

REFERENCES

1. **Bilezekian, J. P., Marcus, R. and Levine, M. A.,** *The Parathyroids: Basic and Clinical Concepts,* Raven Press, New York, 1994.
2. **Kronenberg, H. M., Igarashi, T., Freeman, M. W. and Okazaki, T., Brand, S. J., Wiren, K. M., and Potts, J. T., Jr.,** Structure and expression of the human parathyroid hormone gene, *Recent Prog. Horm. Res.*, 42, 641, 1986.
3. **Kemper, B.,** Molecular biology of parathyroid hormone, *CRC Critical Reviews in Biochemistry,* 19, 353, 1986.

4. **Cohn, D. V., Kumarasamy, R. and Ramp, W. K.,** Intracellular processing and secretion of parathyroid gland proteins, *Vit. Horm.*, 43, 283, 1986.
5. **Habener, J. F., Kemper, B. W., Potts, J. T., Jr. and Rich, A.,** Calcium-independent intracellular conversion of proparathyroid hormone to parathyroid hormone, *Endocr. Res. Commun.*, 1, 239, 1974.
6. **Raisz, L. G., Au, W. Y. W. and Stern, P. H.,** Regulation of parathyroid activity, in *The Parathyroid Glands: Ultrastructure, Secretion, and Function*, Gaillard, P. J., Talmage, R. V. and Budy, A. M. eds., University of Chicago Press, Chicago, 1965.
7. **Brown, E. M., Gamba, G., Riccardi, D., Lombardi, M., Butters, R., Kifor, O., Sun, A., Hediger, M. A., Lytton, J. and Hebert, S. C.,** Cloning and characterization of an extracellular Ca^{2+}-sensing receptor from bovine parathyroid, *Nature*, 366, 575, 1993.
8. **Brown, E. M., Redgrave, J. and Thatcher, J.,** Effect of phorbol ester TPA on PTH secretion: evidence for a role for protein kinase C in the control of PTH release, *FEBS Letters*, 175, 72, 1984.
9. **Kifor, O. and Brown, E. M.,** Relationship between diacylglycerol levels and extracellular Ca^{2+} in dispersed bovine parathyroid cells, *Endocrinology*, 123, 2723, 1988.
10. **Brown, E. M.,** PTH secretion in vivo and in vitro: regulation by calcium and other secretagogues, *Min. Elect. Metab.*, 8, 130, 1982.
11. **Caporale, L. H. and Rosenblatt, M.,** Parathyroid hormone secretion: molecular events and regulation, *Contr. Nephrol.*, 50, 73, 1986.
12. **Sherwood, L. M., Potts, J. T., Jr., Care, A. D., Mayer, G. P. and Aurbach, G. D.,** Evaluation by radioimmunoassay of factors controlling the secretion of parathyroid hormone, *Nature*, 209, 52, 1966.
13. **Mayer, G. P. and Hurst, J. G.,** Sigmoidal relationship between parathyroid hormone secretion rate and plasma calcium concentration in calves, *Endocrinology*, 102, 1036, 1978.
14. **Brown, E. M.,** Four-parameter model of the sigmoidal relationship between parathyroid hormone release and extracellular calcium concentration in normal and abnormal parathyroid tissue, *J. Clin. Endocrinol. Metab.*, 56, 572, 1983.
15. **Brown, E. M., Broadus, A. E., Brennan, M. F., Gardner, D. G., Marx, S. J., Spiegel, A. M., Downs, R. W., Jr., Attie, M. and Aurbach, G. D.,** Direct comparison in vivo and in vitro of suppressibility of parathyroid function by calcium in primary hyperparathyroidism, *J. Clin. Endocrinol. Metab.*, 48, 604, 1979.
16. **Brown, E. M., Wilson, R. E., Eastman, R. C., Pallotta, J. and Marynick, S. P.,** Abnormal regulation of parathyroid hormone release by calcium in secondary hyperparathyroidism due to chronic renal failure, *J. Clin. Endocrinol. Metab.*, 54, 172, 1982.
17. **Martin, K. J., Hruska, K. A., Freitag, J. J., Klahr, S. and Slatopolsky, E.,** The peripheral metabolism of parathyroid hormone, *New Engl. J. Med.*, 301, 1092, 1979.
18. **Segre, G. V., D'Amour, P. and Potts, J. T., Jr.,** Metabolism of radioiodinated bovine parathyroid hormone in the rat, *Endocrinology*, 99, 1645, 1976.
19. **Tregear, G. W., Rietschoten, J. V., Green, E., Keutman, J. T., Niall, N. D., Reit, B., Parsons, J. A. and Potts, J. T., Jr.,** Bovine parathyroid hormone: minimum chain length of synthetic peptide required for biological activity, *Endocrinology*, 93, 1349, 1973.
20. **Puschett, J. B., McGowan, J., Fragola, J., Chen, T. C., Keutmann, H. and Rosenblatt, M.,** Difference between 1-84 parathyroid hormone and the 1-34 fragment on renal tubular calcium transport in the dog, *Min. Elect. Metab.*, 10, 271, 1984.
21. **Goltzman, D., Bennett, H. P. J., Koutsilieris, M., Mitchell, J., Rabbani, S. A. and Rouleau, M. F.,** Studies of the multiple molecular forms of bioactive parathyroid hormone, *Rec. Prog. Horm. Res.*, 42, 665, 1986.
22. **Jüppner, H., Abou-Samra, A.-B., Freeman, M. and Kong, X. F., Schipani, E., Richards, J., Kolakowski, L. F., Jr., Hock, J., Potts, J. T., Jr., Kronenberg, H. M., and Segre, G. V.,** A G protein-linked receptor for parathyroid hormone and parathyroid hormone-related peptide, *Science*, 254, 1024, 1991.
23. **Rizzuoli, R. E.,** Binding of intact parathyroid hormone to rat osteosarcoma cells: major contribution of binding sites for the carboxyl-terminal region of the hormone, *Endocrinology*, 112, 1303, 1983.
24. **Rao, L. G., Murray, T. M., Marx, S. J. and Aurbach, G. D.,** Binding of radioiodinated bovine parathyroid hormone-(1-84) to canine renal cortical membranes, *Endocrinology*, 117, 1632, 1985.
25. **Zull, J. E., Chuang, J. and Yike, I.,** Interaction of parathyroid hormone with its receptors, in *Current Research on Calcium Regulating Hormones*, Cooper, C. W. eds., University of Texas Press, Austin, Texas, 1987.
26. **Talmage, R. V.,** A study of the effect of parathyroid hormone on bone remodelling and calcium homeostasis, *Clin. Orthop. Rel. Res.*, 54, 163, 1967.
27. **Agarwala, N. and Gay, C. V.,** Specific binding of parathyroid hormone to living osteoclasts, *J. Bone Min. Res.*, 7, 531, 1992.
28. **Dempster, D. W., Cosman, F., Parisien, M., Shen, V. and Lindsay, R.,** Anabolic actions of parathyroid hormone on bone, *Endocr. Rev.*, 14, 690, 1993.
29. **Massry, S. G.,** Current status of the role of parathyroid hormone in uremic toxicity, *Contr. Nephrol.*, 49, 1, 1985.
30. **Collip, J. B. and Clark, E. P.,** Further studies on the physiological action of parathyroid hormone, *J. Biol. Chem.*, 64, 484, 1925.

31. **Munson, P. L.,** Biological assay of parathyroid hormone, in *The Parathyroids*, Greep, R. P. and Talmage, R. P. eds., Charles C. Thomas, Springfield, Illinois, 1961.
32. **Chambers, D. J., Dunham, J., Zanelli, J. M., Parsons, J. A., Bitensky, L. and Chayen, J.,** A sensitive bioassay of parathyroid hormone in plasma, *Clin. Endocrinol.*, 9, 375, 1978.
33. **Berson, S. A., Yalow, R. S., Aurbach, G. D. and Potts, J. T., Jr.,** Immunoassay of bovine and human parathyroid hormone, *Proc. Natl. Acad. Sci. USA*, 49, 613, 1963.
34. **Berson, S. A. and Yalow, R. S.,** Immunochemical heterogeneity of parathyroid hormone in plasma, *J. Clin. Endocrinol. Metab.*, 28, 1037, 1968.
35. **Canterbury, J. M., Levey, G. S. and Reiss, E.,** Activation of renal cortical adenylate cyclase by circulating immunoreactive parathyroid hormone fragments, *J. Clin. Inv.*, 52, 524, 1973.
36. **Wood, P. J.,** The measurement of parathyroid hormone, *Ann. Clin. Biochem.*, 29, 11, 1992.
37. **Arnold, A., Staunton, C. E., Gaz, R. D. and Kronenberg, H.,** Origin of parathyroid adenoma- a clonal assessment, in *Calcium Regulation and Bone Metabolism: Basic and Clinical Aspects*, Cohn, D. V., Martin, T. J. and Meunier, P. J. eds., Elsevier Science Publishers, Amsterdam, 1987.
38. **Rubin, L. P., Posillico, J. T., Anast, C. S. and Brown, E. M.,** Circulating levels of biologically active and immunoreactive intact parathyroid hormone in human newborns, *Ped. Res.*, 29, 201, 1991.
39. **Rudnick, M., Thode, J., Jørgenson, T., Heitmann, B. L. and Sørensen, O. H.,** Effects of age, sex, season and diet on serum ionized calcium, parathyroid hormone and vitamin D in a random population, *J. Int. Med.*, 234, 195, 1993.
40. **Logue, F. C., Fraser, W. D., O'Reilly, D. S. J. and Beastall, G. H.,** The circadian rhythm in intact parathyroid hormone (1-84) and nephrogenous cyclic adenosine monophosphate in normal men, *J. Endocrinol.*, 121, R1, 1989.
41. **Herfarth, K., Schmidt-Gayk, H., Graf, S. and Maier, A.,** Circadian rhythm and pulsatility of parathyroid hormone secretion in man, *Clin. Endocrinol.*, 37, 511, 1992.
42. **Nielsen, H. K., Brixen, K., Bouillon, R. and Mosekilde, L.,** Changes in biochemical markers of osteoblastic activity during the menstrual cycle, *J. Clin. Endocrinol. Metab.*, 70, 1431, 1990.
43. **Pitkin, R. M., Reynolds, W. A., Williams, G. A. and Hargis, G. K.,** Calcium-regulating hormones during the menstrual cycle, *J. Clin. Endocrinol. Metab.*, 47, 626, 1978.
44. **Sherman, S. S., Hollis, B. W. and Tobin, J. D.,** Vitamin D status and related parameters in a healthy population: the effects of age, sex, and season, *J. Clin. Endocrinol. Metab.*, 71, 405, 1990.
45. **Davis, O. K., Hawkins, D. S., Rubin, L. P., Posillico, J. T., Brown, E. M. and Schiff, I.,** Serum parathyroid hormone (PTH) in pregnant women determined by an immunoradiometric assay for intact PTH, *J. Clin. Endocrinol. Metab.*, 67, 850, 1988.
46. **Chesney, R. W., Specker, B. L., Mimouni, F. and McKay, C. P.,** Mineral metabolism during pregnancy and lactation, in *Disorders of Bone and Mineral Metabolism*, Coe, F. L. and Favus, M. J. eds., Raven Press, 1992.
47. **Greer, F. R., Lane, J. and Ho, M.,** Elevated serum parathyroid hormone, calcitonin, and 1,25-dihydroxyvitamin D in lactating women nursing twins, *Am. J. Clin. Nutr.*, 40, 562, 1984.
48. **Calvo, M. S., Kumar, R. and Heath, H.,** Persistently elevated parathyroid hormone secretion and action in young women after four weeks of ingesting high phosphorus, low calcium diets, *J. Clin. Endocrinol. Metab.*, 70, 1334, 1990.
49. **Morrissey, J. J. and Cohn, D. V.,** Secretion and degradation of parathormone as a function of intracellular maturation of hormone pools, *J. Cell Biol.*, 83, 521, 1979.
50. **Zull, J. E. and Lev, N. B.,** A theoretical study of the structure of parathyroid hormone, *Proc. Natl. Acad. Sci. USA*, 77, 3791, 1980.

Chapter 12

VITAMIN D

Svein U. Toverud, DMD, Ph.D., John J. B. Anderson, Ph.D., and Sanford C. Garner, Ph.D.

TABLE OF CONTENTS

0-8493-7845-1/95/$0.00+$.50

I. INTRODUCTION

Vitamin D is the major hormonal agent responsible for long-term maintenance of adequate whole-body mineral levels through enhanced intestinal absorption of calcium (Ca) and phosphorus (P). Together with parathyroid hormone, which regulates plasma Ca and P concentrations on a short-term basis, vitamin D stimulates movement of Ca from the bone surface to the extracellular fluid. In addition, vitamin D has an essential role in normal bone formation and mineralization.

Vitamin D represents a unique molecule in human function because its requirements can be met from both dietary sources and skin photobiosynthesis. A combination of these two contributions is provided throughout the life cycle, but the relative amounts of each may vary considerably, depending on the availability of dietary vitamin D, geographic latitude, and atmospheric conditions. Vitamin D fortification of dairy products and vitamin D supplementation are important additional contributions to the total supply of this essential nutrient.

The hormonal form of this cholesterol-derived molecule (see Table 1) is produced by two hydroxylations, the first occurs in the liver at the 25 position (25-hydroxyvitamin D, 25(OH)D), and the second in the kidney at the 1 position (1,25-dihydroxyvitamin D, $1,25(OH)_2D$) (see Figure 1). The tightly regulated synthesis of the $1,25(OH)_2D$ molecule, its presence in low concentrations in the blood, and specific steroid-type receptors have led to its acceptance as a hormone. Historically, vitamin D was discovered as a fat-soluble material that prevented the development of rickets. However, biosynthesis of the molecule through transformation of 7-dehydrocholesterol in skin cells by ultraviolet (UV) light is able to supply vitamin D in humans and other species, and the lack of an absolute nutritional requirement removes vitamin D from the classical definition of a vitamin.

This chapter covers the following topics: functional roles of the hormonal metabolite of vitamin D; circulating concentrations of vitamin D metabolites; modern biology of vitamin D; dietary sources, intakes, and allowances of vitamin D through the lifecycle; age-related skin exposures and skin biosynthesis; age-related changes in vitamin D-driven Ca metabolism; and human deficiency and toxicity.

This chapter is an updated version of a review by Anderson and Toverud.[1]

II. METABOLIC ACTIONS OF $1,25(OH)_2D$

Although vitamin D is obtained from the diet as ergocalciferol (vitamin D_2) or cholecalciferol (vitamin D_3) or synthesized in the skin as cholecalciferol, the biological effects require conversion to the hormonal metabolite, $1,25(OH)_2D$. An exception to this concept may be cases of vitamin D toxicity when serum concentrations of 25(OH)D are increased manyfold over the normal range; the 25(OH)D metabolite may then interact directly with the vitamin D receptor and mimic the actions of $1,25(OH)_2D$, causing hypercalcemia[2] (see later section Human Toxicity of Vitamin D).

TABLE 1
Terminology of Vitamin D Molecules

Common Name	Scientific Name
Vitamin D	Calciferol (general): animal — cholecalciferol (D_3); fungal — ergocalciferol (D_2)
Calcidiol	25-hydroxycholecalciferol or 25-OH-D_3
Calcitriol	1,25-dihydroxycholecalciferol or $1,25(OH)_2D_3$; also Vitamin D hormone
24,25-dihydroxy-cholecalciferol	$24,25(OH)_2D_3$ (low-activity metabolite of unknown function)

From Anderson, J. J. B. and Toverud, S. U., Diet and vitamin D: a review with an emphasis on human function, *J. Nutr. Biochem.*, 5, 58, 1994.

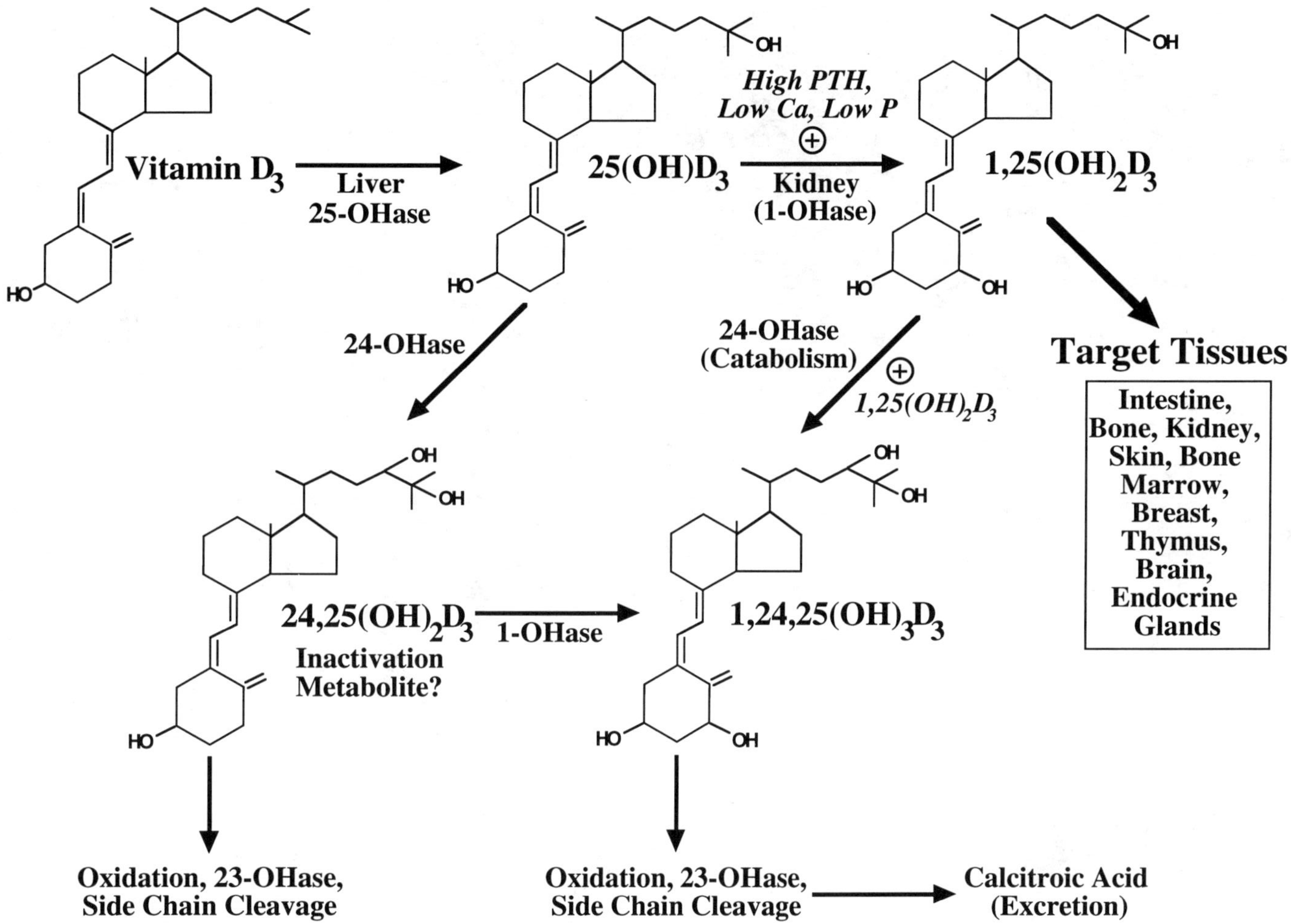

FIGURE 1. Vitamin D Endocrine System. The hormonal form (1,25-dihydroxyvitamin D, 1,25$(OH)_2$D) of this cholesterol-derived molecule is produced by two hydroxylations; the first occurs in the liver at the 25 position (25-hydroxyvitamin D, 25(OH)D), and the second in the kidney at the 1 position. The hydroxylation of 1,25$(OH)_2$D at the 24 position is the major catabolic pathway for the active metabolite. Hydroxylation of 25(OH)D at the 24 position produces 24,25-dihydroxyvitamin D, which may be an inactive metabolite. (Modified from Reference 76)

A. INTESTINAL ABSORPTION

The major effect of 1,25(OH)$_2$D is to increase the efficiency of intestinal absorption of Ca and inorganic phosphate (Pi), and to maintain the blood concentration of these ions for mineralization of bones and teeth. Although most intestinal Ca absorption probably occurs by a passive mechanism, 1,25(OH)$_2$D can stimulate the active transport of Ca ions in the duodenum and to a lesser extent in the ileum. Such active transport, which takes place against a concentration gradient across the mucosal epithelium, is of greatest importance when the dietary Ca intake is low. There is ample evidence in experimental animals, but limited evidence in humans, that a reduced Ca intake leads to increased efficiency of Ca absorption, i.e., a relatively greater fraction of ingested Ca will be absorbed at low Ca intakes, because of increased active transport mediated by an increase in serum 1,25(OH)$_2$D concentration.[3] During periods of ample, or high, Ca intakes, a relatively smaller fraction of the ingested Ca will be absorbed by active transport, and most of the Ca will be absorbed by passive transfer across the jejunum and the ileum. This process of adaptation of Ca absorption to the needs of the organism may not be equally efficient in all individuals and may require variable periods of time. In the elderly, adaptation may be less efficient,[4] but not all reports are in agreement with this finding.[5] Additional details regarding vitamin D action on intestinal Ca absorption can be found in Chapter 4.

B. BONE TISSUE

The hormonal effects of 1,25(OH)$_2$D on bone metabolism are similar to those of parathyroid hormone. It is well documented that the presence of adequate amounts of 1,25(OH)$_2$D is required for normal growth, maturation, and mineralization of bone, and for the maintenance of mature bone tissue. To a large extent these effects of the hormone result from the increased intestinal absorption of Ca and phosphate. The rachitic bone lesion in vitamin D-deficient rats (described later) can be prevented by providing the vitamin D-deficient rats with a diet containing high amounts of Ca and phosphate, indicating that the critical action of vitamin D is to provide an adequate supply of Ca and phosphate to the mineralizing bone.[6] However, 1,25(OH)$_2$D also acts directly on bone. Osteoblasts and their precursors contain receptors for the hormone that mediate synthesis of a bone-specific protein, osteocalcin, that is associated with the bone formation process in a poorly understood manner. Another nonmatrix protein, osteopontin, has also been reported to be under vitamin D regulation.[7] In addition, evidence exists that 1,25(OH)$_2$D stimulates the differentiation of osteoblasts by a direct action.[8] Furthermore, 1,25(OH)$_2$D indirectly stimulates the maturation and activity of osteoclasts. Osteoclasts do not have receptors for the hormone, but they respond to factors released from activated osteoblasts. Superphysiologic concentrations of the hormone produce an increase in the number and activity of osteoclasts, which will result in an increased rate of bone resorption and a net bone loss. The net effect of the hormone on bone is therefore an increase in rates of both bone formation and bone resorption, i.e., an increase in bone turnover.[9]

Morrison and co-workers[10] have recently reported that one vitamin D receptor (VDR) allele in Caucasian women in Australia is associated with low bone density and that another allele correlates with higher bone density, and they suggest that the allele variation can account for a substantial fraction (80%) of the known genetic determination of bone mineral density. Similar observations have been made in a population of postmenopausal women in the United Kingdom.[11] However, a study of Caucasian women in the United States failed to reveal a significant relationship between VDR genotypes and the bone mineral density of the spine.[12] These results, which may have important implications for the etiology of postmenopausal osteoporosis, are presently too conflicting for any conclusive statement.

C. CALCIUM HOMEOSTASIS

A third action of 1,25(OH)$_2$D in bone is that of maintaining Ca homeostasis, i.e., the control of the Ca concentration in serum and extracellular fluid. The minute-to-minute and hour-to-hour regulation of the Ca concentration depends on the transfer of Ca from a pool of readily accessible

Ca ions on the surface of the bone mineral crystals. This transfer appears to be under the control of a subpopulation of osteoblasts, and it is stimulated by $1,25(OH)_2D$, as well as by parathyroid hormone. These hormones appear to function in concert, even though they act by different mechanisms.

D. INHIBITION OF PARATHYROID HORMONE SECRETION

Vitamin D hormone receptors in parathyroid gland cells, when occupied by $1,25(OH)_2D$ or analogs of the hormone such as 22-oxacalcitriol, mediate inhibition of parathyroid hormone secretion. Concentrations as low as 10^{-11} *M* $1,25(OH)_2D$ have been found to reduce parathyroid hormone secretion from primary cultures of bovine parathyroid cells.[13] In clinical studies, administration of $1,25(OH)_2D$ to patients with secondary hyperparathyroidism due to uremia have led to a significant reduction in serum parathyroid hormone concentration.[14] The significance of this inhibitory action of $1,25(OH)_2D$ in normal physiology is uncertain, particularly in view of the observation that lactating rats maintain elevated serum levels of both parathyroid hormone and $1,25(OH)_2D$.[15,16]

E. OTHER ACTIONS

Other effects of $1,25(OH)_2D$ include the stimulation of renal conservation of Ca and phosphate, effects that are not well documented in man.[17] An interaction with the immune system involves the activation of T-lymphocytes. However, the significance of this interaction is not clear because vitamin D-deficient patients have few if any signs of impaired immunity.[8] The hormonal form of vitamin D is also involved in the function of skeletal muscles as evidenced by the presence of $1,25(OH)_2D$ receptors and reports of muscular weakness in patients with severe rickets.[2,18] In the skin $1,25(OH)_2D$ promotes terminal differentiation of keratinocytes. This action is the basis for the topical application of the hormone used experimentally in patients with the hyperproliferative skin disease, psoriasis.[19]

Solar ultraviolet radiation exposure, and thereby vitamin D, has been suggested, on the basis of epidemiologic studies, for protection against prostate cancer[20] and possibly other cancers.[8] Additional evidence for an anticancer action of $1,25(OH)_2D_3$ has been obtained with human breast cancer cell lines that contain vitamin D receptors.[21] Addition of $1,25(OH)_2D$ (10^{-8} to 10^{-10} *M*) to the medium (1) reduced the proliferation of the cell lines regardless of their sex steroid status, (2) opposed the epidermal growth factor (EGF)-induced increase in the proliferation of the cell lines, and (3) reversed the increase in the proliferation rate when the tumor cells were co-cultured with fibroblasts derived from breast tumor biopsies.

F. SUMMARY

In summary, $1,25(OH)_2D$ exerts important roles in intestinal absorption of Ca and phosphate, bone metabolism and mineralization, and Ca homeostasis. Other roles are not yet well understood and include the conservation of Ca and phosphate by the kidney, and the interactions of the hormone with the immune system, skin, and skeletal muscle. Finally, an anticancer role of the hormone is suggested from data in recently published reports.

III. MECHANISMS OF ACTION OF $1,25(OH)_2D$

The mechanism of the physiologically relevant actions of the hormonal form of vitamin D is clearly genomic. However, recent evidence from animal experiments indicates that the hormone may also act by a nongenomic mechanism.

A. GENOMIC ACTION

The specific receptor for $1,25(OH)_2D$ that mediates the genomic action of the hormone, referred to as the vitamin D receptor (VDR), is a protein of approximately 48,000 molecular weight[22] and belongs to the steroid/thyroid hormone receptor superfamily. It is present in specific cells in most tissues of the body,[18] and is localized primarily in the nucleus, but possibly in the cytoplasm as well.[23] The VDR has a specific domain responsible for binding the hormone and another domain that binds the hormone-receptor complex to DNA. The nucleotide sequence of vitamin D response elements (VDRE) on DNA have been identified on the following genes: calbindin D_{9K}, rat osteocalcin, human osteocalcin, and mouse osteopontin.[7,24]

Osteocalcin is found in osteoblasts and the Ca-binding protein, calbindin $D_{9K,}$ in the mucosal cells of the small intestine. Calbindin levels are closely associated with the rate of active Ca transport, and calbindin is believed to be involved in the transcellular movement of Ca.[25] The VDR studies have revealed that $1,25(OH)_2D$ acts in the same manner as other steroid hormones. The clinical significance of the receptor studies is illustrated by the discovery of VDR defects in patients with hereditary vitamin D-dependent rickets type 2, a rare autosomal recessive condition. These defects, which impair the binding of the receptor to the hormone and the binding of the complex to DNA, explain why the patients are unresponsive to both the endogenous hormone as well as to treatment with high doses of the hormone.

B. NONGENOMIC ACTION

Several effects of $1,25(OH)_2D_3$ occur too rapidly to be explained by new protein synthesis following gene activation, i.e., the genomic action of vitamin D. These changes, which include alteration in intracellular pH and Ca concentration, occur within seconds or a few minutes of addition of $1,25(OH)_2D_3$ and are called nongenomic. Of particular interest is the observation that increased absorption of Ca from chick intestine can be observed as early as 5 minutes after administration of the hormone, a phenomenon called transcaltachia (rapid transfer of Ca).[26] In rat colonic epithelial cells, $1,25(OH)_2D_3$ caused the formation of diacylglycerol and 1,4,5-triphosphate, the subsequent activation of protein kinase C, and an increase in intracellular Ca concentration; all these events occurred within seconds to minutes.[27] Rapid effects of the vitamin D hormone on phosphoinosotide metabolism was also detected in rat duodenal mucosal cells, but not prior to the time of nuclear receptor development by young suckling rat pups, which suggests the involvement of cell surface receptors that are similar or identical to the nuclear receptor.[28] However, other data indicate that the postulated D-hormone receptor in the cell membrane is different from the nuclear receptor.[29] Further support for the view that the ligand-binding domains of receptors associated with the genomic and nongenomic responses are different comes from work showing that the hormone analog $1\beta,25(OH)_2D_3$ acts as an antagonist of the hormone action in the transcaltachia assay, but the analog does not antagonize the genomic action of the hormone.[30] Based on studies of the hormone-induced transcription of the osteocalcin gene in osteoblast-like cells in culture, others have suggested that the rapid effect of $1,25(OH)_2D_3$ serves to facilitate the genomic action.[31] The physiological significance of the nongenomic action of the hormone in different cell types remains to be established, in part because the hormone concentration required for some of the rapid *in vitro* effects (10^{-8} *M*) may be superphysiologic. However, recent work has shown that concentrations as low as 3×10^{-10} *M* $1,25(OH)_2D_3$ added to the transcaltachia assay can increase Ca transport within minutes.[30] This concentration is similar to the circulating $1,25(OH)_2D_3$ level in Ca-restricted rats (10^{-9} *M*).[15]

C. SUMMARY

Even though all the classical actions of calcitriol appear to be explained satisfactorily by a genomic mechanism, further research may reveal that only a nongenomic action explains other functions of calcitriol. Certain effects of this active hormonal form of vitamin D may result from a combination of the two mechanisms, as proposed by Baran and co-workers.[31]

IV. SKIN BIOSYNTHESIS AND AGE-RELATED SUN EXPOSURES

Energy from ultraviolet radiation (UV, 290-315 nm) derived from sunlight (and certain artificial lamps) can break the B ring of 7-dehydrocholesterol in the epidermal layer of human skin and that of most other vertebrates to produce vitamin D_3 (cholecalciferol) (see Figure 2). The amount of skin biosynthesis per day is affected by many factors, such as latitude, sun (UV) exposure, dress, season of year, and skin melanin pigmentation (color). It has been estimated that only 15 to 20 minutes of arm and face exposure at mid-day will yield skin production of vitamin D sufficient to meet daily needs, i.e., 5 mg (or 200 IU), of adults living in Boston, Massachusetts.[32] In the elderly, however, almost twice as much time is required to yield the same amount of vitamin D production by the skin.[32] Other environmental conditions can also modify skin biosynthesis of vitamin D.[33,34] Low skin production coupled with an inadequate intake of vitamin D has been attributed as a primary cause of secondary hyperparathyroidism, osteomalacia, and hip fractures of elderly Chinese living in Hong Kong.[35]

Sunlight may also regulate cutaneous production of vitamin D by causing its degradation to presumably inactive photoproducts. However, the wavelengths responsible for this effect are higher than the range required for its production from 7-dehydrocholesterol, i.e., > 315 nm.[36]

V. BIOTRANSFORMATION OF VITAMIN D AND CONCENTRATIONS OF CIRCULATING METABOLITES

The antirachitic factor, cholecalciferol (vitamin D_3), is now considered a part of an endocrine system because it is synthesized in the skin under the influence of UV light and is ultimately converted in the kidney to a hormone, $1,25(OH)_2D$ (calcitriol), which circulates at low concentrations and exerts effects in many target organs.[37]

The precursor in the skin, 7-dehydrocholesterol (also called provitamin D), is converted to an intermediate form, previtamin D_3, by opening the B-ring of the sterol molecule, a process mediated by UV light in the range 290–315 nm[38,39] (see Figure 2). A subsequent rearrangement of the molecule takes place under the influence of skin temperature and leads to the formation of cholecalciferol, which is then slowly released into the blood and binds to the circulating vitamin D-binding protein. In the elderly the epidermal concentration of 7-dehydrocholesterol is diminished, and the rate of conversion to vitamin D_3 is also reduced.[40] When one considers that the elderly usually have reduced sun exposure as well, it becomes clear that they are at increased risk of developing vitamin D insufficiency unless they have an adequate dietary supply of vitamin D.[40]

The next biotransformation step occurs in the liver where vitamin D_3 or D_2 is hydroxylated in the 25-position of the sterol by an enzyme reaction that is not closely controlled,[2] (see Figure 1). In other words, the higher the blood concentration of vitamin D, the greater the amount of 25(OH)D produced. This metabolite circulates mostly bound to the vitamin D-binding protein. The concentration of this metabolite in the blood is the best indicator of the adequacy of the vitamin D supply, whether from the diet or the skin. The final biotransformation step occurs in the kidney where 25(OH)D is hydroxylated further at the 1-position with the formation of the active hormone, $1,25(OH)_2D$. This hydroxylation is tightly regulated, in that the hydroxylase, a cytochrome P450 enzyme, is stimulated by elevated circulating parathyroid hormone concentrations, a fall in serum Ca, or a fall in the serum phosphate level. In the absence of any of these signals, 25(OH)D will be hydroxylated in the 24-position with the formation of $24,25(OH)_2D$, a metabolite that lacks hormonal activity. Synthesis of $1,25(OH)_2D$ is inhibited by elevated circulating $1,25(OH)_2D$ levels and probably also by elevated serum Ca levels. In other words, the hormone is synthesized in response to changes reflecting either Ca or phosphate deficiency, or increased need.

In the presence of an adequate supply of the precursor, 25(OH)D, the circulating hormone level is increased during the pubertal period of rapid growth and during the third trimester of pregnancy, as well as during lactation if milk production is high, as in mothers nursing twins. Alteration in the vitamin D endocrine system in old age, such as a decrease in the circulating $1,25(OH)_2D$ level, has been implicated in the pathogenesis of postmenopausal osteoporosis, because reduced serum $1,25(OH)_2D$ levels have been found in some women afflicted with this condition. However, there is no evidence indicating a general age-related decrease in serum $1,25(OH)_2D$ concentration. A recent study of a large group of healthy Caucasian adults ranging in age from 20 to 94 years revealed

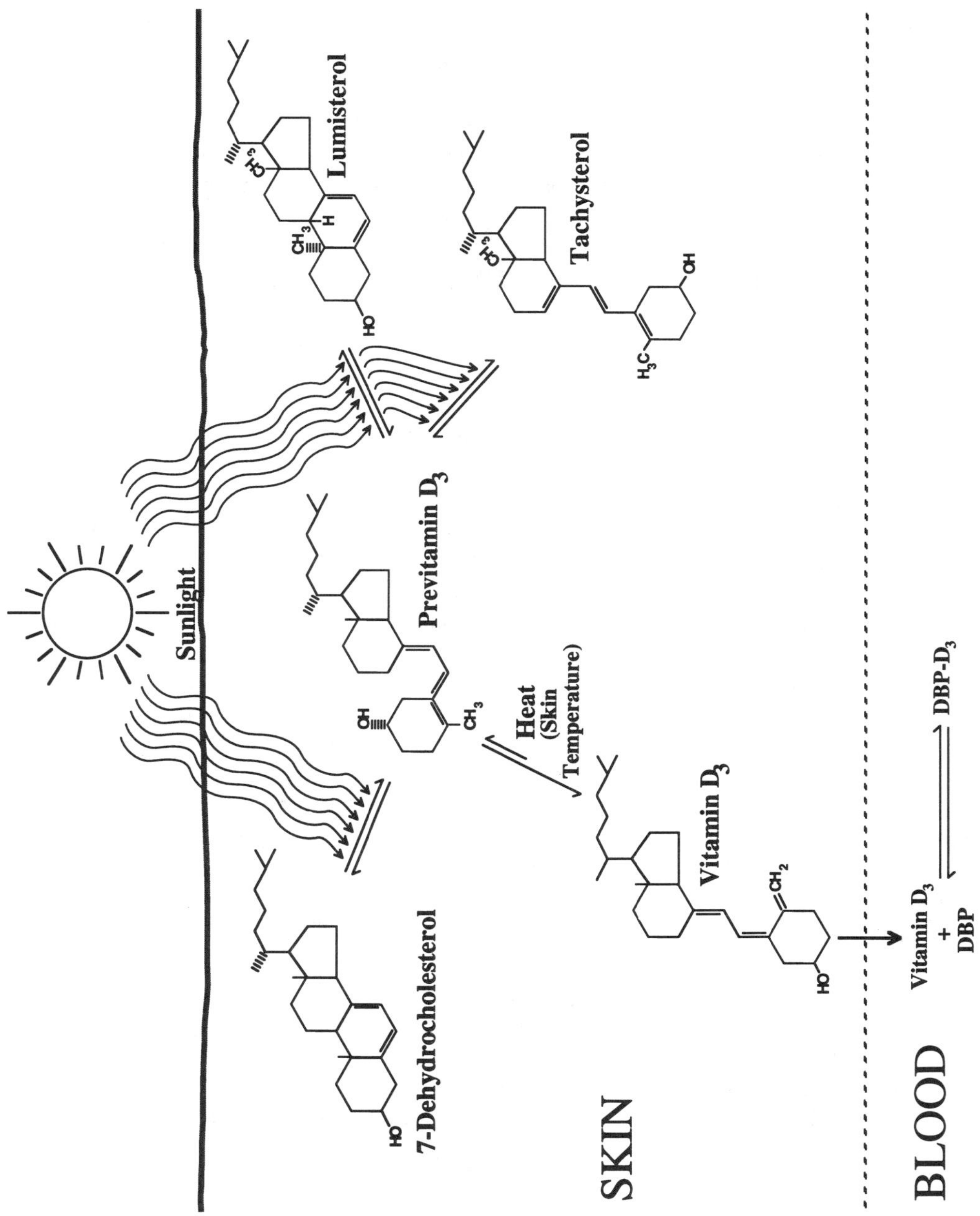
Sunlight
Lumisterol
Tachysterol
Previtamin D_3
Heat (Skin Temperature)
7-Dehydrocholesterol
Vitamin D_3
SKIN
BLOOD
Vitamin D_3 + DBP
DBP-D_3

FIGURE 2. (Facing page) Vitamin D Biosynthesis. Energy from ultraviolet radiation derived from sunlight (and certain artificial lamps) can break the B ring of 7-dehydrocholesterol in the epidermal layer of skin of humans and most other vertebrates to produce previtamin D_3. A subsequent rearrangement of the molecule takes place under the influence of skin temperature and leads to the formation of vitamin D_3 (cholecalciferol), which is then slowly released into the blood and binds to the circulating vitamin D-binding protein (DBP). Continued exposure of skin to the sun promotes photoisomerization of previtamin D_3 to lumisterol and tachysterol, which are biologically inactive forms of the molecule. (Modified from Holick et al.[39])

no decline in serum 25(OH)D or 1,25$(OH)_2$D concentrations in either sex.[41] In another study, involving women between ages 26 and 88 years, serum 1,25$(OH)_2$D levels were actually higher after age 65 than in the youngest subjects, but the rate of intestinal Ca absorption was unaltered, suggesting a decreased responsiveness to the hormone with increasing age followed by a compensatory increase in hormone synthesis.[42]

A. CIRCULATING BLOOD CONCENTRATIONS OF MAJOR VITAMIN D METABOLITES

Blood concentrations of the major vitamin D metabolites, 25(OH)D and 1,25$(OH)_2$D, have a fairly broad range in healthy individuals, but they do vary according to age, sex, dietary intake, or skin biosynthesis of vitamin D. Whereas a seasonal variation exists for 25(OH)D, none has been found for 1,25$(OH)_2$D. Values of the major vitamin D metabolites are similar among African American and white women in the U.S.[43]

Table 2 provides data (means, SDs, and ranges) on circulating vitamin D metabolites by age, i.e., vitamin D status; these data are combined from reports of several different laboratories.

B. VITAMIN D-BINDING PROTEIN (DBP)

A hepatic-produced specific transport protein, DBP, binds large fractions of the circulating metabolites of vitamin D. The binding affinities of DBP for the metabolites are low, but the capacities are high. The qualitative order of affinities of DBP for vitamin D and its metabolites is as follows: 25(OH)D > 24,25$(OH)_2$D > D > 1,25$(OH)_2$D.[44] According to these authors, the binding affinity of DBP for vitamin D is approximately 300 times weaker than for 25(OH)D. As far as is known, DBP is never a limiting factor for carrying these metabolites in healthy individuals, even among the elderly with reasonably good liver function. DBP carries vitamin D or its metabolites from the fat depots (the major store of vitamin D), from skin after biosynthesis, and from the liver and kidney after biotransformations to other tissues. (Orally absorbed vitamin D is transported from the gut along with other lipid-soluble vitamins via chylomicrons.) The greatest quantity of a

TABLE 2
Concentrations of Major Vitamin D Metabolites across the Life Cycle from Reports in the Literature

Age (years)	N	25-Hydroxyvitamin D nmol/L	1,25-Dihydroxyvitamin D pmol/L	Reference
1–16	103	—	103.2 ± 4.8*	Chesney, et al.,[74]
10–20	86	—	132.0 ± 4.3	Rosen and Chesney,[75]
20–35	37	—	67.2 ± 4.3	Rosen and Chesney,[75]
26–88	51	62.2 ± 21.5	77.3 ± 19.4	Eastell et al.,[42] (males only)
>65	22	(1) 40.0 ± 4.2*	(1) 46.0 ± 4.2*	Gloth et al.,[63]
		(2) 83.4 ± 3.2*	(2) 66.2 ± 3.2*	

* SEM
1. Sunlight-deprived elderly.
2. Free-living elderly of the Baltimore Longitudinal Study of Aging.

From Anderson, J. J. B. and Toverud, S. U., Diet and vitamin D: a review with an emphasis on human function, *J. Nutr. Biochem.*, 5, 58, 1994.

circulating metabolite carried by DBP is 25(OH)D, which, in effect, serves as the major readily available store of vitamin D. DBP, in effect, serves as a buffer against toxicity, since the free metabolites of vitamin, 25(OH)D and $1,25(OH)_2D$, are toxigenic.

It should be noted that the transport of vitamin D obtained from food sources via intestinal absorption is largely in chylomicrons that enter the lymphatic circulation prior to joining the venous circulation to the heart. The delivery of vitamin D from chylomicron remnants to the liver is highly efficient compared to exclusive DBP delivery of cutaneously biosynthesized vitamin D.[45] Furthermore, exclusive DBP delivery of vitamin D results in a more gradual and sustained increase in 25(OH)D concentration in blood, since the more rapid elevation following oral delivery also results in less sustained increments in circulating 25(OH)D during fasting periods.[45]

C. ORAL THERAPY WITH VITAMIN D, CALCITRIOL, AND A CALCITRIOL ANALOG

Therapeutic studies of elderly subjects using vitamin D have been conducted over the last couple of decades, but only one controlled investigation has been reported.[46] A review of these and several of his own reports led Gallagher[47] to recommend the use of 800 IU of vitamin D per day for elderly individuals. In Japan vitamin D (or $1,25(OH)_2D_3$ or its analog 1α-OH-D_3) is favored as the therapy for osteoporotic patients.[48] A recent study of osteoporotic women from New Zealand using low doses of calcitriol demonstrated a significant reduction in vertebral fractures after three years, and no serious side-effects.[49]

Oral therapy of 1-α-hydroxy-cholecalciferol has recently been introduced in Japan, and it has been shown to reduce the fracture rate of elderly subjects with low bone mass or fractures.[50,51] The 1-alpha form must be converted in the liver to $1,25(OH)_2D$ by 25-hydroxylation. Dosages are generally low because of concerns about toxic effects. The efficacy of this therapy has not yet been fully evaluated.

VI. DIETARY SOURCES, INTAKES, AND ALLOWANCES OF VITAMIN D THROUGH THE LIFE CYCLE

The major dietary sources of vitamin D in the U.S., Canada, and a few other technologically advanced nations are fortified dairy products (especially milks and infant formulas), eggs, fortified margarines, and fishes, including their oils. In less advanced nations where the consumption of dairy products, eggs, and fish is minimal or nonexistent, vitamin D intakes must be extremely low. For example, foods such as cassava, maize (corn), yams, plantains, and rice, or other grains contain no vitamin D. Thus, subtropical and tropical peoples of the world must depend almost totally on skin biosynthesis to meet their tissue requirements for vitamin D. This section provides data on intakes, allowances, and supplements of vitamin D.

A. INTAKES OF VITAMIN D

In the U.S., all processed cow's milk is fortified with 10 mg (400 IU) of cholecalciferol (or ergocalciferol) per quart (approximately one liter), which exceeds by tenfold the approximately 1 mg/L of human breast milk. Actual estimated intakes by breast-feeding infants in the U.S. would range between 0.5 and 1.5 mg cholecalciferol a day and by formula-fed infants approximately ten times higher for those up to six months of age. Beyond six months, vitamin D intakes of infants and children would relate directly to the amounts of fortified milks consumed. Two cups of milk (about 500 ml) would provide approximately 5 mg of calciferol (as either vitamin D_2 or D_3) per day. Other foods would, of course, supply varying amounts of vitamin D. Adult consumption patterns of vitamin D-fortified dairy products are considerably lower than for infants and children, as assessed in a recent American survey. Intakes are approximately 2 mg cholecalciferol for males and 1.5 mg for females.[52] No other survey data on vitamin D intakes are available in the U.S.

TABLE 3
Recommended Dietary Allowances of Vitamin D, U.S., 1989[53]

Category	Age (years)	Vitamin D, mg*
Infants	0.0–0.5	7.5
	0.5–1.0	10
Children	1–10	10
Males	11–24	10
	25+	5
Females	11–24	10
	25+	5
Pregnant/lactating	—	10

* As cholecalciferol: 10 mg cholecalciferol = 400 IU of vitamin D.

From Anderson, J. J. B., and Toverud, S. U., Diet and vitamin D: a review with an emphasis on human function, *J. Nutr. Biochem.*, 5, 58, 1994.

In the United Kingdom (UK), vitamin D intakes are lower than in the U.S. because milk fortification has been greatly reduced there over the last few decades. The same is true for most of Europe. Scandinavian countries fortify margarine, but not dairy products.

In Japan, fish consumption provides almost 15% of total food energy and, thus, vitamin D intake from diverse fishes by adults would be approximately 1 mg per day. Fortified milk products would add an additional small amount of vitamin D to adult Japanese diets.

Estimates of vitamin D intakes by populations in the developing world are not available.

B. RECOMMENDED DIETARY ALLOWANCES OF VITAMIN D

Recommended intakes of vitamin D, which are based on both sunlight exposure for vitamin D skin biosynthesis and dietary sources, have been and remain extremely difficult to derive. In the U.S. a set of recommended dietary allowances (RDA) has been established since the early 1940s. The most recent, tenth edition of the RDAs[53] has set forth RDAs according to specific ages for both genders (see Table 3).

The vitamin D requirements for pregnant and lactating women have been reviewed and discussed recently by Specker,[54] who emphasizes the importance of sunshine exposure for both lactating mothers and their infants. Even with adequate maternal vitamin D, the vitamin D content of breast milk is low and insufficient for the infant. Only those women who avoid sun exposure and vitamin D-containing foods need a vitamin D supplement to meet the allowance of 400 IU per day[54] (see also Chapter 16).

Vitamin D allowances for other nations are generally lower than those of the U.S., but higher intakes are recommended by nations such as Canada and the former Soviet Union, whose latitudes are significantly removed from the equator.

C. SUPPLEMENTS

In recent years, supplements of vitamin D have been increasingly recommended for the elderly, especially those who have become institutionalized or shut-in because of limited mobility or confining conditions and diseases. Since the elderly have declining capabilities of skin biosynthesis and vitamin D conversion (see earlier discussion), larger doses of vitamin D supplements are being recommended for this segment of the population. This recommendation is supported by low circulating concentrations of 25(OH)D[55] or $1,25(OH)_2D$.[56,57] Low blood levels of the 25-OH-vitamin D metabolite are now being defined as characteristic of vitamin D insufficiency rather than of frank deficiency.

TABLE 4
Clinical Features and Serum Changes in Human Vitamin D Deficiency

Age	Clinical Features	Blood Serum Measurements
Children	Skeletal deformations (Rickets)	Hypocalcemia
	Impaired growth	Hypophosphatemia
		Secondary hyperparathyroidism
		Low 25-Hydroxyvitamin D
		Elevated alkaline phosphatase
Adults	Widened osteoid seams:	Hypocalcemia
	Accumulation of undermineralized	Hypophosphatemia
	bone matrix (Osteomalacia)	Low 25-Hydroxyvitamin D
		Elevated alkaline phosphatase
	Fractures	Elevated osteocalcin*
		Elevated parathyroid hormone

* This finding has not been consistently reported (see Vieth[9]).
From Anderson, J. J. B., and Toverud, S. U., Diet and vitamin D: a review with an emphasis on human function, *J. Nutr. Biochem.*, 5, 58, 1994.

Typical dosages of vitamin D supplements being recommended for elderly subjects in the U.S. are 400 IU per day or more.

A recent report from Finland, where wintertime deficiencies of vitamin D among the elderly become relatively severe, demonstrated that single yearly intramuscular vitamin D injections of 150,000–300,000 IU of ergocalciferol maintained serum levels of 25(OH)D within the normal range and reduced hip fracture incidence.[58] Wintertime supplementation of elderly women in the northern latitudes of the U.S. also resulted in improved 25(OH)D blood levels.[59]

VII. AGE-RELATED CHANGES IN VITAMIN D-DRIVEN CALCIUM METABOLISM

Large numbers of elderly residents in the Northern parts of the U.S. and of Europe have been shown to have depressed circulating levels of 25(OH)D and, in some reports, also low serum concentrations of $1,25(OH)_2D$. Seasonal differences in 25(OH)D have become well established in these geographic regions,[57,60] but $1,25(OH)_2D$ insufficiency without symptoms of a full-scale deficiency have only recently been documented.[42,47,57,58] Because of the increasing lifespans of so many elderly people, especially women, and the residence of large numbers of the elderly in nursing homes or similar facilities which permit little exposure of residents to sunlight, frank deficiency of vitamin D is likely to become more common and even possibly reach epidemic proportions. The public health consequences of osteomalacic bone tissue and increased fracture incidence could become enormous. Thus, some investigators have raised questions about the adequacy of the current allowance of vitamin D, i.e., 200 IU per day, for the elderly.[61-63]

VIII. HUMAN DEFICIENCY OF VITAMIN D

Human vitamin D deficiency may result from inadequate dietary intake and/or insufficient skin biosynthesis of vitamin D. This relatively prevalent deficiency is characterized by the clinical features and laboratory measurements of blood given in Table 4.

The terms rickets and osteomalacia refer to the histologic and radiologic abnormalities seen in a variety of vitamin D deficiency conditions. (Rickets may also, however, develop from inadequate Ca intake in children without a vitamin D deficiency[64]). Rickets describes the disordered growth and mineralization of the growth plate of the long bones.[65] The resulting abnormalities (widening of the growth plate, delayed conversion of the growth plate cartilage to bone, and irregularly arranged bone trabeculae) are only seen when the vitamin D deficiency occurs during childhood or adolescence, i.e., before the growth plates close. Osteomalacia describes the abnormalities resulting from delayed and reduced mineralization of mature bone, whether trabecular or cortical. This mineralization defect leads to a widened area of unmineralized bone matrix, called osteoid, on the bone surface. Osteomalacia is observed at all ages. Biochemical changes in most cases of rickets and osteomalacia include decreased serum Ca and phosphate levels because of insufficient intestinal absorption of these ions, increased serum parathyroid hormone levels as a result of the reduced serum Ca concentration, and elevated serum alkaline phosphatase concentration. In cases of an inadequate vitamin D supply or in chronic severe liver disease associated with fat malabsorption, serum 25(OH)D levels are invariably low, but the levels of 1,25-$(OH)_2D$ may still be normal, depending on the severity of the condition. Kidney disease (when glomerular filtration rate is less than 30% of normal) will invariably lead to low serum 1,25-$(OH)_2D$ levels, although the serum 25(OH)D may be normal.

Infants and young children with vitamin D deficiency suffer from growth retardation, primarily because of the stunted growth of the long bones, and they may become bowlegged because of the reduced mechanical strength of these bones. Skeletal muscle weakness and increased urinary excretion of amino acids may also occur.

Roentgenographic evidence of rickets includes widened growth plate of the long bones of both arms and legs and reduced bone density. In osteomalacia of the adult undermineralization of the bones may show up as pseudofractures, which are radiolucent lines on the roentgenograms that mimic stress fractures. However, the pseudofractures are usually bilateral and often involve non-weight-bearing bones, such as the scapula.[66]

After vitamin D-fortification of foods or the use of cod liver oil was instituted 60 years ago, simple vitamin D deficiency rickets became relatively rare in the U.S., Canada, and Western Europe. However, a recent increase in the number of such cases in these countries appears to result from either strict vegetarianism, i.e., dietary or religious practices that avoid the selection of foods containing vitamin D, or religious dress codes that prevent exposure of the skin to sunlight.[67-69] Furthermore, infants that are exclusively breast-fed and not given a vitamin D supplement have a higher risk of developing rickets,[68] particularly black infants of African descent or of other backgrounds whose mothers have a low vitamin D status.[70]

Rickets or osteomalacia may also result from diseases that may interfere with absorption and biotransformations of vitamin D_3 or D_2 and from conditions leading to decreased tissue responsiveness to the hormone (see Figure 3). Patients suffering from malabsorption of fats may have inadequate absorption of vitamin D from the small intestine. Liver disease may interfere with the conversion of vitamin D to 25(OH)D or lead to increased degradation of this metabolite, both of which will lead to decreased circulating levels of 25(OH)D. Patients whose kidneys have been removed or are severely diseased cannot convert 25(OH)D to the hormone 1,25$(OH)_2D$, and if parathyroid hormone production is inadequate, the vitamin D hormone production will decrease. Finally, three inborn errors of metabolism lead to rickets. Vitamin D-dependent rickets type 1 is caused by a defect in the kidney enzyme, 25(OH)D-1-hydroxylase, which is responsible for the synthesis of 1,25$(OH)_2D$. In vitamin D-dependent rickets type 2, the receptor for 1,25$(OH)_2D$ is defective and cannot mediate the genomic action of the hormone. In the third condition, called hypophosphatemic vitamin D-resistant rickets, defects in the renal synthesis of 1,25$(OH)_2D$ occur as well as in the renal reabsorption of phosphate, leading to low circulating phosphate levels.[71]

IX. HUMAN TOXICITY OF VITAMIN D

Toxicity due to vitamin D or its active metabolite may be caused by an inadvertent intake of excessive amounts of vitamin D-containing preparations, such as vitamin tablets, or it may occur spontaneously in patients treated with high doses of vitamin D_3, replacement doses of 1,25$(OH)_2D$,

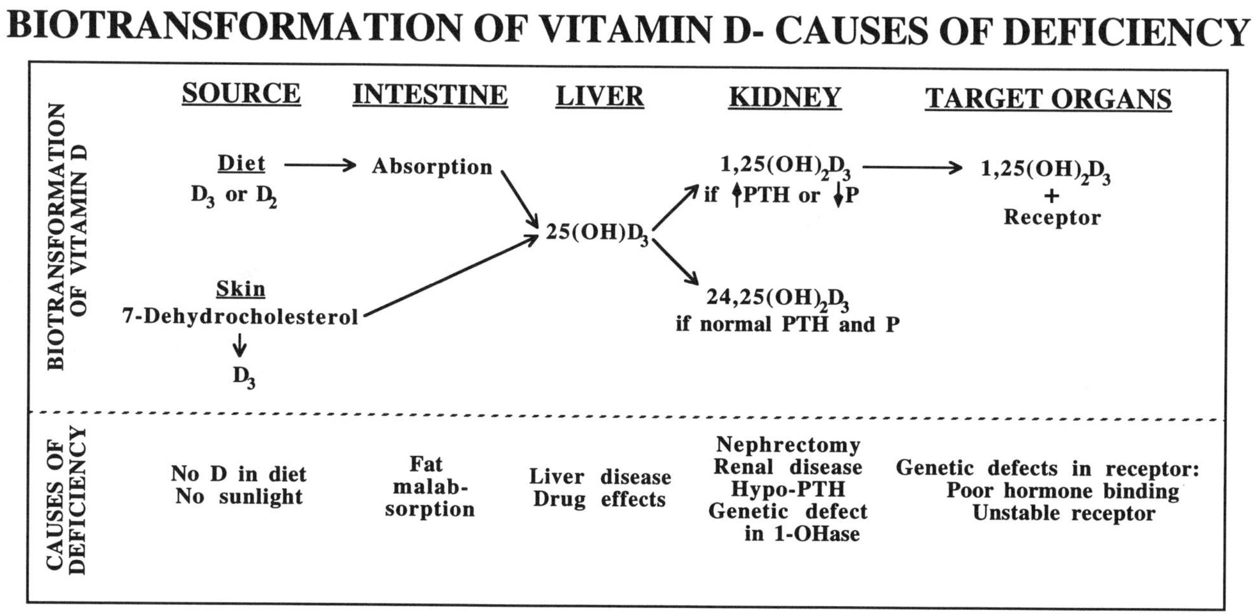

FIGURE 3. Biotransformation of Vitamin D and Causes of Deficiency. Absorption and biotransformation of vitamin D require normal function of the intestine, liver, and kidney, while occupation of active vitamin D receptors in target organs is necessary for biological activity. Rickets or osteomalacia may result from diseases that interfere with absorption or biotransformations of vitamin D_3 or D_2 and conditions leading to decreased tissue responsiveness to the hormone: (1) malabsorption of fats from the small intestine, (2) liver disease or drug effects that interfere with the conversion of vitamin D to 25(OH)D or increase degradation of this metabolite, (3) patients whose kidneys have been removed or are severely diseased cannot convert 25(OH)D to the hormone, $1,25(OH)_2D$, and if PTH production is inadequate, the vitamin D hormone production will decrease, and (4) three inborn errors of metabolism that lead to rickets. (Abbreviations: 1-OHase = $25(OH)D_3$-1-hydroxylase; PTH = parathyroid hormone; Hypo-PTH = hypoparathyroidism; P = serum phosphate)

TABLE 5
Symptoms of Vitamin D Toxicity in Humans

Clinical Features	Blood and Urine Measurements
Soft tissue depositions of mineral (Calcium) salts	Hypercalcemia
	Hypercalciuria
Renal and cardiovascular damage (reversible and irreversible)	Elevated serum 25-hydroxyvitamin D
	Elevated serum 1,25-dihydroxyvitamin D*

* Depending on the cause of the toxicity (see Vieth[9]). A few patients have elevated $1,25(OH)_2D$ when the cause of hypercalcemia is excessive intake of vitamin D_3, but most patients have normal $1,25(OH)_2D$ concentrations.
From Anderson, J. J. B., and Toverud, S. U., Diet and vitamin D: a review with an emphasis on human function, *J. Nutr. Biochem.*, 5, 58, 1994.

or an analog of the latter, 1-OH-D, which is converted in the liver to the active hormone. The human symptoms of vitamin D toxicity (hypervitaminosis D) are, in general, opposite those of deficiency, as detailed in Table 5. The earliest and most consistent symptom of vitamin D toxicity is hypercalcemia, i.e., serum Ca levels above the normal range of 9.5 to 11 mg/dl. The serum phosphate level often remains unaltered, but it may also increase acutely, especially if $1,25(OH)_2D$ is the offending agent. The cause of the hypercalcemia is most likely an increased net Ca efflux from bone, and therefore an extension of the normal physiological action of vitamin D, but increased Ca absorption also occurs, and it may contribute to the hypercalcemia.

A variety of signs and symptoms associated with vitamin D toxicity result from the increased serum Ca level, including anorexia, nausea, vomiting, memory loss, confusion, muscle weakness, constipation (or diarrhea), polyuria, and dehydration. The kidneys are particularly sensitive to an elevation of the serum Ca level. First, there is a decrease in the water-concentrating mechanism in the renal tubules, leading to excessive urinary water excretion. Next, Ca salts may form in the renal tubules, giving rise to kidney stones. Finally, if the hypercalcemic condition persists, Ca salts will be deposited in the renal tissues and cause damage to both the glomeruli and the tubules with subsequent loss of renal function. Ca salts may be deposited in other soft tissues as well, such as the heart, blood vessels, and skeletal muscles. In general, this phenomenon is referred to as metastatic calcification. In long-standing vitamin D toxicity, bone changes characterized by excessive resorption may occur and are referred to as osteitis fibrosa, because part of the bone is replaced by fibrous tissue.[66,72]

The duration of the patient's toxic episode is relatively brief if the administered agent is $1,25(OH)_2D$ because of the relatively short half-life of the hormone, i.e., 4–6 hr. If, however, vitamin D_3 or D_2 has been administered, the episode could last for weeks or months because of the higher lipid solubility and storage of these molecules in fat, leading to longer half-lives. When administered at high dose levels, vitamin D_3 or D_2 will be deposited in body fat and released slowly into the circulation long after dosing is discontinued. Treatment must therefore be continued for a long time to counteract the hypercalcemic response. The treatment includes both drugs to enhance urinary excretion of Ca and drugs to diminish the Ca efflux from bone and the absorption of Ca from the intestine.

The sequence of events leading to the hypercalcemia when excessive amounts of vitamin D_2 or D_3 or 25(OH)D are given is not completely clear. It was previously thought that the high blood levels of 25(OH)D that result from administration of this metabolite or its precursor could result in activation of the $1,25(OH)_2D$ receptor and, thus, mimicking the action of the hormone itself. However, an alternative explanation is based on the known binding affinities of the different metabolites for the D-binding protein.[9] Both vitamin D_3 and 25(OH)D bind more tightly to the binding protein than $1,25(OH)_2D$ does (see earlier subsection on Vitamin D-Binding Protein). Therefore, when the total concentration of 25(OH)D increases manyfold, a certain fraction of the circulating $1,25(OH)_2D$ will be displaced from the binding protein by 25(OH)D and lead to an increase in the free hormone concentration. Thus, the offending agent may be the elevated free hormone concentration, even if the total hormone concentration does not increase. Determination of the free hormone fraction has not yet been made in cases of vitamin D toxicity stemming from high doses of 25(OH)D. Consequently, it remains to be seen if the substance interacting with the $1,25(OH)_2D$ receptor is the hormone itself or 25(OH)D when excessive doses of vitamin D or 25(OH)D are administered.

Some infants and children may be particularly sensitive to the toxic actions of vitamin D and develop toxicity signs and symptoms after doses as low as 4–5 times the recommended daily intake of 400 IU.[73] The toxic dose in otherwise healthy adults is probably closer to 30–40 times the RDA (U.S.).

X. SUMMARY

Vitamin D, either derived from the diet or skin production, has become an increasingly important molecule in human function because of the extended longevity of human populations in many nations. The actual vitamin D requirements of elderly individuals remain difficult to determine, since environmental conditions, especially sunlight exposure, vary so greatly throughout the world. Data are limited on the potential prophylactic benefit of vitamin D or $1,25(OH)_2D$ in metabolic bone diseases, such as osteoporosis, in the absence of vitamin D deficiency. Possible roles of vitamin D or its metabolites in the etiology or treatment of diabetes mellitus, cancer, and hypertension have been reviewed recently by Bikle.[8] An exciting area of research is the recently reported association between expression of a vitamin D receptor allele variant and low bone density in Caucasian women. New information on the functional roles of $1,25(OH)_2D$ on target tissues and the mechanism of action of this key molecule continue to emerge.

REFERENCES

1. **Anderson, J. J. B. and Toverud, S. U.,** Diet and vitamin D: a review with an emphasis on human function, *J. Nutr. Biochem.*, 5, 58, 1994.
2. **Reichel, H., Koeffler, H. P. and Norman, A. W.,** The role of the vitamin D endocrine system in health and disease, *New Engl. J. Med.*, 320, 980, 1989.
3. **Norman, A.,** Intestinal calcium absorption: A vitamin D-hormone-mediated adaptive response, *Am. J. Clin. Nutr.*, 51, 290, 1983.
4. **Slovik, D. M., Adams, J. S., Neer, R. M., Holick, M. F. and Potts, J. T.,** Deficient production of 1,25-dihydroxyvitamin D in elderly osteoporotic patients, *New Engl. J. Med.*, 305, 372, 1981.
5. **Clemens, T. L., Zhou, X.-Y., Myles, M., Endres, D. and Lindsay, R.,** Serum vitamin D_2 and vitamin D_3 metabolite concentrations and absorption of vitamin D_2 in elderly subjects, *J. Clin. Endocrinol. Metab.*, 63, 656, 1986.
6. **Clark, S. A., Boass, A. and Toverud, S. U.,** Effects of high dietary contents of calcium and phosphorus on mineral metabolism and growth of vitamin D-deficient suckling and weaned rats, *Bone Miner.*, 2, 257, 1987.
7. **DeLuca, H. F.,** Vitamin D, *Nutrition Today*, 28, 6, 1993.
8. **Bikle, D. D.,** Clinical counterpoint: Vitamin D: New actions, new analogs, new therapeutic potential, *Endocrine Rev.*, 13, 765, 1992.
9. **Vieth, R.,** The mechanisms of vitamin D toxicity, *Bone Miner.*, 11, 267, 1990.
10. **Morrison, A. N., Qi, C. J., Tokita, A., Kelly, P. J., Crofts, L., Nguyen, T. V., Sambrook, P. N. and Eisman, J. A.,** Prediction of bone density from vitamin D receptor alleles, *Nature (London)*, 67, 284, 1994.
11. **Spector, T. D., Keen, R. W., Arden, N. K., Major, P. J., Baker, J. R., Morrison, N. A., Kelly, P. J., Sambrook, P. N., Lanchbury, J. S. and Eisman, J. A.,** Vitamin D receptor gene (VDR) alleles and bone density in postmenopausal women, *J. Bone Miner. Res.*, 9 (suppl. 1), S143, 1994.
12. **Hustmyer, F. G., Peacock, M., Hui, S., Johnston, C. C. and Christian, J. C.,** Polymorphisms at the vitamin D receptor gene locus and bone mineral density, *J. Bone Miner. Res.*, 9 (Suppl. 1), S142, 1994.

13. **Nishii, Y., Abe, J., Mori, T., Brown, A. J., Dusso, A. S., Finch, J., Lopez-Hilker, S., Morrissey, J. and Slatopolsky, E.,** The noncalcemic analogue of vitamin D, 22-oxacalcitriol, suppresses parathyroid hormone synthesis and secretion, in *Calcium-Regulating Hormones. II. Calcium Transport, Bone Merabolism, and New Drugs, Contrib. Nephrol.*, Morii, H., ed., Karger, Basel, 1991.
14. **Delmez, J. A., Tindira, C., Gromms, P., Dusso, A., Windus, D. W. and Slatopolsky, E.,** Parathyroid hormone suppression by intervenous $1,25(OH)_2D_3$. A role for increased sensitivity to calcium, *J. Clin. Invest.*, 83, 1349, 1989.
15. **Lobaugh, B., Boass, A., Lester, G. E. and Toverud, S. U.,** Regulation of serum 1,25-dihydroxyvitamin D_3 in lactating rats, *Am. J. Physiol.*, 259 (*Endocrinol. Metab.*, 22), E665, 1990.
16. **Garner, S. C., Peng, T.-C., Hirsch, P. F., Boass, A. and Toverud, S. U.,** Increase in serum parathyroid hormone concentration in the lactating rat: effects of dietary calcium and lactational intensity, *J. Bone Miner. Res.*, 2, 347, 1987.
17. **Kawashima, H. and Kurokawa, K.,** Metabolism and sites of action of vitamin D in the kidney, *Kidney Int.*, 29, 98, 1986.
18. **Walters, M. R.,** Newly identified actions of the vitamin D endocrine system, *Endocrine Rev.*, 13, 719, 1992.
19. **Holick, M. F.,** Vitamin D: Cutaneous production and therapeutic effect in psoriasis, in *Eighth Workshop on Vitamin D*, Norman, A. W. eds., (Abstract), Paris, 1991.
20. **Hanchette, C. L. and Schwartz, G. G.,** Geographic patterns of prostate cancer mortality: Evidence for a protective effect of ultraviolet radiation, *Cancer*, 70, 2861, 1992.
21. **Saez, S., Falette, N., Guillot, C., Meggouh, F., Lefebvre, M.-F. and Crepin, M.,** $1,25(OH)_2D_3$ modulation of mammary tumor cell growth in vitro and vivo, *Breast Cancer Res. Treatment*, 27, 69, 1993.
22. **Pike, J. W.,** Vitamin D_3 receptors: Structure and function in transcription, *Ann. Rev. Nutr.*, 11, 189, 1991.
23. **Halloran, B. P. and DeLuca, H. F.,** Appearance of the intestinal cytosolic receptor for 1,25-dihydroxyvitamin D_3 during neonatal development in the rat, *J. Biol. Chem.*, 256, 7338, 1981.
24. **Darwish, H. M. and DeLuca, H. F.,** Identification of a 1,25-dihydroxyvitamin D_3-response element in the 5′-flanking region of the rat calbindin D-9k gene, *Proc. Natl. Acad. Sci. USA*, 89, 603, 1992.
25. **Wasserman, R. H. and Fullmer, C. S.,** Calcium transport proteins, calcium absorption, and vitamin D, *Ann. Rev. Physiol.*, 45, 375, 1983.
26. **Nemere, I. and Norman, A. W.,** Transcaltachia, vesicular calcium transport, and microtubule-associated calbindin-D_{28K}: Emerging views of 1,25-dihydroxyvitamin D_3-mediated intestinal calcium absorption, *Miner. Electrolyte Metab.*, 16, 109, 1990.
27. **Wali, R. K., Baum, C. L., Sitrin, M. D. and Brasitus, T. A.,** $1,25(OH)_2$ vitamin D_3 stimulates membrane phosphoinositide turnover, activates protein kinase C, and increases cytosolic calcium in rat colonic epithelium, *J. Clin. Invest.*, 85, 1296, 1990.
28. **Lieberherr, M., Grosse, B., Duchambon, P. and Drueke, T.,** A functional cell surface type receptor is required for the early action of 1,25-dihydroxyvitamin D_3 on the phosphoinositide metabolism in rat enterocytes, *J. Biol. Chem.*, 264, 20403, 1989.
29. **Norman, A. W., Nemere, I., Zhou, L.-X., Bishop, J. E., Lowe, K. E., Maiyar, A. C., Collins, E. D., Taoka, T., Sergeev, I. and Farach-Carson, M. C.,** $1,25(OH)_2$-vitamin D_3, a steroid hormone that produces biological effects via both genomic and nongenomic pathways, *J. Steroid Biochem. Molec. Biol.*, 41, 231, 1992.
30. **Norman, A. W., Bouillon, R., Farach-Carson, M. C., Bishop, J. E., Zhou, L.-X., Nemere, I., Zhao, J., Muralidharan, K. R. and Okamura, W. H.,** Demonstration that 1β,25-dihydroxyvitamin D_3 is an antagonist of the nongenomic but not genomic biological responses and biological profile of the three A-ring diastereomers of 1α,25-dihydroxyvitamin D_3, *J. Biol. Chem.*, 268, 20022, 1993.
31. **Baran, D. T., Sorensen, A. M., Shalhoub, V., Owen, T., Stein, G. and Lian, J.,** The rapid nongenomic actions of 1α,25-dihydroxyvitamin D_3 modulate the hormone-induced increments in osteocalcin gene transcription in osteoblast-like cells, *J. Cell Biochem.*, 50, 124, 1992.
32. **Webb, A. R., Kline, L. and Holick, M. F.,** Influence of season and latitude on the cutaneous synthesis of vitamin D_3: exposure to winter sunlight in Boston and Edmonton will not promote vitamin D_3 synthesis in human skin, *J. Clin. Endocrinol. Metab.*, 67, 373, 1988.
33. **Stryd, R. P., Gilbertson, T. J. and Brunden, M. N.,** A seasonal variation study of 25-hydroxyvitamin D_3 serum levels in normal humans, *J. Clin. Endocrinol. Metab.*, 48, 771, 1979.
34. **Lawson, D. E. M.,** Metabolism of vitamin D, in *Vitamin D: Molecular Biology and Clinical Nutrition*, Norman, A. E. eds., Marcel Dekker, New York, 1980.
35. **Pun, K. K., Wong, F. H. W., Wang, C., Lau, P., Pun, W. K., Chow, S. P., Cheng, C. L., Leong, C. Y. and Young, R. T. T.,** Vitamin D status among patients with fractured neck of femur in Hong Kong, *Bone*, 11, 365, 1990.
36. **Webb, A. R., DeCosta, B. R. and Holick, M. F.,** Sunlight regulates the cutaneous production of vitamin D_3 by causing its photodegradation, *J. Clin. Endocrinol. Metab.*, 68, 882, 1989.
37. **DeLuca, H. F.,** The metabolism and functions of vitamin D, *Adv. Exper. Med. Biol.: Steroid Hormone Resistance: Mechanisms and Clinical Aspects*, 196, 361, 1986.
38. **Holick, M. F., MacLaughlin, J. A., Clark, M. B., Holick, S. A., Potts, J. T., Jr., Anderson, R. R., Blank, I. H., Parrish, J. A. and Elias, P.,** Photosynthesis of previtamin D_3 in human skin and the physiologic consequences, *Science*, 210, 203, 1980.

39. **Holick, M. F., MacLaughlin, J. A. and Doppelt, S. H.,** Regulation of cutaneous previtamin D_3 photosynthesis in man: Skin pigment is not an essential regulator, *Science*, 21, 590, 1981.
40. **MacLaughlin, J. and Holick, M. F.,** Aging decreases capacity of human skin to produce vitamin D_3, *J. Clin. Invest.*, 76, 1536, 1985.
41. **Sherman, S. S., Hollis, B. W. and Tobin, J. D.,** Vitamin D status and related parameters in a healthy population: the effects of age, sex, and season, *J. Clin. Endocrinol. Metab.*, 71, 405, 1990.
42. **Eastell, R., Yeargey, A., Veiera, N., Cedel, S., Kumar, R. and Riggs, B.,** Interrelationship among vitamin D metabolism, true calcium absorption, parathyroid function, and age in women: evidence of an age-related intestinal resistance to 1,25-dihydroxyvitamin D action, *J. Bone Miner. Res.*, 6, 125, 1991.
43. **Meier, D. E., Luckey, M. M., Wallenstein, S., Clemens, T. L., Orwoll, E. S. and Waslien, C. I.,** Calcium, vitamin D, and parathyroid hormone status in young white and black women: Association with racial differences in bone mass, *J. Clin. Endocrinol. Metab.*, 72, 703, 1991.
44. **Mallon, J. P., Matuszewski, D. and Sheppard, H.,** Binding specificity of the rat serum vitamin D transport protein, *J. Steroid Biochem.*, 13, 409, 1980.
45. **Haddad, J. G., Matsuoka, L. Y., Hollis, B. W., Hu, Y. Z. and Wortsman, J.,** Human plasma transport of vitamin D after its endogenous synthesis, *J. Clin. Invest.*, 91, 2552, 1993.
46. **Chapuy, M. C., Arlot, M. E., Duboeuf, F., Brun, J., Crouzet, B., Arnaud, S., Delmas, P. D. and Meunier, P. J.,** Vitamin D_3 and calcium to prevent hip fractures in elderly women, *New Engl. J. Med.*, 327, 1637, 1992.
47. **Gallagher, J. C.,** Vitamin D metabolism and therapy in elderly subjects, *South. Med. J.*, 85 (suppl 2), 43, 1992.
48. **Fujita, T.,** Vitamin D in the treatment of osteoporosis, *Proc. Soc. Exper. Biol. Med.*, 199, 394, 1992.
49. **Tilyard, M. W., Spears, G. F., Thomson, J. and Dovey, S.,** Treatment of postmenopausal osteoporosis with calcitriol or calcium, *New Engl. J. Med.*, 326, 357, 1992.
50. **Orimo, H., Shiraki, M., Hayashi, T. and Nakamura, T.,** Reduced occurrence of vertebral crush fractures in senile osteoporosis treated with 1a(OH)-vitamin D, *Bone Miner.*, 3, 47, 1987.
51. **Fujita, T.,** Studies of osteoporosis in Japan, *Metabolism*, 39 (suppl 1), 39, 1990.
52. U.S. Department of Agriculture (USDA), H. N. I. S., *Dietary Levels: Households in the United States, Spring 1977. 1977–78 Nationwide Food Consumption Survey*, U.S. Government Printing Office, Washington, D.C., 1985,
53. National Research Council Subcommittee on Dietary Allowances, *Recommended Dietary Allowances, 10th edition*, National Academy Press, Washington, D.C., 1989.
54. **Specker, B. L.,** Do North American women need supplemental vitamin D during pregnancy or lactation? *Am. J. Clin. Nutr.*, 59 (Suppl.), 484, 1994.
55. **Omdahl, J. L., Garry, P. J., Hunsaker, L. A., Hunt, W. C. and Goodwin, J. S.,** Nutritional status in a healthy population: Vitamin D, *Am. J. Clin. Nutr.*, 36, 1225, 1982.
56. **Bouillon, R. A., Auwerx, J. H., Lissens, W. D. and Peleman, W. K.,** Vitamin D status in the elderly: seasonal substrate deficiency causes 1,25-dihydroxycholecalciferol deficiency, *Am. J. Clin. Nutr*, 45, 755, 1987.
57. **Egsmose, C., Lund, B., McNair, P., Storm, T. and Sørensen, O.,** Low serum levels of 25-hydroxyvitamin D and 1,25-dihydroxyvitamin D in institutionalized old people: influence of solar exposure and vitamin D supplementation, *Age Ageing*, 16, 35, 1987.
58. **Heikinheimo, R. J., Inkovaara, J. A., Harju, E. J., Haavisto, M. V., Kaarela, R. H., Kataja, J. M., Kokko, A. M.-L., Kolho, L. A. and Rajala, S. A.,** Annual injection of vitamin D and fractures of aged bones, *Calcif. Tissue Int.*, 51, 105, 1992.
59. **Dawson-Hughes, B., Dallal, G. E., Krall , E. H., Harris, S., Sokoll, L. J. and Falconer, G.,** Effect of vitamin D supplementation in wintertime and overall bone loss in healthy postmenopausal women, *Ann. Int. Med.*, 115, 505, 1991.
60. **Tjellesen, L. and Christiansen, C.,** Vitamin D metabolites in normal subjects during one year. A longitudinal study, *Scand. J. Clin. Lab. Invest.*, 43, 85, 1983.
61. **Parfitt, A. M., Gallagher, J. C., Heaney, R. P., Johnston, C. C., Jr., Neer, R. and Whedon, G. D.,** Vitamin D and bone health in the elderly, *Am. J. Clin. Nutr.*, 36, 1014, 1982.
62. **Webb, A. R., Pilbeam, C., Hanafin, N. and Holick, M. F.,** An evaluation of the relative contributions of exposure to sunlight and of diet to the circulating concentrations of 25-hydroxyvitamin D in an elderly nursing home population in Boston, *Am. J. Clin. Nutr.*, 51, 1075, 1990.
63. **Gloth, F., III, Tobin, J., Sherman, S. and Hollis, B.,** Is the Recommended Daily Allowance for vitamin D too low for the homebound elderly? *J. Am. Geriatr. Soc.*, 39, 137, 1991.
64. **Okonofua, F., Gill, D. S., Alabi, Z. O., Thomas, M., Bell, J. L. and Dandona, P.,** Rickets in Nigerian children: A consequence of calcium malnutrition, *Metabolism*, 40, 209, 1991.
65. **David, L.,** Common vitamin D-deficiency rickets, in *Rickets*, Glorieux, F. H. eds., Raven Press, New York, 1991.
66. **Pitt, M. J.,** Rickets and osteomalacia are still around, *Radiol. Clin. No. Am.*, 29, 97, 1991.
67. **Dagnelie, P. C., Vergote, F. J. V. R. A., vanStaveren, W. A., vandenBerg, H., Dingjan, P. G. and Hautvast, J. G. A. J.,** High prevalence of rickets in infants on macrobiotic diets, *Am. J. Clin. Nutr.*, 51, 202, 1990.
68. **Markestad, T. and Elzouki, A. Y.,** Vitamin D-deficiency rickets in Northern Europe and Libya, in *Rickets*, Glorieux, F. H. eds., Raven Press, New York, 1991.

69. **Key, L. L., Jr.,** Nutritional rickets, *Trends Endocrinol. Metab.*, 2, 81, 1991.
70. **Chang, Y. T., Germain-Lee, E. L., Doran, T. F., Migeon, C. J., Levine, M. A. and Berkovitz, G. D.,** Hypocalcemia in nonwhite breast-fed infants, *Clin. Pediatr.*, 31, 695, 1992.
71. **Glorieux, F. H.,** *Rickets*, Raven Press, New York, 1991.
72. **Jacobus, C. H., Holick, M. F., Shao, Q., Chen, T. C., Holm, I. A., Kolodny, J. M., Fuleihan, G. E.-H. and Seely, E. W.,** Hypervitaminosis D associated with drinking milk, *New Engl. J. Med.*, 326, 1173, 1992.
73. **Jeans, P. C. and Stearns, G.,** The effect of vitamin D on linear growth in infancy. II. The effect of intakes above 1,800 USP units daily, *J. Pediatr.*, 13, 730, 1938.
74. **Chesney, R., Rosen, J., Hamstra, A. and DeLuca, H.,** Serum 1,25-dihydroxyvitamin D levels in normal children and in vitamin D disorders, *Am. J. Dis. Child.*, 134, 135, 1980.
75. **Rosen, J. and Chesney, R.,** Circulating calcitriol concentrations in health and disease, *J. Pediatr.*, 103, 1, 1983.
76. **Haussler, M. R., Mangelsdorf, D. J., Komm, B. S., Terpening, C. M., Yamaoka, K., Allegretto, E. A., Baker, A. R., Shine, J., McDonnel, D. P., Hughes, M., Weigel, N. L., O'Malley, B. W., Pike, J. W.,** Molecular biology of the vitamin D hormone, *Rec. Prog. Hormone Res.*, 44, 263, 1988.

Chapter 13

CALCITONIN

Philip F. Hirsch, Ph.D. and John J. B. Anderson, Ph.D.

TABLE OF CONTENTS

I. INTRODUCTION

Calcitonin (CT) is the most recently discovered hormone that has a significant role in the regulation of serum Ca concentration. Although it has been only a little over three decades since the discovery of CT, the advances in our knowledge of the chemical structures, the molecular biology, embryology, cellular actions, pathology, and therapeutic uses of CT have been extremely rapid.[1-3] The relative significance of CT in normal physiology compared to the other two major Ca-regulating hormones, parathyroid hormone (PTH), and 1,25-dihydroxyvitamin D_3, the active metabolite of vitamin D, is still unknown. Adult humans can function well without the hormone, as demonstrated in thyroidectomized patients who receive adequate replacement therapy with thyroxine; no dysfunction in Ca metabolism is apparent from CT deficiency. Little is known about whether newborns and children function reasonably well without circulating CT. CT may have been more important

0-8493-7845-1/95/$0.00+$.50

physiologically at earlier stages in the evolution of vertebrates; it has a much older evolutionary history than PTH. Although it is possible that CT is now vestigial, its survival as a distinct, identifiable hormone in mammalian thyroid glands and as a normal blood constituent suggests that it has a function not readily discernible under our usual life style.

CT is a peptide hormone of relatively short length, 32 amino acids, that is secreted by cells of the thyroid gland, known variously as C-cells, cells of Nonidez, or parafollicular cells of the thyroid gland. CT has been shown to inhibit osteoclastic activity and bone resorption. These actions of CT have been utilized in the therapy of certain skeletal diseases and conditions with high bone resorption rates and, hence, turnover. In this regard CT is often selected as the drug of choice for the emergency treatment of hypercalcemia, for Paget's disease, and for conserving bone mass in the treatment of osteoporosis.

This chapter reviews the discovery of CT, its chemical structure, and its roles in health and disease. In addition, information is presented on a CT gene-related peptide (CGRP), an alternative product of the CT gene apparently involved in neural transmission or modulation.

II. HISTORICAL ASPECTS OF THE DISCOVERY OF CALCITONIN

The discovery of CT resulted from observations of a blood Ca-lowering factor released by the thyro-parathyroid complex. Although CT was initially thought to be a product of the parathyroid gland, additional research soon demonstrated the thyroid origin of this peptide hormone.

A. DISCOVERY

Two groups of investigators in North America played a major role in the discovery of CT. The first key evidence for the existence of a hypocalcemic hormone was obtained by Copp and his Canadian colleagues. They perfused blood high in Ca concentration through the thyroid-parathyroid gland of dogs. When the perfusate entered the systemic circulation, serum Ca fell. The result could not be ascribed to the inhibition of PTH secretion because the fall in serum Ca was more rapid than after thyroparathyroidectomy. Copp et al.[4] attributed the fall to the release of a hypocalcemic substance, named *calcitonin.* They initially concluded that the parathyroid gland was the source of CT.

Confirmation that a hypocalcemic hormone was secreted by the thyroid-parathyroid complex was obtained the following year by Kumar et al.[5] in experiments with dogs in which hypercalcemic perfusion *in situ* of the thyroid and parathyroid glands led to a rapid lowering of serum Ca. Their experiments did not distinguish between the parathyroid or thyroid glands as the source of the hormone. Earlier, Sanderson et al.[6] had observed that after administration of Ca to dogs, the time required to restore serum Ca to preinjection levels was much slower in thyroparathyroidectomized than in intact dogs; however, they did not consider that a hypocalcemic hormone from the thyroid-parathyroid complex might be involved in the restoration of Ca levels.

At the same time as Copp and colleagues were finding evidence for a hypocalcemic hormone, Hirsch and colleagues in Boston were attempting to explain the more rapid and severe fall in serum Ca in rats that were parathyroidectomized by hot wire cautery than in those treated to the surgical removal of the parathyroid gland. The difference between these two methods of parathyroidectomy, observed much earlier,[7] appeared to be due to a cautery-induced release of a hypocalcemic substance from the thyroid.[8] This explanation was strongly supported when extracts were prepared from thyroid glands from which the parathyroid glands had been removed. These extracts given by subcutaneous injection to intact rats resulted in a significant fall in serum Ca within one hour. The thyroid hypocalcemic agent was originally named *thyrocalcitonin* [8] to distinguish it from Copp's *calcitonin.*[4] Shortly thereafter, Hirsch et al.[9] showed that thyrocalcitonin in rats also resulted in a hypophosphatemic response.

Initially, it was unclear whether thyrocalcitonin was the same or a different hormone than CT. However, within one year the issue was resolved with experiments showing that the hypocalcemic hormone was secreted by the thyroid gland. Results obtained by Talmage et al.[10] demonstrated quite conclusively that hypercalcemia induced in rats by Ca administration was restricted by a hypocalcemic principle from the thyroid rather than the parathyroid gland. Also, experiments were performed on goats[11] and pigs,[12] species in which the parathyroid gland can be perfused separately from the thyroid gland. The results provided convincing evidence that high Ca perfusion of the thyroid gland but not the parathyroid gland resulted in CT secretion. Thus, thyrocalcitonin extracted from the thyroid gland of rats by Hirsch et al.[8] was the same hormone as CT, described by Copp et al.[4] as a second hormone from the parathyroid gland. CT has been accepted for over a decade as the name of choice for the hormone. A detailed historical account of the discovery and the rapid progress achieved during the first seven years after the discovery of CT was published by Hirsch and Munson.[13]

B. CELL OF ORIGIN OF CALCITONIN AND THE EMBRYOLOGY OF THE C-CELLS

Shortly after identifying the thyroid as the source of CT, Pearse showed that CT was localized in the parafollicular cells of the thyroid;[14] these cells are now commonly called the C-cells, but they have also been called the cells of Nonidez,[15] parafollicular cells, and light cells.[16,17] Shortly thereafter, Pearse and Carvalheira[18] provided cytochemical evidence that the thyroid C-cells were of ultimobranchial origin. In lower vertebrates, such as fish, amphibians, and birds, the ultimobranchial body remains as a separate gland,[19] whereas in mammals it merges with the thyroid gland. At a later time Le Dourain and Le Lievre[20] and Pearse and Polak[21] published experiments demonstrating that, during embryogenesis, C-cells were of neural crest origin and migrated from the neural crest to the ultimobranchial body. Neural crest cells with common cytochemical and structural characteristics of endocrine cells produce polypeptide hormones. These cells exhibit cytochemical characteristics shared by a number of apparently unrelated endocrine cells, namely amine precursor uptake and decarboxylation, named the APUD series by Pearse.[22] The neural crest-derived cells migrate to the thyroid and a number of other tissues, including the gastrointestinal tract. Cells of the APUD series are often involved in the pathology of the multiple endocrine neoplasias (MEN) and some are ectopic sources of CT.

C. ULTIMOBRANCHIAL CALCITONIN

Potent hypocalcemic ultimobranchial extracts were prepared simultaneously and independently by Copp et al.[23] from chickens and dogfish and Tauber[24] from chickens. In the summer and fall of 1968 Copp and collaborators collected over 200 pounds of ultimobranchial tissue from salmon, from which CT was purified and its structure determined.[25] Shortly thereafter, salmon CT was synthesized.[26] Because of its longer duration of action and its higher potency than mammalian CTs, including human CT, salmon CT has become the most widely used CT in therapy.

D. SUMMARY

The rapid advances made in understandings of the cells that synthesize and secrete CT and of the physiologic stimuli that elicit the release of CT have been quite remarkable. From the time of its discovery in the early 1960s, its embryological and cellular origins were identified, the hormone was isolated from a number of species, its structure was determined, and an injectable drug was ready for marketing within 15 years. Furthermore, within another five-year period, a nasal CT preparation was developed so that users could avoid injections.

III. CHEMICAL STRUCTURE AND STRUCTURE-ACTIVITY RELATIONSHIPS OF CALCITONINS

All CTs have 32 amino acids with a proline amide at the C-terminus and cysteine at the N-terminus that forms a 1-7 disulfide intrachain ring with another cysteine at position 7. Considerable homology in amino acid sequences exists within the ring structure between CTs from different

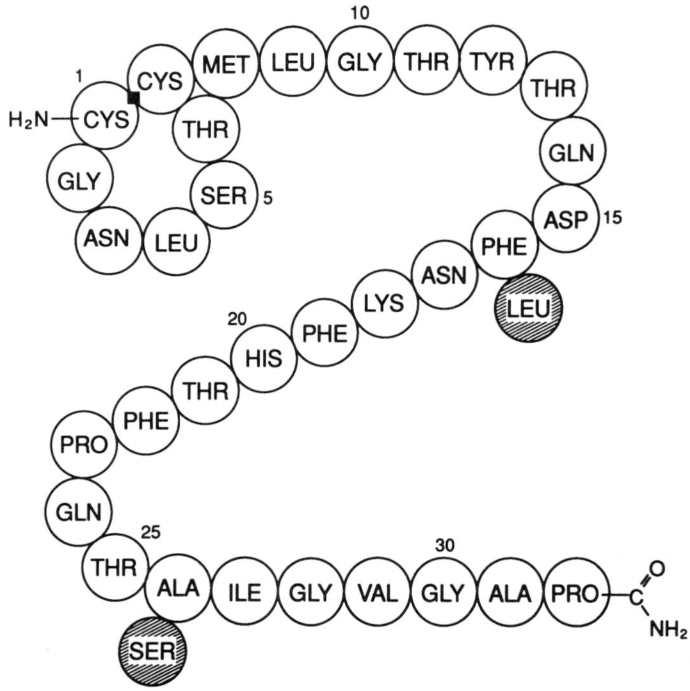

FIGURE 1. The Amino Acid Sequence of Human CT (open circles), as Compared to that of the Rat when LEU and SER (shaded circles) replace PHE and ALA at positions 16 and 26, respectively.

species. Significant differences in the amino acid sequence from positions 8 to 31 occur between unrelated species;[27] however, the sequences in related species, such as ovine, bovine, and porcine, are quite similar. Also, human and rat CTs differ by only two amino acids.[28] Figure 1 shows the amino acid sequence of human CT and the changes in amino acids that occur in rat CT.

The biological activities of the various CTs, measured initially by the hypocalcemic response in rats, differ. Studies of the structure-activity relationship have shown that the loss of just one amino acid results in the loss of almost all activity. However, the disulfide bond forming the ring structure has been replaced in eel CT with a C-C linkage without a loss of activity.[29] Potts has described some of the consequences of substitutions and analogs between residues 8 to 22.[27] Extensive interest has been generated by the finding that receptors for CT, PTH, and many other polypeptide hormones have substantial structural homologies,[30] indicating that these receptors may have evolved from a common ancestral molecule.

In summary, evolutionary changes in the amino acid sequence of CT from fish to mammals have occurred, but without changes in the number of amino acids. Surprisingly, the potency of the fish CTs is greater than that of human CT when examined in many mammalian species.

IV. BLOOD CONCENTRATIONS OF CALCITONIN ACROSS THE LIFE CYCLE

The measurement of CT in blood has been difficult because antibodies used in immunoassays have interacted with molecules other than the CT monomer. The problems encountered in the past have been reviewed.[31-33] As the methods of determination have improved, the measured concentrations of CT in blood have decreased. Many of the problems previously encountered appear resolved by utilizing immunoradiometric assays (IRMA). A comparison of newer methods indicates that the

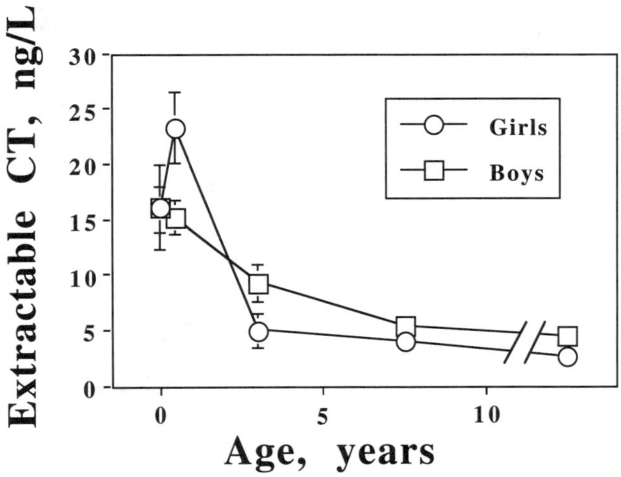

FIGURE 2. The Changes in Serum CT Concentration across the Life Cycle. (Adapted from Table 1 of Body et al.[38])

serum values for CT in healthy subjects are much lower with IRMA methods than with radioimmunoassays.[34] In a recent study by Barbot et al.[35] plasma levels of CT in healthy human subjects measured by IRMA were less than 10 pg/mL. These values are similar to those previously obtained with radioimmunoassays by Body and Heath[36] in silica-extracted plasma and by Bucht and coworkers[37] using acidic alcohol to extract CT from blood.

The concentration of CT in human serum was found to be highest at birth and in infancy, decreasing rapidly within the first year and slowly with increasing age at least to the age of 10 years.[38] Evidence is becoming overwhelming that CT levels in adults are higher in men than in women.[39-41] Whether CT levels decrease with increasing age in adult humans remains controversial. Deftos et al.[39] reported a decrease in CT levels with increasing age, whereas Tiegs et al.[41] did not find a significant change in serum CT with increasing age. Convincing evidence for diurnal rhythms of the monomeric form of CT in human blood is lacking.[42,43] Figure 2 illustrates these life-cycle changes in serum CT concentrations.

V. FUNCTIONS AND ROLES OF CALCITONIN IN CALCIUM METABOLISM

Despite extensive studies since the discovery of CT in the early 1960s, no definitive role for CT in normal physiology has been identified. Several possible functions for CT have been proposed: (1) CT, by working in concert to the well-known Ca-mobilizing PTH, helps to maintain the constancy of blood Ca; (2) CT prevents hypercalcemia; and (3) CT aids in the storage of consumed Ca in bone for periods when exogenous Ca is unavailable. Although these three functions are interrelated, evidence to support the first two as important physiological roles for CT is still lacking.

Improvements in the sensitivity of Ca measurements revealed that blood Ca in rats does not remain constant, but undergoes diurnal rhythms.[44] These rhythms appear to be influenced by diurnal fluctuations in the secretion of CT; when CT levels increase, serum Ca decreases, and vice versa.[45] Thyroidectomized rats with functional parathyroid transplants, however, maintain a relatively normal level of serum Ca, although the patterns of the diurnal rhythms are altered.[46,47] Also, even though CT can protect against hypercalcemia produced by levels of PTH or vitamin D or high dietary Ca, the necessity for such a mechanism is remote and therefore not of major importance. On the other hand, considerable evidence exists in rats showing that CT protects against or helps prevent the excretion of ingested Ca.[48,49] Most impressive are the experiments by Talmage et al.,[49] which demonstrated a sevenfold increase in urinary Ca excretion in thyroidectomized rats with functional parathyroid-transplants after the rats were switched from a Ca-free to a Ca-containing diet. The increase in Ca excretion did not occur in thyroid-intact rats or in thyroidectomized rats treated with CT. The results strongly suggest that CT helps to conserve intestinally absorbed Ca by retaining it in bone.[50]

The mechanisms responsible for the rapid hypocalcemic response to administered CT in rats has been somewhat controversial. *In vitro* experiments have demonstrated that CT inhibits PTH-induced osteoclastic resorption of bone in tissue culture,[51,52] induces changes in the shape of osteoclasts isolated from rats, and inhibits their motility.[53] However, the rapid fall in serum Ca after administration of CT or the typical diurnal changes in blood Ca do not likely result from changes in osteoclasts because of their small existent numbers and limited activity. All bone cells, osteocytes, osteoblasts, and osteoblastic lining cells, are affected by CT.[54,55]

Numerous animal, and a few human, experiments have employed large, i.e., supraphysiologic, doses of CT to demonstrate effects. Although large doses of CT have had effects on the kidney, liver, gut, brain, and other tissues, the importance of these effects at such high levels to the normal function of CT is unknown.

VI. FUNCTIONS AND ROLES OF CALCITONIN IN PHOSPHORUS METABOLISM

CT influences the metabolism of inorganic phosphate (Pi) in a similar way as for Ca. The Ca-lowering effect restricts the transfer of Ca and Pi ions from bone and bone fluid compartments to the extracellular fluid (ECF). Because the rate of bone metabolism in healthy adult humans is low, an injection of CT causes only a modest lowering of the blood concentrations of Ca and phosphorus.[56]

In rats and dogs the administration of CT significantly lowered the plasma Pi levels that had been increased by Ca infusion.[57,58] These and other experiments have led Talmage and colleagues to suggest that one of the primary actions of CT is to increase intracellular Pi[59] and thereby enhance storage of Ca in a labile (metastable) form.[50] Thus, CT secretion at mealtimes helps retain both Ca and Pi for the skeleton. This mechanism supports a physiologically important role of CT to protect the skeleton by conserving Ca during Ca ingestion that can be used to maintain blood Ca during intermeal periods.[50]

VII. CALCITONIN RELEASE BY GASTROINTESTINAL HORMONES

In 1971 Cooper et al.[60] and Care et al.[61] independently presented evidence that gastrointestinal (GI) hormones with the same penultimate carboxy-terminal tetrapeptide found in gastrin and cholecystokinin are potent CT secretagogues. It is possible that gastrin, or related GI hormones, may act as the natural secretagogues that increase CT after oral ingestion of Ca or other food components.[62]

VIII. MEDULLARY THYROID CARCINOMA

Tumors of the CT-secreting C-cells of the thyroid are rare, but medullary carcinoma of the thyroid (MCT) is present in >90% of individuals with multiple endocrine neoplasia (MEN) type IIA or IIB. Patients with MEN are also likely to have pheochromocytomas (MEN IIA and IIB) and hyperplasia of the parathyroid gland (MEN IIA). MCT is a highly metastatic tumor that secretes excessive amounts of calcitonin.[63-65] Although fatal in many instances because of its aggressive metastasis to local lymph nodes or to bone and other tissues, MCT is curable in early stages of development by removal of the thyroid lobe containing the tumor.

Measurement of CT levels in blood is useful in detecting MCT, following the success of surgery, and discovering its recurrence.[66] Even before resting concentrations of CT are increased in MCT, the presence of abnormal C-cells can be detected by a provocative test with Ca and pentagastrin infusion.[67] The observations of the CT-releasing effects of pentagastrin [60,61] and Ca, either alone[68,69] or in combination,[69] led to their use in the detection of MCT. Patients with MCT respond to this test with a manyfold increase in circulating CT. Barbot et al.[35] have recently provided convincing data showing that the pentagastrin stimulation test used in conjunction with a sensitive immunoradiometric assay (IRMA) to measure plasma CT can be used successfully for the early detection of hereditary MCT.

IX. CLINICAL USES OF CALCITONIN AS A DRUG

CT has been used effectively as a drug via parenteral administration to treat patients with hypercalcemias,[70] Paget's disease,[71] postmenopausal osteoporosis,[72] glucocorticoid-induced osteoporosis,[73] and to inhibit pain, especially bone pain.[74,75] Convincing evidence has been published by European and Australian investigators indicating that nasal administration of CT is also effective.[76-78] However, the U.S. Food and Drug Administration has not yet given approval for this route of administration. Because CT inhibits bone resorption, it is highly effective in treating patients with pathologies involving a high rate of bone turnover, such as Paget's disease,[71] and glucocorticoid-induced[73,78] and high turnover osteoporosis (Type II, HTOP).[72,76,77,79]

Although antibodies develop in patients with long-term treatment with CT, they have not been shown to reduce the therapeutic effectiveness of CT to the point where its use must be discontinued. Intermittent use following a period of refractoriness and/or use of alternating treatments appears to be the direction being taken by practitioners.

CT is markedly degraded by the kidney, but other tissues such as the liver and bone may also be involved in the degradation of this peptide. No fragments are known to circulate. Large amounts of CT have been identified in the urine of patients with medullary thyroid carcinoma.[64]

X. CALCITONIN GENE-RELATED PEPTIDE

A second peptide (37 amino acids), referred to as CT gene-related peptide (CGRP), has been identified. CGRP is generated from the CT gene by alternative processing that generates a different mRNA.[80] Whereas the C-cells in the thyroid gland synthesize predominantly CT, neural tissues form predominantly CGRP.[81] A second CGRP, produced via a different gene, has also been found.[82] The mechanism that directs the appropriate mRNA pathway is being actively investigated.[83,84] Like CT, the physiological importance of CGRP is not yet elucidated. It appears to have a neural function either as a neurohormone or as an inhibitor of neural transmission. The evolutionary significance of CT and CGRP as products of a single gene is, as yet, not clear, and is of obvious interest to investigators concerned with the roles of these secretory agents in hormonal and neural regulation.

XI. SUMMARY AND CONCLUSIONS

This brief review of CT reflects three decades of research work since the first publications on this new hormone appeared. The rapid postdiscovery scientific developments of CT as a drug uncovered major actions of this hormone. The actions of CT to inhibit bone resorption, slow bone turnover, and induce analgesia have been utilized in the treatment of bone problems, namely hypercalcemias, Paget's disease, and osteoporosis. Identification of medullary thyroid carcinoma as a CT-producing excess syndrome has made it possible to identify the disease early with provocative tests and assess the success of removing the tumor, and also to detect its recurrence. That CT, an older hormone than PTH, is highly conserved during evolution suggests that it must still retain an important physiological function. However, unlike parathyroidectomy that causes life-threatening hypocalcemia, the absence of CT after thyroidectomy does not impose serious disturbances in Ca metabolism.

Although its medical utility has been remarkable, the elucidation of the physiological importance of CT in human function remains. Despite evidence that CT conserves Ca for the skeleton, its functional importance remains in question. The possibility that this hormone serves an important role in the early stages of the life cycle, including fetal life, still exists.

REFERENCES

1. **Azria, M.,** *The Calcitonins, Physiology and Pharmacology*, Karger, Basel, 1989.
2. **Munson, P. L.,** Parathyroid hormone and calcitonin, in *Endocrinology: People and Ideas*, McCann, S. M., ed., Amercian Physiological Society, Bethesda, 1988.
3. **Austin, L. A. and Heath, H., III,** Calcitonin: physiology and pathophysiology, *New Engl. J. Med.*, 304, 269, 1981.
4. **Copp, D. H., Cameron, E. C., Cheney, B. A., Davidson, A. G. F., and Henze, K. G.,** Evidence for calcitonin-a new hormone from the parathyroid that lowers blood calcium, *Endocrinology*, 70, 638, 1962.
5. **Kumar, M. A., Foster, G. V., and MacIntyre, I.,** Further evidence for calcitonin, a rapid-acting hormone which lowers plasma-calcium, *Lancet*, ii, 480, 1963.
6. **Sanderson, P. H., Marshall, F., and Wilson, R. E.,** Calcium and phosphorus homeostasis in the parathyroidectomized dog; evaluation by means of ethylenediamine tetraacetate and calcium tolerance tests, *J. Clin. Invest.*, 39, 662, 1960.
7. **Munson, P. L.,** Biological Assay of parathyroid hormone, in *The Parathyroids*, Greep, R. O. and Talmage, R. V., eds., C. C. Thomas, Springfield, IL, 1961.
8. **Hirsch, P. F., Gauthier, G. F., and Munson, P. L.,** Thyroid hypocalcemic principle and recurrent laryngeal nerve injury as factors affecting the response to parathyroidectomy in rats, *Endocrinology*, 73, 244, 1963.
9. **Hirsch, P. F., Voelkel, E. F., and Munson, P. L.,** Thyrocalcitonin: hypocalcemic hypophosphatemic principle of the thyroid gland, *Science*, 146, 412, 1964.
10. **Talmage, R. V., Neuenschwander, J., and Kraintz, L.,** Evidence for the existence of thyrocalcitonin in the rat, *Endocrinology*, 76, 103, 1965.
11. **Foster, G. V., Baghdiantz, A., Kumar, M. A., Slack, E., Soliman, H. A., and MacIntyre, I.,** Thyroid origin of calcitonin, *Nature*, 202, 1303, 1964.
12. **Care, A. D.,** Secretion of thyrocalcitonin, *Nature*, 205, 1289, 1965.
13. **Hirsch, P. F. and Munson, P. L.,** Thyrocalcitonin, *Physiol Rev*, 49, 548, 1969.
14. **Pearse, A. G. E.,** The cytochemistry of the thyroid C cells and their relationship to calcitonin, *Proc. Roy. Soc. Lond. B*, 164, 478, 1966.
15. **Nonidez, J. F.,** The origin of the 'parafollicular' cell, a second epithelial component of the thyroid gland of the dog, *Am. J. Anat.*, 49, 479, 1932.
16. **Young, B. A. and Leblond, C. P.,** The light cell as compared to the follicular cell in the thyroid gland of the rat, *Endocrinology*, 73, 669, 1963.
17. **Wissig, S. L.,** The fine structure of parafollicular (light) cells of the rat thyroid gland, in *Electron Microscopy*, Breese, S. S., Jr. ed., Academic Press, New York, 1962.
18. **Pearse, A. G. E. and Carvalheira, A. F.,** Cytochemical evidence for an ultimobranchial origin of rodent thyroid C cells, *Nature*, 214, 929, 1967.
19. **Godwin, M. C.,** Complex IV in the dog with special emphasis on the relation of the ultimobranchial body to interfollicular cells in the postnatal thyroid gland, *Am. J. Anat.*, 60, 299, 1937.
20. **Le Dourain, N. and LeLièvre, C.,** Démonstration de l'origine neurale des cellules à calcitonine du corp ultimobranchial chez l'embryon du poulet, *C. R. Acad. Sci. Paris*, 270, 2857, 1970.
21. **Pearse, A. G. E. and Polak, J. M.,** Cytochemical evidence for the neural crest origin of mammalian ultimobranchial C cells, *Histochemie*, 27, 96, 1971.
22. **Pearse, A. G. E.,** Common cytochemical and ultrastructural characteristics of cells producing polypeptide hormones (the APUD series) and their relevance to thyroid and ultimobranchial C cells and calcitonin, *Proc. Roy. Soc. Lond. B*, 170, 71, 1968.
23. **Copp, D. H., Cockcroft, D. W., and Kueh, Y.,** Calcitonin from the ultimobranchial glands from dogfish and chickens, *Science*, 158, 924, 1967.
24. **Tauber, S. D.,** The ultimobranchial origin of thyrocalcitonin, *Proc. Natl. Acad. Sci. USA*, 58, 1684, 1967.
25. **Niall, H. D., Keutmann, H. T., Copp, D. H., and Potts, J. T., Jr.,** Amino acid sequence of salmon ultimobranchial calcitonin, *Proc. Natl. Acad. Sci. USA*, 64, 771, 1969.
26. **Guttmann, St., Pless, J., Huguenin, R. L., Sandrin, E., Bossert, H., and Zehnder, K.,** Synthese von salm-calcitonin, eineme hochactiven hypocalcamischen hormon, *Helv. Chim. Acta*, 52, 1789, 1969.
27. **Potts, J. T., Jr.,** Chemistry of the calcitonins, *Bone Miner.*, 16, 169, 1992.
28. **Raulais, D., Hagaman, J., Ontjes, D. A., Lundblad, R. L., and Kingdon, H. S.,** The complete amino-acid sequence of rat thyrocalcitonin, *Eur. J. Biochem.*, 64, 607, 1976.
29. **Morikawa, T., Munekata, E., Sakakibara, S., Noda, T. and Otani, M.,** Synthesis of eel-calcitonin and [$Asu^{1,7}$]-eel-calcitonin: contribution of the disulfide bond to the hormonal activity, *Experientia*, 32, 1104, 1976.
30. **Segre, G. V. and Goldring, S. R.,** Receptors for secretin, calcitonin, parathyroid hormone (PTH)/PTH-related peptide, vasoactive intestinal peptide, glucagon-like peptide 1, growth hormone-releasing hormone, and glucagon belong to a newly discovered G-protein-linked receptor family, *Trends Endocrinol. Metab.*, 4, 309, 1993.
31. **Catherwood, B. D. and Deftos, L. J.,** General principles, problems and interpretation in the radioimmunoassay of calcitonin, *Biomed. Pharmacother.*, 38, 235, 1984.

32. **Heath, H. III., Body, J. J., and Fox, J.,** Radioimmunoassay of calcitonin in normal human plasma: problems, perspectives and prospects, *Biomed. Pharmacother.*, 38, 241, 1984.
33. **Moukhtar, M. S.,** Le dosage de la calcitonine humaine par voie radioimmunologique, *Biomed. Pharmacother.*, 38, 257, 1984.
34. **Weissel, M., Kainz, H., Tyl, E., Ogunyemi, E., and Woloszczuk, W.,** Clinical evaluation of new assays for determination of serum calcitonin concentrations, *Acta Endocrinol.*, 124, 540, 1991.
35. **Barbot, N., Calmettes, C., Schuffenecker, I., Saint-André, J. P., Franc, B., Rohmer, V., Jallet, P., and Bigorgne, J. C.,** Pentagastrin stimulation test and early diagnosis of medullary thyroid carcinoma using an immunoradiometric assay of calcitonin: comparison with genetic screening in hereditary medullary thyroid carcinoma, *J. Clin. Endocrinol. Metab.*, 78, 114, 1994.
36. **Body, J. J. and Heath, H., III,** Estimates of circulating monomeric calcitonin: physiological studies in normal and thyroidectomized man, *J. Clin. Endocrinol. Metab.*, 57, 897, 1983.
37. **Bucht, E., Torring, O., and Sjöberg, H. E.,** Gel chromatography of immunoextracted plasma calcitonin in response to the calcium clamp in healthy males, *Acta Endocrinol.*, 110, 421, 1985.
38. **Body, J. J., Chanoine, J. P., Dumon, J. C., and Delange, F.,** Circulating calcitonin levels in healthy children and subjects with congenital hypothyroidism from birth to adolescence, *J. Clin. Endocrinol. Metab.*, 77, 565, 1993.
39. **Deftos, L. J., Weisman, M. H., Williams, G. W., Karpf, D. B., Frumar, A. M., Davidson, B. J., Parthemore, J. G., and Judd, H. L.,** Influence of age and sex on plasma calcitonin in human beings, *New Engl. J. Med.*, 302, 1351, 1980.
40. **Cannarozzi, D. B., Canale, D. D., and Donabedian, R. K.,** Hypercalcitoninemia in infancy, *Clin. Chem. Acta*, 66, 387, 1976.
41. **Tiegs, R. D., Body, J. J., Barta, J. M. and Heath, H., III.,** Secretion and metabolism of monomeric human calcitonin: effects of age, sex, and thyroid damage, *J. Bone Miner. Res.*, 1, 339, 1986.
42. **Manolagas, S. C. and Deftos, L. J.,** No diurnal variations in calcitonin and vitamin D_2, *New Engl. J. Med.*, 312, 122, 1985.
43. **Tiegs, R. D. and Heath, H., III.,** Effects of altered calcium intake on diurnal and calcium-stimulated plasma calcitonin in normal women, *J. Bone. Miner. Res.*, 4, 407, 1989.
44. **Perault-Staub, A. M., Staub, J. F., and Milhaud, G.,** A new concept of plasma calcium homeostasis in the rat, *Endocrinology*, 95, 480, 1974.
45. **Hirsch, P. F. and Hagaman, J. R.,** Feeding regimen, dietary calcium, and the diurnal rhythms of serum calcium and calcitonin in the rat, *Endocrinology*, 110, 961, 1982.
46. **Perault-Staub, A. M., Staub, J. F., and Milhaud, G.,** Constancy and rhythmicity, a dual concept for homeostasis exemplified by 24-hour plasma calcium regulation in the rat, in *Calcium Regulating Hormones*, Talmage, R. V., Owen, M., and Parsons, J. A., eds., Excerpta Medica, Amsterdam, 1975.
47. **Talmage, R. V., Roycroft, J. H., and Anderson, J. J. B.,** Daily fluctuations in plasma calcium, phosphate, and their radionuclide concentrations in the rat, *Calcif. Tissue Res.*, 17, 91, 1975.
48. **Gray, T. K. and Munson, P. L.,** Thyrocalcitonin: Evidence for physiological function, *Science*, 166, 512, 1969.
49. **Talmage, R. V., VanderWiel, C. J., Decker, S. A., and Grubb, S. A.,** Changes produced in postprandial urinary calcium excretion by thyroidectomy and calcitonin administration in rats on different calcium regimes, *Endocrinology*, 105, 459, 1979.
50. **Talmage, R. V., Grubb, S. A., Norimatsu, H., and VanderWeil, C. J.,** Evidence for an important physiological role for calcitonin, *Proc. Natl. Acad. Sci. USA*, 77, 609, 1980.
51. **Friedman, J. and Raisz, L. G.,** Thyrocalcitonin: inhibitor of bone resorption in tissue culture, *Science*, 150, 1465, 1965.
52. **Aliapoulios, M. A., Goldhaber, P., and Munson, P. L.,** Thyrocalcitonin inhibition of bone resorption induced by parathyroid hormone in tissue culture, *Science*, 151, 330, 1966.
53. **Chambers, T. J. and Moore, A.,** The sensitivity of isolated osteoclasts to morphological transformation by calcitonin, *J. Clin. Endocrinol. Metab.*, 57, 819, 1983.
54. **Matthews, J. L., Martin, J.H., Collins, E.J., Kennedy, J.W., III., and Powell, E.L., Jr.,** Immediate changes in the ultrastructure of bone cells following thyrocalcitonin administration, in *Calcium, Parathyroid Hormone, and the Calcitonins*, Talmage, R. V. and Munson, P. L., Eds., Excerpta Medica, Amsterdam, 1972.
55. **Matthews, J. L., Talmage, R. V., and Doppelt, R.,** Response of the osteocyte lining cell complex — the bone cell unit to calcitonin, *Metab. Bone Dis. Res.*, 2, 113, 1980.
56. **Milhaud, G., Tsien-Ming, L., Nesralla, H., Moukhtar, M. S., and Perault-Staub, A. M.,** Studies on the mode of action and the therapeutic use of thyrocalcitonin, in *Calcitonin. Proceedings of the Symposium on Thyrocalcitonin and the C Cells*, Taylor, S. R., ed., Heinemann, London, 1968.
57. **Talmage, R. V., Anderson, J. J. B., and Cooper, C. W.,** The influence of calcitonins on the disappearance of radiocalcium and radiophosphorus from plasma, *Endocrinology*, 90, 1185, 1972.
58. **Anderson, J. J. B. and Talmage, R. V.,** The effect of calcium infusion and calcitonin on plasma phophate in sham-operated and thyroparathyroidecomized dogs, *Endocrinology*, 93, 1222, 1973.

59. **Talmage, R. V., VanderWeil, C. J., and Mathews, J. L.,** Calcitonin and phosphate, *Mol. Cell. Endocrinol.*, 24, 235, 1981.
60. **Cooper, C. W., Schwesinger, W. H., Mahgoub, A. M., and Ontjes, D. A.,** Thyrocalcitonin: stimulation of secretion by pentagastrin, *Science*, 172, 1238, 1971.
61. **Care, A. D., Bruce, J. B., Boelkins, J., Kenny, A. D., Conaway, H., and Anast, C. S.,** Role of pancreozymin-cholecystokinin and structurally related compounds as calcitonin secretagogues, *Endocrinology*, 89, 262, 1971.
62. **Cooper, C. W., Bolman, R. M., III, Linehan, W. M., and Wells, S. A., Jr.,** Interrelationships between calcium calcemic hormones and gastrointestinal hormones, *Rec. Prog. Horm. Res.*, 34, 259, 1978.
63. **Milhaud, G., Tubiana, M., Parmentier, C. and Coutris, G.,** Epithélioma de la thyroïde secretant de la thyrocalcitonine, *C. R. Acad. Sci. Paris*, 266, 608, 1968.
64. **Melvin, K. E. W. and Tashjian, A. H., Jr.,** The syndrome of excessive thyrocalcitonin produced by medullary carcinoma of the thyroid, *Proc. Natl. Acad. Sci. USA*, 59, 1216, 1968.
65. **Cunliffe, W. J., Black, N. M., Hall, R., Johnston, I. D. A., Hudgson, P., Shuster, S., Gudmundsson, T. V., Joplin, G. F., Williams, E. D., Woodhouse, N. J. Y., Galante, L., and MacIntyre, I.,** A calcitonin-secreting thyroid carcinoma, *Lancet*, 2, 63, 1968.
66. **Gharib, H., Kao, P. C., and Heath, H., III,** Determination of silica-purified plasma calcitonin for the detection and management of medullary thyroid carcinoma: comparison of two provocative tests, *Mayo Clin. Proc.*, 62, 373, 1987.
67. **Wells, S. A., Jr., Baylin, S. B., Linehan, W. M., Farrell, R. E., Cox, E. B., and Cooper, C. W.,** Provocative agents and the diagnosis of medullary carcinoma of the thyroid gland, *Ann. Surg.*, 188, 139, 1978.
68. **Hennessy, J. F., Wells, S. A., Jr., Ontjes, D. A., and Cooper, C. W.,** A comparison of pentagastrin injection and calcium infusion as provocative agents for the detection of medullary carcinoma of the thyroid, *J. Clin. Endocrinol. Metab.*, 39, 487, 1974.
69. **Mallette, L. E. and Gagel, R. F.,** Parathyroid hormone and calcitonin, in *Primer on the Metabolic Bone Diseases and Disorders of Mineral Metabolism, Second Edition*, Favus, M. M., ed., Raven Press, New York, 1993.
70. **Bilezikian, J. P.,** Management of acute hypercalcemia, *New Engl. J. Med.*, 326, 1196, 1992.
71. **Bone, H. G. and Kleerekoper, M.,** Clinical review 39: Paget's disease of bone, *J. Clin. Endocrinol. Metab.*, 75, 1179, 1992.
72. **Avioli, L. V. and Gennari, C.,** Calcitonin therapy in osteoporotic syndromes, in *The Osteoporotic Syndrome: Detection, Prevention, and Treatment*, Avioli, L. V., ed., Wiley-Liss, New York, 1993.
73. **Silverman, S. L.,** Editorial: Management of corticosteroid-induced osteoporosis: a clinicians perspective, *Calcif. Tissue Int.*, 50, 101, 1992.
74. **Pecile, A.,** Calcitonin and the relief of pain, *Bone Miner.*, 16, 187, 1992.
75. **Passeri, M., Baroni, M. C., Pedrazzoni, M., and Vescovi, P. P.,** Protocols of treatment of chronic back pain in involutional osteoporosis, *Bone Miner.*, 22 (suppl.), S23, 1993.
76. **Christiansen, C.,** Use of nasally administered salmon calcitonin in preventing bone loss, *Calcif. Tissue Int.*, 49 (suppl. 2), S14, 1991.
77. **Reginster, J. Y.,** Calcitonin for prevention and treatment of osteoporosis, *Am. J. Med.*, 95(suppl. 5A), 445, 44, 1993.
78. **Sambrook, P., Birmingham, J., Kelly, P., Kempler, S., Nguyen, T., Pocock, N., and Eisman, J.,** Prevention of corticosteroid bone loss, *Osteoporosis Int.*, 3 (suppl. 1), 141, 1993.
79. **Civitelli, R., Gonnelli, S., Zacchei, F., Bigazzi, S., Vattimo, A., Avioli, L. V., and Gennari, C.,** Bone turnover in postmenopausal osteoporosis. Effect of calcitonin treatment, *J. Clin. Invest.*, 82, 1268, 1988.
80. **Rosenfeld, M. G., Mermod, J. J., Amara, S. G., Swanson, L. W., Sawchenko, P. E., Rivier, J., Vale, W. W., and Evans, R. M.,** Production of a novel neuropeptide encoded by the calcitonin gene via tissue-specific RNA processing, *Nature*, 304, 129, 1983.
81. **Sundler, F., Ekblad, E., and Håkanson, R.,** Occurrence and distribution of substance P- and CGRP-containing nerve fibers in gastric mucosa: species differences, *Adv. Exp. Med. Biol.*, 298, 29, 1991.
82. **Steenbergh, P. H., Hoppener, J. W. M., Zandberg, J., Lips, C. J. M., and Jansz, H. S.,** A second human calcitonin/CGRP gene, *FEBS Letters*, 183, 403, 1985.
83. **Delsert, C. D. and Rosenfeld, M. G.,** A tissue-specific small nuclear ribonucleoprotein and the regulated splicing of the calcitonin/calcitonin gene-related protein transcript, *J. Biol. Chem.*, 267, 14573, 1992.
84. **Horn, D. A., Suburo, A., Terenghi, G., Hudson, L. D., Polak, J. M., and Latchman, D. S.,** Expression of the tissue specific splicing protein SmN in neuronal cell lines and in regions of the brain with different splicing capacities, *Brain. Res. Mol. Brain. Res.*, 16, 13, 1992.

Chapter 14

THE ROLE OF ESTROGENS AND OTHER STEROID HORMONES IN BONE METABOLISM

David A. Ontjes, M.D.

TABLE OF CONTENTS

0-8493-7845-1/95/$0.00+$.50

I. INTRODUCTION

The naturally occurring steroid hormones are cholesterol derivatives synthesized by the adrenal glands and the gonads. During the reproductive years in women, the principal ovarian steroids are estradiol and progesterone. In men the principal testicular steroid is testosterone. In both sexes the adrenal glands produce cortisol and aldosterone, as well as androstenedione and dehydroepiandrosterone. Estradiol and estrone act physiologically as estrogens, whereas testosterone acts as an androgen. These sex steroids are primarily responsible for female and male secondary sex characteristics, but they also have metabolic effects on many somatic tissues, including bone. Cortisol acts principally as a glucocorticoid, regulating multiple metabolic processes throughout the body.

Once produced by the gonads or the adrenal glands, steroid hormones can be metabolized by other tissues to modify their original biological activities. Weaker androgens such as androstenedione can be converted by the liver and other peripheral tissues into testosterone, a much more potent androgen. Testosterone, in turn, can be converted by peripheral aromatization into estrone. Thus adrenal androgens can give rise to both androgens and estrogens in the peripheral circulation.

In general, sex steroids promote a positive body calcium balance and an increased skeletal mass. Clinically, osteopenic disease tends to develop when estrogens or androgens become deficient. At high physiologic levels glucocorticoids such as cortisol have effects opposite to those of sex steroids, causing a negative calcium balance and a reduced bone mass. Thus clinical osteopenia may also occur in conditions of glucocorticoid excess, whether due to the hypersecretion of cortisol or to the long-term administration of synthetic glucocorticoids as drugs to treat inflammatory or immunologic diseases.

The purpose of this chapter is to describe the basic effects of estrogens, progestins, androgens and glucocorticoids on bone and mineral metabolism, as well as their roles in the etiology and therapy of bone diseases. These steroids all act on one or more of the organs that normally regulate calcium balance. These organs include the gastrointestinal tract, the kidney, and bone itself. As described earlier in this text in Chapter 3, a constant serum level of ionized calcium is maintained primarily by the traditional calciotropic hormones: parathyroid hormone (Chapter 11), calcitonin (Chapter 12), and 1,25-dihydroxyvitamin D (Chapter 14). Sex steroids and glucocorticoids do not play a direct role in calcium homeostasis, nor are they subject to feedback control by alterations in the serum calcium level. They do, however, have important long-term effects on the net retention of calcium by the skeleton. It is these long-term effects on calcium balance that explain the importance of steroid hormones in osteopenic bone disease and its therapy.

II. ESTROGENS

A. BASIC EFFECTS ON CALCIUM METABOLISM

1. Steroid Receptors and Gene Expression

Estrogens, like other steroid hormones, act through specific intracellular receptors that are capable of regulating the expression of specific genes.[1] Figure 1 shows the main steps involved in steroid action at the cellular level. Before acting on the cell, the hormone must first dissociate from a steroid-binding globulin acting as a carrier protein in plasma. The free steroid enters the cell by diffusion and binds to high affinity receptors located in the cytoplasm. Binding of the steroid ligand to the receptor induces conformational changes in the receptor leading to formation of an activated receptor dimer, as depicted in Figure 1. The activated receptor complex then binds to specific sequences of DNA, termed steroid response elements, located in particular genes that are subject to

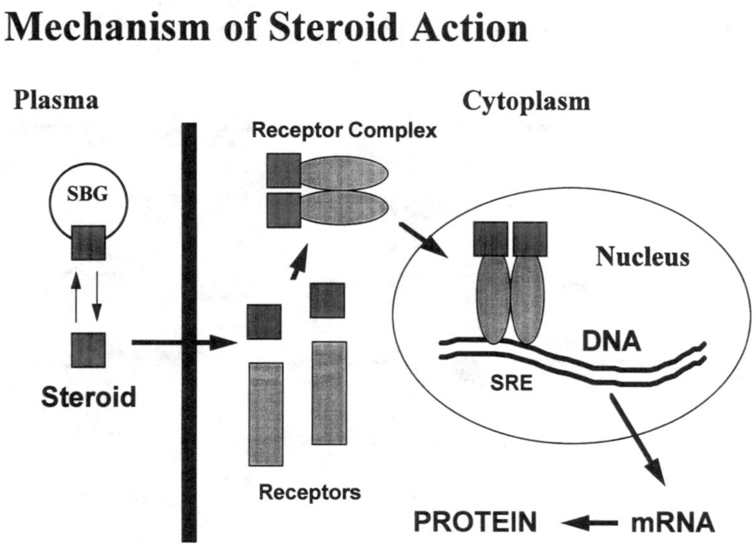

FIGURE 1. General Mechanism of Action for Steroid Hormones. The steroid ligand dissociates from its specific steroid-binding globulin (SBG) in plasma to enter the target cell by diffusion. Once inside the cell, the steroid binds to an intracellular receptor that is specific for each class of steroid hormones. The steroid-receptor complexes associate to form dimers and then enter the cell nucleus where they bind to the DNA of steroid-responsive genes at specific steroid-response elements (SREs.) Binding results in either enhancement or suppression of gene expression, resulting in alterations in the amounts of messenger RNA (mRNA) and protein formed.

regulation by steroids. The steroid response element of the gene is usually adjacent to a promoter region, which serves to regulate the transcription of messenger RNA from DNA sequences further downstream. By regulating the synthesis of mRNA, the steroid also regulates the synthesis of specific proteins within the cell. The biological activities of the steroid-dependent proteins determine the ultimate effects of the steroid on the cell.

The estrogen receptor is a member of a family of steroid hormone receptors having homologous structures as shown in Figure 2. Each receptor type has two functional domains of critical importance.[2] One domain, a steroid binding region, is capable of recognizing steroids of a specific functional class and binding them with high affinity. A second domain is capable of recognizing and binding to specific steroid response elements in particular steroid-responsive genes. Thus the structure of the steroid-binding domain of the estrogen receptor confers specificity for interacting with estrogens, and the DNA binding domain in turn for interacting with estrogen-responsive genes.

2. Estrogen Effects on Bone Cells

High-affinity estrogen receptors have been found in all of the tissues usually considered to be targets for estrogen action. These include the oviduct, the endometrium and the breast. Many of the proteins produced by cells in these tissues are known to be synthesized under estrogenic control.[1] Bone cells also have estrogen receptors. High-affinity estrogen receptors are present in a variety of osteoblast-like cells,[3,4] suggesting that estrogens may promote a positive calcium balance by direct effects on bone itself. However, much less is known concerning which genes and which proteins in bone cells may be subject to estrogen regulation. Gray, et al.,[5] using a cultured line of rat osteosarcoma cells, have demonstrated a variety of direct estrogen effects, including the stimulation of alkaline phosphatase activity and the release of insulin-like growth factors and transforming growth factor into the culture medium. Ernst, et al.[6] have reported similar effects in osteoblastic cells from normal rat calvariae and long bones. In addition, estradiol blocks the usual stimulation of cyclic-AMP production by parathyroid hormone in these cells.

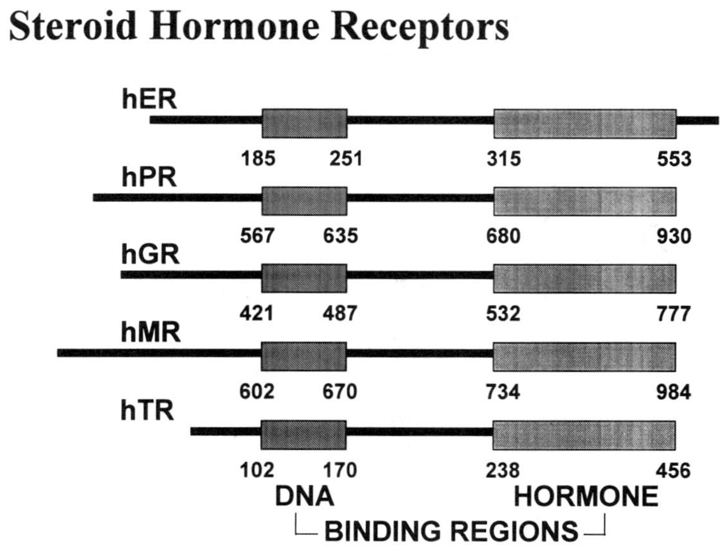

FIGURE 2. Structure of the Family of Steroid Hormone Receptors. The domains responsible for binding to the steroid ligand and to the steroid response elements of genomic DNA are indicated. The structure of the hormone binding domain confers specificity for binding of the steroid class. Human estrogen receptor (hER); human progestin receptor (hPR); human glucocorticoid receptor (hGR); human mineralocorticoid receptor (hMR); and human thyroid hormone receptor (hTR) are shown.

Recently Manolagas and his associates have found that estrogens can inhibit the production of interleukin-6 (IL-6) by cultured murine osteoblast cell lines as well as by normal human bone-cells.[7] Two other cytokines, interleukin-1 (IL-1) and tumor necrosis factor (TNF) normally stimulate the production of IL-6 by these cells, but their stimulatory effects are blocked by the presence of estradiol at concentrations of 10^{-9} *M*. IL-6, in turn, can act as a paracrine factor on nearby osteoclasts, promoting bone resorption through its stimulatory action on osteoclast development and activity. Thus by inhibiting the production of IL-6 by osteoblasts, estrogens may indirectly inhibit osteoclast activity and bone resorption. In mice, ovariectomy is associated with increased IL-6 production by bone marrow cells and increased numbers of osteoclasts in trabecular bone. Administration of either estradiol or an antibody to IL-6 to the ovariectomized animals can prevent these changes.[8]

There is abundant evidence that estrogen replacement reduces rates of bone resorption and bone turnover in estrogen-deficient women as well as in animal models. It is less clear whether estrogens also have a significant effect in promoting bone formation. In the intact individual, estrogen deficiency leads first to an increased rate of bone resorption, followed by a compensatory increase in bone formation. Estrogen replacement, after first reducing the elevated rates of resorption, will eventually also lead to reduced rates of bone formation. Due to the normal linkage between resorption and formation, it is difficult to determine from *in vivo* studies whether estrogens have any direct bone-forming effects. Estrogen supplements tend to be ineffective in increasing bone mass in animals or women who are not already estrogen deficient, and who do not already have increased rates of bone resorption.. However, under appropriate experimental conditions it is possible to show bone-forming effects in the absence of resorption-inhibiting effects. In ovariectomized rats, treatment with a bisphosphonate (3-amino-1-hydroxypropylidene-1-bisphosphonate) can markedly inhibit both bone resorption and bone formation rates. When animals first treated with the bisphosphonate are given physiologic replacement doses of estradiol, bone formation rates, as measured by histomorphometry, increase. There is a corresponding increase in the volume of trabecular but not cortical bone.[9] In spite of such evidence in experimental animals, it is still unclear whether direct bone-forming effects of estrogens are important in women undergoing estrogen replacement.

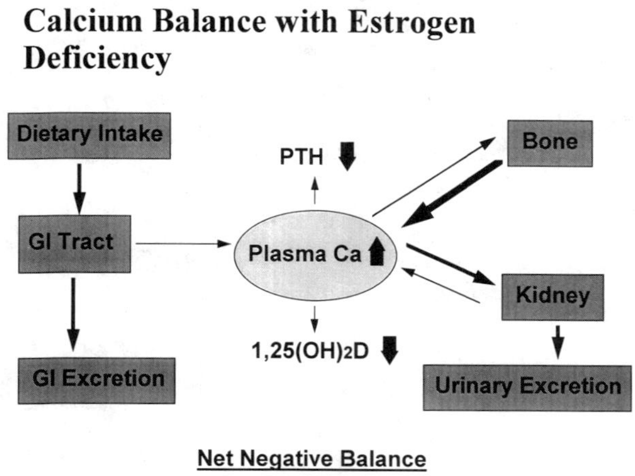

FIGURE 3. Calcium Balance in the Presence of Estrogen Deficiency. Bone resorption is increased, leading to an increased flux of calcium from bone to plasma. Slight increases in plasma calcium lead to increased urinary losses of calcium and reduced levels of parathyroid hormone (PTH). Reduced PTH levels may stimulate less formation of active $1,25(OH)_2D$, leading to decreased gastrointestinal calcium absorption.

3. Estrogen Effects on Dietary Calcium Absorption

The efficiency of gastrointestinal absorption of calcium declines gradually with age. In women there appears to be a small but significant additional decline in calcium absorption with the onset of estrogen deficiency at menopause. Conversely, calcium absorption is increased during pregnancy when estrogens are high. In spite of the evidence suggesting a role for estrogens in promoting absorption, it has not been possible to demonstrate direct estrogen stimulation of either gastrointestinal calcium transport or the formation of 1,25-dihydroxyvitamin D by the kidney. There is likely to be an indirect effect, however, exerted through estrogen inhibition of bone resorption, as discussed next. There is also evidence that estrogens may potentiate the stimulatory effects of vitamin D on the gut by increasing the content of a $1,25(OH)_2D$ receptor protein in intestinal mucosa.[10]

4. Summary of Estrogen Interactions with Calciotropic Hormones

Although there is little evidence that either the parathyroid glands or the kidney are direct targets for estrogen action, estrogens can influence parathyroid hormone and $1,25(OH)_2D$ levels indirectly through inhibiting the movement of calcium from the bone compartment into the bloodstream. The relationships between parathyroid hormone, $1,25(OH)_2D$, and calcium balance are summarized in Figures 3 and 4. With the onset of estrogen deficiency after menopause, bone resorption is increased as shown in Figure 3. Parathyroid hormone levels tend to be suppressed. Consequently there is increased excretion of calcium in the urine due to reduced calcium reabsorption by the renal tubules. Reduced renal production of $1,25(OH)_2D$ and possibly reduced responsiveness to $1,25(OH)_2D$ also tends to reduce gastrointestinal calcium absorption. The overall effect of these multihormonal changes triggered by estrogen deficiency is a negative calcium balance. Estrogen replacement improves calcium balance by the mechanisms shown in Figure 4. Bone resorption is reduced while bone deposition initially remains high, causing a net movement of calcium from the plasma into bone. Parathyroid hormone levels may rise as plasma levels of ionized calcium fall. This leads to decreased excretion of calcium in the urine and increased production of $1,25(OH)_2D$. Higher levels of $1,25(OH)_2D$ can promote more efficient gastrointestinal absorption of calcium. The overall effect is a positive calcium balance.

B. CLINICAL USE AND EFFECTS OF ESTROGENS

1. Normal Sources of Estrogen Before and After Menopause

Circulating estrogens in normal women are derived both from ovarian secretion and from peripheral conversion of steroid precursors as shown in Figure 5. During the reproductive years the

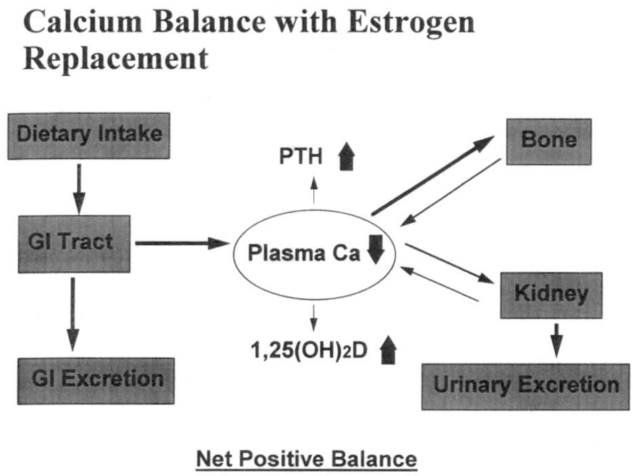

FIGURE 4. Calcium Balance after Estrogen Replacement. Bone resorption and the flux of calcium from bone to plasma are reduced. Consequently, there is a diminished urinary excretion of calcium. Slightly lower plasma levels of calcium may stimulate PTH and $1,25(OH)_2D$ production, thus improving gastrointestinal calcium absorption.

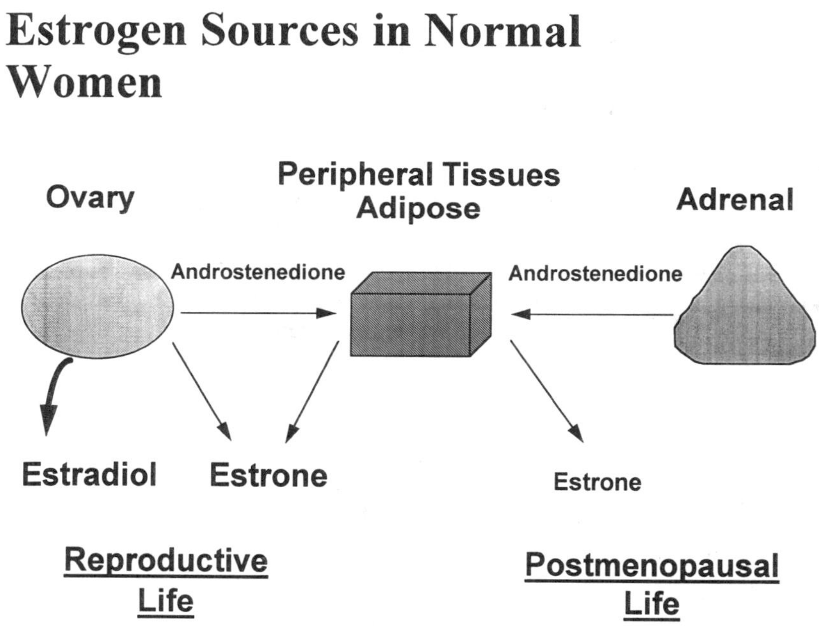

FIGURE 5. Sources of Estrogens in Women before and after Menopause. During the reproductive years, estradiol, secreted directly by the ovary, is the predominant circulating estrogen. In addition, estrone is produced from the peripheral conversion of androstenedione, derived both from the ovary and the adrenals. With ovarian failure at the time of menopause, estradiol secretion ceases. Estrone production from ovarian androstenedione also declines, but production from adrenal androgens continues.

ovaries produce the most potent estrogen, 17β-estradiol, at a rate of 70 to 250 μg per day, depending on the phase of the menstrual cycle. The ovaries also produce estrone, a much weaker estrogen having only 10% of the activity of 17β-estradiol. A secondary source of circulating estrogens is from the conversion of the ovarian and adrenal androgen, androstenedione, to estrone by peripheral tissues, including adipose tissue and liver. In premenopausal women ovarian estradiol accounts for nearly all of the circulating estrogenic activity.

Normal menopause is due to a natural aging process leading to ovarian failure. Prior to menopause, ovulation becomes irregular and rates of ovarian estrogen production begin to fall. Due to the

TABLE 1
Serum Estrogen and Gonadotropin Levels in Women[11]

	Estradiol (pg/mL)	Estrone (pg/mL)	LH (mIU/mL)	FSH (mIU/mL)
Ovulating women				
Basal	20–60	10–40	5–25	5–20
Ovulatory	>200	30–120	25–100	12–30
Postmenopausal women	5–20	10–30	40–80	50–100

lack of negative feedback from estrogens, circulating levels of pituitary gonadotropins begin to rise. As ovarian function continues to decline, menstrual periods cease. Within a few years following natural menopause, ovarian estrogen and androstenenedione production have ceased entirely. However, the peripheral production of estrogens, primarily estrone from adrenal androstenedione, continues (see Figure 5.) Estrone now becomes the principal circulating estrogen. Because it is a relatively weak estrogen, its effects are insufficient to prevent manifestations of estrogen deficiency in a number of estrogen-dependent tissues, including bone. Table 1 shows the range of serum levels of estrogens, luteinizing hormone, and follicle stimulating hormone for normally ovulating young women and postmenopausal women. Note that levels of estrone fall much less than levels of estradiol after menopause. There is evidence that peripheral estrone production depends on adipose tissue mass, as well as on the supply of androstenedione from the adrenals. For this reason estrone levels tend to be higher in obese women than in thin women. This may afford obese women greater protection from complete estrogen deficiency after menopause.

2. Other Causes of Estrogen Deficiency

Ovarian estrogen production may be insufficient due to a number of disease states. Some of these are listed in Table 2. Some diseases affect the ovaries directly, causing primary ovarian failure. Others involve abnormalities of the hypothalamus or pituitary gland leading to failure of gonadotropin production and secondary ovarian failure. The degree of failure may vary in severity with respect to estrogen production. Women who do not ovulate may still produce enough estrogens to allow occasional menstruation, although the quantity of estrogens is usually less than in women who ovulate regularly. Thus young women who have irregular, anovulatory menstrual cycles may have a relative estrogen deficiency. This is a situation sometimes found in women engaging in stringent physical exercise programs, such as marathon-running, or in those who are malnourished for any reason. The abnormality in such cases appears to be deficient stimulation of pituitary gonadotropin production by luteinizing-hormone-releasing hormone (LHRH) from the hypothalamus. Any severe chronic systemic illness can cause functional gonadotropin deficiency through effects on the central nervous system.

Lesions of the pituitary can also cause estrogen deficiency by interfering with gonadotropin function. Small pituitary tumors that secrete prolactin can inhibit gonadotropin production through an inhibitory effect of high prolactin levels on hypothalamic LHRH release. Patients with this problem may present with a syndrome of inappropriate lactation (galactorrhea) and a lack of menstrual periods (amenorrhea.) Removal of the tumor and reduction of prolactin levels may allow restoration of normal pituitary and ovarian function. Lesions that destroy the pituitary gland, such as large pituitary tumors, can cause irreversible gonadotropin deficiency. Gonadotropin secretion can also be blocked by certain LHRH analogs that act as antagonists of LHRH. Inhibitory analogs such as nafarelin and buserelin are used to induce a "chemical castration" by blocking the pituitary-ovarian axis in conditions such as breast cancer or endometriosis, where low levels of estrogens may be therapeutically desirable.

Other abnormal conditions may cause estrogen deficiency through direct effects on the ovaries. Girls with chromosomal abnormalities causing gonadal dysgenesis fail to have normal ovarian development and thus never have menarche. They will have estrogen deficiency throughout their

TABLE 2
Abnormalities Associated with Estrogen Deficiency

Condition	Cause of Abnormality	Gonadotropin Secretion	Estrogen Secretion
Anorexia nervosa	Hypothalamic dysfunction	Low	Low
Excessive physical activity	Hypothalamic dysfunction	Low	Variably low
Chronic systemic illness	Hypothalamic dysfunction	Low	Variably low
Prolactin-producing pituitary tumor	Hypothalamic dysfunction	Low	Low
Large pituitary tumor or lesion	Pituitary destruction	Low	Low
Treatment with LHRH antagonists	Blockade of gonadotropin secretion	Low	Low
Gonadal dysgenesis (Turner's syndrome)	Chromosomal defect causing failure of ovarian development	High	Very low
Spontaneous premature menopause	Usually autoimmune ovarian destruction	High	Very low
Surgical menopause	Surgical removal of ovaries	High	Absent
Chemotherapy with drugs toxic to ovaries	Chemical damage to ovaries	High	Variably low

entire lives unless given replacement therapy. The most easily recognized form of gonadal dysgenesis in females is Turner's syndrome in which one of the female sex chromosomes is missing, giving a 45-X karyotype.

Spontaneous premature menopause is a form of primary ovarian failure occurring before the age of 40 and often is accompanied by typical menopausal symptoms. The cause is often an autoimmune inflammatory disease affecting the ovaries. Premature menopause may be associated with autoimmune disease of other endocrine organs such as the thyroid or the adrenals. Surgical removal of the ovaries for diseases such as cancer or endometriosis can cause a particularly abrupt and severe estrogen deficiency in younger women. Finally, a number of drugs such as cyclophosphamide, used in cancer chemotherapy, have toxic effects on the ovaries, causing a cessation of ovulation and reduced estrogen production.

3. Effects of Estrogen Deficiency

Whether estrogen deficiency is due to normal menopause or to one of the abnormal conditions discussed above, the effects are similar. The uterine lining, or endometrium, and the female external genitalia, including the vulva and vagina, are estrogen dependent, as are the lining of the urethra and the glandular tissue of the breasts. Atrophy of these tissues leads to a number of changes that include thinning of the vaginal and urethral mucosa, and symptoms such as vaginal irritation, painful intercourse, and urinary incontinence. If estrogen levels fall rapidly, due to the abrupt onset of ovarian failure, women tend to experience "hot flashes." These are recurrent episodes of flushing and sweating, and are related to vasomotor instability that occurs in the presence of falling estrogens.

Estrogen deficiency also has profound effects on the function of tissues not ordinarily considered to be estrogen dependent. Notable among such tissues are liver and bone. Estrogen deficiency affects hepatic function in many ways, particularly with regard to the synthesis of certain proteins, including transcortin (CBG), thyroxine-binding globulin (TBG), sex-hormone-binding globulin (SHBG), transferrin, renin substrate, and fibrinogen. The most significant hepatic effects of estrogens, however, involve lipoprotein metabolism. With the advent of estrogen deficiency, there is a small but significant rise in the synthesis of low-density lipoprotein (LDL), and a decline in the synthesis of both high-density lipoprotein (HDL) and triglycerides. The end result is an elevation in plasma levels of LDL and total cholesterol, and a fall in HDL. These changes have the adverse effect of increasing the risk of atherosclerosis in women with estrogen deficiency to levels similar to those seen in men.

The effects of estrogen deficiency on bone can be predicted from the known effects of estrogens on bone cells and calcium balance, as discussed earlier. With the onset of menopause, increased bone resorption results in an accelerated decline in bone mass at rates ranging from 1 to 6% per year, depending upon which areas of the skeleton are measured. Loss tends to be more rapid in trabecular bone, as represented by the vertebral bodies, than in cortical bone, as represented by the proximal radius.[12] Within 10 years after the onset of menopause, rates of bone loss decrease from an early postmenopausal rate of about 2% a year to about 1% a year and remain fairly constant thereafter. Heaney has postulated that about 10–15% of the total skeletal mass is estrogen-dependent.[13] This represents the excess loss, over and above that related to age, occurring in the first 10 years following menopause, when estrogen replacement is not given. Between the ages of 50 and 80 years, a woman's bone density declines by about 30%. Thus, about half of the loss during this period may be attributed to estrogen deficiency.

As bone density declines, fracture rates begin to increase, first in the vertebral bodies and distal radius, and later in the hip. Cummings, et al.,[14] have estimated that the lifetime risk of a 50-year-old white woman in the United States is 15% for distal radius (Colles') fracture, 32% for vertebral fracture, and 16% for hip fracture. The rate for vertebral fracture in women begins to rise steeply in the 6th decade of life, whereas the rate for hip fracture rises only in the 7th and 8th decades.

Women who experience estrogen deficiency at an earlier age, due to one of the abnormalities listed in Table 2, may never achieve an optimum peak bone mass in early adult life. There is evidence that a number of the conditions associated with estrogen deficiency in young women are also associated with a low bone mass. These include anorexia nervosa,[15] gonadal dysgenesis,[16] hyperprolactinemia,[17] and amenorrhea in female athletes[18] or ballet dancers.[19] As the result of having a lower than normal peak bone mass, these women may demonstrate increased rates of fracture even before reaching the usual age of menopause.

4. Forms of Estrogen Replacement Therapy

There are a number of different products available for use in estrogen replacement therapy. Most of these are given orally. Transdermal formulations, capable of being absorbed through the skin, and formulations for intramuscular depot injection are also available. Table 3 lists some of the most commonly used forms.

Natural estrogens such as estradiol and conjugated estrogens are converted largely into less potent estrone in the process of being absorbed from the gastrointestinal tract. Once absorbed, they are carried first to the liver via the hepatic portal circulation. There they are largely metabolized into inactive derivatives before reaching the systemic circulation. Because of this "first pass effect" in the liver, all natural estrogens have low bioavailability and pharmacologic efficacy when administered orally.[12] Synthetic modifications of natural estradiol, such as the introduction of an ethinyl group at carbon atom 17 in the steroid nucleus, can yield derivatives that are resistant to hepatic metabolism, and thus are far more potent. Ethinyl estradiol, a synthetic estrogen used in many oral contraceptives, has approximately 100 times the efficacy of estradiol itself, when given orally.

Bioavailability is greatly improved when estradiol is given transdermally or parenterally. Estradiol is absorbed unchanged through the skin and released directly into the systemic circulation. Similarly, esters of estradiol, when deposited intramuscularly, are gradually de-esterified, allowing release of estradiol over a long period of time. Estradiol cypionate and estradiol valerate are examples of formulations for depot injection. Powers, et al.[20] have compared the effects of several different estrogen preparations on serum levels of estradiol and estrone in postmenopausal women. Table 4 summarizes some of the results of such measurements.

In the doses customarily given for postmenopausal replacement, oral estrogens do not produce serum estradiol levels equivalent to the basal, nonovulatory levels seen in normal premenopausal women (see Table 1.) Estrone levels, however, tend to be higher. Transdermal estradiol more closely replicates the normal premenopausal pattern. Both oral and transdermal estrogens are effective in relieving menopausal symptoms and in preventing accelerated bone loss, as discussed next. Oral

TABLE 3
Forms of Estrogen Used in Replacement Therapy

Generic Name	Mode of Administration	Proprietary Names	Typical Replacement Dose	Dose Range
Conjugated estrogens	Oral	Premarin	0.625 mg/day	0.3–1.25 mg/day
Esterified estrogens	Oral	Estratab	0.625 mg/day	0.3–1.25 mg/day
Esterified estrogens with methyltestosterone	Oral	Estratest	0.625 mg/day +1.25 mg methyltestosterone	Similar to esterified estrogens
Micronized estradiol	Oral	Estrace	1 mg/day	1–2 mg/day
Estrone	Oral	Ogen	1.25 mg/day	0.625–5 mg/day
Ethinyl estradiol	Oral	Demulen, Ortho-Novum, Ovral, and others	0.03 mg/day	0.01–0.05 mg/day
Estradiol	Transdermal	Estraderm	0.05 mg/day	0.05–0.1 mg/day
Estradiol cypionate	Intramuscular injection	E-cypionate and others	2 mg/3–4 wks	2–5 mg/3–4 wks
Estradiol valerate	Intramuscular injection	Menaval	4 mg/2 wks	2–20 mg/2 wks
Estradiol valerate with testosterone enanthate	Intramuscular injection	Testaval	14 mg/2 wks +90 mg testosterone enanthate	Similar to estradiol valerate

TABLE 4
Mean Serum Levels and Ratios of Estradiol and Estrone before and during Therapy with Transdermal and Oral Estrogens

Serum Levels	Before Treatment	Transdermal Estradiol, 0.05 mg/day	Transdermal Estradiol, 0.1 mg/day	Micronized Estradiol, 2 mg/day	Conjugated Estrogens, 1.25 mg/day
Estradiol (pg/ml)	7.4	39	74	66	31
Estrone (pg/ml)	32.3	41	59	334	152
Estradiol: Estrone ratio	0.23	0.95	1.25	0.20	0.20

estrogens, because of the much higher levels reaching the liver, have a relatively greater effect on hepatic protein synthesis and greater effects in modifying serum lipoprotein composition. This may constitute an advantage when lowering the risk of cardiovascular disease is a primary consideration.

5. Effects of Estrogen Replacement on Osteoporosis

There is abundant evidence that estrogen replacement therapy is effective both in preventing the development of osteoporosis and in preventing further progression of established osteoporosis. Because the fractures and skeletal deformities of osteoporosis are generally irreversible once they have occurred, replacement therapy is more effective when given early rather than late. Clinical trials using estrogens to prevent osteoporosis have focused mainly on two end points, bone density and fracture rates. Various biochemical markers of bone metabolism have also been used in some studies as auxiliary end points. Most studies have administered a progestin together with estrogen in order to avoid the increased risk of endometrial cancer from estrogen therapy alone. Although it is possible that the progestin may modify the skeletal effects of the estrogen, such effects are likely to be relatively small, for reasons discussed later.

Bone density is the most frequent end point in randomized clinical trials because measurable differences can occur within a two- to three-year time frame. Fracture rates, which usually entail

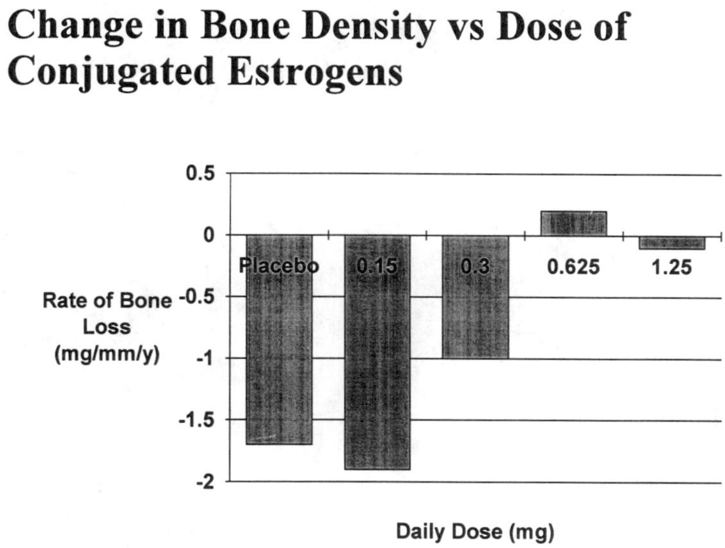

FIGURE 6. Dose Response Effects of Conjugated Estrogens on Metacarpal Mineral Content in Postmenopausal Women. Replacement with the indicated dose of conjugated estrogens was given for two years. (Data from Lindsay et al.[23])

longer periods of measurement, are more often the end point in retrospective and observational studies. Since declining bone density is a reliable predictor of the probability of fracture under most conditions,[21] it is reasonable to assume that a therapy that preserves bone density will ultimately prevent fractures. There have been relatively few randomized, prospective trials of estrogen replacement therapy in which reduced fracture rates have been reported. Such trials are particularly important, because they are more likely to be free of the potential biases inherent in nonrandomized or retrospective studies.[22]

a. Estrogen Effects on Bone Density

When given as replacement therapy to postmenopausal women, estrogens prevent the usual decline in bone mineral density, and may even cause slight increases, depending on which site is measured. In a two-year clinical trial examining dose-response relationships of estrogen replacement on metacarpal bone density, Lindsay, et al.[23] found that doses of at least 0.625 mg of conjugated estrogens were required to prevent bone loss, as shown in Figure 6.

In practice, estrogen replacement therapy is often given in conjunction with dietary supplements of calcium and vitamin D, as well as with a variety of exercise or conditioning programs. There is evidence, based on a limited number of clinical trials that estrogens and calcium can have additive effects. Ettinger, et al. have reported that 0.3 mg of conjugated estrogens together with a calcium intake of 1500 mg per day is as effective as 0.625 mg of conjugated estrogens without calcium supplementation.[24] Most studies comparing estrogen replacement with calcium supplementation alone in postmenopausal women have found estrogens to be more effective. Prince, et al. conducted a trial comparing an exercise program alone, exercise plus a calcium supplement of 1000 mg per day, and exercise plus an estrogen-progestin regimen of 1.25 mg estrone plus 2.5 mg medroxyprogesterone. During the two-year period of the study, distal forearm bone density fell by 2.7% per year in control subjects, by 2.6% in subjects receiving exercise alone, and by 0.5% in subjects receiving exercise plus calcium. In subjects receiving exercise plus estrogen, density rose by 2.7% per year.[25] Aloia, et al.[26] conducted a three-year trial in early postmenopausal women who were within 6 years of menopause, comparing calcium supplementation (to 1700 mg per day) with calcium plus estrogen-progestin replacement (0.625 mg conjugated estrogens per day plus 10 mg of medroxyprogesterone on days 16 to 25 of each monthly cycle). Rates of change in bone mineral at various sites are shown below in Figure 7.

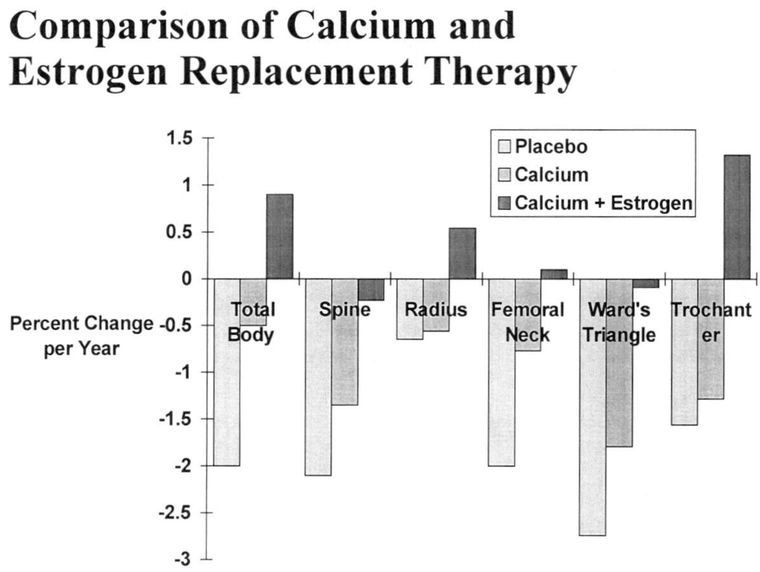

FIGURE 7. Rates of Change in Bone Mineral Density at Various Skeletal Sites with Calcium Supplementation Alone or Combined Calcium and Estrogen Replacement in Postmenopausal Women. Hormone replacement consisted of 0.625 mg of conjugated estrogens per day plus a cyclical progestin. Calcium supplementation was 1700 mg per day. The study period was 3 years. (Data from Aloia et al.[26])

Estrogens are also effective in preserving or increasing bone mass in elderly women who already have established osteoporosis. Lindsay and Tohme[27] compared the effects of calcium supplementation with calcium plus estrogens (0.625 mg conjugated estrogens) in women over 60 years of age with low bone density and preexisting vertebral compression fractures. In the women receiving calcium alone, bone density decreased over two years in both the lumbar spine and femoral neck, whereas in women receiving calcium plus estrogen, density increased modestly at both sites. It appeared that the gain in bone density with estrogens was positively correlated with the number of years post menopause. That is, the older the subject, the greater the gain achieved with estrogen replacement. Results from the Framingham Study, in which bone density was surveyed in a population of women 68 to 75 years of age, showed that in women who had previously taken postmenopausal estrogens for at least 7 years, bone density at all sites averaged 11.2% greater than in women who had never taken estrogens.[28] In an older population 75 to 96 years of age, the difference was only 3.2%. In women who had taken estrogens for fewer than 7 years, there was no difference in bone density between previous estrogen users and controls. These findings suggest that for long-term preservation of bone density, postmenopausal estrogen replacement must be continued for at least 7 years.

b. Estrogen Effects on Fractures

A number of studies have shown convincingly that estrogens can also reduce the risk of fractures involving the hip, distal radius, and spine.[29-33] Most of the published evidence has been derived from case-control or retrospective cohort investigations, but a few confirmatory prospective trials with oral estrogens have also been reported in women with early surgical menopause[34] and natural menopause.[35] Transdermal estrogens can reduce fracture rates in the spine,[36] and will most likely prove to reduce hip fractures as well, because they improve bone density in the femoral trochanter. The magnitude of the reduction in fracture risk due to estrogens has ranged from a relative risk of 0.75 to 0.17 in various studies.[37] There is likely to be a greater effect in reducing spinal compression fractures than hip fractures. No other intervention has thus far been shown to reduce fracture risk in both the hip and the spine.[12]

TABLE 5
Untoward Effects of Estrogen Replacement Therapy

Untoward Effect	Excess Frequency	Comments
Vaginal bleeding	25–40%	Diminished by continuous progestin administration
Breast tenderness	30–45%	Declines after 6–12 months of therapy
Fluid retention, bloating	5–15%	Usually mild
Migraine headaches	<5%	May increase frequency of migraine attacks
Hypertension	<5%	Blood pressure is unchanged in most women
Cholestasis, cholecystitis	<5%	Risk may increase twofold
Endometrial cancer	2–5%	Risk may increase eightfold. Prevented by concurrent progestin administration
Breast cancer	1–3%	Risk may increase from 10–50%. No protection with progestin administration

6. Other Benefits of Estrogen Therapy

Estrogen replacement therapy is effective in relieving common menopausal symptoms, including hot flashes, painful intercourse, and sleeplessness.[25,37,38] There is a widely held clinical impression that estrogen replacement also alleviates some of the more subjective psychological symptoms associated with menopause. Some placebo-controlled clinical trials have reported improved memory and decreased irritability and anxiety.[39]

The effects of estrogens on hepatic lipoprotein metabolism were described earlier. These effects are associated with a reduced risk for the development of coronary atherosclerosis and death from myocardial infarction. A 50-year-old white woman has a 46% probability of developing coronary artery disease during her lifetime and a 31% chance of dying from coronary heart disease.[40] Almost all epidemiological studies of post menopausal estrogen use and coronary heart disease have reported a protective effect. Meta-analyses have yielded pooled estimates of relative risk of 0.55 to 0.65. Prolonged estrogen replacement is probably more beneficial than short-term use, since atherosclerosis develops over a period of years. One study reported a relative risk of 0.5 for women using estrogens for 15 years or longer compared with a relative risk of 0.9 in those using them for fewer than 3 years.[41] The benefits of estrogen replacement appear to be greatest in those women who are at greatest risk of dying from coronary artery disease. Sullivan, et al. have reported an observational cohort study in which estrogen replacement reduced ten-year mortality by over 80% in women with angiographically documented coronary disease.[42]

7. Untoward Effects of Estrogen Therapy

Estrogen replacement is associated with several undesirable side effects as well as a limited number of more serious potential complications. These are listed in Table 5. The most frequent side effects are intermittent vaginal bleeding and breast discomfort.[25,37,38] These symptoms occur in roughly one-third of women within 6 months of starting estrogen replacement and tend to decline with continuing use. Other more sporadic side effects include fluid retention and bloating, increased frequency of migraine headaches, and increased blood pressure in some individuals. The relative risk for stroke is probably not increased.

More serious diseases that may be associated with postmenopausal estrogen use include cholecystitis, endometrial cancer, and breast cancer. The relative risk for cholecystitis or gall bladder surgery may increase approximately twofold.[40] Endometrial hyperplasia, which can be a precursor to the development of endometrial carcinoma, occurs in approximately 30% of women given estrogens alone, but may be prevented entirely by the administration of a progestin.[38] Hyperplasia causes irregular vaginal bleeding that leads to an increased need for repeated endometrial biopsy and the increased likelihood of hysterectomy. Only a small proportion of women with estrogen-related endometrial hyperplasia actually develop endometrial carcinoma. However, the relative risk for this uncommon disease is increased approximately eightfold.[40]

Potentially the most serious untoward effect of estrogen replacement is an increased incidence of breast cancer. This is because breast cancer is common. A 50-year-old white woman has a 10% probability of developing breast cancer during her lifetime and a 3% chance of dying from the disease.[40] Numerous epidemiologic studies have been done to assess whether estrogen replacement therapy might be associated with breast cancer, and the results of such studies have varied widely. Several meta-analyses have been performed on the available data, with estimates of relative risk ranging from 1.1 to 1.5.[40] This small increase in risk probably applies only to women using estrogens for longer periods of time, in excess of 8 years. Concurrent progestin therapy appears to have no protective effect.

8. Issues of Selection and Compliance

The attitudes of physicians and patients towards estrogen replacement are changing gradually as the wider benefits and risks are better understood. Today, the majority of postmenopausal women do not receive estrogen replacement therapy for a long enough time to reduce the risks of osteoporosis and coronary artery disease. One survey of women aged 45 to 55 years in the U.S. indicated that among women beginning therapy for the first time, 20% stopped within 9 months, 10% used estrogens only intermittently, and 20–30% never had their prescriptions filled because they were not convinced of the benefits or safety of the therapy.[43] Surveys in the UK among patients of general practitioners have indicated that only 9% of eligible women aged 40–64 years were receiving hormones.[44] Fear of cancer was a major reason for avoiding therapy. Other reasons included undesirable vaginal bleeding or other side effects.

Women who will benefit most from long-term estrogen replacement therapy include those who are at higher risk for osteoporosis or coronary artery disease at the time of menopause. Many physicians advocate an assessment of these risks as part of the process of helping the individual patient to decide whether to take estrogens or not. Such an assessment should include a careful history of manifestations of skeletal and cardiovascular disease, measurement of serum lipids, and measurement of bone mineral density.[21] There is evidence that knowledge of an abnormally low bone density provides effective motivation to undertake replacement therapy and increases the likelihood of long-term compliance.[45]

9. Effects of Estrogen Antagonists on Bone Metabolism

As one might expect, drugs that block the secretion of estrogens, either through effects on the pituitary or on the ovary, will increase the rate of bone loss. For example, the long-term administration of LHRH antagonists, such as leuprolide, to premenopausal women can induce estrogen deficiency and reduce bone density. "Add-back" estrogen replacement can prevent bone loss under these conditions.[46]

The estrogen antagonist, tamoxifen, is widely used in the adjunctive chemotherapy of breast cancer. When given to premenopausal women, tamoxifen can induce symptoms of estrogen deficiency such as hot flashes. However, when given to postmenopausal women, tamoxifen actually mimics some of the effects of estrogen. Love, et al. found that in postmenopausal women with a history of breast cancer, tamoxifen caused an increase in bone mineral density over a two-year treatment period, compared with a placebo group, where bone mineral density decreased.[47] In a similar group of women, tamoxifen also caused an increase in serum levels of high-density lipoprotein and a decrease in levels of low-density lipoprotein and cholesterol.[48] Thus in the absence of high levels of endogenous estrogen, tamoxifen can act as an estrogen substitute with respect to bone and lipoprotein metabolism. In postmenopausal women with a history of breast cancer, where the administration of estrogens may be contraindicated, tamoxifen may be a useful substitute for treating osteoporosis.

10. Summary of Estrogen Replacement Therapy

Estrogen deficiency in women, regardless of the cause, is associated with a negative calcium balance, decreased bone mineral density, and increased rates of fracture. Estrogen replacement can improve bone mineral density and reduce fracture rates when given long-term to estrogen-deficient patients. In addition to these skeletal effects, estrogen replacement provides a number of other beneficial effects including relief of menopausal symptoms, improvement in serum lipoprotein patterns, and reduction in the risk of cardiovascular disease. Possible adverse effects of estrogen replacement therapy include increased risk of endometrial and breast cancer. The risk of endometrial cancer may be prevented by concurrent administration of a progestin. Oral, parenteral, and transdermal forms of estrogen are all effective. Orally administered conjugated estrogens are used most frequently in postmenopausal women.

III. PROGESTINS

A. BASIC EFFECTS ON CALCIUM METABOLISM

Progestins are deficient, together with estrogens, in women with gonadal failure. Information about the effects of progesterone on bone is relatively scarce, but there is some evidence that progesterone may exert a trophic effect of its own on bone metabolism.[49] In several *in vitro* bone tissue systems, progesterone appears to act as an antiglucocorticoid. Glucocorticoid receptors are found in the cytoplasm of osteoblast cell lines and cells from fetal rat calvaria. Progesterone is more effective than cortisol in displacing labeled glucocorticoids, such as dexamethasone, from these receptors. Dexamethasone and other glucocorticoids generally inhibit the growth of these cells, and progesterone can block these inhibitory effects.[50] In contrast to progesterone, other gonadal steroids, including estradiol and testosterone, have little ability to displace dexamethasone or block its actions.

In certain *in vivo* models of bone formation, progesterone appears to be stimulatory. One model for matrix-induced bone formation involves implantation of demineralized bone matrix over the thorax of castrated rats, who are then treated with gonadal steroids. In this system, progesterone independently increases alkaline phosphatase production, and acts synergistically with estrogen in stimulating ^{3}H-thymidine incorporation into bone cells. Estrogen alone has little effect on this system.[51] To date, progesterone has not been found to increase thymidine incorporation or collagen production in any bone-cell system when added alone. The significance of possible synergistic effects with estrogens or other steroids remains uncertain.

B. CLINICAL USE AND EFFECTS OF PROGESTINS

1. Forms of Progesterone and Common Therapeutic Uses

Natural progestins are 21-carbon steroids related in structure to progesterone, and having in common the ability to induce the maturation of a secretory endometrium and to maintain pregnancy. Some synthetic progestins are closely related to progesterone in structure, but others are 19-carbon steroids related to 19-nortestosterone. These compounds have greater androgenic and anabolic activities and do not support pregnancy in animals. Some of the pharmacological properties of commonly used progestins are summarized in Table 6. All progestins share with estrogens the ability to suppress gonadotropin secretion and endogenous ovarian function. For this reason their most frequent clinical use is for the purpose of contraception, either combined with estrogens, or alone.

Progestins are also used to induce regular withdrawal bleeding in women who are not ovulating but who still produce enough estrogens to stimulate endometrial growth. As discussed in the section on estrogens, unopposed estrogen action on the uterus leads to endometrial hyperplasia and an increased incidence of endometrial cancer. This is a concern whether the estrogens are produced by the ovaries or are taken as a medication. Cyclical administration of a progestin can prevent endometrial hyperplasia and obviate the risk of endometrial cancer.[38] In postmenopausal women who do not desire to have withdrawal bleeding, the same benefits may be obtained with continuous administration of lower doses of the progestin. For example, continuous administration of a daily dose of 2.5 to 5 mg of medroxyprogesterone together with an estrogen is usually sufficient to avoid endometrial hyperplasia. Most women treated in this way will have intermittent vaginal bleeding only for the first several months of therapy. As therapy continues, bleeding tends to stop, and endometrial biopsy most often reveals an inactive, atrophic endometrium.[52]

TABLE 6
Progestins Available for Clinical Use

Compound	Formulations	Typical Dose	Uses and Comments
Progesterone and related derivatives			
Progesterone	Injectable	150 mg IM daily	Short duration of action limits use
Medroxyprogesterone acetate	Depot injection	100 mg IM monthly	For suppression of ovulation
	Oral	5–10 mg daily on days 16–25 of each menstrual cycle	For induction of regular withdrawal bleeding
Megestrol acetate	Oral	40–320 mg daily	For antitumor effects in endometrial and breast cancer
19-Nortestosterone derivatives			
Norethynodrel	Oral	5–10 mg daily	With estrogen for induction of regular withdrawal bleeding
Norethindrone	Oral	0.5–1 mg daily	With estrogen or alone for oral contraception
Ethynodiol diacetate	Oral	1–2 mg daily	With estrogen for oral contraception
Norgestrel	Oral	0.075–0.5 mg daily	With estrogen or alone for oral contraception
	Pellet for subcutaneous implantation	0.010 mg per day released over several years	Very long-acting contraceptive

Like estrogens, progestins have multiple effects outside of the reproductive system. They affect protein synthesis in the liver, particularly of lipoproteins. In general their hepatic actions are counter to those of estrogens. They tend to reduce high-density lipoprotein synthesis, whereas low-density lipoprotein synthesis may be increased, especially with the more androgenic derivatives. Triglyceride synthesis is decreased. Glucose tolerance and the effectiveness of insulin on peripheral tissues may be decreased.

2. Effects of Progestins on Osteoporosis

Few clinical trials have been conducted to determine the effects of progestins alone on osteoporosis. Generally, progestins seem to add little to the strongly positive effects of estrogens when the two are given together, but they may have positive effects, at least on bone density, when administered by themselves. Medroxyprogesterone, a 21-carbon analog of progesterone, is the most frequently used progestin for replacement therapy in the U.S. It may also be given as a long-acting depot injection for contraception. In the high doses used for contraception, it actually suppresses endogenous estrogen production. Cundy, et al. examined bone densities in a group of premenopausal women who had used depot medroxyprogesterone for contraception for at least 5 years and found them to be lower than those in premenopausal controls. This suggested that any positive effects of medroxyprogesterone itself on bone density were insufficient to make up for the loss of estrogens resulting from ovarian suppression.[53] In a two-year clinical trial in postmenopausal women, Gallagher, et al. compared the effects of oral medroxyprogesterone, 20 mg per day, with conjugated estrogens, 0.6 mg per day, on bone density and total body calcium. They found that compared to a placebo, medroxyprogesterone reduced the rate of loss in cortical areas of the skeleton, whereas conjugated estrogens reduced the rate of loss in both cortical and trabecular areas. A combination of conjugated estrogens with 10 mg medroxyprogesterone was not superior to conjugated estrogens alone.[54] Grecu, et al. administered medroxyprogesterone to male asthma patients with steroid-induced osteoporosis and observed increases in serum osteocalcin and serum alkaline phosphatase, both of which are considered to be biological markers of osteoblastic activity.[55] The same investigators also found that medroxyprogesterone in high doses could increase bone density in patients with steroid-induced osteoporosis.

There is evidence that the 19-nortestosterone-related progestins can also have positive effects on the skeleton. Christiansen, et al. examined the effects of cyclical norethisterone acetate on biochemical markers of bone metabolism when added to an estrogen replacement regimen. They found that serum alkaline phosphatase and serum osteocalcin both increased during progestin administration. They hypothesized that this might be due to a stimulatory effect of the progestin on bone formation, apart from the antiresorptive effects of the estrogen.[56] Other clinical studies suggest that the effects of norethisterone may be primarily antiresorptive, similar to those of estrogens. In one clinical trial in which norethisterone was given alone without an accompanying estrogen, the predominant action was reduction of bone resorption, as evidenced by decreasing urinary hydroxyproline and calcium excretion.[57] Norethindrone also has an antiresorptive effect when given to postmenopausal women with mild primary hyperparathyroidism. Here it reduces urinary hydroxyproline and calcium excretion and leads to an increase in forearm bone mineral density.[58]

In summary, clinical trials of progestins as sole agents in treating postmenopausal women with high bone turnover suggest an antiresorptive effect. This benefit may be overshadowed in premenopausal women by the suppressive effects of progestins on endogenous estrogen secretion. There is little evidence that the addition of progestins to an estrogen replacement regimen provides significant additional benefits in terms of increased bone density or decreased fracture rates. Because of their ability to compete for binding to the glucocorticoid receptor, progestins may have a role in the prevention of glucocorticoid-induced osteoporosis.

IV. ANDROGENS AND ANABOLIC STEROIDS

A. BASIC EFFECTS ON CALCIUM METABOLISM

Androgens have effects on bone that are similar to those of estrogens, but less is known about their mechanism of action. Androgen receptors have been described in human osteoblast-like cells,[59] and androgens directly stimulate the proliferation of bone cells *in vitro*.[60] This suggests that androgens have a direct effect on bone, either to increase bone formation or to decrease bone resorption. A part of this effect may be mediated by androgen stimulation of IGF-I formation.[61] Androgens may also promote a positive calcium balance by stimulating the production of 1,25-dihydroxyvitamin D by the kidney. Francis, et al., found that administration of testosterone to hypogonadal men increased levels of 1,25-dihydroxyvitamin D and improved gastrointestinal calcium absorption, as measured by radiocalcium absorption and calcium balance techniques.[62]

There is evidence from several sources that androgens are important determinants of bone density in men. Testosterone, or a metabolite, appears to be a major determinant of the increase in both cortical and trabecular bone mass occurring at puberty in males. Men have higher bone densities than women at any age.[63] Bone density is decreased in men with hypogonadism of any cause, whether due to lack of stimulation by gonadotropins at puberty or to primary gonadal failure due to chromosomal abnormalities such as Klinefelter's syndrome.[64] Spinal bone density decreases at an accelerated rate after surgical orchiectomy.[65]

There is currently uncertainty whether testosterone itself, or a metabolite, may be the active steroid affecting bone metabolism. In many androgen target tissues, the action of testosterone is mediated by dihydrotestosterone (DHT). DHT formation can take place in target tissues by the conversion of testosterone to DHT by the enzyme 5-α reductase. In some target tissues, especially prostate and skin, DHT appears to be the final mediator of androgen action. The drug, finasteride, is a specific inhibitor of 5-α reductase that is currently used for the treatment of benign prostatic hypertrophy. Matzkin, et al. have reported that prolonged finasteride treatment does not decrease bone density in men, even though it significantly reduces serum levels of DHT.[66] Thus it appears that DHT is not the active hormone in bone metabolism. Testosterone can also be converted by peripheral tissues into estradiol. The possibility remains that some of the positive effects of androgens on bone *in vivo* may actually be the result of the estrogens that are produced. This view

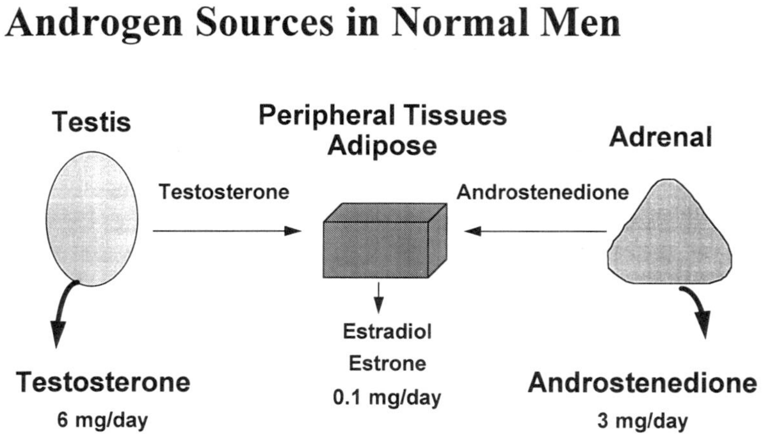

FIGURE 8. Sources of Androgens in Normal Men. Testosterone, the predominant androgen, is secreted directly by the testis. Small additional amounts of testosterone are produced in peripheral tissues by the conversion of adrenal androgens, mainly androstenedione. Further conversion of these androgens to small amounts of estradiol and estrone also take place peripherally.

is supported by the report that osteoporosis can be a complication in men who lack functioning estrogen receptors,[67] even though their androgen receptor function is normal.

Some evidence suggests that androgen production may influence the development of osteoporosis in women as well as men. The weak adrenal androgens, dehydroepiandrosterone and androstenedione, appear to be correlated with maintenance of bone density in aging women.[68] These weak androgens probably act on bone via their peripheral conversion to estrone, as previously discussed.

B. CLINICAL USE AND EFFECTS OF ANDROGENS

1. Normal Sources of Androgens and Causes of Androgen Deficiency

Testosterone production by the testis begins to rise at puberty under the influence of pituitary gonadotropins, particularly luteinizing hormone (LH). Figure 8 illustrates the normal sources of androgens in men. In the normal adult male, testosterone production by the testes averages 5-8 mg per day. The adrenal glands normally contribute only a small proportion of the circulating pool of testosterone through production of androstenedione, which is converted peripherally into small quantities of the more potent androgen. Testosterone itself may be converted peripherally either to DHT or to estradiol, as shown in Figure 8. With aging, men do not experience an abrupt decline in androgens comparable to the decline in estrogen experienced by women at menopause. In healthy elderly men, average circulating levels of testosterone may decline moderately, but usually remain within the normal range.[69]

Table 7 outlines some of the causes of androgen deficiency in men. Androgen deficiency may result early in life from developmental disorders such as isolated gonadotropin deficiency or Klinefelter's syndrome. More commonly, androgen deficiency arises during adult life as a result of acquired testicular, pituitary, or hypothalamic disease. A wide variety of chronic systemic illnesses are associated with reduced testicular function and low circulating levels of testosterone. These include chronic liver disease, kidney disease, and sickle cell anemia, as well as the use of certain drugs such as alkylating agents causing direct testicular damage, or high-dose adrenal corticosteroids, causing suppression of the hypothalamic-pituitary axis.[69]

2. Indications for Androgen Replacement and Forms Available for Therapy

Androgens are used medically for replacement therapy in men with all forms of hypogonadism. They are also used, sometimes inappropriately, for their anabolic effects on muscle or bone in individuals of both sexes who do not have androgen deficiency. They are used illegally by athletes

TABLE 7
Some Abnormalities Associated with Androgen Deficiency

Condition	Cause of Abnormality	Gonadotropin Secretion	Testosterone Secretion
Isolated gonadotropin deficiency	Hypothalamic defect; deficient LHRH	Low	Low at puberty
Prolactin producing pituitary tumor	Hypothalamic-pituitary dysfunction	Low	Low
Glucocorticoid excess	Hypothalamic-pituitary dysfunction	Low	Low
Chronic systemic illness or malnutrition	Hypothalamic-pituitary dysfunction	Low	Low
Hemochromatosis	Pituitary dysfunction	Low	Low
Large pituitary tumor or lesion	Pituitary destruction	Low	Low
Klinefelter's syndrome	Testicular developmental defect	High	Low at puberty
Trauma or surgical orchiectomy	Testicular removal	High	Very low
Viral orchitis	Testicular injury	High	Variably low
Radiation and alkylating drug therapy	Testicular injury	High	Variably low

TABLE 8
Androgens Used for Replacement Therapy and as Anabolic Steroids

Generic Name	Mode of Administration	Proprietary Name	Clinical Use
Testosterone	Transdermal	Testoderm	Replacement therapy
Testosterone cypionate	Intramuscular injection	DEPO-testosterone	Replacement therapy
Testosterone enanthate	Intramuscular injection	Testaval, others	Replacement therapy
Methyltestosterone	Oral, sublingual	Android, Metandren	Replacement therapy
Fluoxymesterone	Oral	Halotestin	Replacement, anabolic steroid
Nandrolone	Intramuscular injection	Durabolin	Anabolic steroid
Oxandrolone	Oral	Anavar	Anabolic steroid
Oxymetholone	Oral	Androl	Anabolic steroid
Stanozolol	Oral	Winstrol	Anabolic steroid

and body builders in the belief that they will increase not only muscle mass, but strength and athletic performance. Because of this potential for abuse, androgens and anabolic steroids are considered controlled substances by the U.S. Food and Drug Administration, and their use has been banned by national and international athletic organizations.

Table 8 lists some of the androgen preparations available for clinical use. Testosterone itself is not effective when given orally because of its rapid breakdown by the liver in a "first pass" effect after it is absorbed from the gastrointestinal tract. For this reason, parenteral forms of testosterone, primarily esters of enanthate and cypionate, are the mainstay of replacement therapy. These insoluble ester derivatives are given as depot injections and are absorbed slowly over 2 to 4 weeks. Like estradiol, testosterone can be absorbed transdermally in active form. The area of skin with the highest efficiency of absorption is the scrotum. Testosterone transdermal patches are available for scrotal application, but they must be applied daily and are more expensive than the depot injections. Another potential disadvantage is that much of the testosterone in the patches is converted to DHT by 5-α reductase in the scrotal skin, so that circulating levels of DHT tend to be disproportionately high.[65] Because the androgen receptor in the prostate is primarily responsive to DHT, this may predispose to prostatic hypertrophy.

Chemical modifications of the natural testosterone structure can produce derivatives that escape inactivation by the liver and are active when taken by mouth. Introduction of alkyl groups on carbon-17 of the steroid nucleus has this effect. An example is methyltestosterone. The main disadvantage of such compounds for androgen replacement is their greater toxicity. The 17-alkyl derivatives all tend to cause hepatic injury, ranging from mild liver enzyme abnormalities to fatal hepatitis. Another disadvantage is that it is difficult to monitor their effects by measurement of testosterone levels in the blood, because they are not measured by the usual plasma immunoassays for testosterone.[69]

Other chemical modifications involve alteration of the ring structure of the steroid nucleus yielding derivatives that are generally marketed as "anabolic steroids." These compounds all retain their androgenic properties, but many of them cannot be converted into estrogens, as can the natural testosterone products. They are not used for androgen replacement in hypogonadal men, but are used to attempt to induce a positive nitrogen balance in patients with chronic illnesses associated with catabolic states. Their effectiveness for this purpose is usually modest.

3. Effects of Androgen Therapy

The aim of replacement therapy in hypogonadal men is to restore normal male secondary sex characteristics as well as normal male sexual potency and behavior. Androgens usually have a positive effect on male libido and the frequency of erections. They do not restore fertility in most men with hypogonadism, however. Spermatogenesis is not increased, although there is an increase in the volume of ejaculate derived from the prostate and seminal vesicles. When testosterone is given in full replacement doses to men with normal gonadal function, gonadotropin levels fall, sperm production decreases by 90% or more, and testicular size decreases by 20%.

A secondary goal in androgen replacement therapy is often to achieve positive anabolic effects on muscle, bone, and other tissues. Androgen administration to hypogonadal men, as well as to normal women and children, causes a positive nitrogen balance and an overall weight gain, due to an increase in skeletal and muscle mass. The enlargement of muscles is due to the formation of new myofilaments along the myofibrils and to the division of enlarging myofibrils.[69] Androgen administration in pharmacological doses to normal men causes only a transient increase in the nitrogen balance if food intake is constant. Because androgens also increase appetite, they may improve the nitrogen balance and increase weight in some subjects who are undernourished or debilitated, but not hypogonadal. Their efficacy as anabolic agents in such settings is limited, however. Several controlled studies have shown no significant benefits in terms of weight or strength.[70,71]

There is only limited information available about the clinical effects of androgen replacement on the skeleton and even less relating to fracture rates. This is because androgen replacement in males is used far less frequently than estrogen replacement in postmenopausal women. Several investigators have shown that testosterone replacement can increase bone mineral density in hypogonadal males. Devogelaer, et al.[72] gave testosterone esters to 16 young males with varying types of hypogonadism for periods up to 120 months. The average bone mineral density in the radius of these subjects was approximately 1.5 standard deviations below those of normal controls. In those having fused epiphyses at the outset of the study, the bone mineral content of the distal radius increased by an average of 5.7% per year whereas that of the midshaft radius increased by only 0.9% per year. Thus it appeared that the beneficial effects were mainly on trabecular bone. Isaia, et al. measured changes in vertebral bone mineral content as well as several biochemical indicators of bone metabolism in a small group of young men with either Klinefelter's syndrome or hypogonadotrophic hypogonadism. Prior to therapy, the lumbar bone mineral content was significantly lower than in controls. With therapy for only 3 months, lumbar bone mineral content rose significantly. Serum levels of osteocalcin also rose, as did the calcitonin response to a hypercalcemic challenge. There was no change in mean levels of immunoreactive PTH or in urinary hydroxyproline or calcium excretion.[73]

Testosterone or anabolic steroids are sometimes given to women, along with estrogens, for the treatment of osteoporosis. Some of the combination estrogen/androgen products available are listed in Table 3. When given together with estradiol in a percutaneous implant, testosterone confers no additional bone-sparing effect in postmenopausal women. Garnett, et al. found that the increase in femoral neck density in women treated for one year with implants containing either estradiol or estradiol plus testosterone correlated with the serum levels of estradiol achieved but were not affected by testosterone.[74] The addition of an anabolic steroid such as nandrolone to an estrogen replacement regimen also provides no benefits over estrogen replacement alone. Birkenhager, et al. in a two-year clinical trial, found that nandrolone decanoate, given as a monthly intramuscular injection, caused no further improvement in bone density when added to a regimen of oral estrogen and medroxyprogesterone.[75] These negative studies suggest that there is no reason for adding androgens to established estrogen regimens in treating postmenopausal osteoporosis in women. In the presence of adequate estrogens, androgens provide no further skeletal benefits, but they may still cause undesirable side effects such as virilization. They may also have an undesirable effect on serum lipids, opposing the effects of estrogens by raising LDL-cholesterol and lowering HDL-cholesterol.

In summary, from the limited information available it is clear that androgen replacement can improve bone density in hypogonadal men, but it is uncertain whether bone metabolism can be fully restored to normal, or whether fracture rates can ultimately be decreased. Androgens cause virilization when given to women and appear to provide no added skeletal benefits when added to estrogen replacement therapy.

V. ADRENAL CORTICOSTEROIDS

The adrenals secrete several types of steroids, including glucocorticoids, mineralocorticoids, and androgens. Adrenal androgens have already been discussed in the sections on estrogens and androgens. The glucocorticoids, typified by cortisol, are essential for life because of their role at physiological concentrations in supporting vital functions such as vascular responsiveness and energy metabolism. At higher concentrations they play a role in the response of the body to stress. High levels of glucocorticoids suppress the inflammatory and immune responses of the body to a wide variety of injurious stimuli. Since inflammation and immunity play a role in the progression of some diseases, adrenal glucocorticoids are widely used as anti-inflammatory and immunosuppressive drugs. It is in this capacity that glucocorticoids are important contributors to the risk of osteoporosis through their negative effects on bone density and bone strength.

A. BASIC EFFECTS ON CALCIUM METABOLISM

At high levels, glucocorticoids tend to have inhibitory or catabolic effects on bone and connective tissues. At low or physiological levels certain connective tissue functions may actually be enhanced. Glucocorticoid receptors have been described in both osteoblasts and fibroblasts, indicating that direct effects are likely. However, indirect effects, mediated through local cytokines and growth factors as well as traditional calciotropic hormones, are also important.

At high physiological concentrations glucocorticoids inhibit both type I and type III collagen production by fibroblasts. They also inhibit glycosaminoglycan production. The actions of cortisol on the synthesis of collagen have been studied in detail in isolated human fibroblasts.[76] Cortisol at high physiological concentrations reduces cellular accumulations of mRNAs for the procollagen peptide chains involved in the formation of mature collagen. This effect is not due to a decrease in gene transcription, but to an increase in the rate of degradation of the specific mRNAs. The effect may be mediated by a steroid-induced increase in ribonuclease activity.

Supraphysiological levels of glucocorticoids continued for extended periods of time result in progressive bone loss. Receptors for glucocorticoids have been identified in osteoblast-like bone cells and may also be present in osteoblasts.[77] Although high levels of glucocorticoids are associated with an overall increase in bone resorption and a decrease in bone formation, these effects are dose-related. Low concentrations of cortisol actually increase the production of collagen by fetal rat bone. At higher concentrations there is a dose-dependent suppression of the synthesis of types I and III collagen, as well as of noncollagen proteins.[78] One specific osteoblast protein whose synthesis is suppressed by glucocorticoids is osteocalcin. In normal human subjects, serum osteocalcin levels show a diurnal rhythm in which the peak coincides with the nadir of diurnal cortisol production.

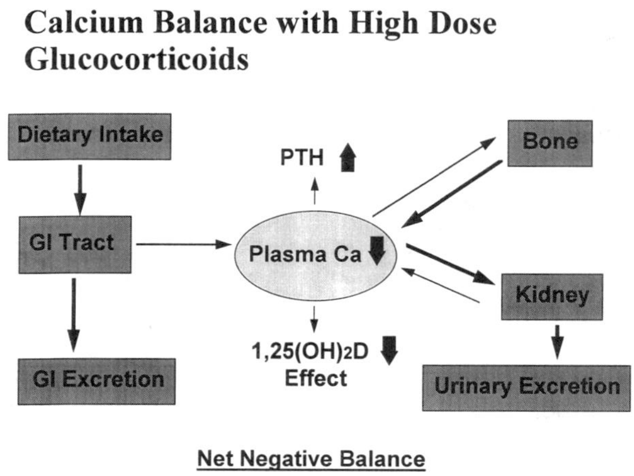

FIGURE 9. The Effects of Glucocorticoid Excess on Calcium Balance. Calcium deposition in bone declines due to the direct inhibitory effect of glucocorticoids on osteoblast number and activity. The action of $1,25(OH)_2D$ on the gastrointestinal tract is also impaired, leading to a reduced absorption of dietary calcium. Mild secondary hyperparathyroidism and possibly suppressed levels of calcitonin lead to increased bone resorption. Urinary calcium excretion is increased.

Single small doses of glucocorticoid, given just before peak levels of serum osteocalcin are reached, can reverse the rise.[79] The osteocalcin gene is subject to control by both glucocorticoids and 1,25-dihydroxyvitamin D. The activated vitamin D receptor normally binds to a DNA sequence in the promoter region of the osteocalcin gene and stimulates the transcription of osteocalcin mRNA. The activated glucocorticoid receptor also interacts with the gene, inhibiting its expression and blocking the effects of vitamin D.[80]

Several of the effects of glucocorticoids on bone are indirect. With high doses there is a negative total body calcium balance, as shown in Figure 9. The intestinal absorption of calcium is decreased. Glucocorticoids have direct suppressive effects on calcium transport in the gut, where they again oppose the actions of vitamin D. This effect may be due to reduced synthesis of an intestinal calcium-binding protein.[81] Glucocorticoids also promote increased urinary excretion of calcium and phosphorus. The characteristic hypercalciuria seen with glucocorticoid excess probably represents a direct glucocorticoid effect on the kidney. Conversely, glucocorticoid deficiency can cause impaired renal calcium clearance and predispose to hypercalcemia.

In patients treated with large doses of glucocorticoids, parathyroid hormone levels tend to be high, possibly secondary to a decreased influx of calcium from the gastrointestinal tract and an increased urinary calcium excretion. Calcitonin levels, on the other hand, tend to be suppressed.[78] The combination of elevated PTH and reduced calcitonin secretion probably contributes to the increased rates of bone resorption associated with high-dose glucocorticoid therapy. High-dose glucocorticoids also suppress gonadotropin secretion in both men and women, leading to reduced circulating levels of sex steroids in some patients. The resulting state of hypogonadism further interferes with maintenance of the calcium balance. Thus, through a combination of effects including increased bone resorption, decreased osteoblast function, and decreased bone formation, high-dose glucocorticoid therapy leads to a net negative calcium balance through the mechanisms illustrated in Figure 9.

B. CLINICAL EFFECTS OF GLUCOCORTICOIDS ON BONE

Glucocorticoid excess occasionally results from the endogenous overproduction of cortisol by the adrenals (Cushing's syndrome), but is more commonly due to the administration of high doses of synthetic glucocorticoids in treating inflammatory or autoimmune diseases. Glucocorticoids are among the most frequently prescribed drugs in the U.S., and their long-term side effects have been thoroughly reviewed.[82,83]

1. Skeletal Complications of High-Dose Glucocorticoid Therapy

Bone loss and pathologic fractures are among the most common and distressing side effects of corticosteroid therapy, as well as of spontaneous Cushing's syndrome. The incidence of atraumatic fractures in patients on long-term treatment has been estimated at 30% to 50%.[84] Trabecular bone is more affected than cortical bone. Glucocorticoid doses exceeding the equivalent of 30 mg of hydrocortisone (cortisol) or 7.5 mg of prednisone per day are associated with diminished bone density. The extent of bone loss increases with the cumulative dose of glucocorticoid.[85] Effects on lumbar bone mineral density may be seen as early as 20 weeks after the initiation of prednisone therapy at 20 mg per day. If corticosteroids are discontinued at this point, recovery of bone density occurs.[86] Short-term longitudinal studies suggest that the rate of bone loss is most rapid during the first 6 months of corticosteroid therapy. After that, the rate slows and approaches the rate seen in untreated subjects after one to two years.[78] Bone loss leads to fractures only after a critically low mineral density is reached. Thus patients who already have relatively low bone densities at the outset of corticosteroid therapy will be more likely to suffer fractures. Older patients, especially postmenopausal women, are at highest risk.

2. Prevention and Treatment of Steroid-Induced Osteoporosis

The diminished bone density associated with a long course of glucocorticoid therapy usually persists after glucocorticoid administration is stopped. Thus most strategies to ameliorate the problem are directed at slowing the rate of loss during ongoing steroid therapy. Lowering the dose of glucocorticoid to the minimum amount required and shortening the course of therapy as much as possible will help to minimize the problem. Assurance of an adequate dietary calcium intake of at least 1000 mg per day and a vitamin D intake of at least 400 units per day is prudent in all patients.[84] Thiazide diuretics may be given to reduce urinary calcium excretion if hypercalciuria is present. Estrogen replacement should be given to all postmenopausal women receiving glucocorticoids unless estrogens are contraindicated by other medical problems. Luckert, et al. found that women receiving 0.625 mg of conjugated estrogens daily, plus cyclical medroxyprogesterone, were protected against excessive bone loss for at least one year while taking prednisone in doses ranging from 5–15 mg per day.[87] Other agents that decrease bone resorption have also been effective in limited clinical trials in reducing steroid-induced bone loss. Short-term administration of salmon calcitonin,[88,89] or repeated infusions of the bisphosphonate, pamidronate,[90,91] have also been found to increase bone density moderately in glucocorticoid-treated patients. Whether these agents will also be effective in lowering fracture rates in such patients is unknown.

Perhaps the best approach to diminishing the impact of corticosteroid-induced osteoporosis lies in better application of pharmacokinetic principles in the therapy of chronic steroid-responsive diseases. Topical or regional administration of a corticosteroid is often sufficient to control a regional disease, thus avoiding the complications of systemic therapy. For example, the inhaled glucocorticoid, beclomethasone dipropionate, is available as an alternative to systemic glucocorticoids in the treatment of asthma and other obstructive lung diseases. Corticosteroids administered by aerosol to the bronchial tree have local anti-inflammatory effects but minimal systemic effects when administered in the usual doses.[92]

In summary, bone loss cannot be entirely avoided in patients who must be treated with large doses of adrenal corticosteroids. There are a number of measures, however, that may be taken to ameliorate steroid-induced osteoporosis. These are summarized below in Table 9.

VI. SUMMARY

The steroid hormones, as a group, have profound effects on bone metabolism. Estrogens and androgens both promote a positive calcium balance and increased bone mass and strength. Estrogen deficiency, commonly occurring at menopause in women, contributes to more rapid bone loss and an increase in the incidence of fractures. Androgen deficiency, although it is less common, has

TABLE 9
Measures for Decreasing the Skeletal Complications of High Dose Corticosteroid Therapy

Preventive Measures	Specific Applications
Maintain physical activity	
Maintain optimal nutritional status	Calcium intake at least 1000 mg/day
	Vitamin D intake at least 800 IU/day
Replace gonadal hormones if deficient	Estrogens in postmenopausal or amenorrheic women
	Testosterone in hypogonadal men
Minimize dose and duration of therapy with glucocorticoids	Use regional or topical glucocorticoids when possible
Therapeutic Measures when Low Bone Mineral Density is Present	
Administration of salmon calcitonin	50–100 units per day, sc
Administration of pamidronate	30 mg, i.v., every 60–90 days or 100 mg per day, by mouth

similar effects in men. Estrogen replacement therapy in hypogonadal women and androgen replacement in men are both beneficial in reversing bone loss. Both estrogens and androgens have multiple extraskeletal effects that must be taken into account when one is considering replacement therapy.

Adrenal glucocorticoids, in contrast to sex steroids, have largely negative effects on the calcium balance. High doses of glucocorticoids, commonly used to suppress inflammatory and immunologically mediated diseases, almost invariably lead to osteoporosis if therapy is continued long enough. Strategies to prevent glucocorticoid-induced osteoporosis include concurrent administration of estrogens or androgens, supplementation with calcium and vitamin D, and the use of antiresorptive agents such as calcitonin and the bisphosphonates.

REFERENCES

1. **Clark, J. H., Schrader, W. T., and O'Malley, B. W.,** Mechanisms of action of steroid hormones, in *Textbook of Endocrinology*, 8th edition, Wilson, J. D. and Foster, D. W., eds., W.B. Saunders Co., Philadelphia, 1992.
2. **Evans, R. M.,** The steroid and thyroid hormone receptor superfamily, *Science*, 240, 889, 1988.
3. **Komm, B. S., Terpening, C. M., Benz, D. J., Graeme, K. A., Gallegos, A., Kore, M., Greene, G. L., O'Malley, B. W., and Haussler, M. R.,** Estrogen binding, receptor mRNA, and biologic response in osteoblast-like osteosarcoma cells, *Science*, 241, 81, 1988.
4. **Eriksen, E. R., Colvard, D. S., Berg, N. J., Graham, M. L., Mann, K. G., Spelsberg, T. C., and Riggs, B. L.,** Evidence of estrogen receptors in normal human osteoblast-like cells, *Science*, 241, 84, 1988.
5. **Gray, T. K.,** Estrogens and the skeleton: cellular and molecular mechanisms, *J. Steroid Biochemistry*, 34, 285, 1989.
6. **Ernst, M., Heath, J. K., and Rodan, G. A.,** Estradiol effects on proliferation, messenger ribonucleic acid for collagen and insulin-like growth factor-1, and parathyroid hormone-stimulated adenylate cyclase activity in osteoblastic cells from calvariae and long bones, *Endocrinology*, 125, 825, 1989.
7. **Girasole, G., Jilka, R. L., Passeri, G., Boswell, S., Boder, G., Williams, D. C., and Manolagas, S. C.,** 17β-estradiol inhibits interleukin-6 production by bone marrow-derived stromal cells and osteoblasts in vitro: a potential mechanism for the antiosteoporotic effect of estrogens, *J. Clin. Invest.*, 89, 883, 1992.
8. **Jilka, R. L., Hangoc, G., Girasole, G., Passeri, G., Williams, D.C., Abrams, J. S., Boyce, B., Broxmeyer, H., and Manolagas, S. C.,** Increased osteoclast development after estrogen loss: mediation by interleukin-6, *Science*, 257, 88, 1992.
9. **Chow, J., Tobias, J. H., Colston, K. W., and Chambers, T. J.,** Estrogen maintains trabecular bone volume in rats not only by suppression of bone resorption but also by stimulation of bone formation, *J. Clin. Invest.*, 89, 74, 1992.
10. **Miller, R. A., Russell, J. E., and Birge, S. J.,** Quantitation of the receptor proteins for $1,25(OH)_2D$ in the intestine of the aging rat. *Calcif. Tissue Int.*, 35, 697a, 1983.
11. **Carr, B. R.,** Disorders of the ovary and female reproductive tract, in *Textbook of Endocrinology*, 8th edition, Wilson, J. D. and Foster, D. W., eds., W.B. Saunders Co., Philadelphia, 1992.

12. **Compston, J. E.,** HRT and osteoporosis, *Br. Med. J.*, 48, 309, 1992.
13. **Heaney, R. P.,** Estrogen-calcium interaction in the postmenopause: a quantitative description, *Bone Min.*, 11, 67, 1990.
14. **Cummings, S. J., Black, D. M., and Rubin, S. M.,** Lifetime risks of hip, Colles' or vertebral fracture and coronary heart disease among white postmenopausal women, *Ann. Int. Med.*, 149, 2445, 1989.
15. **Rigotti, N. A., Nussbaum, S. R., Herzog, D. B., and Neer, R. M.,** Osteoporosis in women with anorexia nervosa, *New Engl. J. Med.*, 311, 1601, 1984.
16. **Shore, R. M., Chesney, R. W., Mazess, R. B., Rose, P. G., and Bergman, G. J.,** Skeletal demineralization in Turner's syndrome, *Calcif. Tissue Int.*, 34, 519, 1982.
17. **Klibanski, A. and Greenspan, S. L.,** Increase in bone mass after treatment of hyperprolactinemic amenorrhea, *New Engl. J. Med.*, 315, 542, 1986.
18. **Drinkwater, B. L., Nilson, K., Chestnut, C. H., Bremmer, W. J., Shainholtz, S., and Southworth, M. B.,** Bone mineral content of amenorrheic and eumenorrheic athletes, *New Engl. J. Med.*, 311, 277, 1984.
19. **Frusztajer, N. T., Dhuper, S., Warren, M. P., Brooks-Gunn, J., and Fox, R. P.,** Nutrition and the incidence of stress fractures in ballet dancers, *Am. J. Clin. Nutr.*, 51, 779, 1990.
20. **Powers, M. S., Schenkel, L., Darley, P. E., Good, W. R., Balestra, J. C., and Wallace, V. A.,** Pharmacokinetics and pharmacodynamics of transdermal dosage forms of 17β-estradiol: comparison with conventional oral estrogens used for hormone replacement, *Am. J. Obstet. Gynecol.*, 152, 1099, 1985.
21. **Johnston, C. C., Jr. and Melton, L. J., III,** Bone density measurement and the management of osteoporosis, in *Primer on the Metabolic Bone Diseases and Disorders of Mineral Metabolism*, 2nd edition, M. J. Favus, ed., Raven Press, 1993.
22. **Barrett-Conner, E.,** Postmenopausal estrogen and prevention bias, *Ann. Int. Med.*, 115, 455, 1991.
23. **Lindsay, R., Hart, D. M., and Clark, D. M.,** The minimum effective dose of estrogen for prevention of postmenopausal bone loss, *Obstet. Gynecol.*, 63, 759, 1984.
24. **Ettinger, B., Genant, H. K., and Cann, C. E.,** Postmenopausal bone loss is prevented by treatment with low-dosage estrogen with calcium, *Ann. Int. Med.*, 106, 40, 1987.
25. **Prince, R. L., Smith, M., Dick, I. M., Price, R. I., Webb, P. G., Henderson, N. K., and Harris, M. M.,** A comparative study of exercise, calcium supplementation and hormone-replacement therapy, *New Engl. J. Med.*, 325, 1189, 1991.
26. **Aloia, J. F., Vaswani, A., Yeh, J. K., Ross, P. L., Flaster, E., and Dilmanian, F. A.,** Calcium supplementation with and without hormone replacement therapy to prevent postmenopausal bone loss, *Ann. Int. Med.*, 120, 97, 1994.
27. **Lindsay, R. and Tohme, J. F.,** Estrogen treatment of patients with established postmenopausal osteoporosis, *Obstet. Gynecol.*, 76, 290, 1990.
28. **Felson, D. T., Zhang Y., Hannan, M. T., Kiel, D. P., Wilson, P. W. F., and Anderson, J. J.,** The effect of postmenopausal estrogen therapy on bone density in elderly women, *New Engl. J. Med.*, 329, 1141, 1993.
29. **Weiss, N. S., Ure, C. L., Ballard, J. H., Williams, B. A., and Daling, J. A.,** Decreased risk of fractures of the hip and lower forearm with postmenopausal use of estrogen, *New Engl. J. Med.*, 303, 1195, 1980.
30. **Paganini-Hill, A., Ross, R. K., Gerkins, V. R., Henderson, B. E., Arthur, M., and Mack, T. M.,** Menopausal estrogen therapy and hip fractures, *Ann. Int. Med.*, 95, 28, 1981.
31. **Kreiger, N. S., Kelsey, J. L., Holford, T. R., O'Connor, T.,** An epidemiological study of hip fracture in postmenopausal women, *Am. J. Epidemiol.*, 116, 141, 1982.
32. **Ettinger, B., Genant, H. K., and Cann, C. E.,** Long-term estrogen replacement therapy prevents bone loss and fractures, *Ann. Int. Med.*, 102, 319, 1985.
33. **Kiel, D. P., Felson, D. T., Anderson, J. J., Wilson, P. W. F., and Moskowitz, M. A.,** Hip fracture and the use of estrogens in postmenopausal women: the Framingham study, *New Engl. J. Med.*, 317, 1169, 1987.
34. **Lindsay, R., Hart, D. M., Forrest, C., and Baird, C.,** Prevention of spinal osteoporosis in oophorectomised women, *Lancet*, ii, 1151, 1980.
35. **Naessen, T., Persson, I., Adami, H.-O., Bergstrom, R., and Bergkvist, L.,** Hormone replacement therapy and risk for first hip fracture, *Ann. Int. Med.*, 113, 95, 1990.
36. **Lufkin, E. G., Wahner, H. W., O'Fallon, W. M., Hodgson, S. F., Kotowicz, M. A., Lane, A. W., Judd, H. L., Caplan, R. H., and Riggs, B. L.,** Treatment of postmenopausal osteoporosis with transdermal estrogen, *Ann. Int. Med.*, 117, 1, 1992.
37. **Ettinger, B.,** Overview of the efficacy of hormonal replacement therapy, *Am. J. Obstet. Gynecol.*, 156, 1298, 1987.
38. **Whitehead, M. I., and Fraser, D.,** Controversies concerning the safety of estrogen replacement therapy, *Am. J. Obstet. Gynecol.*, 156, 1313, 1987.
39. **Campbell, S., and Whitehead, M.,** Oestrogen therapy and the postmenopausal syndrome, *Clin. Obstet. Gynaecol.*, 4, 1, 1977.
40. **Grady, D., Rubin, S. M., Petitti, D. B., Fox, C. S., Black, D. Ettinger, B., Ernster, V. L., and Cummings, S. R.,** Hormone therapy to prevent disease and prolong life in postmenopausal women, *Ann. Int. Med.*, 117, 1016, 1992.
41. **Henderson, B. E., Paganini-Hill, A., and Ross, R. K.,** Decreased mortality in users of estrogen replacement therapy, *Arch. Int. Med.*, 151, 75, 1991.

42. **Sullivan, J. M., Vander Zwaag, R., Hughes, J. P., Maddock, V., Kroetz, F. W., Ramanathan, K. B., and Mirvis, D. M.,** Estrogen replacement and coronary artery disease. Effect on survival in postmenopausal women, *Arch. Int. Med.*, 150, 2557, 1990.
43. **Ravnikar, V. A.,** Compliance with hormone therapy, *Am. J .Obstet. Gynecol.*, 156, 1332, 1987.
44. **Coope, J., and March, J.,** Can we improve compliance with long-term HRT?, *Maturitas*, 15, 151, 1992.
45. **Rubin, S. M., and Cummings, S. R.,** Results of bone densitometry affect women's decisions about taking measures to prevent fractures, *Ann. Int. Med.*, 116, 990, 1992.
46. **Leather, A. T., Studd, J. W. W., Watson, N. R., and Holland E. F. N.,** The prevention of bone loss in young women treated with GnRH analogues with "add-back" estrogen therapy, *Obstet. Gynecol.*, 81, 104, 1993.
47. **Love, R. R., Mazess, R. B., Barden, H. S., Epstein, S., Newcomb, P. A., Jordan, V. C., Carbone, P. P., and DeMets, D. L.,** Effects of tamoxifen on bone mineral density in postmenopausal women with breast cancer, *New Engl. J. Med.*, 326, 852, 1992.
48. **Love, R. R., Wiebe, D. A., Newcomb, P. A., Cameron, L., Leventhal, H., Jordan V. C., Feyzi, J., and DeMets, D. L.,** Effects of tamoxifen on cardiovascular risk factors in postmenopausal women, *Ann. Int. Med.*, 115, 860, 1991.
49. **Prior, J. C.,** Progesterone as a bone-trophic hormone, *Endocr. Rev.*, 11, 386, 1990.
50. **Chen, T. L., Aronow, L., and Feldman, D.,** Glucocorticoid receptors and inhibition of bone cell growth in primary culture, *Endocrinology*, 100, 619, 1977.
51. **Burnett, C. C., and Reddi, A. H.,** Effect of sex steroids on bone collagen synthesis *in vitro*, *Calcif. Tissue Int.*, 35, 609, 1983.
52. **Leather, A. T., Savvas, M., and Studd, J. W. W.,** Endometrial histology and bleeding patterns after 8 years of continuous combined estrogen and progestogen therapy in postmenopausal women, *Obstet. Gynecol.*, 78, 1008, 1991.
53. **Cundy, T., Evans, M., Roberts, H., Wattie, D., Ames, R., and Reid, I. R.,** Bone density in women receiving depot medroxyprogesterone acetate for contraception, *Br. Med. J.*, 303, 13, 1991.
54. **Gallagher, J. C., Kable, W. T., and Goldgar, D.,** Effect of progestin therapy on cortical and trabecular bone: comparison with estrogen, *Am. J. Med.*, 90, 171, 1991.
55. **Grecu, E. O., Simmons, R., Baylink, D. J., Haloran, B. P., and Spencer, M. E.,** Effects of medroxyprogesterone acetate on some parameters of calcium metabolism in patients with glucocorticoid-induced osteoporosis, *Bone Min.*, 13, 153, 1991.
56. **Christiansen, C., Riis, B. J., Nilas, L., Rodbro, P., and Deftos, L.,** Uncoupling of bone formation and resorption by combined oestrogen and progestagen therapy in post menopausal osteoporosis, *Lancet*, ii, 800, 1985.
57. **Abdalla, H. I., Hart, D. M., Lindsay, R., Leggate, I., and Hooke, A.,** Prevention of bone mineral loss in postmenopausal women by norethisterone, *Obstet. Gynecol.*, 66, 789, 1985.
58. **Horowitz, M., Wishart, J., Need, A. G., Norris, H., Philcox, J., and Nordin, B. E. C.,** Treatment of postmenopausal hyperparathyroidism with norethindrone, *Arch. Int. Med.*, 147, 681, 1987.
59. **Colvard, D. S., Eriksen, E. F., Keeting, P. E., Wilson, E. M., Lubahn, D. B., French, F. S., Riggs, B. L., and Spelsberg, T. C.,** Identification of androgen receptors in normal human osteobalst-like cells, *Proc. Natl. Acad. Sci. USA*, 86, 854, 1989.
60. **Kasperk, C. H., Wergedal, J. D., Farley, J. R., Kinkhart, T. A., Turner, R. T., and Baylink D. J.,** Androgens directly stimulate proliferation of bone cells *in vitro*, *Endocrinology*, 124, 1576, 1989.
61. **Zapf, J., Schmid, C., and Froesch, E. R.,** Biological and immunological properties of insulin-like growth factors (IGF), *Clin. Endocrinol. Metab.*, 13, 3, 1984.
62. **Francis, R. M., Peacock, M., Aaron, J. E., Selby, P. L., Taylor, G. A., Thompson, J., Marshall, D. H., and Horsman, A.,** Osteoporosis in hypogonadal men: role of decreased plasma 1, 25-dihyroxyvitamin D, calcium malabsorption, and low bone formation, *Bone*, 7, 261, 1986.
63. **Mosekilde, L. and Mosekilde, L.,** Sex differences in age-related changes in vetebral body size, density and biomechanical competence in normal individuals, *Bone*, 11, 67, 1990.
64. **Seeman, E., Melton, L. J., O'Fallon, W. M., and Riggs, B. L.,** Risk factors for spinal osteoporosis in men, *Am. J. Med.*, 75, 977, 1983.
65. **Bhasin, S.,** Clinical review 34; androgen treatment of hypogonadal men, *J. Clin. Endocrinol. Metab.*, 74, 1221, 1992.
66. **Matzkin, H., Chen, J., Weisman, Y., Goldray, D., Pappas, F., and Braf, Z.,** Prolonged treatment with finasteride (a 5-αreductase inhibitor) does not affect bone density and metabolism, *Clin. Endocrinol.*, 37, 432, 1992.
67. **Smith, E. P., Boyd, J., Frank, G. R., et al.,** Estrogen resistance caused by a mutation in the estrogen-receptor gene in a man, *New Engl. J. Med.*, 331, 1056, 1994.
68. **Wild, R. A., Buchanan, J. R., Myers, C., and Demers, L. M.,** Declining adrenal androgens: an association with bone loss in aging women, *Proc. Soc. Exp. Biol. Med.*, 186, 355, 1987.
69. **Griffen, J. E., and Wilson, J. D.,** Disorders of the testes and male reproductive tract, in *Textbook of Endocrinology*, 8th edition, J. D. Wilson and D. W. Foster, eds., W.B. Saunders Co., 1992.
70. **Watson, R. N., Bradley, M. H., Callahan, R., Peters, B. J., and Kory, R. C.,** A six month evaluation of an anabolic drug, norethandrolone, in underweight persons, *Am. J. Med.*, 26, 238, 1959.
71. **Kopera, H.,** The history of anabolic steroids and a review of experience with anabolic steroids, *Acta Endocrinol.*, (suppl) 271, 11, 1985.

72. **Devogelaer, J. P., De Cooman, S., and Nagant de Deuxchaisnes, C.,** Low bone mass in hypogonadal males; effect of testosterone substitution therapy, a densitometric study, *Maturitas,* 15, 17, 1992.
73. **Isaia, G., Musetta, M., Pecchio, F., Sciolla, A., di Stefano, M., and Molinatti, G. M.,** Effect of testosterone on bone in hypogonadal males, *Maturitas,* 15, 47, 1992.
74. **Garnett, T., Studd, J., Watson, N., Savvas, M., and Leather, A.,** The effects of plasma estradiol levels on increases in vertebral and femoral bone density following therapy with estradiol and estradiol with testosterone implants, *Obstet. Gynecol.,* 79, 968, 1992.
75. **Birkenhager, J. C., Erdtsieck, R.J., Zeelenberg, J., van Kuik, C., van Veen, L. C. P., Birkenhäger-Frenkel, D. H., and Luiken, G. P. M.,** Can nandrolone add to the effect of hormonal replacement therapy in postmenopausal osteoporosis?, *Bone Min.,* 18, 251, 1992.
76. **Hamalainen, L., Dikarinen, J., and Kivirikko, K. I.,** Synthesis and degradation of type I procollagen mRNA's in cultured human skin fibroblasts and the effect of cortisol, *J. Biol. Chem.,* 260, 720, 1985.
77. **Chen, T. L., Aronow, L., and Feldman, D.,** Glucocorticoid receptors and inhibition of bone cell growth in primary culture, *Endocrinology,* 100, 619, 1977.
78. **Gennari, C.,** Glucocorticoids and bone, In *Bone and Mineral Research, Volume 3,* W.A. Peck, ed., Elsevier Science Publishers, 1985.
79. **Nielsen, H. K., Charles, P., and Mosekilde, L.,** The effect of single oral doses of prednisone on the circadian rhythm of serum osteocalcin in normal subjects, *J. Clin. Endocrinol. Metab.,* 67, 1025, 1988.
80. **Morrison, N. A., Shine, J., Fragonas, J-C., verKest, V., McMenemy, M. L., and Eisman, J. A.,** 1,25-dihydroxy-vitamin D-responsive element and glucocorticoid repression in the osteocalcin gene, *Science,* 246, 1158, 1989.
81. **Feher, J. V., and Wasserman, R. H.,** Intestinal calcium-binding protein and calcium absorption in cortisol-treated chicks: effects of vitamin D_3, *Endocrinology,* 104, 547, 1979.
82. **Seale, J. P. and Compton, M. R.,** Side effects of corticosteroid agents, *Med. J. Australia,* 144, 139, 1986.
83. **Ontjes, D. A.,** The adrenocortical steroids, in *Principles of Pharmacology: Basic Concepts and Clinical Applications,* P.L. Munson, G. Breese and R. Mueller, eds., Chapman and Hall, New York, 1995.
84. **Luckert, B. P., and Raisz, L. G.,** Glucocorticoid-induced osteoporosis: pathogenesis and management, *Ann. Int. Med.,* 112, 352, 1990.
85. **Dykman, T. R., Gluck, O. S., Murphy, W. A., Hahn, T. J., and Hahn, B. H.,** Evaluation of factors associated with glucocorticoid-induced osteopenia in patients with rheumatic diseases, *Arthr. Rheum.,* 28, 361, 1985.
86. **Laan, R. F. J. M., van Riel, P. L. C. M., van de Putte, L. B. A., van Erning, L. J. T. O., van't Hof, M. A., and Lemmens, J. A. M.,** Low-dose prednisone induces rapid reversible axial bone loss in patients with rheumatoid arthritis, *Ann. Int. Med.,* 119, 963, 1993.
87. **Luckert, B. P., Johnson, B. E., and Robinson, R. G.,** Estrogen and progesterone replacement therapy reduces glucocorticoid-induced bone loss, *J. Bone Min. Res.,* 7, 1063, 1992.
88. **Ringe, J. D., and Welzel, D.,** Salmon calcitonin in the therapy of corticoid-induced osteoporosis, *Eur. J. Clin. Pharmacol.,* 33, 35, 1987.
89. **Montemurro, L., Schiraldi, G., Fraioli, P., Tosi, G., Riboldi, A., and Rizzato, G.,** Prevention of corticosteroid-induced osteoporosis with salmon calcitonin, *Calcif. Tiss. Int.,* 49, 71, 1991.
90. **Reid, I. R., King, A. R., Alexander, C. J., and Ibbertson, H. K.,** Prevention of steroid-induced osteoporosis with (3-amino-1-hyroxypropylidine)-1,1-bisphosphonate (APD), *Lancet,* 1, 143, 1988.
91. **Gallacher, S. J., Fenner, J. A. K., Anderson, K., Bryden, F. M., Banham, S. W., Logue, F. C., Cowan, R. A., and Boyle, I. T.,** Intravenous pamidronate in the treatment of osteoporosis associated with corticosteroid dependent lung disease: an open pilot study, *Thorax,* 47, 932, 1992.
92. **Utiger, R. D.,** Differences between inhaled and oral glucocorticoid therapy, *New Engl. J. Med.,* 329, 1731, 1993.

Section IV.

CALCIUM AND PHOSPHORUS METABOLISM ACROSS THE LIFE CYCLE

In this section, the demands for calcium (Ca) and phosphorus (P) by the organism during various stages of the life cycle are reviewed. First, challenges of the major reproductive phases to Ca and P homeostasis, namely pregnancy (Chapter 15) and lactation (Chapter 16), are detailed. The demands for Ca in pregnancy and, especially, lactation contribute to increased bone remodeling transients and, thus, to increased bone resorption, with loss of bone mineral, at least temporarily. These chapters are followed by one that highlights bone changes across the life cycle and reviews the major environmental factors that influence bone mass throughout life (Chapter 17). Ethnic differences in bone are also covered. Chapter 18 attempts to unravel the effects of alcohol (ethanol) on Ca homeostasis and bone, in particular, and to provide an understanding of the mechanisms through which ethanol acts. In essence, osteoblastic activity is depressed whereas osteoclasts remain essentially unchanged by alcohol. Chapter 19 provides a conceptual framework for the beneficial effects of aerobic and strength activities on bone mass. This chapter points out the difficulties of producing improved bone mass in chronic exercise studies. Chapter 20 details the changes in bone mass during the late years of life and the potential influences of nutrients and life-style factors on bone turnover of the elderly. Emphasis in this chapter is placed on the beneficial effects of vitamin D and Ca supplements on bone density and reduction of fractures in elderly subjects.

This section sets the stage for the development of pathologic changes in bone tissue, as expressed in the disorder/disease osteoporosis, which will be outlined in the final section of this text.

Chapter 15

CALCIUM AND BONE METABOLISM DURING PREGNANCY

Sanford C. Garner, Ph.D. and John J. B. Anderson, Ph.D.

TABLE OF CONTENTS

I. INTRODUCTION

The regulation of calcium metabolism and bone development during pregnancy involves complex interactions among the maternal organism, the placenta, and the growing fetus. The mother must supply all nutrients to the fetus for proper development, and, therefore, the nutritional status of the mother is particularly important. Inadequate intake of some nutrients by the mother may be offset, at least in part, by the removal of needed elements or molecules from the mother's own body tissue. The mother will remove calcium (Ca) and phosphorus (P) from her skeleton to provide these elements for fetal skeletal growth. The hormonal regulation of calcium

0-8493-7845-1/95/$0.00+$.50

metabolism during pregnancy and lactation has been reviewed by Garel[1] and Pitkin.[2] Sowers has reviewed the associations of epidemiologic risk factors, including dietary Ca, with bone changes during reproductive events.[3]

Although the homeostasis of fetal Ca and inorganic P (Pi) are dependent on a supply of these nutrients from the mother, it is evident that regulation of these ions by the fetus itself also occurs. The fetus maintains a higher Ca concentration than exists in the maternal circulation. The hormonal mechanisms responsible for this difference have not been completely explained, but it is possible that a parathyroid hormone-like molecule (parathyroid hormone-related peptide or PTHrP) may be active in fetal Ca homeostasis.[4]

The transfers of Ca and Pi, along with other nutrients and oxygen, across the placenta from the mother to the fetus are essential for fetal growth and development within normal limits. These transfers remain primarily unidirectional throughout gestation, although the capability for reverse flow, i.e., fetal to maternal circulation, always remains possible. The placental transfers of Ca and Pi are both uphill, which means that active transport mechanisms exist because of the higher total serum concentrations of each mineral ion on the fetal side of the placenta. In essence, significant amounts of energy (ATP) are required to drive the placental transport mechanisms, which reasonably assure optimal skeletal and dental development of fetal tissues.

This chapter reviews maternal and fetal homeostatic processes that govern plasma Ca and Pi concentrations in their respective circulations, separated by the placental barrier. In addition, changes in maternal skeletal tissue and bone mass during the gestation period are highlighted. Finally, fetal bone development and mineral (Ca and Pi) accretion are discussed under conditions of nutritional sufficiency and insufficiency.

II. MATERNAL CALCIUM HOMEOSTASIS DURING PREGNANCY

The fetal demand for Ca becomes significant during the third month of pregnancy (weeks 9 to 12) and this demand continues to increase until the last few weeks of gestation, when it levels off. The Ca that is transferred across the placenta to the fetus is derived from both the current dietary Ca and from the maternal skeletal tissue. If the dietary supply is not adequate, skeletal tissue will be resorbed in order to meet the fetal demands. Because of typically suboptimal intakes of Ca by many adolescent and young adult women, the maternal burden of resorbing their own bone to meet fetal Ca needs can be great in these women. Although experiments in animal models, primarily rats, have shown that pregnancy can be successfully completed in mothers receiving very low calcium diets, rats maintained continuously on a calcium-deficient diet eventually showed evidence of reproductive failure.[5,6]

Historically, low Ca intakes by mothers during successive pregnancies (and lactations) have contributed to high rates of bone resorption, low bone mass (observed by X-ray in the past), and even fractures. In Asian countries especially, women may have had such extensive alveolar bone loss in their jaws that the loss of one or more teeth per baby was not considered unusual. (An old wive's tale still exists today that for each child born, a tooth is lost!)

Dr. Isidore Snapper described the severe deficiency of calcium and vitamin D in the diets of women seen at the clinics of the Peiping (Beijing) Union Medical College.[7] He also discussed the osteomalacia that was frequent among women in Beijing, with pregnancy and lactation exacerbating the condition. Women often showed the first symptoms of osteomalacia during their first lactation and suffered relapses during subsequent pregnancies. More recently, Gruber, et al. have described the osteoporosis associated with pregnancy and lactation in three patients.[8]

Total Ca concentrations of plasma decline during lactation; however, parallel decreases in both P and albumin occur,[9] and the net result is little if any change in ionized Ca.[10] Changes in the total amount of Ca ions in the circulation are necessary to maintain ionized Ca concentration in the normal range as dilution occurs because of the plasma volume expansion that accompanies pregnancy. Urinary Ca excretion is also significantly increased in pregnant women, probably as a result of increased glomerular filtration rates.

Intestinal Ca absorption is increased in late pregnancy. Kent and co-workers used a nonradioactive Ca isotope[11] and an oral Ca load[12] to measure the fractional absorption of Ca during the last trimester of pregnancy and in established lactation. They found that intestinal Ca absorption was significantly increased in late pregnancy, but not in established lactation.

The regulation of maternal Ca and Pi metabolism is carried out by the same calcium-regulating hormones covered in earlier chapters. Brief descriptions of the roles of the three major hormones, parathyroid hormone (PTH), $1,25(OH)_2D$, and calcitonin (CT) are presented next.

A. PARATHYROID HORMONE

An increase in plasma PTH during pregnancy has been postulated as a likely response of the maternal Ca homestatic system to the demands on plasma Ca; i.e., plasma volume expansion, increased urinary Ca loss, and transfer of maternal Ca to the developing fetus. A concept of "physiologic hyperparathyroidism" was proposed in the past, based on increases in C-terminal fragments of PTH. However, more recent studies using assays specific for the intact PTH molecule have cast doubt on increased plasma PTH during pregnancy,[13-16] and have even suggested a decrease in plasma PTH during pregnancy.[15]

B. VITAMIN D

The same reasoning that suggests that plasma PTH should be increased during pregnancy also leads one to expect an increase in plasma $1,25(OH)_2D$ concentrations. The increased demand for Ca ions to replace those lost to urinary excretion and placental transfer would best be met by enhanced intestinal absorption of dietary Ca. An increase in intestinal Ca absorption has been documented in pregnant women.[17] An increase in $1,25(OH)_2D$ occurs during pregnancy, which results in a doubling of plasma levels compared to nonpregnant women. This increase appears to be the result of increased synthesis of $1,25(OH)_2D$ by the kidney (1α-hydroxylation) rather than of increased circulating 25-OH-vitamin D, which does not change during pregnancy.

The report of Whitehead et al.[13] characterizes plasma $1,25(OH)_2D$ levels in pregnant women at 10–12, 20–22, 30–32, and 36–40 weeks of pregnancy. Plasma $1,25(OH)_2D$ concentrations were already elevated at 10–12 weeks of gestation with a gradual, modest rise to 36–40 weeks. Although Whitehead, et al. and others have proposed that the increase in plasma $1,25(OH)_2D$ may be responsible for the increased efficiency of intestinal Ca absorption to provide adequate Ca for fetal calcification, the majority of fetal Ca needs occur late in gestation, primarily in the third trimester. Thus, the increase in $1,25(OH)_2D$ is already present in a period of pregnancy when the calcium demands of the developing fetus are quite small, i.e., <10 mg per day. Although the availability of adequate vitamin D levels during pregnancy is necessary for proper fetal growth and calcification (see later section, Effects of Maternal Nutrition on Fetal Skeletal Development), the physiologic role for the $1,25(OH)_2D$ metabolite of this vitamin in enhancing intestinal Ca absorbtion remains to be determined.[11,12]

C. CALCITONIN

The role of CT in normal human physiology remains undefined (see Chapter 13), although its effects to decrease bone resorption are consistent with a skeleton-protecting action. Because the maternal skeleton may be required to supply Ca and P when dietary intakes are inadequate, an increased plasma CT concentration during pregnancy has been suggested as a likely protective response. The findings of several investigators on changes in plasma CT with pregnancy, however, are contradictory. CT levels have been found to rise during pregnancy[18] and, therefore, to be higher at the end of pregnancy than in nonpregnant women.[19,20] However, other longitudinal studies have indicated no consistent rise in CT from early to late gestation.[21]

D. SUMMARY

The adjustments in maternal Ca homeostasis during pregnancy appear to be rather small. Although total plasma Ca decreases significantly during pregnancy, the decrease in the ionized Ca concentration is minimal. The reported increase in maternal intestinal Ca absorption appears to be related to an increase in plasma 1,25$(OH)_2$D levels. Changes in PTH and CT that might be expected to stimulate and inhibit bone turnover, respectively, have not been found consistently by researchers in this area. Thus, the demands of the growing fetus for adequate Ca and Pi for skeletal mineralization may be met without dramatic alteration in Ca homeostatic mechanisms when the mother is reasonably well nourished.

III. PLACENTAL TRANSFER OF CALCIUM AND PHOSPHORUS

The maintenance of a higher ionized Ca concentration in the fetal circulation compared to that of the mother supports the contention that the transplacental transfer of Ca ions must be an active process. The maternal-fetal plasma Pi relationship is not as well documented, but data suggest that the fetal plasma Pi concentration is higher than that of the mother. The actual mechanism by which Ca and Pi are transferred across the placenta has not been established, but a Ca^{2+}-activated ATPase has been isolated from human placenta.[22] Studies with isolated, perfused guinea pig placentas suggest that the placental transport of Pi may be regulated, at least in part, by the maternal ionized Ca concentration, with increasing Ca leading to increasing Pi transport.[23]

IV. FETAL CALCIUM HOMEOSTASIS DURING PREGNANCY

Despite the total dependence of the fetus on the mother as a source of minerals and other nutrients, fetal calcium, both total and ionized, concentrations are significantly higher than maternal levels during late gestation. Therefore, the fetus or fetal-placental unit is able to maintain fetal calcium homeostasis somewhat independently of the mother.

A. PARATHYROID HORMONE AND PARATHYROID HORMONE-RELATED PROTEIN

Studies with isotopically labeled PTH indicate that intact PTH molecules do not cross the placental barrier. Therefore, fetal regulation of plasma Ca is dependent on the endogenous secretion of PTH (or a PTH-like molecule), in addition to the ready supply of Ca ions from the mother. The fetal parathyroid gland develops early in gestation, and parathyroid cells are immunoreactive for PTH beginning at 10 weeks of gestational age.[24]

The parathyroid hormone-related protein (PTHrP) was first characterized as the systemic factor in many cases of hypercalcemia of malignancy. Subsequently, examination of expression of this molecule has indicated that its expression and function are regulated in normal tissue, including the lactating mammary gland and smooth muscle cells of blood vessels and the gastrointestinal tract. Both the fetal parathyroid and the placenta have been reported to synthesize and secrete this hormone-related molecule.[4] The regulation of PTHrP secretion by Ca in the fetal parathyroid, however, has not been investigated. Thus, whether fetal Ca is regulated in part or in whole by PTHrP is not known.

B. VITAMIN D

The maternal and fetal concentrations of both 25(OH)D and 1,25$(OH)_2$D correlate well, suggesting that transplacental transfer of these molecules regulates the fetal plasma concentrations. Direct evidence from experiments with radiolabeled (^{3}H, tritium) 25(OH)D and 1,25$(OH)_2$D has confirmed the movement of vitamin D metabolites from mother to fetus.

In addition to the maternal supply of 1,25$(OH)_2$D, the placental tissue also has 1α-hydroxylating capability and may provide 1,25$(OH)_2$D to the fetus.

C. CALCITONIN

The CT-secreting C-cells of the thyroid develop early in gestation. By the 14th week, CT can be detected by immunostaining of fetal thyroids.[25] Most investigators have reported higher CT concen-

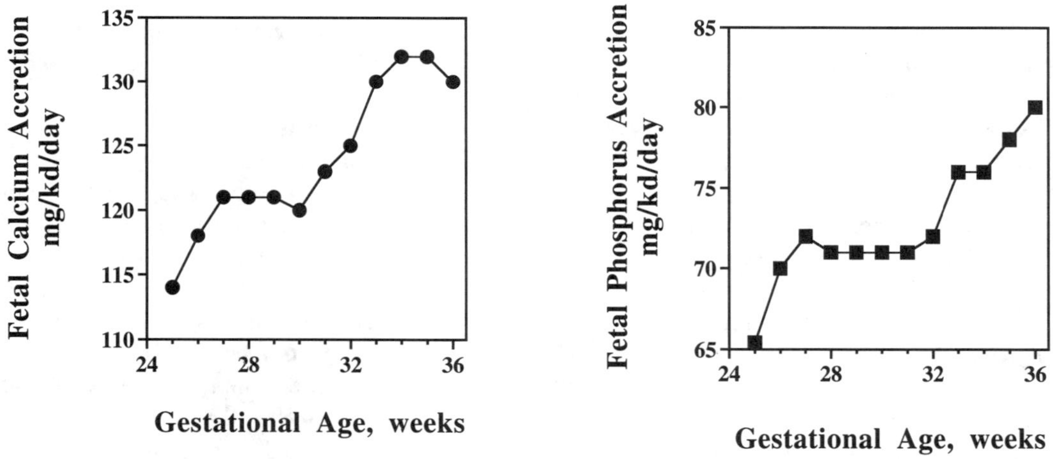

Figure 1. Fetal Accretion of Calcium and Phosphorus During the Third Trimester. These graphs are based on data summarized by Greer and Tsang from original data for the accretion of calcium (Panel A) and phosphorus (Panel B) obtained from body composition studies of stillborn fetuses.[33]

trations in the circulation of fetal blood compared to maternal blood, consistent with the relative hypercalcemia of the fetus. The fetal thyroid gland in rhesus monkeys responded to a hypercalcemic challenge with an elevation in CT secretion.[26] Despite the presence of CT in the fetal circulation, however, we cannot assign a definite physiologic function.

D. SUMMARY

A striking finding in fetal physiology is the hypercalcemia and hyperphosphatemia relative to the maternal circulation. Although the maintenance of higher Ca and Pi concentrations may be due, at least in part, to the active transport of both ions by the placenta, the fetus also is able to synthesize and secrete both PTH and CT from an early stage of development. The fetal supply of vitamin D and its metabolites is regulated mainly by the placental transfer of these molecules from the mother or by the placental synthesis of $1{,}25(OH)_2D$.

V. CHANGES IN MATERNAL BONE DURING PREGNANCY

Changes in maternal bone mineral status during pregnancy are potentially important because of the need for continued adequate supplies of Ca if lactation follows and the possible cumulative effects of multiple pregnancy and lactation cycles (multiparity) on bone health in future postmenopausal years. The RDAs for Ca for women between 25 and 50 years of age are increased from 800 to 1200 mg/day during pregnancy and lactation.[27] No increase has been given, however, in the RDAs of 1200 mg/day for women between the ages of 11 and 24 years who are pregnant or lactating. At this age, peak bone mass (PBM) at all sites has probably not yet been achieved, and the potential for an adverse impact on the maternal skeleton in young women who have not reached PBM may be great if they fail to reach, or at least approach, the consumption of Ca at the RDA.

A. LOSS OF BONE

The amount of Ca accrued by the fetal skeleton over a full 280-day gestation, ~30 g, is supplied by the mother mostly during a period covering the last one-half to two-thirds of her pregnancy, i.e., approximately 4–6 months. As shown in Figure 1, the average daily accumulation of Ca does not exceed 150 mg. One would, therefore, expect that fetal Ca needs could be met by dietary Ca at intakes approximating the RDA of 1200 mg/day. In general, examination of maternal skeletal mineral content supports the idea that little or no loss of maternal bone is necessary for the support of fetal calcification. The information currently available on changes in bone mass during pregnancy is limited to comparisons between pregnant women and matched nonpregnant controls, or to prospective studies in which women are recruited before pregnancy and bone mineral content is measured before pregnancy and immediately postpartum.

A recent prospective study by Sowers et al.[28] found that there was no significant change in femoral bone mineral density in 32 white women aged 20–40 years. In another prospective study by Tylavsky et al.,[29] a group of well-nourished young adult women were followed through pregnancy. Bone measurements by single-photon absorptiometry (SPA) of the distal and mid radius, and by dual-photon absorptiometry (DPA) of the lumbar vertebrae, were made prior to conception and within 3 weeks after delivery of singleton offspring. In the trabecular-rich sites of the lumbar spine and distal radius, less than 1% of bone mineral content was lost. The midshaft of the radius lost between 2 and 3% of the baseline (preconception) bone mineral content. In contrast, Lamke et al.[30] found that pregnant women lost trabecular, but not cortical, bone between the first or early-second trimester and one week postpartum.

Goldsmith and Johnston[31] reported that women at age 35 years who had been through pregnancy but had not lactated had a higher bone mineral content than nulliparous (never pregnant) women.

Gruber et al.[8] reported on cases of three young women who developed vertebral fractures and other skeletal complications during pregnancy and/or lactation. Although there were severe decrements in bone mass postpartum, with three to nine vertebral fractures, no further fractures were observed during more than 5 years of follow-up in two of the three women.

Drinkwater and Chesnut[32] examined the bone mineral density (BMD) of six women before and during pregnancy by DPA and SPA. Although Ca intake during pregnancy was >1500 mg/d in these women, losses of BMD both in the femoral neck and radial shaft were observed. In constrast, the BMD of the midtibia increased.

In summary, the available studies on bone mineral changes across the course of a normal pregnancy in well-nourished young women support the idea that very small changes in total bone mass occur during fetal development. Since participants in these studies were consuming Ca at levels near or exceeding RDAs, the possible detrimental effects of pregnancy accompanied by inadequate Ca intakes were not addressed.

B. EFFECTS OF NUTRITION

Very few studies of maternal bone changes during pregnancy have been reported, and those that are available have generally omitted any estimation of Ca intake. Sowers et al.[28] collected data on maternal Ca intake from both diet and supplements; however, their subjects had substantial Ca intakes. They did not report any correlation between bone changes that were quite small and Ca intakes. Anecdotal reports of postpregnancy osteoporosis have suggested that some women may develop symptoms of osteoporosis at the end of pregnancy or in the early postpartum period. The role of Ca nutrition in this gestational loss of bone has not been established (Tylavsky, F. A. and Anderson, J. J. B., unpublished data).

C. SUMMARY

The requirements of the fetus for Ca total only about 30 g, approximately 3–4 % of the maternal skeletal stores of this element. The well-nourished pregnant women who have been the subjects of most of the published studies on bone loss during pregnancy have not lost significant bone mineral. However, the possibility remains that women consuming amounts of Ca far below the RDA may experience a net loss of bone during pregnancy, which may be exacerbated by the greater drain of lactation.

VI. DEVELOPMENT OF FETAL BONE DURING PREGNANCY

Mineralization of the fetal skeleton occurs primarily during the third trimester, when the rate of placental transfer of calcium in humans and several experimental animal models has been observed to increase by twofold or more. Approximately 80% of the Ca and P in the skeleton of newborns is accrued from 25 weeks of gestation to full term. Premature infants, therefore, will have less mineral in their skeletons in proportion to the number of weeks less than full term, i.e., 40 weeks. The quantitative deposition of Ca and Pi in newly mineralizing fetal bone tissue has also been shown to increase exponentially until near parturition.[33] By full term, a neonate will contain approximately 28 g of Ca and 16 g of P.[34] The fetal accretion of Ca and P between 24 and 36 weeks of gestation under conditions of eunutrition is illustrated in Figure 1.

A. INITIATION OF CALCIFICATION IN THE FETAL SKELETON

During the fetal period, the skeleton undergoes both development and growth. Development implies an orderly progression of changes in cell and matrix structures and relationships from the primitive embryonic beginnings to mature tissues or organs. In the case of bone tissues, the final mature structure may not be completed until well after birth, even though the basic skeletal structure is present in the newborn.[35] In contrast to development, growth may be defined simply as an increase in the mass of a preexisting structure through an increase in cell size, cell number, and/or accumulation of extracellular matrix, all of which occur in bone. The developmental processes forming fetal bone are the same as those described in Chapter 7, i.e., intramembranous and endochondral bone formation.

Development is initiated at different times for different parts of the skeleton during fetal development. The first development of structures that will become part of the skeleton occurs during the second week of gestation with formation of the notochord. The limb buds develop at 4–5 weeks after fertilization.

All bone formation begins with mesenchymal cells condensing to form either a site of membranous bone formation or a cartilaginous model that is later calcified (endochondral bone formation). Initiation of calcification of membranous bones and the appendicular skeleton occurs within the first trimester of pregnancy, but the time of this event differs for various parts of the skeleton (Table 1). The calcification of the cartilaginous models procedes by two stages; the first involves the formation of a primary osseous collar around the cartilage that is followed by vascular invasion resulting in a primary ossification center that will become the diaphysis and metaphysis. The secondary ossification center forms within the epiphyseal cartilage and generally occurs after birth. An important exception to this sequence is in the distal femoral ossification center, which is formed in utero and is considered an indicator of a full-term pregnancy.

B. RATE OF BONE MINERAL ACCRETION DURING FETAL DEVELOPMENT

Mineralization of the fetal skeleton is accomplished primarily during the third trimester. Estimates of fetal calcium and phosphorus accretion rates for weeks 24 through 36 are shown in Figure 1.

C. EFFECTS OF MATERNAL NUTRITION ON FETAL SKELETAL DEVELOPMENT

Maternal nutrition influences fetal skeletal development, but only in rather severe general undernutrition is the development of organic matrix significantly reduced because the mother mobilizes much of her own tissues to at least partially compensate for poor nutrient intakes. Under the specific conditions of inadequate mineral intake, namely that of Ca and/or P, maternal skeletal stores are resorbed to maintain a steady, but depressed, flux of these minerals across the placenta to the highly avid developing skeleton of the fetus. (Ca ions essentially flow only in one direction across the placenta from the maternal side to the fetus. If Ca, or Ca and vitamin D, replacement of malnourished mothers up to the recommended intake levels of human mothers or of animal models follows, then the fetal skeleton responds with increased Ca transfer across the placenta and greater bone mineral content, as has been reported for human neonates.[36-38] Although providing extra calcium and/or vitamin D to poorly nourished mothers is likely to have a favorable outcome for neonatal mineralization, the effect of supplementing the diets of adequately nourished mothers with additional calcium and vitamin D has not been documented.

TABLE 1
Onset of Ossification in Various Bones during Fetal Development

Bone	Onset of Ossification, Postovulatory Age
Facial bones:	
Mandible	6.0 weeks
Maxilla	6.5 weeks
Nasal	8.5 weeks
Lacrimal	10.0 weeks
Calvarial bones:	
Frontal	7.5 weeks
Parietal	8.5 weeks
Thoracic bones:	
Sternum	27.0 weeks or after
Ribs	9.5–13 weeks
Vertebrae	11–21 weeks
Upper Limb:	
Clavicle	6–7 weeks
Humerus	7.0 weeks
Radius	7–8 weeks
Ulna	8.0 weeks
Scapula	8.0 weeks
Phalanges	8–12 weeks
Lower Limb:	
Femur	8.0 weeks
Tibia	8.0 weeks
Fibula	8–9 weeks
Ilium	8.0 weeks
Phalanges	10.0 weeks-birth

Note: The bones of the fetal skeleton initiate ossification at different times that are characteristic for each bone.[39]

D. SUMMARY

The development of skeletal structures and the initiation of calcification are relatively well defined for the human fetus, although we are lacking information on the effect of maternal malnutrition on these processes. However, since the fetus must derive all of its nutritional needs from the maternal circulation via the placenta, we may expect that decreased intakes of Ca, Pi, and other essential nutrients by the mother may lead to a reduction in fetal growth and calcification. By ensuring adequate intakes of Ca and other nutrients by pregnant women, we should enhance the development and growth of the skeleton *in utero*.

VII. SUMMARY AND CONCLUSIONS

The maternal supply of adequate amounts of Ca and Pi for normal fetal growth and development represents a significant challenge to homeostatic regulatory mechanisms. This challenge especially looms large in the face of inadequate dietary provision of Ca and Pi by the mother. Although the amount of mineral transfered from mother to fetus is small compared to the skeletal reserves, the amount of Ca needed daily represents an amount similar to that absorbed from normal dietary intakes.

Although the fetus utilizes maternal nutrient supplies in order to meet its own needs for *in utero* development, it does not behave as a perfect parasite. Hence, under conditions of marginal nutrition of the mother (or dam of experimental rodents), the fetal supply of nutrients may be modestly compromised and bone development only slightly reduced, but under conditions of severe undernutrition, fetal development is typically greatly decreased.

The bone density of neonates has been found to reflect the nutritional status of the mother. Although a lack of other nutrients, such as protein and even total calories, may contribute to poor bone development, supplementation of undernourished mothers with either calcium or vitamin D has been shown to significantly increase fetal bone mineral density.

REFERENCES

1. **Garel, J.-M.,** Hormonal control of calcium metabolism during the reproductive cycle in mammals, *Physiological Reviews*, 67, 1, 1987.
2. **Pitkin, R. M.,** Human maternal-fetal calcium homeostasis, in *Perinatal Calcium and Phosphorus Metabolism*, Holick, M. F., Gray, T. K. and Anast, C. S. eds., Elsevier Science Publishers, 1983.
3. **Sowers, M. R. and Galuska, D. A.,** Epidemiology of bone mass in premenopausal women, *Epidemiol. Rev.*, 15, 374, 1993.
4. **Rodda, C. P., Kubota, M., Heath, J. A., Ebeling, P. R., Moseley, J. M., Care, A. D., Caple, I. W. and Martin, T. J.,** Evidence for a novel parathyroid hormone-related protein in fetal lamb parathyroid glands and sheep placenta: comparisons with a similar protein implicated in humoral hypercalcemia of malignancy, *J. Endocrinol.*, 117, 261, 1988.
5. **Simmonds, N.,** Reproduction and rearing of young by rats as influenced by diet, *Am. J. Hyg.*, 4, 1, 1924.
6. **Cox, W. M. and Imboden, M.,** The role of calcium and phosphorus in determining reproductive success, *J. Nutr.*, 11, 145, 1936.
7. **Snapper, I.,** *Chinese Lessons to Western Medicine: A Contribution to Geographical Medicine from the Clinics of Peiping Union Medical College*, Grune & Stratton, New York, 1965.
8. **Gruber, H. E., Gutteridge, D. H. and Baylink, D. J.,** Osteoporosis associated with pregnancy and lactation: bone biopsy and skeletal features in three patients, *Metab. Bone Dis. Rel. Res.*, 5, 159, 1984.
9. **Pitkin, R. M.,** Calcium metabolism in pregnancy: a review, *Am. J. Obstet. Gynecol.*, 121, 724, 1975.
10. **Pitkin, R. M. and Gebhardt, M. P.,** Serum calcium concentrations in human pregnancy, *Am. J. Obstet. Gynecol.*, 127, 775, 1977.
11. **Kent, G. N., Price, R. I., Gutteridge, D. H., Rosman, K. J., Smith, M., Allen, J. R., Hickling, C. J. and Blakeman, S. L.,** The efficiency of intestinal calcium absorption is increased in late pregnancy but not in established lactation, *Calcif. Tissue Int.*, 48, 293, 1991.
12. **Kent, G. N., Price, R. I., Gutteridge, D. H., Allen, J. R., Blakeman, S. L., Bhagat, C. I., St. John, A., Barnes, M. P., Smith, M. and Evans, D. V.,** Acute effects of an oral calcium load in pregnancy and lactation: findings on renal calcium conservation and biochemical indices of bone turnover, *Miner. Electrol. Metab.*, 17, 1, 1991.
13. **Whitehead, M., Lane, G., Young, O., Campbell, S., Abeyasekera, G., Hillyard, C. J., MacIntyre, I., Phang, K. G. and Stevenson, J. C.,** Interrelationships of calcium-regulating hormones during normal pregnancy, *Br. Med. J.*, 283, 10, 1981.
14. **Pederson, E. B., Johannesen, P., Kristensen, S., Rasmussen, A. B., Emmertsen, K., Moller, J., Lauritsen, J. G. and Wohlert, M.,** Calcium, parathyroid hormone and calcitonin in normal pregnancy and preeclampsia, *Gynecol. Obstet. Inv.*, 18, 156, 1984.
15. **Davis, O. K., Hawkins, D. S., Rubin, L. P., Posillico, J. T., Brown, E. M. and Schiff, I.,** Serum parathyroid hormone (PTH) in pregnant women determined by an immunoradiometric assay for intact PTH, *J. Clin. Endocrinol. Metab.*, 67, 850, 1988.
16. **Mimouni, F., Tsang, R. C., Hertzberg, V. S., Neumann, V. and Ellis, K.,** Parathyroid hormone and calcitriol changes in normal and insulin-dependent diabetic pregnancies, *Obstet. Gynecol.*, 74, 49, 1989.
17. **Heaney, R. P. and Skillman, T. G.,** Calcium metabolism in normal human pregnancy, *J. Clin. Endocrinol.*, 33, 661, 1971.
18. **Stevenson, J. C., Hillyard, C. J., MacIntyre, I., Cooper, H. and Whitehead, M. I.,** A physiological role for calcitonin: protection of the maternal skeleton, *Lancet*, ii, 769, 1979.
19. **Woloszczuk, W., Kovarik, J. and Pavelka, P.,** Calcitonin in pregnant women and in cord blood, *Gynecol. Obstet. Invest.*, 12, 272, 1981.
20. **Samaan, N. A., Hill, C. S., Jr., Beceiro, J. R. and Schultz, P. U.,** Immunoreactive calcitonin in medullary carcinoma of the thyroid and in maternal and cord serum, *J. Lab. Clin. Med.*, 81, 671, 1973.
21. **Pitkin, R. M., Reynolds, W. A., Williams, G. A. and Hargis, G. K.,** Calcium metabolism in normal pregnancy: a longitudinal study, *Am. J. Obstet. Gynecol.*, 133, 781, 1979.

22. **Miller, R. K. and Berndt, W. O.,** Evidence for Mg^{2+}-dependent, Na^+ + K^+-activated ATPase and Ca^{2+}-ATPase in the human term placenta, *Proc. Soc. Exp. Biol. Med.*, 143, 118, 1973.
23. **McKercher, H. G., Derewlany, L. O. and Radde, I. C.,** Free calcium concentrations in Krebs-Ringer bicarbonate buffer: effects of ^{45}Ca- and ^{32}P-transport across the perfused guinea pig placenta, *Biochem. Biophys. Res. Commun.*, 105, 841, 1982.
24. **Leroyer-Alizon, David, L., Anast, C. S. and Dubois, P. M.,** Immunocytochemical evidence for parathyroid hormone in human fetal parathyroid glands, *J. Clin. Endocrinol. Metab.*, 52, 513, 1981.
25. **Leroyer-Alizon, David, L. and Dubois, P. M.,** Evidence for calcitonin in the thyroid gland of normal and anencephalic human fetuses: immunocytological localization, radioimmunoassay, and gel filtration of thyroid extracts, *J. Clin. Endocrinol. Metab.*, 50, 316, 1980.
26. **Reynolds, W. A., Pitkin, R. M., Williams, G. A., Bauman, A. F., Hargis, G. K., Beluhan, F. Z. and Kawahara, W.,** Calcitonin responsiveness in the primate fetus, *J. Clin. Endocrinol. Metab.*, 51, 595, 1981.
27. National Research Council, Subcommittee on Dietary Allowances, *Recommended Dietary Allowances, 10th edition.*, National Academy Press, Washington, D.C., 1989.
28. **Sowers, M., Crutchfield, M., Jannausch, M., Updike, S. and Corton, G.,** A prospective evaluation of bone mineral change in pregnancy, *Obstet. Gynecol.*, 77, 841, 1991.
29. **Tylavsky, F. A., Curtis, R. C., Anderson, J. J. B. and Metz, J. A.,** Changes in radial and vertebral bone mass due to pregnancy and lactation in humans, *J. Bone Min. Res. (suppl. 1)*, 4, S414, 1989.
30. **Lamke, B., Brundin, J. and Moberg, P.,** Changes of bone mineral content during pregnancy and lactation, *Acta Obstet. Gynecol. Scand.*, 56, 217, 1977.
31. **Goldsmith, N. F. and Johnston, J. O.,** Bone mineral: effects of oral contraceptives, pregnancy, and lactation, *J. Bone Joint Surg.*, 57-A, 657, 1975.
32. **Drinkwater, B. L. and Chesnut, C. H., III,** Bone density changes during pregnancy and lactation in active women: a longitudinal study, *Bone Min.*, 14, 153, 1991.
33. **Greer, F. and Tsang, R. C.,** Calcium, phosphorus, magnesium, and vitamin D requirements for the preterm infant, in *Vitamin and Mineral Requirements in Preterm Infants*, Tsang, R. C. eds., Marcel Dekker, New York, 1985.
34. **Ziegler, E. E., O'Donnell, A. M., Nelson, S. E. and Fomon, S. J.,** Body composition of the reference fetus, *Growth*, 40, 329, 1976.
35. **Ogden, J. A. and Grogan, D. P.,** Prenatal development and growth of the musculoskeletal system, in *The Scientific Basis of Orthopaedics*, Albright, J. A. and Brand, R. A. eds., Appleton & Lange, Norwalk, Connecticut, 1987.
36. **Krishnamachari, K. A. V. R. and Iyengar, L.,** Effect of maternal malnutrition of bone density of the neonates, *Am. J. Clin. Nutr.*, 28, 482, 1975.
37. **Raman, L., Rajalakshmi, K., Krishnamachari, K. A. V. R. and Sastry, J. G.,** Effect of calcium supplementation to undernourished mothers during pregnancy on the bone density of the neonates, *Am. J. Clin. Nutr.*, 31, 466, 1978.
38. **Brooke, O. G., Brown, I. R. F., Bone, C. D. M., Carter, N. D., Cleeve, H. J. W., Maxwell, J. D., Robinson, V. P. and Winder, S. M.,** Vitamin D supplements in pregnant Asian women: effects on calcium status and fetal growth, *Br. Med. J.*, 280, 751, 1980.
39. **Gardner, E.,** Osteogenesis in the human embryo and fetus, in *The Biochemistry and Physiology of Bone, vol. III*, Bourne, G. H. eds., Academic Press, New York, 1971.

Chapter 16

HORMONAL CONTROL OF CALCIUM METABOLISM IN LACTATION

Svein U. Toverud, D.M.D., Ph.D. and Agna Boass, Ph.D.

TABLE OF CONTENTS

0-8493-7845-1/95/$0.00+$.50

I. INTRODUCTION

Lactation represents a physiological state in which alteration in the regulation of the mother's calcium (Ca) metabolism appears to have two major goals: to provide adequate amounts of milk with a relatively constant concentration of Ca and inorganic phosphate (Pi) for the offspring, and to maintain the Ca homeostasis of the mother. To meet the Ca demands of milk secretion, additional Ca enters the circulation either through increased intestinal Ca absorption, increased rate of bone resorption, or by increased renal tubular reabsorption of Ca. Maintenance of Ca homeostasis in the face of the significant loss of Ca in the milk is of great importance, not only for Ca-dependent maternal functions, but also for the maintenance of milk production. Severe maternal hypocalcemia tends to diminish the volume of milk produced rather than affect the Ca concentration in the milk.

Current knowledge of the mechanisms involved in the adaptive changes in intestinal Ca absorption, urinary Ca excretion, bone resorption, and Ca homeostasis are discussed in this chapter. The exact hormonal signals involved in these adaptive changes are yet to be elucidated.

II. OVERVIEW OF CHANGES IN HUMAN LACTATION

The daily amount of Ca output in the milk of nursing women may be no greater than the urinary Ca loss, i.e., 150–300 mg. This human output is in contrast to the much greater relative milk Ca output in the lactating rat, which may be 100 times that of the urinary Ca loss. Not unexpectedly, only relatively modest adaptive changes in Ca metabolism are seen in lactating women. Consistent changes include net loss of bone after several months of breast feeding and a small decrease in urinary Ca excretion. The efficiency of intestinal Ca absorption is not increased. When the lactational intensity is increased, as in women nursing twins, adaptive increases in the circulating levels of parathyroid hormone, calcitriol and calcitonin have also been observed. Based on evidence for increased bone formation rate as well as net bone loss, bone remodeling is probably markedly increased in the lactating woman.

III. REGULATION OF SERUM CALCIUM CONCENTRATION IN LACTATION

Maintenance of Ca homeostasis during lactation poses a special problem when the Ca drain into the milk is high, such as in dairy cows and rats. The sudden high efflux of Ca immediately postpartum in certain cows leads to the potentially fatal hypocalcemia of parturient paresis (milk fever) in which the salient feature is a fall in serum Ca with ensuing tetany.[1] This reproductive disorder is an example of the failure of the homeostatic mechanisms, especially parathyroid hormone, to respond quickly to the falling serum Ca concentration. In rats a lower circulating Ca concentration invariably exists during lactation than in nonlactation, but the level is never low enough to cause tetany in the intact rat. Two of the Ca-regulating hormones, parathyroid hormone (PTH) and calcitriol, are clearly of special importance during lactation, whereas the role of calcitonin remains less certain. Table 1 shows changes in serum hormone and Ca concentrations of lactating rats relative to those of nonmated rats.

A. PARATHYROID HORMONE

In the lactating rat, removal of the parathyroid glands will lead to a more rapid fall in the serum Ca concentration than in the nonlactating rat, and such an operation will be fatal unless the rat is given a high-Ca diet preoperatively.[2] The rapid fall in serum Ca is not due to the enhanced disappearance of PTH from the circulation,[3] but is rather a reflection of the greater need for the hormone during lactation. This view is supported by the finding of elevated circulating PTH levels in lactating rats,[4] as well as in women nursing twins (Table 2).[5] Recent studies using a new immunoradiometric assay specific for rat PTH indicate that circulating PTH levels are severalfold

TABLE 1
Serum Hormone and Calcium Levels during Lactation in Rats Consuming a Diet with 0.4% Ca

	Fold Elevation above the Level for Nonmated Rats (NM)		
	Weeks of Lactation		
Hormone	**1**	**2**	**3**
Parathyroid hormone	1	1.5	2–4
Calcitriol	1.5	2	3–4
Calcitonin	ND	ND	2–3
Serum Ca, % of NM	100	95	90

Note: ND = not determined
The numbers represent an approximation of data combined from several publications referenced in this chapter.[4,6,12-14,20,25,26]

TABLE 2
Serum Hormone Concentrations in Fifteen Women Nursing Twins at 6, 12, and 26 Weeks Postpartum

	Fold Elevation above Value for Mothers Nursing Single Infant:			
Hormone	**6 weeks**	**12 weeks**	**26 weeks**	**Above Normal Range for Non-Nursing Women**
Parathyroid hormone	1.7	1.7	2.1	Yes
Calcitriol	2.0	1.4*	1.4*	Yes
Calcitonin	2.3	3.1	1.5^NS	No
Serum Ca	1.1	1.1	1.0	No

Note: Values without a superscript are significantly different from those for mothers of a single infant at P <0.02
Note: NS = not significant
* Significant at P <0.1
Modified from Reference 5.

higher in lactating than in nonlactating rats.[6] In view of this observation it may seem surprising that rats maintain a significantly lowered serum Ca concentration during lactation. Are even the markedly elevated serum PTH levels insufficient for the Ca demand? This possibility was tested by large doses of PTH given to both intact and thyroidectomized lactating rats. Only in those lactating rats lacking calcitonin was there a significant increase in serum Ca.[7] The low normal serum Ca level in lactating rats appears therefore not to be due to PTH insufficiency, but rather to a combination of the antihypercalcemic effect of calcitonin and the high rate of Ca transfer to the mammary glands. Nevertheless, PTH is clearly of increased importance for Ca homeostasis during lactation in rats.

B. VITAMIN D — CALCITRIOL

Vitamin D deficiency will invariably lead to hypocalcemia during lactation. Studies by Liu et al. of lactating Chinese women with low vitamin D status revealed severe hypocalcemia and other evidence of osteomalacia.[8] In the rat even a two-week-long period of vitamin D deprivation during lactation led to significant hypocalcemia, even though the diet contained an adequate amount of Ca and phosphorus (A. Boass and S. U. Toverud, unpublished observations). Vitamin D deprivation, started at the beginning of pregnancy, caused marked hypocalcemia during lactation, resulting in hypocalcemic tetany and death of many rats, particularly those of low body weight.[9] When dietary vitamin D was withheld from rats for several months prior to pregnancy, serum Ca values as low as 4 mg/dL were obtained. However, the milk secreted by these rats had a reduced water content, and litter weight gains were greatly reduced, indicating impaired milk secretion as a consequence of the severe hypocalcemia.[7]

Vitamin D deprivation of rats from the beginning of pregnancy and throughout lactation will affect the suckling pups adversely. By the time of weaning at 3 weeks of age, the pups are hypocalcemic and hypophosphatemic and show histological evidence of rickets, including widening of the hypertrophic cartilage zone of the epiphyseal growth plate and irregular width and arrangement of the metaphyseal bone trabeculae.[10]

Hypocalcemia after vitamin D deprivation is related to the circulating calcitriol levels. In one experiment lactating rats, deprived of vitamin D from the beginning of pregnancy, were hypocalcemic and had calcitriol levels no higher than those of nonlactating vitamin D-sufficient rats, but the lactating vitamin D-sufficient rats had calcitriol levels 3–4-fold higher.[11] Elevated circulating calcitriol levels are therefore required for Ca homeostasis during lactation in rats. A similar elevation of serum calcitriol in lactating rats was shown by Halloran et al.[12] A subsequent time-course study indicated that the elevation of calcitriol is dependent on the stage of lactation and the Ca demand placed on the mother. Circulating calcitriol was increased at the end of pregnancy; it decreased immediately after parturition; it was elevated again by the end of the first week of lactation, and it remained elevated until the end of lactation, when it fell quickly to a level below that of nonlactating controls.[13]

In lactating women no consistent elevation of circulating calcitriol has been found[5,14] unless the women are nursing twins, in which case the calcitriol level is significantly elevated for at least 26 weeks of lactation (Table 2).[5]

As will be discussed below, active Ca absorption in the duodenum is still elevated in the vitamin D-deprived lactating rat, indicating that other factors besides calcitriol can stimulate active Ca transport in lactation as part of a compensatory mechanism. Hypocalcemia is, therefore, the most sensitive indicator of vitamin D insufficiency during lactation in both rats and humans.

C. CALCITONIN

Several groups have demonstrated that calcitonin secreted from the thyroid gland can prevent a rise in the serum Ca level after the administration of a parenteral or oral Ca load in both young and adult nonmated rats.[15-18] It was therefore tempting to speculate that this antihypercalcemic action of calcitonin could be particularly important during lactation because of the greatly increased influx of Ca from the intestine (see Section on Intestinal Ca Absorption during Lactation). A series of experiments with intact and acutely thyroparathyroidectomized lactating rats did indeed show that calcitonin, whether released endogenously or injected, was more effective in preventing a rise in serum Ca in lactating than in nonlactating rats.[19] A dose of calcitonin, injected into thyroparathyroidectomized lactating rats given an oral Ca load, completely prevented a large increase in serum Ca (a rise from 8 to 12 mg/dL in vehicle-injected controls), whereas the same calcitonin dose given to nonlactating rats did not affect the serum Ca compared with that of the vehicle-injected controls. Thus, the effectiveness of calcitonin to lower blood Ca appears to be greatly enhanced during lactation in rats for reasons that are not clear. In addition, circulating calcitonin levels are elevated during lactation in rats,[20,21] ewes,[22] and in women nursing twins.[5] However, in spite of the increased effectiveness of calcitonin and the increased serum levels of the hormone, the physiological importance of calcitonin secretion in lactation is still uncertain.[23]

D. SUMMARY

In the rat, clear evidence exists that both parathyroid hormone and calcitriol are of increased importance for Ca homeostasis during lactation. In the absence of either hormone, potentially fatal hypocalcemia ensues more quickly during lactation than in the nonlactating state. In rats, as well as in women nursing twins, circulating parathyroid hormone and calcitriol concentrations are elevated during lactation, presumably as a reflection of the greater need for these hormones to maintain Ca homeostasis. Circulating calcitonin concentrations are elevated during lactation not only in rats, but also in ewes and women nursing twins. However, the physiological significance of the action of calcitonin to attenuate hypercalcemia is not clear.

IV. REGULATION OF CIRCULATING HORMONE CONCENTRATIONS IN LACTATION

A. PARATHYROID HORMONE (PTH)

What is the mechanism underlying the elevated circulating PTH level in lactation? Is it solely the persistently low serum Ca level that stimulates the increase in PTH secretion during well-established lactation? Answers to these questions have not been clearly established. Other unidentified factors appear to be involved as well, because lactating rats maintained on a diet with a high Ca/Pi ratio (1.2%/0.4%), which resulted in an elevated serum Ca level, had elevated serum PTH levels as well.[3] Efforts to suppress these high serum PTH levels by injecting Ca failed, suggesting that the ability of Ca to suppress PTH secretion is diminished during lactation, or that the action(s) of other secretagogues mask(s) the suppression of PTH by Ca.[3] Hormones that have been shown to stimulate PTH secretion in nonmated rats include catecholamines, secretin, and corticosterone, but the extent to which their actions are of physiological significance is not clear. Because all three hormones circulate at elevated levels during lactation, one or more of them may conceivably play an important part in PTH secretion during lactation.

Another observation suggesting the participation of other secretagogues is the finding of elevated serum PTH levels during the first several days of lactation in rats eating a low-Ca diet before any significant fall in serum Ca can be detected.[24] One could speculate that a mechanism is needed by which PTH secretion is elevated early in lactation in anticipation of the heavy drain on the blood Ca content during mid and late lactation.

Regulation of PTH secretion during lactation clearly includes the action of a fall in serum Ca to stimulate hormone secretion. However, evidence exists that other stimulatory factors, not yet identified, are also involved in maintaining elevated circulating PTH levels in lactating rats.

B. CALCITRIOL

Circulating calcitriol levels in lactating rats vary inversely with the Ca content of the diet, as they also do in nonlactating rats, but during lactation this relationship is accentuated. Markedly elevated serum calcitriol concentrations are seen in lactating rats maintained on a low-Ca (0.1%) diet for several days, as shown in Figure 1.[25] A high-Ca diet (1.6%), on the other hand, can suppress the circulating calcitriol level to values similar to those of nonlactating rats given the high-Ca diet.

The diet-induced alterations in serum calcitriol correlate well with changes in the V_{max} of the 25-hydroxyvitamin D-1-hydroxylase in the kidney that mediates the final step in the biosynthesis of calcitriol.[26] The increase in the V_{max} of this enzyme in response to a low-Ca diet is also accentuated during lactation, based on the observations of a 20-fold higher increase in the V_{max} of the 1-hydroxylase, and a 5-fold higher increase in serum calcitriol than in nonlactating rats eating the same diet. Thus, it is not lactation itself, but factors associated with lactation, such as the drain on circulating Ca, that result in the marked stimulation of renal calcitriol synthesis. As stated above, both hypocalcemia and elevated serum parathyroid hormone concentrations are hallmarks of lactation in rats, and either of these signals could be expected to stimulate the renal 1-hydroxylase. A study was conducted in which the intensity of lactation, and, therefore, the magnitude of the changes in serum Ca and serum PTH as well, was altered by allowing rats to suckle litters of 3, 6, or 12 pups. It was found that only the serum Ca level, and not the serum phosphate or PTH concentrations, correlated significantly with the renal 1-hydroxylase V_{max}.[27] Thus, as the intensity of lactation increases, the decline in serum Ca appears to stimulate renal synthesis of calcitriol as part of the feedback regulatory system.

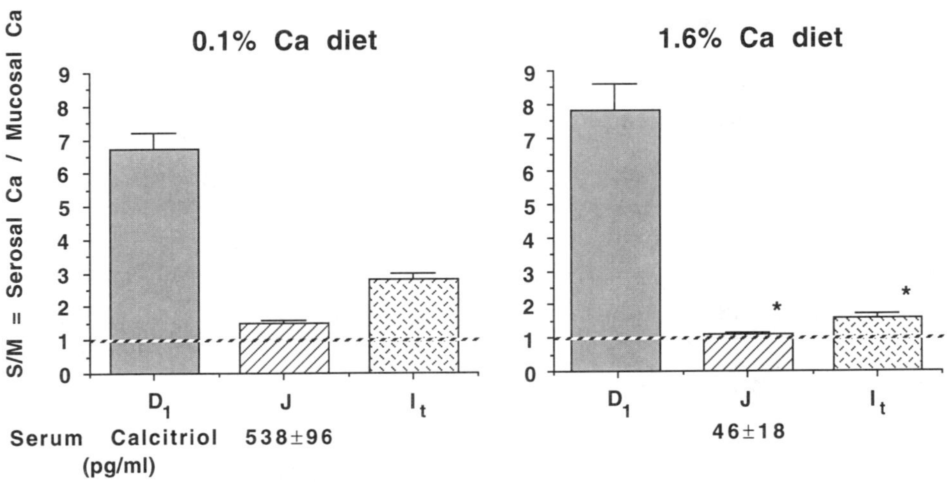

FIGURE 1. Ca Transport Ratio for Everted Sacs of Proximal Duodenum (D_1), Midjejunum (J), and Terminal Ileum (I_t) from Lactating Rats. The data represent groups of 7–10 rats at 16–23 days of lactation. The rats had been consuming the low Ca diet (0.1% Ca and 0.4% P) or the high Ca diet (1.6% Ca and 1.4% P) since 3 days before parturition. (*)Significantly different from the value for the same segment from rats consuming the 0.1% Ca diet, P <0.01. (Modified from Reference 25)

These results raised the question of the relationship of PTH to the renal 1-hydroxylase: does PTH perhaps serve only a permissive role in activating this enzyme during lactation? The answer is yes; stimulation of the 1-hydroxylase by hypocalcemia does require the presence of the parathyroid glands (or parathyroid hormone). After the removal of the parathyroid glands of lactating rats, even severe hypocalcemia did not cause stimulation of the renal 1-hydroxylase, whereas intact lactating rats had the expected marked increase in the renal 1-hydroxylase in response to a fall in serum Ca.[28]

In women nursing twins, in whom both serum PTH and serum calcitriol levels were elevated, PTH, rather than serum Ca, may play the primary role in stimulating calcitriol synthesis, because there was no evidence of concurrent hypocalcemia.[5]

In conclusion, during lactation the main physiological stimulator of increased synthesis of calcitriol appears to be a fall in serum Ca in the presence of a threshold PTH concentration. This conclusion is based entirely on work with rats, because regulation of calcitriol synthesis during lactation has not been directly investigated in other species.

C. CALCITONIN

Maintenance of elevated circulating calcitonin levels during lactation in the rat appears to be closely related to eating, based on the following observations. After a 20-hour fast, both lactating and nonlactating rats had the same low circulating calcitonin level, but after a 2-hour refeeding period the level increased threefold in the lactating rats, but remained essentially unchanged in the nonlactating rats.[19] A repeat of this experiment with larger numbers of rats would undoubtedly have shown a small rise in calcitonin in nonlactating rats as well as a larger increase in lactating rats, in view of the finding of feeding-induced increases in serum calcitonin in nonmated rats.[29] The food constituents involved in this phenomenon include glucose[30] and triglycerides,[31] as well as Ca. In the lactating rat the effect of these constituents may be accentuated, or the higher food consumption may allow stimulation by these constituents over a much longer period of time. The response to an increase in Ca concentration is also altered in lactation. Thyroid glands from lactating and nonlactating rats incubated in a high-Ca medium (2.5 m*M*) released the same amount of calcitonin. However, when the medium Ca concentration was low (1.0 m*M*), C-cells of the thyroid glands from the lactating rats released three times as much calcitonin as the glands from nonlactating rats.[32]

The enhanced release of calcitonin at low-Ca concentrations may explain in part why lactating rats in the fed state maintain higher circulating calcitonin levels than nonlactating rats in spite of their lower circulating Ca level. The elevated serum calcitonin levels in lactating rats may, therefore, result from a combination of the greatly increased food consumption and a higher sensitivity of the thyroid C-cells to the stimulatory action of serum Ca concentrations in the low end of the normal range.

D. ESTROGEN

Serum estrogen concentration falls to very low levels after parturition, and in the rat it remains low until the third week of lactation,[33] after which it increases to levels no higher than those during diestrus, and far lower than during proestrus.[34] A combination of the high prolactin levels and the suckling-induced afferent impulses to the hypothalamus contribute to the decreased estrogen secretion during the first half of lactation. Ovariectomy of rats 1–2 days after parturition does not preclude a normal course of lactation, including normal litter weight gain and the usual fall in maternal serum Ca.[35,36] Thus, estrogen does not appear to play an important role during lactation.

E. SUMMARY

When serum PTH levels are elevated in lactation, as in rats and in women nursing twins, unidentified factors, other than a fall in serum Ca, are probably involved in stimulating PTH secretion. In rats, but not in women, a hypocalcemic signal is also present. Stimulation of calcitriol synthesis in lactating rats appears to be due to a fall in serum Ca during which PTH plays a permissive role. In contrast, increased serum calcitriol levels in women nursing twins are only associated with a rise in serum PTH levels, but not with a fall in serum Ca. Increased serum calcitonin levels in lactating rats appear to be related to increased food consumption; in women nursing twins, no evidence exists for such a relationship, and the cause of the increased calcitonin levels in these women remains unknown.

V. INTESTINAL CALCIUM ABSORPTION DURING LACTATION

A. NET CALCIUM ABSORPTION

Both total amount of Ca absorbed by the intestine and the amount absorbed relative to dietary Ca intake (fractional absorption or absorption as percent of intake) are increased in the lactating rat.[1,7] During lactation, food intake gradually increases until peak lactation (14–18 days), when it may be more than five-fold higher than in nonlactating controls. The increase in the total amount of Ca absorbed is partly due to increased Ca intake and partly due to increased efficiency of the absorption, which is particularly apparent in rats given a low-Ca diet. When Fournier and Susbielle restricted their rats to an intake of only 27 mg of Ca per day, the rats absorbed almost 100% of the ingested Ca during lactation, in contrast to only a 20–40% absorption before and during the early part of pregnancy.[37] When rats are given diets containing either a moderate (0.4%) or high (1.1%) amount of Ca, lactation leads respectively, to a fourfold or twofold, increase in Ca absorbed (as percent of intake) compared to that of nonlactating controls.[7]

The increased efficiency of absorption associated with lactation disappears within a few days after the litters are removed from the mother. The weaning-induced decline in absorption efficiency is delayed when rats have been severely Ca restricted, as in the study of Fournier and Susbielle cited above.[37]

Enhanced intestinal Ca absorption has also been observed in lactating cows and sheep at least at one stage of lactation.[1,7] Lactating women, on the other hand, do not appear to have increased efficiency of Ca absorption.[38,39] Fractional Ca absorption was positively correlated with serum calcitriol concentration in one study, but neither parameter was significantly increased during lactation.[39] Increased absorption efficiency during pregnancy was first shown by Heaney and Skillman[40] and confirmed by Kent et al.[38] The difference in absorption efficiency between pregnancy and lactation may be related to the Ca drain (up to 400 mg/day) on the maternal organism during the last month of human pregnancy that is greater than at any time during lactation, which is less than 300 mg/day, even at 6 months postpartum.[7]

B. SATURABLE CALCIUM TRANSPORT

It was assumed that the increased efficiency of Ca absorption for the intestine as a whole, as just described, was due to enhanced active Ca transport in the duodenum, the only site of active Ca transport in the adult rat. Several studies have indeed confirmed that duodenal active Ca transport is increased in the lactating rat.[9,25,41-43] Using the everted gut sac technique, in which a duodenal sac is incubated in medium containing 0.4 m*M* Ca facing the mucosal surface, these investigators have found that at the end of the incubation period, the ratio of Ca concentration on the serosal side versus the concentration on the mucosal side is much higher for duodenum from lactating rats than for duodenum from nonlactating rats. This Ca concentration ratio may be as high as 8–10 during the last 2–3 days of pregnancy and the first few days of lactation. During peak lactation, ratios of 6–8 have been observed, in contrast to a ratio of only 3–4 for the duodenal transport in nonlactating rats, indicating a marked increase in the ability of the duodenum to move Ca against a concentration gradient (Figure 2).[43] Enhancement of the capacity for active Ca transport clearly can explain, at least in part, the increased efficiency of overall intestinal Ca absorption, as described previously.

The mechanism of the increased active Ca transport during lactation has not been delineated. A concurrent increase in the duodenal content of calbindin (the 9 Kd vitamin D-dependent Ca-binding protein) has also been observed during lactation, which would seem to indicate that the increased circulating calcitriol level is the mediator of the increased active Ca transport.[25] However, lactating rats maintained on a high (1.6%) Ca diet have active Ca transport ratios as high as those of Ca-restricted rats, in spite of circulating calcitriol levels only 10% of those seen in the Ca-restricted rats.[25] Thus, it appears that neither the enhanced active Ca transport nor the increased duodenal calbindin levels require the elevated serum calcitriol concentrations observed in lactation. In addition, rats with undetectable serum calcitriol, because of long-term vitamin D deprivation, have increased active Ca transport ratios during lactation.[42] The efficiency of overall intestinal Ca absorption (fractional Ca absorption) is also increased in lactating rats with undetectable circulating calcitriol.[44]

Factors other than calcitriol can probably stimulate active Ca transport in the lactating rat, but the identity of such factors is not known. Potential stimulators of active Ca transport in lactation include prolactin, because it circulates at elevated levels in lactation, and because prolactin has been shown to increase such transport in male rats with undetectable serum calcitriol.[45] However, serum prolactin levels decrease gradually during lactation, and the active Ca transport ratio increases as lactation proceeds.[43] Such discordant time courses do not support a primary role of prolactin in intestinal Ca absorption during lactation.

Active Ca transport during lactation can also be detected in the ileum and jejunum, although at much lower levels than in the duodenum.[25,43] The Ca transport ratio in the jejunum, determined with the everted gut sac technique, was only slightly, but significantly, higher than 1.0 in lactating rats consuming a diet with 0.1% Ca, suggesting that active transport in this segment is of little physiological significance.[25] The Ca transport ratio in the ileum, on the other hand, was in the range 2–3 and is assumed to be of some importance, particularly in view of the much longer transit time of the intestinal contents in this segment than in the duodenum.[25,43] The ileal Ca transport ratio, as well as the calbindin content, were directly related to the circulating calcitriol level in an experiment in which lacerating rats were given either a low-Ca or a high-Ca diet to achieve a 10-fold range of serum calcitriol concentrations.[25] Thus, during lactation in rats, active Ca transport in the ileum, appears to require a higher circulating calcitrol concentration than that in the duodenum.

C. NONSATURABLE CALCIUM TRANSFER

In the adult nonlactating rat, in which active Ca transport can be detected only in the duodenum, Ca absorption in the remainder of the small intestine presumably takes place by a passive nonsaturable process. Such nonsaturable Ca transfer was studied in lactating and nonlactating rats using the *in vivo* ligated-loop technique, in which different amounts of Ca are introduced into ligated loops of the duodenum, jejunum, or ileum of anesthetized rats. After one hour the remaining Ca content of

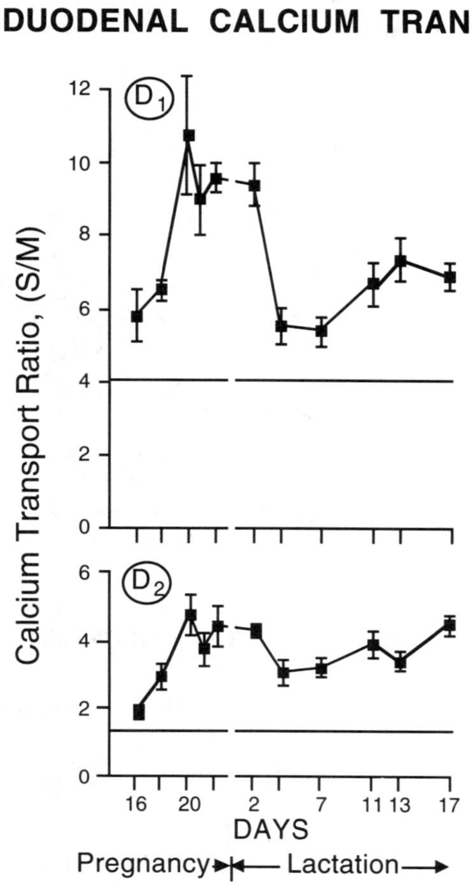

FIGURE 2. Calcium Concentration Ratios (Serosal/Mucosal = S/M) in the First (D_1) and Second (D_2) Segments of the Duodenum Obtained with the Everted Gut Sac Technique. Each segment was 3.5–4 cm long, and D_2 may have extended into the upper jejunum. The symbols represent the mean ± SE of 6–14 pregnant or lactating rats (except for D_2 for 20 d pregnant with n = 3). The horizontal line represents the mean of 31 nonmated rats, 2 or 3 of which were included in every assay with pregnant or lactating rats. The SE for the nonmated rats was 0.2 for D_1 and 0.1 for D_2. For D_1 the mean at pregnancy day 20 is significantly different (P <0.035) from the day 18 mean; the mean at lactation day 4 is significantly different (P <0.01) from the preceding mean, and the mean at day 13 is significantly different from the mean at day 7 (P <0.01). For D_2 the means at pregnancy day 20 and lactation day 4 are significantly (P <0.03) different from the immediately preceding means, respectively; the means at 7 and 17 days of lactation were significantly (P <0.01) different from each other. (From Boass, A., Lovdal, J. A., and Toverud, S. U., Pregnancy- and lactation-induced changes in active intestinal calcium transport in rats, *Am. J. Physiol.*, 263 (*Gastrointest. Liver Physiol.*, 26), G127, 1992)

the loop fluid is determined to allow an estimate of the amount of Ca absorbed per hour per length of intestine. An analysis of the regression of Ca absorbed on Ca introduced yields a value of the slope of the regression line, which is then an expression of the efficiency of nonsaturable Ca absorption. Lactating rats were found to have a higher slope of nonsaturable Ca absorption in the jejunum but not in the duodenum compared to nonlactating rats.[46] The mechanism of such enhanced nonsaturable Ca absorption during lactation is not clear. The increase is not seen until the second week of lactation; it can then be observed in the ileum as well, and it appears to be specific for Ca, because the absorption of magnesium or strontium does not appear to be increased (Boass and Toverud, unpublished observations). The increased efficiency of nonsaturable Ca absorption in the jejunum and ileum during lactation probably makes a greater contribution to overall intestinal Ca absorption than does the enhanced active Ca transport in the duodenum and ileum, unless the rats are given a low-Ca diet.

No increase in the efficiency of intestinal Ca absorption in lactating women nursing a single infant has been reported.

D. SUMMARY

In lactating women the efficiency of intestinal Ca absorption is not increased, even though the efficiency is enhanced during the later part of gestation. Absorption of Ca in women nursing twins has not been determined. In lactating rats, not only is the efficiency of overall intestinal Ca absorption enhanced, but active transport in the duodenum and ileum, as well as nonsaturable Ca absorption in the jejunum and ileum, are also increased. The stimuli for the increased active transport and nonsaturable transfer have not been identified. These phenomena in the rat constitute important aspects of adaptation to the increased Ca demands of lactation.

VI. URINARY CALCIUM EXCRETION DURING LACTATION

The amount of Ca excreted in the urine is determined mostly by the filtered load (i.e., circulating Ca concentration) and the serum PTH concentration through its action to enhance tubular reabsorption of Ca. The lower the serum Ca level and the higher the serum parathyroid hormone level, the lower the urinary Ca excretion (see Chapter 5). A small stimulating effect of calcitriol on the tubular reabsorption of Ca has been documented,[47] but its physiological significance remains unclear.

During lactation, urinary Ca excretion is reduced in cows, ewes, and rats.[7] Such findings are not surprising, because lactation usually leads to a fall in the serum Ca level and an increase in serum PTH. In lactating rats the daily loss of Ca in the urine is quite low, 2–5 mg, which is lower than in the nonlactating rat,[9] but it represents only a minute fraction of the daily loss of at least 100 mg Ca in the milk. In the vitamin D-deprived hypocalcemic lactating rat, urinary Ca excretion is even lower than in vitamin D-replete lactating rats,[9] suggesting that the lack of any vitamin D stimulation of renal tubular reabsorption of Ca is overshadowed by the low filtered Ca load.

Data from the older clinical literature suggest that urinary Ca excretion is reduced in women during lactation.[7] A recent study shows that urinary Ca loss is indeed decreased in lactating women; a 20% decrease was documented in women who had lactated for 6 months, compared with a group of age-matched nonlactating women.[48] Enhanced renal Ca conservation in lactating women was confirmed in a study of responses to an oral Ca tolerance test.[49] A reduction of 40 mg Ca per day from the approximately 200 mg loss in the urine of nonlactating women could play a significant role in the Ca balance of lactating women with a daily loss of 200–300 mg Ca in their milk. The mechanism of the enhanced renal tubular Ca reabsorption during lactation is not clear because, in contrast to the lactating rats, the breast-feeding mothers had unaltered serum Ca, parathyroid hormone, and calcitriol concentrations.[48]

Regardless of mechanism, renal Ca conservation appears to be one of the two major adaptive phenomena affecting calcium conservation during human lactation, the other being Ca mobilization from bone via an increased rate of bone resorption.

VII. LACTATION-MEDIATED BONE LOSS

A. LACTATING RATS

Pregnancy in rats is associated with increased weight of femur and femur ash. Miller et al. found a 10–12% increase in both parameters by 14 days of pregnancy in rats consuming a diet with an adequate Ca content (0.6%).[50] The increased bone weight appeared to be due to an increased bone formation rate.[50] Lactation in rats, on the other hand, invariably leads to a net loss of bone. The same authors found a 20–25% decrease in femur weight and femur ash weight after 3 weeks of lactation. Thus, at the end of lactation the rats had lost far more bone than they had gained during pregnancy. According to analyses of lumbar vertebrae, the bone formation rate in rats is increased during lactation,[50] but the bone resorption rate must therefore be increased even more in order to account for the net loss of bone mass. The extent of the bone loss is greater the lower the Ca content of the diet. Rats given a diet with 0.04% or 0.02% Ca had a significantly greater loss of bone mass than rats on a diet with 0.4% or 0.5% Ca,[4,35] confirming results from earlier investigations.[7] Little if any loss takes place until the second week of lactation when most of the loss occurs; a smaller loss is seen during the third and last week of lactation.[4,51] Litter size, through its effect on lactational intensity, can affect the amount of bone loss, as indicated by a doubling of the bone mineral loss when dams with 7–11 pups were compared with dams with 2–3 pups at the end of lactation.[52] The latter authors showed that several mechanical properties of lactating rat bone correlate well with the bone ash content, indicating that, with increasing bone loss, bone strength diminishes and the risk of fracture increases.

Efforts to prevent lactation-induced bone loss by increasing the Ca content of the diet up to 1.4% in the presence of 0.3% phosphorus, or to 1.2% with 1.2% phosphorus were not successful,[35] but when a diet with 1.6% Ca and 1.2% phosphorus was combined with Ca and added to the drinking water, bone loss could be prevented.[25] However, the latter regimen provides the rats with a daily Ca intake of over 1100 mg, which is extreme and clearly superphysiological. The amount of Ca absorbed when lactating rats are given a diet with moderately high Ca content (1.2%) exceeds by far the amount of Ca lost in the milk and the small amount of Ca lost in the urine (A. Boass and S. U. Toverud, unpublished results), indicating that the bone loss takes place in spite of a positive Ca balance. Thus, perhaps in all species, lactation-mediated bone loss appears to be a normal, physiological process that can be modulated, but not prevented, except by increasing the Ca and phosphorus intake to extreme levels.

The mechanism of lactation-induced bone loss has not yet been elucidated. Surprisingly, PTH is not required for this process, based on the finding of no significant alteration in bone loss in lactating rats deprived of their parathyroid glands.[2,53] Severe vitamin D deficiency, ovariectomy,[36] or adrenalectomy did not prevent or alter the magnitude of the lactation-mediated bone loss in rats.[35] The lack of an ovariectomy effect is not surprising, because the circulating estrogen levels remain very low during the second week of lactation, when most of the bone loss takes place. Efforts to prevent the bone loss by raising the circulating estradiol level, with hormone injections, to that of nonmated rats at diestrus only decreased the bone loss by a third (i.e., from 30% to 20%).[54] Thus, the low circulating estrogen concentration during lactation cannot be the major cause of the bone loss.

Endogenous calcitonin has a slight protective effect against the bone loss in lactating rats, but this effect is no greater than in nonlactating control rats.[55] This conclusion is based on the observation that thyroidectomized rats with transplanted parathyroid glands and replacement doses of thyroxine (calcitonin-deficient rats) had the same small, but significant, reduction in bone weight and ash content compared to thyroid-intact rats over a three-week period, whether they were lactating or not.

The sites of bone loss appear to be primarily the trabeculae of the vertebrae and the metaphyses of tibias and femurs and, to a lesser extent, the endosteal surfaces of the diaphyses of the long bones.[49,55-57] These observations have been obtained by a variety of techniques, such as chemical, histological, and scanning electron microscopic (SEM) techniques, but also with the less disruptive procedure of single-photon absorptiometry (SPA).[57,58] The SPA technique has the advantage of allowing scanning of the intact, anesthetized rat femur so that repeated measurements of bone density at different sites of the femur can be obtained from the same rat at different stages of lactation. Preliminary observations (J. R. Hagaman and A. Boass, unpublished results) obtained with this procedure revealed a significantly greater degree of bone density loss in the femurs of lactating rats consuming a diet with 0.4% Ca than in the femurs of lactating rats given diet with 1.6% Ca. At the end of lactation most, if not all, of the lost bone is replenished over a few weeks, whether the rat becomes pregnant immediately after the lactation period or undergoes a rest period.[57,59]

B. LACTATING WOMEN

Net bone loss in lactating women has been documented in several recent studies. Wardlaw and Pike found a 15% lower bone mass at the ultradistal site of the forearm (containing primarily trabecular bone) in women who had breast-fed each of 3 children for approximately 11 months compared with women who had breast-fed each of 3 children for an average of only 3 months.[60] The lower bone mass in the long-term breast-feeding mothers occurred in spite of a mean daily Ca intake of 1600 mg while they were pregnant and lactating, and 1150 mg while they were nonpregnant. It is not clear how soon after the last lactation the bone mass was determined, and it is possible that the women were in the process of replenishing their bone loss, as will be discussed below in connection with a more recent study.

Hayslip et al.[61] found a significant 6.5% loss of mineral content from the lumbar spine, a trabecular-rich site, after 3 and 6 months of exclusive breast-feeding by 19 women. Kent et al. examined women who had lactated for 6 months, and found a 7% loss of bone mineral density in the most distal site of the forearm.[48] According to markers of bone formation rate (serum alkaline phosphatase) and bone resorption rate (urinary hydroxyproline after overnight fast), bone resorption appeared to be increased more than bone formation, which is consistent with the observation of net bone loss.[48] Similarly, in a calcium kinetic study of a small group of women who had nursed for 5–9 weeks, the increase in bone resorption rate (V_0-) was significantly greater than the increase in the bone accretion rate (V_0+).[39] According to the study by Kent et al.,[48] recovery of the lost bone appeared to have occurred within 6 months after weaning, during which time the increase in bone formation rate persisted, whereas the bone resorption rate had decreased compared to the rates measured during different stages of lactation. Another study of women breast-feeding for different lengths of time revealed that those breast-feeding for less than 5 months had no significant bone loss at any time. Measurements made at 6 months postpartum of women providing breast milk for at least 5 months showed losses of bone mineral density of approximately 5% at the lumbar spine and femoral neck compared to baseline values; at the femoral neck a 4% loss was seen at 4 months postpartum in this group of women.[62] However, a return towards baseline values at 12 months postpartum occurred in women who continued to breast-feed beyond 6 months. A complete return to baseline values would undoubtedly have been observed if the women who continued to nurse for the full 12 months had been eliminated from the comparison.

The significant bone loss in women breast-feeding more than 6 months occurred in spite of a relatively high Ca intake, 1600 mg/day, which may or may not replenish the mothers' Ca losses in urine and milk, depending on the intestinal Ca absorption efficiency, which was not determined in this study.[62] However, using the authors' estimate of 20% efficiency and assuming 200–250 mg of Ca lost in the milk per day, the net amount of Ca absorbed, 320 mg, would not be sufficient to cover the loss in both the milk and the urine. The latter has been found to be in the same range as the loss in the milk for women.[7] These women may, therefore, have been in a negative Ca balance, which would be conducive to enhancement of bone resorption. On the other hand, if the intestinal Ca absorption efficiency were higher than the 20% estimate, the women may have been in a positive Ca balance. The reason for the bone loss by lactating women, as well as by rats given diets with moderately high Ca contents, remains unknown.

The long-term consequences of lactation-mediated bone loss have not been well defined. If the loss is replenished within several months postlactation, even repeated pregnancies and lactations would not be expected to have adverse skeletal consequences, unless periods of prolonged lactation coincided with pregnancies. Because the bone loss during lactation is the result of a normal process, and not a pathological phenomenon, the possibility exists that the concomitant increase in the rate of bone formation, albeit less than the increase in the rate of bone resorption, may be of benefit for subsequent bone metabolism and perhaps reduce the risk of postmenopausal osteoporosis. The enhanced remodeling of bone during lactation could provide a significant amount of new and qualitatively superior bone. The consequences of lactation for the bone mass in postmenopausal women were examined in over 2300 women by bone mineral density measurements of the distal radius (60% cortical and 40% trabecular bone).[63] Over 60% of the women had breast-fed an average of 1.9 children for a total of 7.4 months. Breast-feeding appeared to have provided a 1% increase (not statistically significant) in bone mineral density. A review of the literature by Fox et al. indicated that most studies failed to reveal a significant effect of lactation on bone mass by the time the women were postmenopausal.[63]

C. SUMMARY

Women who breast-feed for a minimum of 6 months appear to lose between 5 and 15% of their bone mass, according to bone mineral density determinations of the distal forearm, lumbar spine, or femoral neck. These sites contain more trabecular than cortical bone. Most, if not all, of the lost bone is replenished over a period of months after lactation ceases. When measurements were made in postmenopausal women late in life, the majority of studies in developed nations revealed no significant adverse effects of multiple lactations on bone mineral mass compared to that of similarly aged nulliparous women.

Rats gain bone at the end of pregnancy, but lose an even greater amount during lactation. The bone loss, mainly trabecular, is related to lactational intensity (litter size) and can be prevented only by supplying diets that are extremely high in Ca and phosphorus. The stimulus for the bone loss remains unknown; neither PTH, vitamin D, nor ovarian or adrenal hormones appear to be required for the bone loss. Essentially all of the lost bone is replenished during the postlactational period if adequate amounts of dietary Ca and Pi are supplied.

VIII. CALCIUM AND VITAMIN D IN MILK

The total vitamin D content of breast milk represents a source of antirachitic activity for the offspring. The other source is cholecalciferol generated from 7-dehydrocholesterol in the skin under the influence of ultraviolet (UV) radiation. However, many newborn infants may not get sufficient exposure to the sun to protect them adequately against rickets. Milk as a source of vitamin D may therefore play an important role in the growth and development of the offspring. However, the amount of vitamin D activity in breast milk is low even when the mother's vitamin D status is adequate (see below).

If pregnant rats are deprived of dietary vitamin D and UV light exposure, rat pups at 2–3 weeks of age will show evidence of human-type rickets, including hypocalcemia and hypophosphatemia, widening of the hypertrophic cartilage zone of the growth plate, irregular arrangement and thickening of the bony trabeculae, reduced bone ash, and undetectable serum 25-OHD_3 level.[10] Reduced placental transfer of vitamin D activity to the fetuses may also have contributed to the pups' vitamin D deficiency. Further evidence that maternal vitamin D status can affect the milk vitamin D activity was obtained when vitamin D-replete lactating rats were given doses of vitamin D high enough to cause hypercalcemia in the mother as well as in the pups.[64] Analysis of the milk revealed the presence of mostly vitamin D, a smaller amount of 25-OHD_3, and only minute amounts of calcitriol. However, when calcitriol was given to the lactating rats in amounts sufficient to cause maternal hypercalcemia, the pups showed no elevation of serum Ca or other evidence of toxicity.[64] Thus, very little calcitriol is conveyed to the offspring through the milk, even in the face of toxic concentrations of the hormone in the mother.

Bovine and human milk contain an amount of vitamin D activity that reflects the maternal vitamin D status.[1] Superphysiological doses of vitamin D given to lactating women resulted in high concentrations of vitamin D in the milk, which is similar to observations in rats described previously. Whereas the major metabolite in rat milk is vitamin D_3, bovine and human milk contain mostly 25-OHD_3. Both bovine and human milk have far lower total vitamin D activity per liter than the recommended dietary allowance (RDA) of vitamin D for infants and children (400 IU = 10 m g).[65,66] Bovine milk sold commercially in the U.S. is therefore fortified with vitamin D to contain 400–500 IU/L. However, the actual vitamin D content may be far lower (or substantially higher, as well) than the stated amount. A recent survey of milk samples from 10 states in the U.S. revealed that 14% of the samples had undetectable amounts, and another 37% had between 5–80% of the stated amount of vitamin D.[67]

In spite of the low vitamin D content of human milk (approximately 25 IU/L), term infants rarely develop rickets, and vitamin D supplementation may not be necessary for those infants who are breast-fed for 6 months or less and whose mothers have adequate vitamin D intake or sun exposure. However, rickets is more prevalent when the mother has a low vitamin D/Ca status or the infant is shielded from sun exposure. Many pediatricians will, therefore, recommend additional vitamin D for all breast-fed infants.[68]

The Ca and Pi contents of milk relative to total milk solids appear to remain quite constant in spite of marked changes in serum Ca and phosphorus concentrations.[2] PTH does not affect the Ca content of the milk directly. However, after removal of the parathyroid glands, the ensuing hypocalcemia will lead to reduction in the water content of the milk, but if normocalcemia can be maintained by an increase of the Ca/Pi ratio in the diet, the water content will remain unaltered.[2] Hypocalcemia following vitamin D deprivation will also cause a reduction in the milk water content. Hypophosphatemia, on the other hand, does not affect milk composition. Thus, the only influence of parathyroid hormone and vitamin D on the Ca and phosphorus contents of milk is through their effects on the serum Ca concentration.

IX. PARATHYROID HORMONE-RELATED PEPTIDE

Parathyroid hormone-related peptide (PTHrP) is synthesized in milk-secreting mammary glands and is present in high concentrations in the milk of many species, including women. However, PTHrP is discussed only briefly, because its physiological role, if any, is not clear.[69] PTHrP is a peptide of 140 amino acids with moderate homology with PTH in the 1-34 N-terminal region. PTHrP interacts with PTH receptors in many tissues and can therefore mimic the effect of PTH on bone to increase the serum Ca concentration and on kidney to enhance urinary phosphate excretion. PTHrP was discovered as the substance that mediates the manifestations of humoral hypercalcemia of malignancy.

The relationship of this peptide to lactation was established in 1988 by Thiede and Rodan, who detected mRNA for PTHrP in mammary tissue of actively suckled rats.[70] Evidence for a stimulatory effect of prolactin on PTHrP message was subsequently reported.[71] PTHrP has also been found in high, nanomolar concentrations in the milk of cows, humans,[72] and rats.[73] Efforts to detect PTHrP in the circulation of lactating rats were unsuccessful, until Miller et al. found detectable levels after extracting and concentrating the plasma.[74] A recent clinical study reported detectable circulating PTHrP levels in the range 2–8 pmol/L in 12 of 19 breast-feeding mothers compared to undetectable levels (<2 pmol/L) in all of 16 bottle-feeding mothers and in all but one of 18 pregnant women.[75] The serum PTHrP concentration in the breast-feeding mothers was similar to their circulating PTH concentration (mean: 2.3 pmol/L). Barlet et al. found in lactating dairy cows prompt, but transient, rises in PTHrP concentrations in mammary venous blood plasma during morning and evening milking.[76] This milking-induced release of PTHrP into the circulation was followed by an increase in renal phosphate clearance, suggesting that the mammary-produced PTHrP exerted an endocrine effect on the kidneys. The physiological significance of this response to PTHrP and a similar suckling-induced phosphaturia in lactating rats[77] is not clear.

In addition to a potential endocrine role of suckling-induced PTHrP release, this peptide may also exert a paracrine action on the mammary gland to increase the blood flow to the gland, based on evidence in ewes,[78] the ability of PTHrP to mediate vasodilation,[79] and on the increased expression of PTHrP mRNA in vascular smooth muscle in inguinal vessels next to the mammary gland in connection with suckling.[80] Other suggestions for the role of mammary-produced PTHrP include actions in the offspring, perhaps in Ca homeostasis.[81]

X. SUMMARY AND CONCLUSIONS

Adaptations of Ca metabolism to the increased demands of lactation appear to differ among the species discussed here. The key to these differences may be the Ca loss in the milk relative to other Ca losses, particularly that in the urine. A comparison between rats and women reveals that rats secrete milk with a Ca content almost 10 times that of women, the hourly Ca loss in the milk relative to body weight is 60 times higher in the rat, and the ratio of Ca loss in the milk relative to the Ca loss in the urine is over 100-fold in the rat compared to a ratio of nearly 1 in women. That fewer lactation-induced changes are seen in women than in rats should, therefore, not be surprising. Changes noted in rats, but not in women breast-feeding a single infant, include increases in serum concentrations of all three Ca-regulating hormones and increased efficiency of intestinal Ca absorption. One could argue that the much lower relative mammary Ca demand in women obviates the need for enhanced Ca absorption and the need for increased secretion of PTH and calcitriol to maintain Ca homeostasis. However, as was noted in the study of women nursing twins,[5] the increased Ca demand was associated with significantly higher circulating concentrations of all three Ca-regulating hormones relative to women nursing a single infant. Whether intestinal Ca absorption is enhanced in these women, who often produce more than two liters of milk per day, is not yet known. Thus, greater similarity exists between lactating women and rats than what at first may appear. Lactational intensity, as determined by the number of offspring nursed, was shown to be positively correlated with serum PTH and calcitriol concentrations in the rat, and the same correlation appears to hold in nursing women as well.

Returning to the comparison between the more usual milk demand of a single human infant and a litter of 10–14 rat pups, both species of mothers of these offspring experience net bone loss even in the presence of a presumed positive Ca balance. Based on studies in the rat, the bone loss appears to be unrelated to vitamin D, PTH, or adrenal or ovarian hormones. The other similarity between the two species is a reduction in urinary Ca excretion. However, the consequence of this reduction is markedly different in the two species. In the rat, which excretes very little Ca in the urine, this reduction makes only a very small contribution to the Ca balance. In women, on the other hand, who lose approximately as much Ca in the urine as in the milk during lactation, even a 20% reduction in urinary Ca makes a significant contribution to the Ca economy.

Many questions concerning the regulation of bone and Ca metabolism during lactation remain unanswered.

- What is the signal for increased bone remodeling and net bone loss?
- Why is urinary Ca excretion reduced during human lactation?
- What stimulates intestinal Ca absorption in lactating rats?
- Are there lactation-associated secretagogues for PTH in addition to hypocalcemia in rats?
- Is calcitonin important during lactation?

Because human lactation studies are difficult to initiate and conduct, answers are more likely to come from animal studies.

Note in proof: In a study of 10 women urinary Ca excretion during lactation was significantly lower than during pregnancy, but not lower than during the prepregnant period. (Cross, N. A., Hillman, L. S., Allen, S. H., Krause, G. F., and Vieira, N. E., Calcium homeostasis and bone metabolism during pregnancy, lactation, and postweaning: a longitudinal study, *Am. J. Clin. Nutr.*, 61, 514, 1995).

REFERENCES

1. **Garel, J.-M.,** Hormonal control of calcium metabolism during the reproductive cycle in mammals, *Physiol. Rev.*, 67, 1, 1987.
2. **Garner, S. C., Boass, A., and Toverud, S. U.,** Parathyroid hormone is not required for normal milk composition or secretion or lactation-associated bone loss in normocalcemic rats, *J. Bone Miner. Res.*, 5, 69, 1990.
3. **Garner, S. C., Boass, A., and Toverud, S. U.,** Hypercalcemia fails to suppress elevated serum parathyroid hormone concentrations during lactation in rats, *J. Bone Miner. Res.*, 4, 577, 1989.
4. **Garner, S. C., Peng, T.-C., Hirsch, P. F., Boass, A., and Toverud, S. U.,** Increase in serum parathyroid hormone concentration in the lactating rat: effects of dietary calcium and lactational intensity, *J. Bone Miner. Res.*, 2, 347, 1987.

5. **Greer, F. R., Lane, J., and Ho, M.,** Elevated serum parathyroid hormone, calcitonin, and 1,25-dihydroxyvitamin D in lactating women nursing twins, *Am. J. Clin. Nutr.*, 40, 562, 1984.
6. **Schultz, V. L., Garner, S. C., Lavigne, J. R., and Toverud, S. U.,** Determination of bioactive rat parathyroid hormone concentrations *in vivo* and *in vitro* by a 2-site homologous immunoradiometric assay, *Bone Miner.*, 27, 121, 1994.
7. **Toverud, S. U. and Boass, A.,** Hormonal control of calcium metabolism in lactation, *Vitamins and Hormones,* 37, 303, 1979.
8. **Liu, S., Su, C. C., Wang, C. W., and Chang, K. P.,** Calcium and phosphorus metabolism in osteomalacia. VI. The added drain of lactation and beneficial action of vitamin D, *Chin. J. Physiol.*, 11, 271, 1937.
9. **Boass, A., Toverud, S. U., Pike, J. W., and Haussler, M. R.,** Calcium metabolism during lactation: enhanced intestinal calcium absorption in vitamin D-deprived hypocalcemic rats, *Endocrinology*, 109, 900, 1981.
10. **Boass, A., Ramp, W. K., and Toverud, S. U.,** Hypocalcemic, hypophosphatemic rickets in rat pups suckling vitamin D-deprived mothers, *Endocrinology*, 109, 505, 1981.
11. **Boass, A., Toverud, S. U., McCain, T. A., Pike, J. W., and Haussler, M. R.,** Elevated serum levels of 1a, 25-dihydroxycholecalciferol in lactating rats, *Nature (London)*, 267, 630, 1977.
12. **Halloran, B. P., Barthell, E. M., and DeLuca, H. F.,** Vitamin D metabolism during pregnancy and lactation in the rat, *Proc. Natl. Acad. Sci., USA*, 76, 5549, 1979.
13. **Pike, J. W., Parker, J. B., Haussler, M. R., Boass, A., and Toverud, S. U.,** Dynamic changes in circulating 1,25-dihydroxyvitamin D during reproduction in rats, *Science*, 204, 1427, 1979.
14. **Hillman, L., Sateesha, S., Haussler, M., Wiest, W., Slatopolsky, E., and Haddad, J.,** Control of mineral homeostasis during lactation: interrelationships of 25-hydroxyvitamin D, 24,25 dihydroxyvitamin D, 1,25 dihydroxyvitamin D, parathyroid hormone, calcitonin, prolactin, and estradiol, *Am. J. Obstet. Gynecol.*, 139, 471, 1981.
15. **Munson, P. L. and Gray, T. K.,** Function of thyrocalcitonin in normal physiology, *Fed. Proc. Fed. Am. Soc. Exp. Biol.,* 29, 1200, 1970.
16. **Harper, C. and Toverud, S. U.,** Ability of thyrocalcitonin to protect against hypercalcemia in adult rats, *Endocrinology*, 93, 1354, 1973.
17. **Perault-Staub, A. M., Staub, J. F., and Milhaud, G.,** A new concept of plasma calcium homeostasis in the rat, *Endocrinology*, 95, 480, 1974.
18. **Talmage, R. V., Doppelt, S. H., and Cooper, C. W.,** Relationship of blood concentrations of calcium phosphate, gastrin and calcitonin to the onset of feeding in the rat, *Proc. Soc. Exp. Biol. Med.*, 149, 855, 1975.
19. **Toverud, S. U., Harper, C., and Munson, P. L.,** Calcium metabolism during lactation: enhanced effects of thyrocalcitonin, *Endocrinology*, 99, 371, 1976.
20. **Toverud, S. U., Cooper, C. W., and Munson, P. L.,** Calcium metabolism during lactation: elevated blood levels of calcitonin, *Endocrinology*, 103, 472, 1978.
21. **Besnard, P. and Garel, J.-M.,** Concentrations plasmatiques de calcitonine immunoreactive chez la ratte au cours de la lactation, *C. R. Seances Acad. Sci. Ser. III Sci. Vie,* 299, 311, 1984.
22. **Barlet, J.-P. and Garel, J.-M.,** Physiological role of calcitonin in pregnant goats and ewes, in *Calcium-Regulating Hormones*, Talmage, R. V., Owen, M., and Parsons, J. A., eds., Exerpta Med., Amsterdam, 1975.
23. **Talmage, R. V., Cooper, C. W., and Toverud, S. U.,** The physiological significance of calcitonin, in *Bone and Mineral Research, Annual 1*, Peck, W. A., ed., Excerpta Medica, Princeton, 1983.
24. **Garner, S. C., Peng, T.-C., and Toverud, S. U.,** Modulation of serum parathyroid hormone and ionized calcium concentrations during reproduction in rats fed a low calcium diet, *J. Bone Miner. Res.*, 3, 319, 1988.
25. **Bruns, M. E., Boass, A., and Toverud, S. U.,** Regulation by dietary calcium of vitamin D-dependent calcium-binding protein and active calcium transport in the small intestine of lactating rats, *Endocrinology*, 121, 278, 1987.
26. **Lobaugh, B., Boass, A., Lester, G. E., and Toverud, S. U.,** Regulation of serum 1,25-dihydroxyvitamin D_3 in lactating rats, *Am. J. Physiol.*, 259 (*Endocrinol. Metab.*, 22), E665, 1990.
27. **Lobaugh, B., Boass, A., Garner, S., C., and Toverud, S. U.,** Intensity of lactation modulates renal 1a-hydroxylase and serum 1,25-dihydroxyvitamin D in the rat, *Am. J. Physiol.*, 262 (*Endocrinol. Metab.*, 25), E840, 1992.
28. **Lobaugh, B., Garner, S. C., Lovdal, J. A., Boass, A., and Toverud, S. U.,** Parathyroidectomy abolishes the increase of renal 25-hydroxyvitamin D-1a-hydroxylase in lactating rats, *Am. J. Physiol.*, 264 (*Endocrinol. Metab.*, 27), E981, 1993.
29. **Peng, T.-C. and Garner, S. C.,** Serum calcium and calcitonin in fed and fasted rats of different ages, *Fed. Proc. Fed. Am. Soc. Exp. Biol.*, 37, 887, 1978.
30. **Cooper, C. W. and Obie, J. F.,** Hypocalcemia and increased serum calcitonin in baby rats given glucose orally, *Proc. Soc. Exp. Biol. Med.*, 157, 374, 1978.
31. **Garel, J.-M. and Besnard, P.,** Milk factors controlling the plasma calcitonin level in the newborn rat, *Endocrinology*, 104, 1617, 1979.
32. **Toverud, S. U., Becker, D. I., Boass, A., Cooper, C. W., Hirsch, P. F., Ontjes, D. A., Peng, T.-C., and Ramp, W. K.,** Hormonal control of calcium metabolism in lactation, in *Endocrinology of Calcium Metabolism*, Copp, D. H. and Talmage, R. V., eds., Exerpta Med. Found., Amsterdam, 1978.

33. **Smith, M. S. and Neill, J. D.,** Inhibition of gonadotropin secretion during lactation in the rat: relative contribution of suckling and ovarian steroids, *Biol. Reprod.*, 17, 255, 1977.
34. **Smith, M. S., Freeman, M. E., and Neill, J. D.,** The control of progesterone secretion during the estrous cycle and early pseudopregnancy in the rat: prolactin, gonadotropin and steroid levels associated with rescue of the corpus luteum of pseudopregnancy, *Endocrinology,* 96, 219, 1975.
35. **Brommage, R. and DeLuca, H. F.,** Regulation of bone mineral loss during lactation, *Am. J. Physiol.,* 248 (*Endocrinol. Metab.,* 11), E182, 1985.
36. **Anderson, J. J. B., Garner, S. C., Mar, M.-H., Boass, A., Toverud S. U., and Parikh, I.,** The ovariectomized, lactating rat as an experimental model for osteopenia: calcium metabolism and bone changes, *Bone Miner.,* 11, 43, 1990.
37. **Fournier, P. and Susbielle, H.,** Les echanges de calcium chez le rat au cours de la gestation, de la lactation et du sevrage. 2- Influence d'un regime pauvre en calcium, *J. Physiol. (Paris),* 44, 575, 1952.
38. **Kent, G. N., Price, R. I., Gutteridge, D. H., Rosman, K. J., Smith, M., Allen, J. R., Hickling, C. J., and Blakeman, S. L.,** The efficiency of intestinal calcium absorption is increased in late pregnancy but not in established lactation, *Calcif. Tissue Int.*, 48, 293, 1991.
39. **Specker, B. L., Vieira, N. E., O'Brien, K. O., Ho, M. L., Heubi, J. E., Abrams, S. A., and Yergey, A. L.,** Calcium kinetics in lactating women with low and high calcium intakes, *Am. J. Clin. Nutr.*, 59, 593, 1994.
40. **Heaney, R. P. and Skillman, T. G.,** Calcium metabolism in normal human pregnancy, *J. Clin. Endocrinol. Metab.*, 33, 661, 1971.
41. **Kostial, K., Grunden, N., and Durakovic, A.,** Intestinal absorption of calcium-47 and strontium-85 in lactating rats, *Calcif. Tissue Res.*, 4, 13, 1969.
42. **Halloran, B. P. and DeLuca, H. F.,** Calcium transport in small intestine during pregnancy and lactation, *Am. J. Physiol.*, 239 (*Endocrinol. Metab.*, 2): E64, 1980.
43. **Boass, A., Lovdal, J. A., and Toverud, S. U.,** Pregnancy- and lactation-induced changes in active intestinal calcium transport in rats, *Am. J. Physiol.*, 263, (*Gastrointest. Liver Physiol.*, 26), G127, 1992.
44. **Brommage, R., Baxter, D. C., and Gierke, L. W.,** Vitamin D-independent intestinal calcium and phosphorus absorption during reproduction, *Am. J. Physiol.*, 259 (*Gastrointest. Liver Physiol.,* 22), G631, 1990.
45. **Pahuja, D. N. and DeLuca, H. F.,** Stimulation of intestinal calcium transport and bone calcium mobilization by prolactin in vitamin D-deficient rats, *Science,* 214, 1038, 1981.
46. **Boass, A. and Toverud, S. U.,** Lactation in rats leads to enhanced nonsaturable calcium absorption in the jejunum, in *Vitamin D: Chemical, Biochemical and Clinical Endocrinology of Calcium Metabolism. Proceedings of the 5th Workshop on Vitamin D,* Norman, A. W., Schaefer, K, v. Herrath, D., and Grigoleit, H.-G., eds., de Gruyter, Berlin, 321, 1982.
47. **Kawashima, H. and Kurokawa, K.,** Metabolism and sites of action of vitamin D in the kidney, *Kidney Int.*, 29, 98, 1986.
48. **Kent, G. N., Price, R. I., Gutteridge, D. H., Smith, M., Allen, J. R., Bhagat, C. I., Barnes, M. P., Hickling, C. J., Retallack, R. W., Wilson, S. G., Devlin, R. D., Davies C., and St. John, A.,** Human lactation: forearm trabecular bone loss, increased bone turnover, and renal conservation of calcium and inorganic phosphate with recovery of bone mass following weaning, *J. Bone Miner. Res.*, 5, 361, 1990.
49. **Kent, G. N., Price, R. I., Gutteridge, D. H., Allen, J. R., Blakeman, S. L., Bhagat, C. I., St. John, A., Barnes, M. P., Smith, M., and Evans, D. V.,** Acute effects of an oral calcium load in pregnancy and lactation: findings on renal calcium conservation and biochemical indices of bone turnover, *Miner. Electrolyte Metab.*, 17, 1, 1991.
50. **Miller, S. C., Shupe, J. G., Redd, E. H., Miller, M. A., and Omura, T. H.,** Changes in bone mineral and bone formation rates during pregnancy and lactation in rats, *Bone*, 7, 283, 1986.
51. **Peng, T.-C., Kusy, R.P., Garner, S. C., Hirsch, P. F., and de Blanco, M. C.,** Influence of lactation and pregnancy plus lactation on mechanical properties and mineral content of the rat femur, *J. Bone Miner. Res.*, 2, 249, 1987.
52. **Peng, T.-C., Garner, S. C., Kusy, R.P., and Hirsch, P. F.,** Effect of number of suckling pups and dietary calcium on bone mineral content and mechanical properties of femurs of lactating rats, *Bone Miner.*, 3, 293, 1988.
53. **Hodnett, D. W., DeLuca, H. F., and Jorgensen, N. A.,** Bone mineral loss during lactation occurs in absence of parathyroid tissue, *Am. J. Physiol.*, 262 (*Endocrinol. Metab.*, 25), E233, 1992.
54. **Garner, S. C., Anderson, J. J. B., Mar, M.-H., and Parikh, I.,** Estrogens reduce bone loss in the ovariectomized, lactating rat model, *Bone Miner.,* 15, 19, 1991.
55. **Hirsch, P. F. and Hagaman, J. R.,** Reduced bone mass in calcitonin-deficient rats whether lactating or not, *J. Bone Miner. Res.*, 1, 199, 1986.
56. **Rasmussen, P.,** Calcium deficiency, pregnancy, and lactation in rats, *Calcif. Tissue Res.*, 23, 87, 1977.
57. **Hagaman, J. R., Ambrose, W. W., and Hirsch, P. F.,** A scanning electron microscopic and photon absorptiometric study of the development, prolongation, and pattern of recovery from lactation-induced osteopenia in rats, *J. Bone Miner. Res.*, 5, 123, 1990.
58. **Hagaman, J. R., Sanchez, T. V., and Myers, R. C.,** The effect of lactation on the mineral distribution profile of the rat femur by single photon absorptiometry, *Bone*, 6, 301, 1985.
59. **Ellinger, G. M., Duckworth, J., Dalgarno, A. C., and Quenouille, M. H.,** Skeletal changes during pregnancy and lactation in the rat: effect of different levels of dietary calcium, *Br. J. Nutr.*, 6, 235, 1952.

60. **Wardlaw, G. M. and Pike, A. M.,** The effect of lactation on peak adult shaft and ultra-distal forearm bone mass in women, *Am. J. Clin. Nutr.*, 44, 283, 1986.
61. **Hayslip, C. C., Klein, T. A., Wray, H. L., and Duncan, W. E.,** The effects of lactation on bone mineral content in healthy postpartum women, *Obstet. Gynecol.*, 73, 588, 1989.
62. **Sowers, M. F., Corton, G., Shapiro, G., Jannausch, M. L., Crutchfield, M., Smith, M. S., Randolph, J. F., and Hollis, B.,** Changes in bone density with lactation, *J. Am. Med. Assoc.*, 269, 3130, 1993.
63. **Fox, K. M., Magaziner, J., Sherwint, R., Scott, J. C., Plato, C. C., Nevitt, M., and Cummings, S.,** Reproductive correlates of bone mass in elderly women, *J. Bone Miner. Res.*, 8, 901, 1993.
64. **Dostal, L. A., Boass, A., and Toverud, S. U.,** Effects of high doses of vitamin D_3 and 1,25-dihydroxyvitamin D_3 in lactating rats on milk composition and calcium homeostasis of the suckling pups, *Endocrinology*, 112, 1631, 1983.
65. **Pittard, W. B., III, Geddes, K. M., Hulsey, T. C., and Hollis, B. W.,** How much vitamin D for neonates?, *Am. J. Dis. Child.*, 145, 1147, 1991.
66. **Anderson, J. J. B. and Toverud, S. U.,** Diet and vitamin D: a review with an emphasis on human function, *J. Nutr. Biochem.*, 5, 58, 1994.
67. **Chen, T. C., Heath, H., III, and Holick, M. F.,** An update on the vitamin D content of fortified milk from the United States and Canada, *New Engl. J. Med.*, 329, 1507, 1993.
68. **Bhowmick, S. and Johnson, K.,** Call for clarification of vitamin D recommendations, *Am. J. Dis. Child.*, 146, 14, 1992.
69. **de Papp, A. E. and Stewart, A. F.,** Parathyroid hormone-related protein: a peptide of diverse physiologic functions, *Trends Endocrinol. Metab.*, 4, 181, 1993.
70. **Thiede, M. and Rodan, G.,** Expression of a calcium-mobilizing parathyroid hormone-like peptide in lactating mammary tissue, *Science*, 242, 278, 1988.
71. **Thiede, M.,** The mRNA encoding a parathyroid hormone-like peptide is produced in mammary tissue in response to elevations in serum prolactin, *Mol. Endocrinol.*, 3, 1443, 1989.
72. **Ratcliffe, W. A., Green, E., Emly, J., Norbury, S., Lindsay, M., Heath, D. A., and Ratcliffe, J. G.,** Identification and partial characterisation of parathyroid hormone-related protein in human and bovine milk, *J. Endocrinol.*, 127, 167, 1990.
73. **Budayr, A., Halloran, B., King, J., Diep, D., Nissenson, R., and Strewler, G.,** High levels of a parathyroid hormone-like protein in milk, *Proc. Natl. Acad. Sci. USA*, 86, 7183, 1989.
74. **Miller, S. C., Bagi, C. M., and Bowman, B. M.,** Increased serum levels of parathyroid hormone-related protein correlate the activation of bone resorption and remodelling during early lactation in rats, *Calcif. Tissue Int.*, 48 (suppl.), A13, 1991.
75. **Grill, V., Hillary, J., Ho, P. M. W., Law, F. M. K., MacIsaac, R. J., MacIsaac, I. A., Moseley, J. M., and Martin, T. J.,** Parathyroid hormone-related protein: a possible endocrine function in lactation, *Clin. Endocrinol.*, 37, 405, 1992.
76. **Barlet, J.-P., Abbas, S. K., Care, A. D., Davicco, M.-J., and Rouffer, J.,** Parathyroid hormone-related peptide and milking-induced phosphaturia in dairy cows, *Acta Endocrinol.*, 129, 332, 1993.
77. **Yamamoto, M., Duong, L. T., Fisher, J. E., Thiede, M. A., Caulfield, M. P., and Rosenblatt, M.,** Suckling-mediated increases in urinary phosphate and 3′,5′-cyclic adenosine monophosphate excretion in lactating rats; possible systemic effect of parathyroid hormone-related protein, *Endocrinology, 129*, 2614, 1991.
78. **Davicco, M.-J., Rouffet, J., Durand, D., Lefaivre, J., and Barlet, J.-P.,** Parathyroid hormone-related peptide may increase mammary blood flow, *J. Bone Miner. Res.*, 8, 1519, 1993.
79. **Nickols, G. A., Nana, A. D., Nickols, M. A., DiPette, D. J., and Asimakis, G. K.,** Hypotension and cardiac stimulation due to the parathyroid hormone-related protein, humoral hypercalcemia of malignancy factor, *Endocrinology*, 125, 834, 1989.
80. **Thiede, M. A., Grasser, W. A., and Petersen, D. N.,** Regulated expression of parathyroid hormone-related protein in mammary blood flow, in *Calcium Regulating Hormones and Bone Metabolism: Basic and Clinical Aspects*, Vol. 11, Cohn, D. V., Gennari, C., Tashjian, A. H., Brandi, P. D., Krane, S. M., eds., Elsevier, Amsterdam, 1992.
81. **Ratcliffe, W. A.,** Role of parathyroid hormone-related protein in lactation, *Clin. Endocrinol.*, 37, 402, 1992.

Chapter 17

DEVELOPMENT AND MAINTENANCE OF BONE MASS THROUGH THE LIFE CYCLE

John J. B. Anderson, Ph.D.

TABLE OF CONTENTS

I. INTRODUCTION

Genetic factors and environmental determinants both contribute to the development of the skeleton, including the complement of mineralized tissue, i.e., bone mass (or bone mineral content), achieved at peak development. Genetic factors, however, dominate to a large extent over the more "passive" environmental factors, which tend to be less powerful. During periods of severe undernutrition, the environmental factors may become the critical determinants of bone growth.[1] Hereditary factors exert a great influence on skeletal development during the first two decades of life, and their influence continues, but at a lower power, during the remainder of the life cycle as environmental factors become more potent.[2-8] Genetic factors are responsible for an estimated 70–80 % of bone mass during early skeletal development in the first decade or two of life; the remainder is determined by environmental and life-style factors, including nutrition.[6,9]

0-8493-7845-1/95/$0.00+$.50

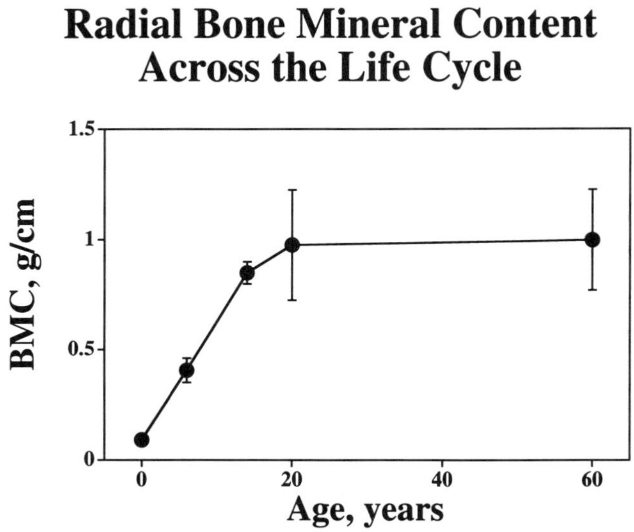

FIGURE 1. Lifetime BMC Measurements. These estimates of bone mass of males and females across the life cycle show the relative changes in radial BMC through skeletal development up to age 20 years and the rather steady maintenance of BMC thereafter to the menopause in women and to approximately age 60 years in men. (Adapted from Greer.[124])

This chapter focuses on females rather than males because the problem of osteoporotic fractures, especially hip fractures, is twice as prevalent among females as males. In addition, this chapter takes a life cycle approach to the early bone development and the later bone loss, a concept first established by Garn.[10] Data on diverse racial/ethnic groups will be reviewed whenever possible.

The promotion of bone health and the prevention of osteopenia (low bone mass) and osteoporosis-associated fractures by females need to be initiated early in the prepubertal years and continued throughout life. Healthy early-life behaviors contribute to greater bone mineral accumulation by approximately age 20 and, presumably, to the optimal achievement of peak bone mass (PBM) by ages 30 to 35 years in women.[11,12] Reports from our laboratory[13-15] and from other institutions[7,16-22] of the effects of dietary calcium (Ca) and/or physical activity in adolescent and young adult females consistently support the conclusion that routinely adequate intakes of nutrients, in particular Ca, and regular physical activities lead to improved bone mineral content (BMC) or bone mineral density (BMD). (Bone mass is an equivalent term for BMC.) The only caveat relates to excessive exercise that may result in primary or secondary amenorrhea and subsequent loss of BMD.[23-27] The skeletal effects of other adverse behaviors, such as cigarette smoking and alcohol consumption, have not been adequately investigated in adolescent or young adult populations of females, but these behaviors remain potentially significant factors in the accrual of PBM. Another factor not adequately researched is the adverse effect of weight loss, i.e., dieting, on bone mass.[28]

Females have a narrow window of approximately six years, four after menarche, for robust incorporation and retention of Ca in the skeleton. Because of this narrow window of opportunity for maximizing skeletal mass, and the well-established resistance of adolescent girls to messages related to improving health behaviors, nutrition educators and other health professionals must be more creative in gaining acceptance of the importance of messages linking dietary Ca and physical activity to bone health. The typical lifetime patterns of development and losses of bone mass (or BMC) by females and males are illustrated in Figure 1. Several environmental factors, often called risk factors, influence bone mass at different stages of the life cycle.[29]

BMC is the mineral mass of bone in units of mg per cm as measured by single-photon or dual-photon absorptiometry (or by similar X-ray absorptiometric machines) (see Chapter 7). Since these measurements are made across a bone in a linear fashion, the BMD value is then calculated by dividing BMC by the width of the bone traversed by the machine. Of these two measurements, now

TABLE 1
Skeletal Accumulation of Calcium during the First Two Decades of Life by Females and Males (Estimated Amounts)

Age, years	Calcium Gain g per year F	Calcium Gain g per year M	Calcium Gain mg per day F	Calcium Gain mg per day M	Cumulative Calcium g F	Cumulative Calcium g M
0–1	75	75	190	190	75	75
1–2	65	65	180	180	140	140
2–8	25	25	60	60	290	290
8–10	60	55	200	150	410	400
10–14	85	90	160	200	750	760
14-20	50	80	100	250	1050	1240

Adapted from Greer.[124]

widely used by bone researchers, BMC seems to be the more useful parameter for assessing bone growth up to age 20 years, whereas BMD appears to be more appropriate for comparing adults through the remainder of the life cycle. Often, researchers will use the terms interchangeably, but they do not have the same meaning.

Starting *in utero,* bone formation and growth is governed by genes responsible for cell proliferation and differentiation. After birth, the continuing bone development is under the control of genes that "model" bones with specific structural organizations that permit them to grow in a controlled pattern and to function according to the grand design of the species. Finally, after the model is completed, i.e., at the end of adolescent growth (in height), remodeling of each bone begins. Remodeling involves the coupling of resorption first and formation second in an organized sequence of cellular activities, and it results from strains or the lack of strains on the skeleton at different sites. Remodeling is primarily an adaptive mechanism that maintains bone health, while also serving as one of the mechanisms providing Ca ions for extraskeletal cellular functions (see Chapter 7). Early in the adult portion of the life cycle, remodeling involves efficient coupling of resorption and formation. In early postmenopause and later years, however, remodeling becomes uncoupled, and this uncoupling results in a net loss of bone. The rate of the bone loss varies, depending on levels of several circulating hormones, physical activity, and other factors.

Recent reviews of the relationships between dietary Ca and bone mass provide additional background information across the life cycle.[30-34]

II. EARLY LIFE DEVELOPMENT OF BONE MASS

This section examines several phases of bone mass development in early life. Ca accumulation by the skeleton remains the critical factor for increments in bone mass, but other nutrients are also required, and hence important for bone development. Infants and young children who have been chronically undernourished for several months with respect to all nutrients have depressed rates of bone turnover compared to recovery periods, as measured by urinary cross-link derivatives of collagen.[35] The approximate amounts of Ca retained by the whole skeleton are given in Table 1 for both well-nourished boys and girls from birth (full term) to 20 years of age.

According to conventional usage, the neonatal period lasts for the first 28 days after parturition, and infancy encompasses the first 12 months after birth.

A. NEONATAL AND INFANT DEVELOPMENT

Skeletal development during the first year of life depends on a balanced nutrient intake, which is provided by breast milk or simulated milk for approximately the first six months. The introduction

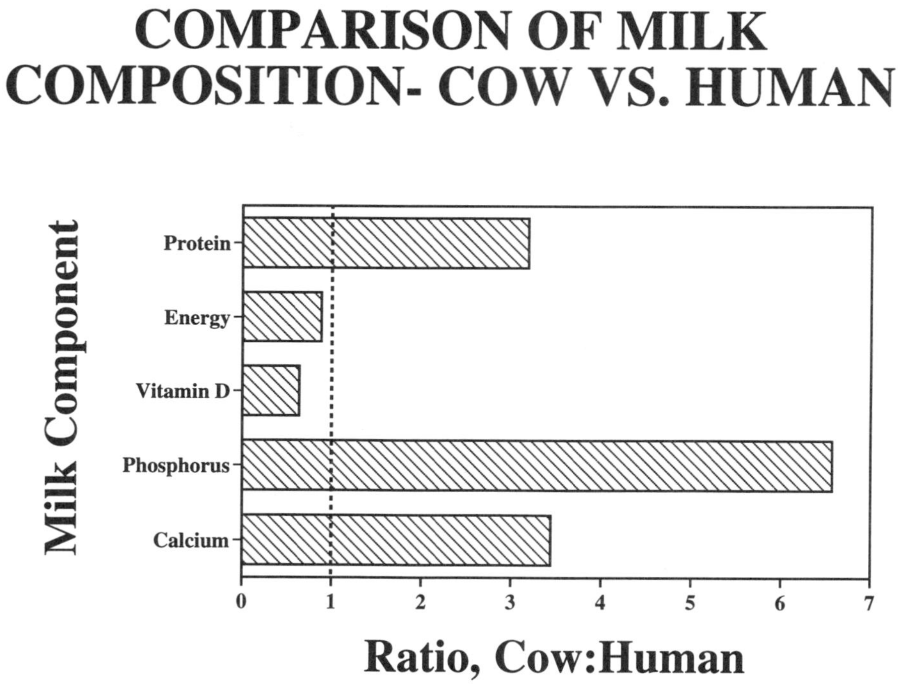

FIGURE 2. Ratios of Nutrients in Cow vs. Human Milk. The ratio of each nutrient or energy in cow's milk compared to human milk is shown here. Note the higher ratio of Ca to P in human compared to cow's milk, but the absolute quantities of Ca and P are much greater in cow's milk than in human milk. Each liter of mature human milk contains 340 mg of calcium, 140 mg of phosphorus, 22 IU of vitamin D, 750 kcal of energy, and 11 g of protein.[125]

of solid foods, either at six months of age or earlier, may have a profound effect either positively or negatively, depending on the acceptance of the foods and whether or not the usual intake of nutrients remains balanced. In general in the U.S., nutritional deficiencies of Ca and phosphorus (P) are extremely rare because of the use of milks, either human-simulated or cow's milk, after six months in practically all children. Even infants raised on soy milk by strict vegetarian parents do quite well in terms of skeletal development, and they achieve length growth at the 50% percentile, which implies no deficiencies of these two minerals.

Human breast milk composition displays a wide variability between subjects and within a subject from early to late lactation.[36] The maximal Ca concentration in milk occurs by approximately 150–200 days of lactation.[36] The concentrations of ionic Ca and free P (as inorganic phosphate or Pi) of human milk are approximately 270–320 and 130–150 mg per L, respectively, which yields a ratio of roughly 2:1. These values are contrasted with those of cow's milk, which has a Ca:P ratio of 1.3:1 (Figure 2). These concentrations of the minerals in milk remain largely independent of the dietary intake of the mother. If a nursing mother's diet is severely deficient in Ca, she will remove much of the needed Ca for milk production from her skeletal stores. Hence, the truly deficient lactating mother could be removing as much as 250 mg Ca a day from her bone tissue in order to produce milk with a minimal concentration of 270 mg of Ca per L.

Racial and ethnic differences in bone mass measurements begin early in the life cycle. A report by Venkataraman and Duke[37] showed that significant differences in radial BMC between blacks and whites were evident by 1 year of age. Significant gender differences in midradial BMC do not generally appear, however, until approximately the age of puberty (see later).

B. CHILDHOOD DEVELOPMENT

Bone growth during childhood occurs by modeling. During this period bone formation occurs first, followed by resorption to maintain the model or shape of each specific bone. Also, during this

TABLE 2
Comparative Mid Radial Bone Mineral Content (BMC) Values of Black and White Infants and Children from Birth to 21 Years as Measured by Single-Photon Absorptiometry

		Mid Radial BMC mg/cm			
Age, yr	**Sex**	**Black**	**White**	**Significance**	**Reference**
Birth*	M/F	91	94	NS	Venkataraman et al.[37]
1–3	M/F	186	160	<0.05	Li et al. 1989[40]
10	M/F	570	520	<0.05	Wakefield et al. 1980[38]
18–22	F	907	840	<0.05	Tylavsky and Anderson†
21	F	908	821	<0.05	Adeleke, 1993[64]

* Approximately 1–7 d of age
† Unpublished data of Tylavsky, F. A. and Anderson, J. J. B.

time, formation greatly exceeds resorption, according to the genetically determined pattern of the human species. The actual amount of bone growth is great during the first two years of life, i.e., the rate of growth is high, but then the amounts of mineral and the rates of growth tend to level off after the second year of life until the two years immediately preceding puberty. Prior to puberty the growth rate again accelerates, and the rate then decays again within a few years after puberty, earlier in girls than in boys. During these important years for growth and development of the skeleton, adequate nutrition is critical for optimal growth. Other environmental factors also exert their effects on bone development, but less is known about these other determinants of bone growth. Gender and racial differences also become prominent during childhood and the peripubertal period.

Virtually all comparative black-white studies in North America show that black females have approximately 10% greater radial BMC and 5% greater radial BMD than white females at the same measurement sites when matched for age, the differences appearing as early as 1 year of age.[37-42] Using quantitative computed tomography (QCT) to measure vertebral BMD, two groups of investigators[43-44] found no difference in BMD between black and white girls up to the time of puberty, but racial differences did appear after puberty. Black males also exhibit greater bone mass than white males at practically every stage of the life cycle. In contrast, white females have greater bone mass than Asian females, although adjustments for body weight, height, or body mass index tend to eliminate these differences. These adjustments do not, however, modify the differences in bone variables between blacks and whites.

Table 2 provides a summary of data on comparative single-photon absorptiometric (SPA) measurements of BMC and BMD of the midshaft of the radius, a nonweight-bearing bone of the forearm, across the life cycle of black and white females. Female bone mass changes in the two ethnic groups occur in parallel across the life cycle; radial BMC increases from birth until some time between ages 20 and 40 years, and declines significantly after approximately age 50, near the average age of the menopause, in both ethnic groups. Males have a slightly different pattern of BMC development; their mean values only begin to exceed female values during the pubertal transition, and their BMC remains greater for the remainder of the life cycle. Mean BMD does not differ so much between the two genders, and late in life they become essentially the same.

Several studies have shown that puberty is not only a crucial time of bone formation in both black and white children, but also that puberty marks a significant divergence between the races in vertebral bone mass accumulation. Vertebral BMD, which is a highly cancellous bone tissue, was measured using QCT in an equal number (75) of black and white females between ages 2 and 20 years.[43] No difference in BMD was observed between the two groups up to the time of puberty. The pubertal increase in BMD, however, was much greater in black females than in white females (34% vs. 11%). This investigation supports the strong contribution of genetic determinants to increases in

TABLE 3
Recommendations for Dietary Calcium during the Life Cycle: RDAs for Both Sexes

Age, years	Calcium, mg per day
0–0.5	400
0.5–1	600
1–10	800
11–24	1200
25–on	800

Recommended Dietary Allowances, 10th ed., 1989.[48]

BMD during pubertal development, independent of dietary Ca intake. Genetic control of the synthesis of proteins involved in osteoid (matrix) production, or of other cellular products involved in bone formation, must be considered as the dominating factor governing adolescent bone development, but racial differences nevertheless persist during peripubertal growth.

The contribution of physical activity to the development of skeletal mass in children has been examined in a study of 118 boys and girls between 5 and 14 years old.[45-46] Increments in skeletal mass were suggested by the authors to result favorably from physical activities and sports, but they could not show that inactivity, i.e., excessive television watching, negatively impacted on BMD at several skeletal sites, including the hip. These investigators also showed that nonweight-bearing activities such as biking and swimming were negatively correlated with all bone sites measured. (They did not provide BMC data in their report.) A recent report from this same group has demonstrated that the bone density of physically active prepubertal children is enhanced over a period of three years by specific activities.[46] Basing their conclusions on the results of their study, Welten and colleagues[47] even went so far as to state that weight-bearing physical activity was more important than Ca intake in the development of PBM.

C. SUMMARY

The development of skeletal mass by infants and children proceeds if adequate nutrition, including both macronutrients and micronutrients, is provided and other environmental determinants of bone mass remain reasonably normal. Dietary Ca must be consumed in amounts that meet the requirements for accumulation of Ca by the skeleton. The current Recommended Dietary Allowances (RDAs, 1989)[48] appear to be adequate to satisfy these needs (see Table 3). Regular physical activities by children have been shown to be beneficial for the accumulation of BMC. Racial differences in bone mass become prominent during childhood, and gender differences begin to be discernible.

III. PERIPUBERTAL DEVELOPMENT OF BONE MASS

Compared to any other period of the life cycle, the greatest amount of Ca incorporated into the skeleton occurs during the peripubertal period of skeletal development of boys and girls. Almost 50% of total bone mineral is deposited from roughly 9 to 18 years of life in a female and 10 to 20 in a male. Puberty is a crucial time for new bone formation and mineral accumulation in children. The retention of mineral by the skeleton is highly correlated with the hormonal changes of puberty, which actually begin to increase during the immediate 2–3 years before puberty when growth acceleration starts. The hormonal milieu dominates by the time of menarche in girls (and the equivalent Tanner stage in boys), after which the need for the nutritional delivery of Ca actually may lessen, although adequate amounts of this mineral remain important for continued bone development.

The first parts of this section are divided into prepubertal, peripubertal (pubertal transition), and adolescent (postpubertal) skeletal accrual of mineral, especially Ca, in order to highlight each of these critical time frames of development. The latter parts of this section deal with the effects of body composition and with the influence of amenorrhea on bone mass during these developmental stages.

A. PREPUBERTAL DEVELOPMENT

The consumption of Ca by prepubertal boys and girls for a period of 2–3 years up to the onset of puberty may be more critical than for any other time during the first 20 years of life. Girls, and probably boys, in the U.S. typically consume more Ca than the RDA suggests during this short prepubertal period, when they are efficiently adding Ca to the skeleton at maximal rates of approximately 200–300 mg per day for girls and 350–450 mg per day for boys. For girls in the U.S. in the 1980s and 1990s, this critical age is between 9 and 12 years, whereas for boys it is roughly between 11 and 15 years at the equivalent Tanner developmental stages. After puberty is established, the needs for Ca may actually decrease somewhat below the RDA for girls of 1200 mg per day, but the amount of Ca needed by males each day probably meets or even exceeds the RDA of 1200, according to data from our laboratory.[49] Our own data would suggest that males may need up to 1500 mg per day during their adolescent growth spurt, since they are adding more Ca in their skeletons each day than females and for a longer period of post-pubertal years, i.e., 6–8 for males versus 3–4 for females, before epiphyseal closures in the long bones are essentially completed.

Increases in sex hormones during the 2- to 3-year prepubertal period have a positive effect on Ca accumulation by the skeleton.[50] Testosterone administration to prepubertal boys resulted in increased skeletal retention of Ca.[51] Presumably, estrogen has the same positive effect on Ca incorporation into the bone of prepubertal girls, although data to support this contention have not been published. After puberty has been established, estrogens remain potent contributors to bone mass accumulation by girls.[52-54]

B. PUBERTAL TRANSITION

Environmental determinants of bone mass, including dietary and other life-style factors, have greater importance prior to puberty than during the pubertal transition in both boys and girls, and the effect of Ca is perhaps most significant during the two years immediately preceding puberty, according to Johnston et al.[20] These authors observed a greater increase in bone mass at three different skeletal sites in prepubertal twins receiving a Ca supplement of 1000 g per day for two years than in similarly treated postpubertal twins. This increase was independent of sex and age of onset of puberty, but it was directly related to the Tanner developmental stage. Radial bone density in this and many other studies was more responsive to Ca supplementation than were the vertebrae and hips.

In the QCT study of Gilsanz et al.[43] the magnitude of the pubertal increase in vertebral BMD was found to be much greater in black than in white females (34% vs. 11%). This study, in particular, supports the strong contribution of genetic determinants to increases in BMD, probably because of increased sex hormone-driven osteoid synthesis during pubertal development, almost independent of dietary Ca intake. Glastre et al.[53] reported similar findings in white French children. Genetic control of bone development, as expressed through testosterone/estrogen stimulated growth hormone secretion, appears to override almost any environmental factor during this period of rapid growth and bone mass accumulation.

By age 18 virtually all females, and by age 22 practically all males in nations with adequate food supplies, have completed their growth in height. Maximum growth is dependent on sufficient amounts of energy and protein in the diet.[1,55] Some investigators support the concept that dietary Ca and exercise patterns play important roles in the development of peak bone mass during the early to mid periods of adolescence.[13,56] It has been concluded that growth ceases in most girls by age 16 to 17 years in western nations, approximately four years after menarche.[57,58] In studies of girls living in Switzerland, 100% of the level of BMC of their parents' generation at the lumbar spine and the proximal femur was reached by approximately age 16. Hence, Ca intake may have an important effect on bone development prior to this age, and on the achievement of peak bone mass during the last four years of the second decade of life.[12,18-20] (Ca is now generally considered a threshold nutrient, as suggested by Matkovic and Heaney,[59] which means that once an age-dependent level of intake is achieved, little or no additional skeletal accumulation of mineral occurs.)

Other evidence from a mother-daughter study suggests that the 18-year-old daughters still must gain almost 10% more radial BMC, and slightly greater than 5% of BMD, to equal their mothers' mean values.[60] A strong familial resemblance in BMD was also demonstrated in a three-generation study, which also examined children of both sexes.[61]

In young adult males, environmental factors appear to influence bone development as well as bone maintenance after the completion of the achievement of peak bone mass. During the early years of the third decade of life in males, the level of dietary Ca has a significant impact on radial bone mass.[11] During middle adult life, other environmental factors may affect the loss of bone mass in males.[5,7,62]

C. LATE ADOLESCENT AND EARLY ADULT LIFE BONE MASS

Genetic and ethnic factors continue to have powerful effects on bone mass accumulation during adolescence, as in early life.[2,63] It has been estimated that hereditary factors account for 70–80 % or more of the contributions to bone mass up to approximately 20 years of age. Dietary and other life-style factors probably determine much of the remainder of bone mass. Beyond age 20 environmental factors may take on greater importance in influencing the mass of this slowly dynamic tissue.[9,11]

Ca intakes by adolescent females in the U.S. continue the decline that typically begins at or just prior to puberty. Males, however, may actually increase their Ca consumption from foods, almost 75% of it from dairy products, and continue this high intake level until their early 20s. Thus, mean Ca intakes of late adolescent females fall to roughly 60–65% of the RDA, whereas male intakes remain at the RDA or even slightly higher (see Table 3). The Ca intakes by adult women older than 24 years continue to be much lower than the age-specific RDA of 800 mg per day, but these mean intakes are relatively good compared to those of women younger than 25 because their RDA for Ca is higher by 400 mg a day!

Although modest differences in nutrient intakes have been shown by several investigators to exist between blacks and whites in the U.S., these differences cannot explain the greater bone mass of blacks. It is especially noteworthy that blacks have a significantly lower Ca intake early in life, as well as throughout the remainder of the life cycle. However, among both young black and white females, those females with chronically low Ca intakes have lower bone mass than high-Ca consumers.[13,64] These differences in BMC between the high and the low Ca consuming young adult women are usually statistically significant.

Studies on twins and parent-offspring pairs provided much of our current knowledge of the contribution of hereditary and environmental factors to bone mass and density. Several investigators[3,4,7,65] have found significantly greater correlations between bone density measurements at different skeletal sites in monozygotic twins than in dizygotic twins and less intrapair variance in these bone measurements.

D. EFFECT OF BODY COMPOSITION ON BONE MASS

In children and early adolescents, height was found to be the best predictor of bone mass.[66] In females at 20 years of age and older, a body mass index seems to be as good a predictor as any anthropometric variable, if not superior.[13,21,67] Racial and ethnic differences in bone mass and density are based on genetic determinants that also express differences in body composition of the lean and/or fat compartments as well. Any anthropometric indicator of a large body mass (body weight, skinfold thickness, body mass index, midarm circumference) is inversely related to the rate of fractures in elderly women, according to a report based on the NHANES Epidemiological Follow-up Study.[68] The more robust anthropometric variables, especially of muscle or lean body mass, of black women are quite highly correlated with bone mass,[69,70] but not with fat mass.[71] Because blacks, therefore, differ from whites in mean compartment values of body composition, they would be expected to differ also in bone mass measurements. Both low body weight and low lean body mass have been shown to be important risk factors for hip fractures in both black and white women.[69,70]

E. EFFECT OF AMENORRHEA ON BONE MASS

Amenorrhea, for whatever reason, contributes to reductions in bone mass over time. In fact, secondary amenorrhea, i.e., cessation of menstrual periods, for as short a period as six consecutive months, will lead to a significant loss of BMC and BMD in young adult women, whether they are athletic or not. Excessive exercise may result in secondary amenorrhea and subsequent loss of BMD, as has been shown for long-distance runners and ballet dancers.[23,24,27] Although exercise more commonly contributes to secondary amenorrhea, it has also been reported to delay menarche and puberty in young gymnasts, and thereby contribute to primary amenorrhea.

The reason for reduced values of BMC and BMD measurements relates to the cessation of estrogen production by the ovaries, which can result from several factors, including heavy exercise, significant weight loss, anorexia nervosa, and some diseases. Estrogen production is necessary for the maintenance of bone tissue, so prolonged interruption of the estrogen supply will result in increased bone resorption rates. The early cessation of menses in an otherwise healthy female will contribute to a similar amount of bone loss as that during the menopausal transition.

F. SUMMARY

Peripubertal skeletal development depends on many environmental and life-style factors. Of these determinants, the effect of Ca consumption, which has been studied more extensively than other factors, is critical for optimizing PBM development, especially during the two years preceding the onset of menses in females. (In general, an optimal intake with respect to all nutrients favors optimal retention of Ca by the skeleton.) Physical activity also appears to be a critical factor during peripubertal skeletal development, but this determinant has not been adequately investigated in prospective studies of girls and boys. Another major contributor to PBM development during this important growth period is body weight (or some other aspect of increased body composition, i.e., body fat or lean body mass compartment). Body weight and body mass index have both been found to be strongly associated with greater bone mass during this developmental period. Other potentially important factors for bone mass accumulation by females have not been adequately studied, but evidence is clear that maintenance of normal reproductive cycles by postpubertal girls strongly supports continued bone development. Further prospective investigations are needed to evaluate the relative importance of oral contraceptive agents, adolescent pregnancy, cigarette smoking, and alcohol consumption on bone development of females during their teens and early 20s.

IV. ATTAINMENT OF PEAK BONE MASS (PBM)

The timing of PBM development in women has not been clearly established for major skeletal sites, although considerable data suggest that the final phase of PBM development occurs between 20 and 30 years of age. (In men it probably occurs a few years later than in women.) Although a few prospective studies of skeletal development of young white women exist, they do not yet clarify this issue. Few data are available on PBM development in blacks. Because osteoporotic fractures in late life are highly correlated with low bone mass, it appears reasonable for adolescent and young adult women to optimize their PBM in order to prevent or delay the serious public health problem of osteoporotic fractures. Fractures may, however, actually result more from other factors, such as microarchitectural defects or fragility, than from low bone mass per se, but low bone mass is a prerequisite. The current status of our understanding of PBM development in white females, and the dietary and lifestyle factors that influence it, are briefly reviewed. Several experimental approaches have been followed to try to establish the precise timing of PBM accumulation. The differences reported in the age at which PBM completion has been estimated in various reports relates both to the choice of bone sites, e.g., radius versus lumbar spine, and to the experimental design and methodology employed in measurement.

For certain bone sites, such as lumbar vertebrae and the proximal femur, PBM development may cease at 20 years of age or earlier. Findings that have been recently published[57,58] on bone mass accumulation by girls demonstrate that, by approximately age 16, girls living in Switzerland have already reached the 100% level of BMC of their parents' generation at the lumbar spine and the proximal femur. Peak vertebral bone mass, for example, is generally accepted to be achieved by about 18 years of age, i.e., at the end of the female adolescent growth phase.[72] In the cross-sectional investigation of Riggs et al.[72] no increase in vertebral bone mass was detected in white women beyond age 20. Geusens et al.[73] found in a cross-sectional population of Belgian women that lumbar vertebral bone mass, but not radial bone mass, began to decline in early premenopausal adulthood, perhaps as early as the 20s. In contrast, Recker et al.[74] reported an increase in vertebral bone mass of white females during the decade of the 20s in a prospective study. Femoral bone mass was found not to change in women beyond age 20 in a cross-sectional investigation.[75] Thus, reports in the literature provide differing findings, showing both a decrease and an increase in bone mass at skeletal sites other than the radius in women during the adult decades preceding the menopause. Further prospective studies are needed to detect important antecedent-consequence relationships. Clarification of this issue is important for the prevention or delay of late-life osteoporotic fractures.

One approach to assessing genetic contributions to bone mass has made use of mother-daughter (offspring) intrapair correlational analyses. In general, these reports have demonstrated quite high intrapair correlations between mothers and daughters. Mothers with low bone mass typically have daughters with low bone mass.[8,18,60,76-79]

In a study of 18-year-old daughters and their 44-year-old premenopausal mothers, heritability estimates between bone variables of mothers and daughters suggested a strong familial component, on the order of 50% at both the distal (50% trabecular tissue) and mid-shaft (95% cortical tissue) sites of the radius.[60]

Additional cross-sectional findings on the same radial sites of white females between ages 20 and 50 years suggest that bone mass increases at these two sites up to approximately age 40. The results of the mother-daughter study of Tylavsky et al.[60] suggest that the mothers represented a health-conscious, physically active group of women who continued to accumulate radial bone mass during their 30s and early 40s because of these bone-enhancing behaviors. The 10% greater amount of bone mass of the mothers compared to their daughters suggests that, if the daughters follow similarly healthy lifestyles and have at least one baby, they too will be able to achieve values of bone mass similar to those of their mothers when they reach 44 years of age (Figure 3). Therefore, it appears that several other factors or events occurring during the third and fourth decades of life must have positive impacts on PBM development.

In early adulthood bone mass accumulation may still occur, but at low rates. A prospective two- to four-year study by Recker et al.[74] of women in their early to late twenties demonstrated that small amounts of bone mass were accrued throughout the decade of the 20s by these young women with their usual Ca intakes. The rate of gain was estimated by these researchers to be approximately 0.5% per year or 5% per decade. Using a cross-sectional research approach, Metz et al.[15] examined young adult women in their mid-twenties and showed that usual intakes of Ca at adequate levels, i.e., approximating the age-specific RDA, had positive effects on bone mass, whereas low intakes were detrimental. Similarly, relatively high intakes of P and protein also had adverse effects on bone mass. Physical activity had benefits for bone mass, as demonstrated in earlier studies from the same laboratory. Bone density measurements at the same skeletal sites in each of these studies showed the same relationships between the nutrient variables and measurements of bone density.

A few life-style and reproductive variables have been identified to increase bone mass; these are pregnancies and lactations, regular physical activities, and upper body lifting of infants and children

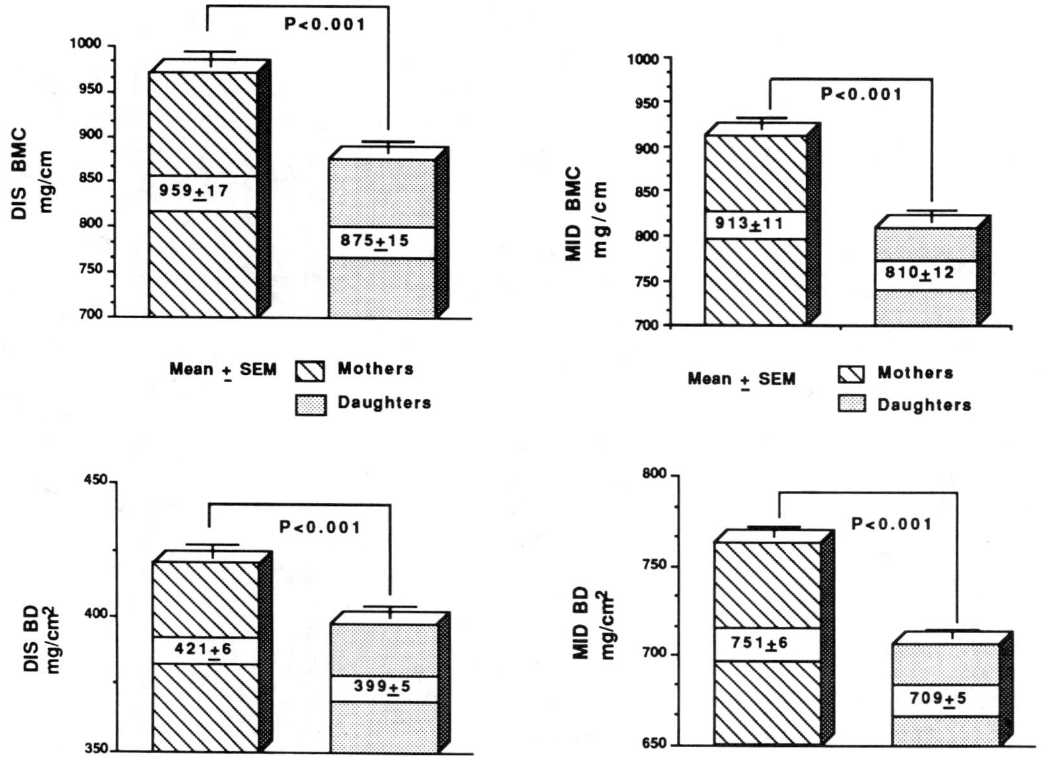

FIGURE 3. Mean Mother-Daughter Radial BMC and BMD Values. If the daughters (18 years old) are to accumulate bone mass over the next two and a half decades, as their mothers (44 years old) had, they will need to gain approximately 10% in BMC and 5% in BMD at each radial bone site to reach their mothers' values. (From Tylavsky, F. A., Bartz, A. D., Hancock, R. L., and Anderson, J. J. B., Familial resemblance of radial bone mass between premenopausal mothers and their college-age daughters, *Calcif. Tissue Int.,* 45, 265, 1989. With permission.)

by mothers.[11,14,52,68,80,81] In addition, good usual intakes of Ca may also improve bone mass,[14,17,74,81,82] as long as the Ca level of the diet reaches or approaches the age-specific RDA, i.e., the threshold. A few groups of researchers could not, however, show a benefit of dietary Ca on bone measurements.[75,83,84] Finally, a greater body size or body mass index also has been shown by several research groups to contribute to greater BMC and BMD in adult women.[17,67,69,70,85-87] Gains in body composition, i.e., both lean and fat mass, with increasing adult years may be the most consistently favorable variable related to increased BMC and BMD in premenopausal women. This same conclusion holds for both black and white adult women,[71] and the differentials in BMC and BMD established in childhood between black and white females continues up to and even beyond the menopause for at least two decades.

Also, dietary Ca, physical activity, and anthropometric variables contribute significantly to the bone mass at both the distal and mid radius.[14,67] Recker et al.[74] reported data from a prospective study of women in their third decade of life that showed similar increases in bone mass of the radius. They also estimated a gain in lumbar vertebral bone mass in women between 20 and 30 years of age. Other investigators,[75,83,84] however, did not find an increase in radial bone mass, or increases at other sites, in their cross-sectional or prospective investigations of white women between 20 and 50 years of age. Furthermore, the latter researchers could not demonstrate a contributory role for physical activity on bone mass. A cross-sectional study by Metz et al.[15] of a small sample of 24–28-year-old white women showed positive effects of dietary Ca and physical activity and negative effects of dietary protein and P on radial bone mass at two sites. Thus, for the forearm (radial) bone, especially at the distal site, data from most cross-sectional reports and one prospective study of young adult white women suggest that PBM development continues to approximately age 30, and that dietary Ca and physical activity, but no other lifestyle factors, may contribute in a positive way to this consolidation of radial bone mass. Increasing body weight or BMI also was found to be associated with greater bone mass. Adverse effects of some dietary variables, such as high intakes of protein, P and sodium, have also been found in studies of young adult women (Metz et al., unpublished data).[15]

The associations of dietary Ca and other nutrients, physical activity, reproductive events, and other life-style variables with bone density during PBM development also need to be explored in a prospective manner in order to assess the contributions of these potentially important determinants to bone consolidation. For example, in the study of Recker et al.[74] both radial and vertebral bone mass continued to increase between 20 to 30 years of age, but the mean Ca intakes of these young women were less than the RDA of 1200 mg per day (19 to 24 years of age) or 800 mg per day (25 years and older). Thus, it has not yet been established whether or not an intake nearer the age-specific RDA will, over a period of several years, contribute to a greater PBM than a low intake of less than 50% of the age-specific RDA. Similar prospective approaches can be used to assess the importance of contributions of regular physical activity and of other variables to bone mass at different skeletal sites.

Few reports of investigations of young adult black women have appeared, but the data of Adeleke[64] have shown that the bone mass or density measurements of blacks are always significantly greater than for white females at any given adult age between 20 and 30 years. Other life-style factors, such as physical activity, also positively influenced bone mass, as did body mass index, in young adult black women. Furthermore, little information has been published on life-style and other environmental factors that contribute to PBM development in blacks.

In summary, PBM development in young adult women has been inadequately investigated. For white females, PBM accrual is completed by approximately age 30, but it could be as late as 35 years of age for the radius. Prospective studies of women who are white, black, or members of other ethnic groups are needed to establish more precisely what factors influence PBM. For example, the fact that many women undergo multiple pregnancies and lactations has not been factored into the normal prospective sequence of bone changes among adult women, nor have their associated child-care activities been considered as important contributors to PBM accumulation. Many of these women carry their children, a significant bone-loading strain, and perform work activities that require considerable upper body strength. Neither have these physical activities been taken into consideration in experimental studies with prospective designs. The precise timing of PBM, therefore, has not been adequately established.

V. BONE MASS MAINTENANCE DURING THE PREMENOPAUSAL DECADES

Multiple factors contribute to bone mass maintenance during the premenopausal decades. These factors, which are practically the same ones involved in PBM accrual, include hereditary, endocrine/reproductive, nutritional, and lifestyle/environmental determinants. These four classes of variables are further divided into more specific factors that affect bone negatively, as listed in Table 4. Most of these factors are reviewed in this section, but emphasis is placed on usual dietary Ca intakes and physical activities of women during their 30s and 40s.

The maintenance of bone mass (or bone density) by women during the fourth and fifth decades of life (30–49 years of age) is probably enhanced by regular physical activity, such as tennis, walking, and other activities, since a slow steady bone loss over these premenopausal decades has been shown for nonexercising women in a few cross-sectional studies.[14,88-91] The role of regular physical activity in increasing bone mass seems to be even more potent than that of usual dietary

TABLE 4
Classes of Risk Factors Related to Osteopenia and Osteoporosis

Class	Specific Risk Factors
Hereditary (non-behavioral)	White/Asian race, female, family history (+), lactose intolerance, milk allergy
Endocrine/Reproductive (partly behavioral)	Estrogen deficiency (amenorrhea, anorexia, natural or surgical menopause)
Nutritional (behavioral)	Low body composition (fat and lean mass), inadequate calcium, excess phosphorus, excess sodium, inadequate vitamin D, excess protein, excess caffeine, inadequate vitamin K, inadequate trace minerals
Lifestyle/Environmental (behavioral)	Physical inactivity, cigarette smoking, excessive alcohol, excessive soft drinks, drugs (diuretics, antacids, barbiturates, corticosteroids, others)

Ca. Only a few studies have examined the effects of aerobic or weight-loading exercises on the BMC or BMD in adolescent girls, and these have not been consistent. Retrospective assessments of the influence of physical activity on bone mass, however, have been almost uniformly positive, at least in our experience.[13,14] This area of research reflects a paucity of data on adolescent and young adult females.

Vertebral bone loss rates may be greater than for other skeletal sites, as demonstrated in an investigation by Baran et al.[82] in which dairy product supplementation was given to one group of women in their mid-thirties for two years and no supplement to another. The supplemented group showed much less bone loss over the period of study compared to the unsupplemented group.

Other environmental and life-style factors also influence the development and maintenance of bone, and most of these are adverse, such as cigarette smoking, excessive alcohol consumption, and prescription and over-the-counter drugs, but published reports are very limited. Usage of oral contraceptive agents (OCA) by young women is considered to be a weak positive factor, but studies have not been conclusive in demonstrating a significant effect of OCA use on measurements of bone mass.[92] In general, relatively few investigations of these risk factors have been undertaken with adolescent and young adult women.

Reproductive/endocrine factors have already been mentioned, but whenever estrogen deficiency occurs, such as in athletic amenorrhea or anorexia nervosa, bone loss will occur. BMC measurements reported for females with hypoestrogenism typically are significantly lower than for healthy eumenorrheic females.[27]

The continuation of normal menstrual cycling (9–10 cycles per year) in premenopausal women remains one of the most positive factors for the maintenance of bone mass. The ovarian production of estrogens is unquestionably very important for bone health, and any condition or life-style behavior that interferes with ovarian function or the efficacy of estrogens will lead to reductions in bone mass. The long-term study of Heaney and co-workers[93] of perimenopausal women has demonstrated the benefits of a healthy life-style on Ca metabolism, and therefore, by inference, on BMD.

In cross-sectional studies of white women between ages 20 and 50 years, analyses showed consistently positive associations between body mass index, body fat mass or estimated lean body mass, and bone measurements.[14,70] Several reports have documented the positive effect of body weight on BMC and BMD in both black and white women.[62,94,95]

In summary, two major risk factors for low bone mass have been shown by researchers to be amenable to modifications that can lead to improvements in BMC and BMD, and therefore, presumably, to PBM achievement. These factors are adequate intake of Ca, preferably from foods, and regular physical exercise in some activities that are aerobic and others that contribute to upper body strength. These optimal bone-enhancing behaviors must be continued indefinitely.

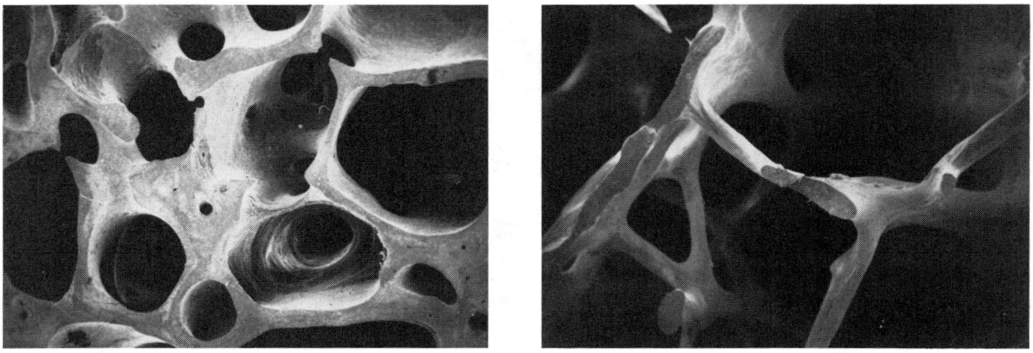

FIGURE 4. Scanning Electron Micrographs of Normal and Osteoporotic Human Cancellous Bone Tissue. Normal cancellous bone (A) has thick trabecular plates with extensive interconnections. Osteoporotic cancellous bone (B) has greatly reduced numbers of connections between trabeculae, as well as thinning of trabecular plates. (Original micrographs reproduced from Dempster, D. W., Shane, E., Horbert, W., and Lindsay, R., A simple method for correlative light and scanning electron microscopy of human iliac crest bone biopsies: qualitative observations in normal and osteoporotic subjects, *J. Bone Min. Res.*, 1, 15, 1986. With permission.)

VI. BONE MASS IN THE POSTMENOPAUSAL AND LATE ADULT YEARS: MENOPAUSAL AND AGE-RELATED BONE LOSSES

The menopausal transition has a significant adverse effect on the bone mass of practically all women at approximately age 50 years or somewhat later, on the average, in the U.S. The cessation of estrogen production by the ovaries has a major adverse effect on the skeletal mass of practically all women. Ca balance becomes significantly negative at this time,[93] which reflects bone loss associated with the loss of estrogens (Figure 4). Only estrogen replacement therapy (ERT) has been found to be successful in slowing the bone loss that normally accompanies the first five or more years following the menopause.[96] Ca supplementation has essentially no effects at this time, but it does after the fifth year or so following the menopause.[97] (Women not placed on ERT, however, typically gain weight and increase their fat stores during the first postmenopausal decade.)

Changes in bone mass and density in women following the menopause are greater in terms of the rate of loss than at any other time during the latter part of life, i.e., roughly 30 years for women whose average life expectancy is 80 years. These late-life changes in bone of elderly women, especially of the vertebrae, which result in loss of height, are illustrated in Figure 5. Note that the reduction in height contributes to the protrusion (or bunching up) of tissues in the back (Dowager's hump) and the abdomen. The length of the legs remains unaffected by the compaction of the vertebral column, but the internal dimensions of the shafts of the legs and their long bones undergo change because of endosteal bone resorption, which results in an enlarged marrow cavity (Figure 6). Thus, both cortical and cancellous bone tissues are significantly affected by the aging process, independent of Ca intake per se (see also Chapter 19 for a review of bone changes of the elderly.)

Bone mass changes during the latter part of the life cycle are still affected by hereditary factors, although these determinants diminish in importance. For example, in women the age of menopause is determined by genetic factors, although it can be affected by environmental variables, especially diet. In the last 50 years, the mean age of menopause of American women has increased from the last half of the fifth decade of life to the first half of the sixth decade, primarily because of an improvement in the overall nutritional status of women. Genetic factors probably contribute to the rapid loss of bone in some women, i.e., the "fast losers," in the early postmenopausal years. The loss of ovarian estrogen production is considered the major contributor to bone loss in women following the menopause, but it is possible that changes in other hormonal factors, such as adrenal corticosteroids and androgens, affect bone turnover. Little information has been published on the genetic determinants of hormonal changes at the menopause, but hereditary factors must make important

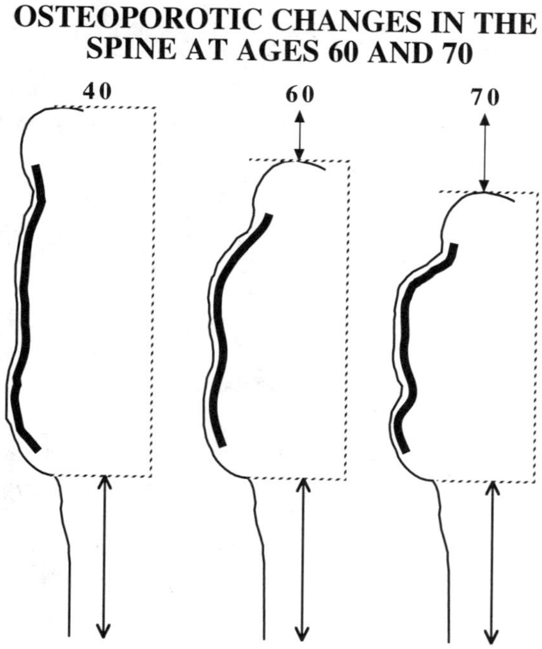

FIGURE 5. Late-Life Changes in Bone of Elderly Women. Compression fractures of the vertebrae result in loss of height. Note that the reduction in height contributes to the protrusion (or bunching up) of tissues in the back, i.e., Dowager's hump. The length of the legs remains unaffected by the compaction of the vertebral column.

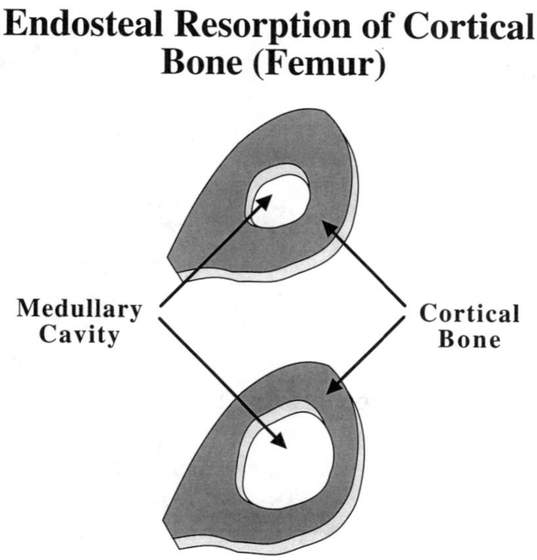

FIGURE 6. Endosteal Bone Resorption of Long Bone Shaft. These diagrams illustrate the increased overall width of bone which occurs with years, and the increased width of the marrow cavity, which also increases with years of life. The net effect is to decrease the width of the remaining cortical bone in the shaft of elderly subjects.

contributions to several parameters of Ca metabolism other than bone, according to a report by Peacock et al.[98]

Body weight, or in general, body fat mass represents another important variable that contributes to greater bone mass. In adults the increases in body weight with age occurs primarily because of increases in fat stores, rather than in lean body mass. Anthropometric measurements and estimates of body fat mass by new techniques have clearly demonstrated the powerful effect that increased weight has on promoting bone health and preventing fractures. Several researchers have found that a high body mass index or body weight are protective of bone mass.[85,86,99-101] Lacey et al.[102] and Tsunerani and co-workers[103] also found a positive association between bone mass and fat mass (or body weight) of older Japanese women.

The correlation between fat mass and bone mass is greater for females than males, an observation made for Caucasians,[86] Asian Japanese[103] and Chinese.[104] The explanation for this difference is not clear, but Felson and colleagues[105] speculate that the peripheral conversion of androstenedione to estrogens is more extensive in females. Also, because of a greater number of estrogen receptors in the bone cells of females, they may conserve bone mass more effectively than males. Thus, obese postmenopausal women who have a higher level of circulating estrogen, maintain bone mass more effectively than lean women, who have basal circulating levels of estrogens.

Women with low circulating concentrations of androstenedione or other adrenal steroids (androgens) and low body fat mass may be at risk for osteoporosis because of a low peripheral conversion of these steroids to estrogens in fat or other tissues. (It would be desirable to have an index of obesity or peripheral fat distribution for the assessment of androstenedione conversion to estrone.) Several investigators have suggested that greater fat distribution conveys a benefit to some women in preventing or delaying osteoporosis, but it is not clear whether the type of fat distribution (apple type of fat distribution vs. pear type) makes a difference in the circulating levels of sex steroids.

In addition to the benefits conferred by fatty tissue on the hormonal maintenance of bone mass by postmenopausal women,[105] body fat is protective against hip fractures from falls, especially backward falls.[106] An upper body fat mass provides a greater gravitational load at the most fracture-susceptible bone site, i.e., the hip, and therefore may further help protect against fractures by increasing bone formation at this site over a period of years to decades.

Blacks differ from whites in body composition, especially muscle (lean tissue) mass and skeletal mass, though not in fat mass.[71] The report on elderly women in the NHANES Epidemiological Follow-up Study[68] indicates that any anthropometric indicator of a large body mass (body weight, skinfold thickness, body mass index, midarm circumference) was inversely related to the rate of fractures. Low body weight was demonstrated by Pruzansky et al.[69] and low fat mass by Lindsay et al.[70] to be important risk factors for hip fractures in both black and white women. Low body fat in elderly Asian female populations[103,104] also has been associated with an increased rate of hip fractures.

Asian women with a high body mass index, body weight, or fat mass as estimated by skinfolds, also have greater bone mass.[102,104] The traditionally low-Ca diet consumed by elderly Japanese does not seem to be as great a risk factor for this population with approximately half the hip fracture rate of western women.[107] Thus, body mass index and other variables in body composition, especially the maintenance of select muscle groups, must be considered in evaluating the significance of differences in bone mass in diverse ethnic groups. In a comparative study of bone measurements of adult and elderly Japanese subjects living in Japan and of Japanese descendants living in Hawaii, however, adjusting BMC by dividing by bone width (i.e., BMD) increased the mean difference between the two groups.[108] Life-style and dietary variables have been offered as the major determinants of differences in bone mass among Japanese migrants to mainland U.S.[109]

In summary, bone losses during the postmenopausal and later adult years are related to declines of circulating concentrations of sex hormones, especially estrogens and androgens. Fat mass synthesis of these hormones, however, may help to counter the loss of bone mass in obese women. Declining levels of physical activity and lean body mass, in general, also contribute to losses of bone mass. The precise role of dietary Ca in helping to slow bone mass losses late in life remains unclear because intakes of Ca at either adequate or low levels appear to have no effect in slowing the rate of bone loss in women approaching 80 years of age in one study.[110] It may be important that the elderly also have good intakes of vitamins D and K as well as of all other nutrients to help retain bone mass. (See Chapter 12 and Chapter 19).

VII. CALCIUM NEEDS AND THE RDAS THROUGH THE LIFE CYCLE

Several points about the current RDAs for Ca need to be made because of the important relationship between the Ca nutritional status and bone mass of girls and adult women. Recall that Ca is found in relatively few foods in the amounts needed to meet age-specific Recommended Dietary Allowances (RDAs, 1989),[48] which are listed in Table 3. Secondly, the RDAs for Ca are now considered to be somewhat underestimated with respect to young girls between ages 8 and 11 years, and they are probably set at too high a level for young adult women between ages 20 and 25. The explanations for these statements relate to the earlier prepubertal skeletal development and incorporation of Ca by girls than in previous generations, and the threshold behavior of Ca at any age of the life cycle.[59] The relative lack of response to Ca supplementation (to amounts greater than the RDAs) of postpubertal girls and boys in a twin study which lasted three years demonstrated that healthy children consuming Ca at less than the RDA had just as good bone measurement values after three years as those receiving Ca at approximately 150% of the age-specific RDA.[20]

The Ca RDAs for pre- and postmenopausal women appear to be set at reasonable levels if Ca needs are met by intake from foods, either fortified or not. If the requirements for Ca are greatly increased among elderly women (and men) beyond the current RDA of 800 mg per day, then supplements of Ca are almost assuredly needed to meet the higher demands. (Not enough food energy can be consumed by the inactive elderly to satisfy Ca needs beyond 800 mg in a single day.) Understandings of the Ca requirements, and probably also the needs of vitamin D, of the elderly are still unfolding.[111]

Furthermore, Ca intakes need to be high enough to counterbalance the potentially negative effects of the high amounts of P in the diets of virtually everyone in the U.S., and the presumed adverse effects of excessive intakes of protein by practically all individuals (see Chapter 2). Because of the generally high absorption of P, the increase in serum Pi, which peaks at approximately one hour after the meal, produces a modest Ca-lowering effect because of the Pi-induced action of calcitonin on osteoclasts.[112] A few reports have shown that low-Ca and high-P diets fed to women for several weeks led to persistently elevated parathyroid hormone levels in the blood, which presumably remove mineral from bone.[113,114] Calvo[115] has put forth convincing evidence that the current consumption of P by Americans may be underestimated because of the increased addition of phosphates to processed foods, especially to carbonated beverages, and the preference of the American population for these foods and drinks, while other researchers have suggested that high phosphate diets may contribute to increases in osteopenia and fractures among the elderly.[116]

The adverse effects of high protein intakes on Ca retention may contribute to low bone mass through mechanisms that increase excessive urinary losses of Ca. Thus, usual protein consumption at high levels may negatively impact on bone mineral density and potentially contribute to increased fracture rates of the hip.[117] The acute and short-term effects of protein in increasing urinary Ca losses in human subjects have been demonstrated under diverse experimental conditions.[118] Several human studies have been reanalyzed in a type of meta-analysis by Kerstetter and Allen[119] who concluded that, with the exception of one report, all investigations showed adverse effects of high-protein intakes on Ca through hypercalciuria. Human experimental evidence using a long-term prospective design has not yet shown that excessive dietary protein leads to osteopenia and osteoporotic fractures.[120]

A review of the reported data on Ca intakes by women in the U.S. reveals that they must be better informed and must become more sophisticated about their diets in order to assure adequate intakes of all essential nutrients in amounts that approach their age-specific RDAs, not just those for Ca. The RDAs remain the best guides for establishing nutritional adequacy across the life cycle[121] (Table 3). Adequate Ca intake, compared to low consumption, has been shown in two distinct Croatian populations to contribute to greater bone mass by age 30 years and to lower fractures rates.[16] In a reanalysis of Ca balance data from several published studies over the past 50 years, Matkovic demonstrated that young adults (ages 18 to 30 years) were able to maintain their Ca balance at median intakes of approximately 750 mg of Ca a day.[122] Therefore, overselling the importance of Ca needs, up to 1500 mg a day as recommended by some researchers, may undermine the long-standing fundamental principle of obtaining nutritional balance from a variety of foods according to the basic food guide or pyramid, even if some of these foods are fortified with Ca. Young women find it very difficult to obtain 800 mg of Ca on a daily basis from foods, and to obtain higher amounts would almost require the use of Ca supplements by the vast majority of the young adult female population. The consumption of fortified foods may help many young women. Several foods, fortified up to 300 mg per serving, are now available to allow consumers to obtain adequate amounts of Ca each day.[123] Supplementation still has a place, but it should remain primarily a therapeutic measure because of potential adverse effects of high intakes of Ca as a supplement on the absorption of a few trace minerals.[123]

VIII. SUMMARY AND CONCLUSIONS

The early-life gains and the late-life losses of bone mineral content (and density) have been detailed with illustrations of effects of both hereditary and environmental/life-style determinants (Figure 7). Bone mass is favorably impacted at practically all stages of the life cycle by adequate intakes of most nutrients, especially Ca, regular physical activity, and higher body weight (or other variables of body composition), but it is unfavorably influenced by high or excessive intakes of other nutrients, especially P and protein, and by several other adverse behaviors, such as excessive alcohol ingestion, cigarette smoking, selected drug usage, and physical inactivity. In addition, bone mass is generally considered to be improved in women by lactation and by child care and lifting. In Asian countries, the performance of many everyday activities on the floor probably also contributes to improved bone mass of the hips through the regular usage of muscle groups of the legs and lower back. Much information has been published on the bone-related variables, but better designed prospective investigations are needed to pinpoint PBM accruals at different bone sites among diverse ethnic and racial groups. The impact of lactation on BMC and BMD losses and gains during the course of a single lactation of six months or longer also needs to be established.

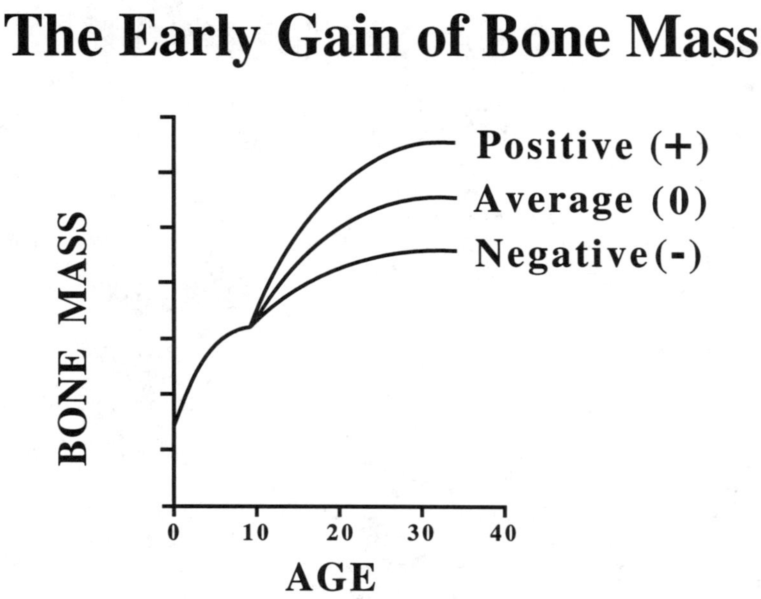

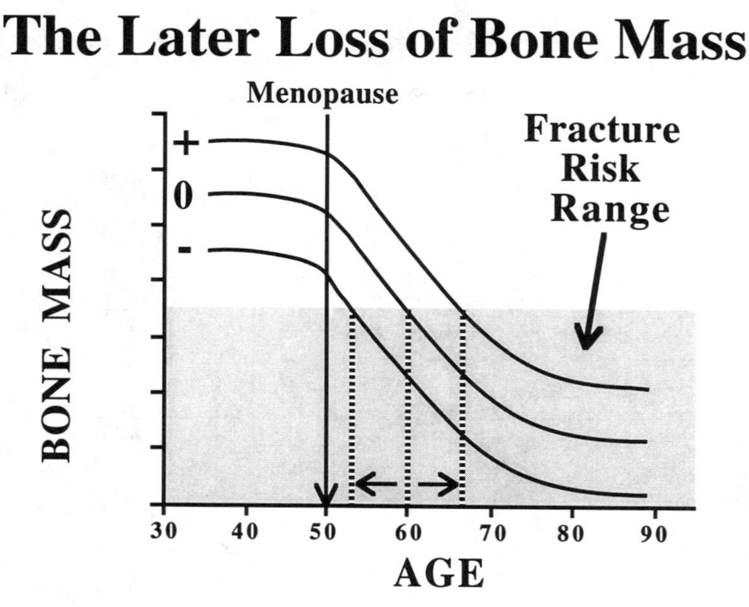

FIGURE 7. The Early Gain and Later Loss of Bone Mass by Women. During the first few decades of life (up to about age 35) bone accumulation results in peak bone mass (PBM). Optimal environmental conditions (Positive, +) maximize PBM for individuals. Conversely, suboptimal conditions (Negative, –) contribute to lower than average (Mean, 0) PBM. The later loss of bone mass tends to track according to the PBM attained early in life, i.e., before the menopause.

REFERENCES

1. **Anderson, J. J. B.,** The role of nutrition in the functioning of skeletal tissue, *Nutr. Rev.*, 50, 388, 1992.
2. **Pollitzer, W. A. and Anderson, J. J. B.,** Ethnic and genetic differences in bone mass: a review with an hereditary vs. environmental perspective, *Am. J. Clin. Nutr.*, 50, 1244, 1989.
3. **Pocock, N. A., Eisman, J. A., Hopper, L., Yeates, M. G., Sambrook, P. N., and Ebert, S.,** Genetic determinants of bone mass in adults, A twin study, *J. Clin. Invest.*, 80, 706, 1987.

4. **Christian, J. C., Yu, P.-L., Slemenda, C. W., and Johnston, C. C., Jr.,** Heritability of bone mass: a longitudinal study in aging male twins, *Am. J. Human.Genet.*, 44, 429, 1989.
5. **Kelly, P. J., Hopper, J. L., Macaskill, G. T., Pocock, N. A., Sambrook, P. N., and Eisman, J. A.,** Genetic factors in bone turnover, *J. Clin. Endocrinol. Metab.*, 72, 808, 1991.
6. **Slemenda, C. W., Christian, J. C., Williams, C. J., Norton, J. A., and Johnston, C. C., Jr.,** Genetic determinants of bone mass in adult women, *J. Bone Miner. Res.*, 6, 561, 1991.
7. **Slemenda, C. W., Christian, J. C., Reed, T., Reister, T. K., Williams, C. J., and Johnston, C. C., Jr.,** Long-term bone loss in men: effects of genetic and environmental factors, *Ann. Int. Med.*, 117, 286, 1992.
8. **Hansen, M. A., Hassager, C., Jensen, S. B., and Christiansen, C.,** Is heritability a risk factor for postmenopausal osteoporosis? *J. Bone Miner. Res.*, 7, 1037, 1992.
9. **Johnston, C. C., Jr. and Slemenda, C. W.,** Changes in skeletal tissue during the aging process, *Nutr. Rev.*, 50, 385, 1992.
10. **Garn, S. M.,** The earlier gain and the later loss of cortical bone: in *Nutritional Perspective*, C. C. Thomas Publ., Springfield, IL, 1970.
11. **Anderson, J. J. B., Tylavsky, F. A., Halioua, L., and Metz, J. A.,** Determinants of peak bone mass in young adult women: a review, *Osteoporosis Int.*, 3 (supp 1), S32, 1993.
12. **Anderson, J. J. B. and Metz, J. A.,** Contributions of dietary calcium and physical activity to primary prevention of osteoporosis in females, *J. Am. Coll. Nutr.*, 12, 378, 1993.
13. **Tylavsky, F. A., Anderson, J. J. B., Talmage, R. V., and Taft, T.,** Are calcium intakes and physical activity patterns during adolescence related to radial bone mass of white college-age females? *Osteoporosis Int.*, 2, 232, 1992.
14. **Halioua, L. and Anderson, J. J. B.,** Lifetime calcium intake and physical activity habits: independent and combined effects on the radial bone of healthy premenopausal Caucasian women, *Am. J. Clin. Nutr.*, 49, 534, 1989.
15. **Metz, J., Anderson, J. J. B., and Gallagher, P. N., Jr.,** Intakes of calcium, phosphorus, protein and level of physical activity are related to radial bone mass in young adult women, *Am. J. Clin. Nutr.*, 58, 537, 1993.
16. **Matkovic, V., Kostial, K., Simonovic, I., Buzina, R., Brodarec, A., and Nordin, B. E. C.,** Bone status and fracture rates in two regions of Yugoslavia, *Am. J. Clin. Nutr.*, 32, 540, 1979.
17. **Picard, D., Ste.-Marie, L. G., Coutu, D., Carrier, L., Chartrand, R., Lepage, R., Fugere, P., and D'Amour, P.,** Premenopausal bone mineral content relates to height, weight and calcium intake during early adulthood, *Bone Miner.*, 4, 299, 1988.
18. **Matkovic, V., Fontana, D., Tomineac, C., Goel, P., and Chesnut, C.H., III,** Factors that influence peak bone mass formation: a study of calcium balance and the inheritance of bone mass in adolescent females, *Am. J. Clin. Nutr.*, 52, 878, 1990.
19. **Sentipal, J. M., Wardlaw, G. M., Mahan, J., and Matkovic, V.,** Influence of calcium intake and growth indexes on vertebral bone mineral density in young females, *Am. J. Clin. Nutr.*, 54, 425, 1991.
20. **Johnston, C. C., Jr., Miller, J. Z., Slemenda, C. W., Reister, T. K., Christian, J. C., and Peacock, M.,** Calcium supplementation and increases in bone mineral density in children, *New Engl. J. Med.*, 327, 82, 1992.
21. **Fehily, A. M., Coles, R. J., Evans, W. D., and Elwood, P. C.,** Factors affecting bone density in young adults, *Am. J. Clin. Nutr.*, 56, 579, 1992.
22. **Lloyd, T., Andon, M. B., Rollings, N., Martel, J. K., Landis, J. R., Demers, L. M., Eggli, D. F., Kieselhorst, K., and Kulin, H. E.,** Calcium supplementation and bone mineral density in adolescent girls, *J. Am. Med. Assoc.*, 270, 841, 1993.
23. **Drinkwater, B. L., Bruemner, B., and Chesnut, C. H., III,** Athletic amenorrhea in girls or young adult women, *J. Am. Med. Assoc.*, 263, 545, 1990.
24. **Warren, M. P., Brooks-Gunn, J., Fox, R. P., Lancelot, C., Newman, D., and Hamilton, W. G.,** Lack of bone accretion and amenorrhea: evidence for a relative osteopenia in weight-bearing bones, *J. Clin. Endocrinol. Metab.*, 72, 847, 1991.
25. **Myerson, M., Gutin, B., Warren, M. P., Wang, J., Lichtman, S., and Pierson, R. N., Jr.,** Total body bone density in amenorrheic runners, *Obstet. Gynecol.*, 79, 973, 1992.
26. **Hetland, M. L., Haarbo, J., and Christiansen, C.,** Running induces menstrual disturbancers but bone mass is unaffected, except in amenorrheic women, *Am. J. Med.*, 95, 53, 1993.
27. **Young, N., Formica, C., Szmukler, G., and Seeman, E.,** Bone density at weight-bearing and nonweight-bearing sites in ballet dancers: the effects of exercise, hypogonadism, and body weight, *J. Clin. Endocrinol. Metab.*, 78, 449, 1994.
28. **Compston, J. E., Laskey, M. A., Croucher, P. I., Coxon, A., and Kreitzman, S.,** Effect of diet-induced weight loss on total body bone mass, *Clin. Sci.*, 82, 429, 1992.
29. **Heaney, R. P.,** Calcium, bone health and osteoporosis. *Bone and Mineral Research 4*, Peck, W. A., ed., Excerpta Medica, Amsterdam, 1986.
30. **Arnaud, C. D. and Sanchez, S. D.,** Calcium and phosphorus, in *Present Knowledge in Nutrition*, 6th ed., Brown, M.L., ed., Nutrition Foundation, Washington, 1990.
31. **Krall, E. A., and Dawson-Hughes, B.,** Osteoporosis, in *Modern Nutrition in Health and Disease*, 8th ed., Shils, M. E., Olson, J.A. and Shike, M., eds., Lea & Febiger, Philadelphia, 1994.

32. **Allen, L. H. and Wood, R. J.,** Calcium and phosphorus, in *Modern Nutrition in Health and Disease*, 8th ed., Shils, M. E., Olson, J. A., and Shike, M., eds., Lea & Febiger, Philadelphia, 1994.
33. **Avioli, L. V.,** Calcium and phosphorus, in *Modern Nutrition in Health and Disease*, 7th ed., Lea & Febiger, Shils, M. E and Young, V., eds., Philadelphia, 1989.
34. **Hegsted, D. M.,** Calcium and phosphorus, in *Modern Nutrition in Health and Disease*, Goodhart, R. S. and Shils, M. E., eds., 5th ed., Lea & Febiger, Philadelphia, 1973.
35. **Branca, F., Robins, S. P., Ferro-Luzzi, A., and Golden, M. H. N.,** Bone turnover in malnourished children, *Lancet*, 340, 1493, 1992.
36. **Allen, J. C., Keller, R. P., Archer, P., and Neville, M. C.,** Studies in human lactation: milk composition and daily secretion rates of macronutrients in the first year of lactation, *Am. J. Clin. Nutr.*, 54, 69, 1991.
37. **Venkataraman, P. S. and Duke, J. C.,** Bone mineral content of healthy, full-term neonates: effect of race, gender, and maternal cigarette smoking, *Am. J. Dis. Child.*, 145, 1310, 1991.
38. **Wakefield, T., Disney, G. W., Mason, R. L., and Beauchene, R. E.,** Relationships among anthropometric indices of growth and creatinine and hydroxyproline excretion in preadolescent black and white girls, *Growth*, 44, 192, 1980.
39. **Mayor, G. H., Sanchez, T. V., and Garn, S. M.,** Adjusting photon-absorptiometry norms for whites to the black subject, in *Fourth International Conference on Bone Measurement*, Mazess, R. B., ed., NIH Publ. No. 80-1938, 1980.
40. **Li, J.-Y., Specker, B. L., Ho, M. L., and Tsang, R. C.,** Bone mineral content in black and white children 1 to 6 years of age: early appearance of race and sex differences, *Am. J. Dis. Child.*, 143, 1346, 1989.
41. **Bell, N. H., Shary, J., Stevens, J., Garza, M., Gordon, L., and Edwards, J.,** Demonstration that bone mass is greater in black than in white children, *J. Bone Miner. Res.*, 6, 719, 1991.
42. **Mazess, R. B. and Cameron, J. R.,** Growth of bone in school children: comparison of radiographic morphometry and photon absorptiometry, *Growth*, 36, 77, 1972.
43. **Gilsanz, V., Roe, T. F., Mora, S., Costin, G., and Goodman, W. G.,** Changes in vertebral bone density in black girls and white girls during childhood and puberty, *New Engl. J. Med.*, 325, 1597, 1991.
44. **McCormick, D. P., Ponder, S. W., Fawcett, H. D., and Palmer, J. L.,** Spinal bone mineral density in 335 normal and obese children and adolescents: evidence for ethnic and sex differences, *J. Bone Miner. Res.*, 6, 507, 1991.
45. **Slemenda, C. W., Miller, J. Z., Hui, S. L., Reister, T. K., and Johnston, C. C., Jr.,** Role of physical activity in the development of skeletal mass in children, *J. Bone Miner. Metab.*, 6, 1227, 1991.
46. **Slemenda, C. W., Reister, T. K., Hui, S. L., Miller, J. Z., Christian, J. C., and Johnston, C. C., Jr.,** Influences on skeletal mineralization in children and adolescents: evidence for varying effects of sexual maturation and physical activity, *J. Pediatr.*, 125, 201, 1994.
47. **Welten, D. C., Kemper, H. C. G., Post, G. B., Van Mechelen, W., Twisk, J., Lips, P., and Teule, G. J.,** Weight-bearing activity during youth is a more important factor for peak bone mass than calcium intake, *J. Bone Miner. Res.*, 9, 1089, 1994.
48. *Recommended Dietary Allowances, 10th ed.*, Subcommittee on the Recommended Dietary Allowances, Food and Nutrition Board, Commission on Life Sciences, National Research Council, National Academy Press, Washington, D.C., 1989.
49. **Anderson, J. J. B., Bennett, L., Curtis, R. C., Metz, J. A., Adeleke, V. M., Tylavsky, F. A., Taft, T. N., and Koch, G. G.,** Radial bone mass in healthy young adult white males: effects of calcium intake and exercise, 1994. (manuscript in preparation)
50. **Krabbe, S., Christiansen, C., Rodbro, P., and Transbol, I.,** Effect of puberty on rates of bone growth and mineralisation: with observations in male delayed puberty, *Arch. Dis. Child.*, 54, 950, 1979.
51. **Mauras, N., Haymond, M. W., Darmaun, D., Vieira, N. E., Abrams, S. A., and Yergey, A. L.,** Calcium and protein kinetics in prepubertal boys: positive effects of testosterone, *J. Clin. Invest.*, 93, 1014, 1994.
52. **Buchanan, J. R., Myers, C., Lloyd, T., Leuenberger, P., and Demers, L. M.,** Determinants of peak trabecular bone density in women: the role of androgens, estrogen, and exercise, *J. Bone Miner. Res.*, 3, 673, 1988.
53. **Glastre, C., Braillon, P., David, L., Cochat, P., Meunier, P. J., and Delmas, P. D.,** Measurement of bone mineral content of the lumbar spine by dual energy X-ray absorptiometry in normal children: correlations with growth parameters, *J. Clin. Endocrinol. Metab.*, 70, 1130, 1990.
54. **Lloyd, T., Rollings, N., Andon, M. B., Demers, L. M., Eggli, D. F., Kieselhorst, K., Kulin, H., Landis, J. R., Martel, J. K., Orr, G., and Smith, P.,** Determinants of bone density in young women. I: relationships among pubertal development, total body bone mass, and total body bone mineral density in premenarcheal females, *J. Clin. Endocrinol. Metab.*, 75, 383, 1992.
55. **Anderson, J. J. B. and Henderson, R. C.,** Dietary factors in the development of peak bone mass. In *Nutritional Aspects of Osteoporosis: Serono Symposium Publications*, Vol. 85, Burckhardt, P. and Heaney, R. P., eds., Raven Press, New York, 1991.
56. **Sandler, R. B., Slemenda, C. W., LaPorte, R. E., Cauley, J. A., Schramm, M. M., Barresi, M. L., and Kriska, A. M.,** Postmenopausal bone density and milk consumption in childhood and adolescence, *Am. J. Clin. Nutr.*, 42, 270, 1985.
57. **Bonjour, J. P., Theintz, G., Buchs, B., Slosman, D,. and Rizzoli, R.,** Critical years and stages of puberty for spinal and femoral bone mass accumulation during adolescence, *J. Clin. Endocrinol. Metab.*, 73, 555, 1991.

58. **Theintz, G., Buchs, B., Rizzoli, R., and Bonjour, J.-P.,** Longitudinal monitoring of bone mass accumulation in healthy adolescents: evidence for a marked reduction after 16 years of age at levels of lumbar spine and femoral neck in female subjects, *J. Clin. Endocrinol. Metab.*, 75, 1060, 1992.
59. **Matkovic, V. and Heaney, R. P.,** Calcium balance during human growth: evidence for threshold behavior, *Am. J. Clin. Nutr.*, 55, 992, 1992.
60. **Tylavsky, F. A., Bortz, A. D., Hancock, R. L., and Anderson, J. J. B.,** Familial resemblance of radial bone mass between premenopausal mothers and their college-age daughters, *Calcif. Tissue Int.*, 45, 265, 1989.
61. **McKay, H. A., Bailey, D. A., Wilkinson, A. A., and Houston, C. S.,** Familial comparison of bone mineral density at the proximal femur and lumbar spine, *Bone Miner.*, 24, 95, 1994.
62. **Meier, D. E., Luckey, M. M., Wallenstein, S., Clemens, T. L., Orwoll, E. S., and Waslien, C. I.,** Calcium, vitamin D, and parathrroid hormone status in young white and black women: association with racial differences in bone mass, *J. Clin. Endocrinol. Metab.*, 72, 703, 1991.
63. **Anderson, J. J. B. and Pollitzer, W. S.,** Ethnic and environmental determinants of peak bone mass. in *Advances in Nutritional Research*, vol. 9, Draper, H. H., ed., Plenum Press, New York, 1995, 129–149.
64. **Adeleke, V. M.,** *Determinants of Bone Mass in Young Adult Black and White Women*, Master's Thesis, University of North Carolina, Chapel Hill, NC, 1993.
65. **Eisman, J. A., Sambrook, P. N., Kelly, P. J., and Pocock, N. A.,** Exercise and its interaction with genetic influences in the determination of bone mineral density, *Am. J. Med.* (suppl 5B), 5S, 1991.
66. **Miller, J. Z., Slemenda, C. W., Meaney, F. J., Reister, T. K., Hui, S., and Johnston, C. C., Jr.,** The relationship of bone mineral density and anthropometric variables in healthy male and female children, *Bone Miner.*, 14, 137, 1991.
67. **Halioua, L. and Anderson, J. J. B.,** Age and anthropometric determinants of radial bone mass in premenopausal caucasian women: a cross-sectional study, *Osteoporosis Int.*, 1, 50, 1990.
68. **Farmer, M. E., Harris, T., Madans, J. H., Wallace, R. B., Cornoni-Huntley, J. R., and White, L. R.,** Anthropometric indicators and hip fractures: The NHANES I Epidemiological Follow-up Study, *J. Am. Geriatr. Soc.*, 37, 9, 1989.
69. **Pruzansky, A., Turano, M., Luckey, M., and Senie, R.,** Low body weight as a risk factor for hip fracture in both black and white women, *J. Orthop. Res.*, 7, 192, 1990.
70. **Lindsay, R., Cosman, F., Herrington, B. S., and Himmelstein, S.,** Bone mass and body composition in normal women, *J. Bone Miner. Res.*, 7, 55, 1992.
71. **Ortiz, O., Russell, M., Daley, T. L., Baumgartner, R. N., Waki, M., Lichtman, S., Wang, J., Pierson, R. N., Jr., and Heymsfield, S. B.,** Differences in skeletal muscle and bone mineral mass between black and white females and their relevance to estimates of body composition, *Am. J. Clin. Nutr.*, 55, 8, 1992.
72. **Riggs, B. L., Wahner, H. W., Dunn, W. L., Mazess, R. B., Offord, K. P., and Melton, L. J., III,** Differential changes in bone mineral density of the appendicular and axial skeleton with aging, *J. Clin. Invest.*, 67, 328, 1981.
73. **Geusens, P., Dequeker, J., Verstraeten, A., and Nijs, J.,** Age-, sex-, and menopause-related changes of vertebral and peripheral bone: population study using dual and single photon absorptiometry and radiogrammetry, *J. Nucl. Med.*, 27, 1540, 1986.
74. **Recker, R. R., Davies, M., Hinders, S. M., Heaney, R. P., Stegman, M. R., and Kimmel, D. B.,** Bone gain in young adult women, *J. Am. Med. Assoc.*, 268, 2403, 1992.
75. **Mazess, R. B. and Barden, H. S.,** Bone density in premenopausal women: effects of age, dietary intake, physical activity, and birth-control pills, *Am. J. Clin. Nutr.*, 53, 132, 1991.
76. **Lutz, J.,** Bone mineral, serum calcium, and dietary intakes of mother/daughter pairs, *Am. J. Clin. Nutr.*, 44, 99, 1986.
77. **Sowers, M. F. R., Burns, T. L., and Wallace, R. B.,** Familial resemblance of bone mass in adult women, *Genet. Epidemiol.*, 3, 85, 1986.
78. **Seeman, E., Hopper, J. L., Bach, L. A., Cooper, M. E., Parkinson, E., Mckay, J., and Jerums, G.,** Reduced bone mass in daughters of women with osteoporosis, *New Engl. J. Med.*, 320, 554, 1989.
79. **Lutz, J. and Tesar, R.,** Mother-daughter pairs: spinal and femoral bone densities and dietary intakes, *Am. J. Clin. Nutr.*, 52, 872, 1990.
80. **Talmage, R. V. and Anderson, J. J. B.,** Bone density loss in women: effects of childhood activity, exercise, calcium intake and estrogen therapy, *Calcif. Tissue Res.*, 36 (suppl 2), S52, 1984.
81. **Kanders, B., Dempster, D. W., and Lindsay, R.,** Interaction of calcium nutrition and physical activity on bone mass in young women, *J. Bone Miner. Res.*, 3, 145, 1988.
82. **Baran, D., Sorensen, A., Grimes, J., Lew, R., Karellas, A., Johnson, B., and Roche, J.,** Dietary modification with dairy products for preventing vertebral bone loss in premenopausal women: a three-year study, *J. Clin. Endocrinol. Metab.*, 70, 264, 1989.
83. **Riggs, B. L., Wahner, H. W., Melton, L. J., Jr., Richelson, L. S., Judd, A. J., and O'Fallon, W. M.,** Dietary calcium intake and rates of bone loss in women, *J. Clin. Invest.*, 80, 979, 1987.
84. **Sowers, M. R., Clark, M. K., Hollis, B., Wallace, R. B., and Jannowski, M.,** Radial bone mineral density in pre- and perimenopausal women: a prospective study of rates and risk factors for loss, *J. Bone Miner. Res.*, 7, 647, 1992.
85. **Slemenda, C. W., Hui, S. L., Williams, C. J., Christian, J. C., Meaney, F., and Johnston, C. C., Jr.,** Bone mass and anthropometric measurements in adult females, *Bone Miner.*, 11, 101, 1990.

86. **Reid, I. R., Plank, L. D., and Evans, M. C.,** Fat mass is an important determinant of whole body bone density in premenopausal women but not in men, *J. Clin. Endocrinol. Metab.*, 75, 779, 1992.
87. **Tremollieres, F. A., Pouilles, J.-M., and Ribot, C.,** Vertebral postmenopausal bone loss is reduced in overweight women: a longitudinal study in 155 early postmenopausal women, *J. Clin. Endocrinol. Metab.*, 77, 683, 1993.
88. **Jacobson, P. C., Beaver, W., Grubb, S. A., and Talmage, R. V.,** Bone density in women: college athletes and older athletic women, *J. Orthop. Res.*, 2, 328, 1984.
89. **Talmage, R. V., Stinnett, S. S., Landwehr, J. T., Vincent, L. M., and McCartney, W. H.,** Age-related loss of bone mineral density in non-athletic and athletic women, *Bone Miner.*, 1, 115, 1986.
90. **Buchanan, J. R. , Myers, C., Lloyd, T., and Greer, R. B., III,** Early vertebral trabecular bone loss in normal premenopausal women, *J. Bone Miner. Res.*, 3, 583, 1988.
91. **Zhang, J., Feldblum, P. J., and Fortney, J. A.,** Moderate physical activity and bone density among perimenopausal women, *Am. J. Public Health*, 82, 736, 1992.
92. **Lindsay, R., Tohme, J., and Kanders, B.,** The effect of oral contraceptive use on vertebral bone mass in pre- and post-menopausal women, *Contraception*, 34, 333, 1986.
93. **Heaney, R. P., Recker, R. R., and Saville, P. D.,** Menopausal changes in calcium balance performance, *J. Lab. Clin. Med.*, 92, 964, 1978.
94. **Liel, Y., Edwards, J., Shary, J., Spicer, K. M., Gordon, L., and Bell, N. H.,** The effects of race and body habitus on bone mineral density of the radius, hip and spine in premenopausal women, *J. Clin. Endocrinol. Metab.*, 66, 1247, 1988.
95. **Luckey, M. M., Meier, D. E., Mandeli, J. P., DaCosta, M. C., Hubbard, M. L., and Goldsmith, S. J.,** Radial and vertebral bone density in white and black women: evidence for racial differences in premenopausal bone homeostasis, *J. Clin. Endocrinol. Metab.*, 69, 762, 1989.
96. **Riis, B. J., Thomsen, K., and Christiansen, C.,** Does calcium supplementation prevent postmenopausal bone loss? *New Engl. J. Med.*, 316, 173, 1987.
97. **Dawson-Hughes, B., Dallal, G. E., Krall, E. A., Sadowski, L., Sahyoun, N., and Tannenbaum, S.,** A controlled trial of the effect of calcium supplementation on bone density in postmenopausal women, *New Engl. J. Med.*, 323, 878, 1990.
98. **Peacock, M., Johnston, C. C., Jr., and Christian, J. C.,** Inheritance of calcium absorption, calcium-regulating hormones and bone turnover, in *Calcium Regulating Hormones and Bone Metabolism*, Cohn, D. V., Gennari, C., and Tashjian, A. H., Jr., eds., Elsevier Science Publishers, Excerpta Medica, Amsterdam, 1992.
99. **Ribot, C., Tremollieres, F., Pouilles, J.-M., Bonneau, M., Germain, F., and Louvet, J.-P.,** Obesity and postmenopausal bone loss: the influence of obesity on vertebral density and bone turnover in postmenopausal women, *Bone*, 8, 327, 1988.
100. **Bevier, W. C., Wiswell, R. A., Pyka, G., Kozak, K. C., Newhall, K. M., and Marcus, R.,** Relationship of body composition, muscle strength, and aerobic capacity to bone mineral density in older men and women, *J. Bone Miner. Res.*, 4, 421, 1989.
101. **Hassager, C. and Christiansen, C.,** Influence of soft tissue body composition on bone mass and metabolism, *Bone*, 10, 415, 1989.
102. **Lacey, J. M., Anderson, J. J. B., Fujita, T., Fukase, M., Tsuchie, S., and Koch, G. G.,** Correlates of cortical bone mass among premenopausal and postmenopausal Japanese women, *J. Bone Miner. Res.*, 6, 651, 1991.
103. **Tsunenari, T., Tsutsumi, M., Ohno, K., Yamamoto, Y., Kawakatsu, M., Shimogaki, K., Negishi, H., Sugimoto, T., Fukase, M., and Fujita, T.,** Age- and gender-related changes in body composition in Japanese subjects, *J. Bone Miner. Res.*, 8, 397, 1993.
104. **Lau, E. M. C., Woo, J., Leung, P. C., and Swaminathan, R.,** Low bone mineral density, grip strength and skinfold thickness are important risk factors for hip fracture in Hong Kong Chinese, *Osteoporosis Int.*, 3, 66, 1993.
105. **Felson, D. T., Zhang, Y., Hannan, M. T., and Anderson, J. J.,** Effects of weight and body mass index on bone mineral density in men and women: the Framingham Study, *J. Bone Miner. Res.*, 8, 567, 1993.
106. **Cummings, S. R. and Nevitt, M. C.,** A hypothesis: the causes of hip fractures, *J. Gerontol.*, 44, M107, 1989.
107. **Fujita, T. and Fukase, M.,** Comparison of osteoporosis and calcium intake between Japan and the United States, *Proc. Soc. Exp. Biol. Med.*, 200,149, 1992.
108. **Ross, P. D., Orimo, H., Wasnich, R. D., Vogel, J. M., MacLean, C. J., Davis, J. W., and Nomura, A.,** Methodological issues in comparing genetic and environmental influences on bone mass, *Bone Miner.*, 7, 67, 1989.
109. **Kin, K., Lee, J. H. E., Kushida, K., Sartoris, D. J., Ohmura, A., Clopton, P. L., and Inoue, T.,** Bone density and body composition on the Pacific rim: a comparison between Japan-born and U.S.-born Japanese-American women, *J. Bone Miner. Res.*, 8, 861, 1993.
110. **Reed, J. A., Anderson, J. J. B., Tylavsky, F. A., and Gallagher, P. N., Jr.,** Comparative changes in radial-bone density of elderly female lactoovovegetarians and omnivores, *Am. J. Clin. Nutr.*, 59 (suppl), 1197S, 1994.
111. **Chapuy, M. C., Arlot, M. E., Duboeuf, F., Brun, J., Crouzet, B., Arnaud, S., Delmas, P. D., and Meunier, P. J.,** Vitamin D_3 and calcium prevent hip fractures in elderly women, *New Engl. J. Med.*, 327, 1637, 1992.
112. **Anderson, J. J. B.,** Nutritional biochemistry of calcium and phosphorus, *J. Nutr. Biochem.*, 2, 300, 1991.

113. **Calvo, M. S., Kumar, R., and Heath, H., III.,** Persistently elevated parathyroid hormone secretion and action in young women after four weeks of ingesting high phosphorus, low calcium diets, *J. Clin. Endocrinol. Metab.*, 70, 1334, 1990.
114. **Barger-Lux, J. and Heaney, R. P.,** Effects of calcium restriction on metabolic characteristics of premenopausal women, *J. Clin. Endocrinol. Metab.*, 76, 103, 1993.
115. **Calvo, M. S.,** Dietary phosphorus, calcium metabolism and bone, *J. Nutr.*, 123, 1627, 1993.
116. **Anderson, J. J. B., and Barrett, C. J. H.,** Dietary phosphorus: the benefits and the problems, *Nutr. Today*, 27, 29, 1994.
117. **Abelow, B. J., Holford, T. R., and Insogna, K. L.,** Cross-cultural association between dietary animal protein and hip fracture: a hypothesis, *Calcif. Tissue Int.*, 150, 14, 1992.
118. **Schuette, S. A. and Linkswiler, H. M.,** Effects on Ca and P metabolism in humans by adding meat, meat plus milk, or purified proteins plus Ca and P to a low protein diet, *J. Nutr.*, 112, 338, 1982.
119. **Kerstetter, J. E. and Allen, L. H.,** Dietary protein increases urinary calcium, *J. Nutr.*, 120, 134, 1990.
120. **Orwoll, E. S.,** The effects of dietary protein insufficiency and excess on skeletal health, *Bone*, 13, 343, 1992.
121. **Anderson, J. J. B.,** Dietary calcium and bone mass through the lifecycle, *Nutr. Today*, 25, 9, 1990.
122. **Matkovic, V.,** Calcium metabolism and calcium requirements during skeletal modeling and consolidation of bone mass, *Am. J. Clin. Nutr.*, 54, 245S, 1991.
123. **Anderson, J. J. B. and Allen, J. C.,** Nutrition of macrominerals and trace elements, in *Functional Foods*, Goldberg, I., ed., Chapman and Hall, New York, 1994.
124. **Greer, F. R.,** Pediatric calcium needs and metabolism beyond infancy, in *Calcium Nutriture for Mothers and Children*, Tsang, R. C. and Mimouni, F., eds., Glendale/Raven Press, New York, 1992.
125. **Fomon, S. J.,** *Infant Nutrition*, 2nd ed., W.B. Saunders, Philadelphia, 1974.
126. **Dempster, D.W., Shane, E., Horbert, W., and Lindsay, R.,** A simple method for correlative light and scanning electron microscopy of human iliac crest bone biopsies: qualitative obervations in normal and osteoporotic subjects, *J. Bone Min. Res.*, 1, 15, 1986.

Chapter 18

EFFECTS OF ALCOHOL ON CALCIUM HOMEOSTASIS AND BONE

Philip F. Hirsch, Ph.D. and Tai-Chan Peng, M.D.

TABLE OF CONTENTS

I. INTRODUCTION

Excessive alcohol consumption in both men and women is a serious medical problem associated with osteopenia and an increased incidence of osteoporotic fractures. Several recent reviews have focused on the relationship between excessive alcohol abuse and bone.[1-6] Almost all human studies, however, have been cross-sectional. In one type of study, data on groups of individuals for whom bone density has been measured have been analyzed against an estimated consumption of ethanol. Alternatively, the bone density of subjects who have a known history of alcoholism has been compared to the bone density of control subjects who either consume only moderate amounts of ethanol or are abstainers. Although both types of analyses have generally demonstrated deleterious effects of excessive ethanol consumption on bone, these approaches do not distinguish between the direct effects of ethanol on bone or on calcium (Ca) metabolism, nor do they report the effects of

0-8493-7845-1/95/$0.00+$.50

other health problems and behaviors that also undoubtedly contribute to the low bone mass and/or fractures.

Poor nutritional habits typically accompany alcoholism. Chronic alcoholics, who consume a large fraction of their daily caloric intake as alcohol, consume few calories and other nutrients from food, and they invariably suffer from malnutrition. Thus, they are more likely to have inadequate daily intakes of Ca, other minerals, and vitamins, particularly vitamin D. Alcoholics also typically reduce their physical activity. Finally, alcoholics are more likely to suffer falls and other accidents while intoxicated, an important factor in the increased incidence of fractures.

The questions of cause and effect between alcohol consumption and decreased bone mass are best answered in prospective studies in which the bone health of individuals with known levels of ethanol intake can be followed in parallel with control subjects abstaining from alcohol. Obvious problems exist with such studies, such as recruiting and following subjects long enough for bone changes to be detectable and resolving the ethical issues involved. These complicating factors make it extremely difficult to establish the changes in bone resulting from the consumption of ethanol per se.

The difficulties inherent in this research arena have been addressed to some extent by the use of an experimental rat model. By providing carefully controlled liquid diets that provide adequate protein, minerals, and vitamins for growth and development of rats,[7] investigators have largely been able to rule out the effects of inadequate nutrient intakes. By substituting ethanol for glucose or sucrose as a component of the diet, investigators can maintain dietary intakes isocaloric to those of alcohol consumption. The consumption of such diets as the sole source of nutrients and water ensures that animals will consume sufficient amounts of ethanol to maintain elevated blood levels.

II. ALCOHOL AND CALCIUM HOMEOSTASIS

Alcohol affects Ca metabolism in several ways through the action of ethanol on diverse body tissues, both directly and indirectly.

A. EFFECTS OF ACUTE ALCOHOL CONSUMPTION ON CALCIUM AND CALCEMIC HORMONES

Research results from both animal models and human studies are reviewed here.

1. Studies in an Animal Model

Peng et al. found that a single dose of alcohol, ranging from 2 to 8g/kg, produced rapid hypocalcemia in both rats and dogs.[8] The onset of hypocalcemia occurred within 30 minutes and it lasted at least 5 hours. In a later study Peng and Gitelman[9] confirmed the Ca-lowering effect of ethanol in rats, showing that serum ionic Ca as well as total serum Ca fell. They also found that serum magnesium increased. Evidence was also presented demonstrating that ethanol inhibited the Ca-mobilizing activity of parathyroid hormone (PTH). Thus, even if PTH secretion were increased, it is unlikely that PTH could mobilize sufficient Ca from bone to restore serum levels to normal. Shah et al.[10] reported an increase in PTH that accompanied the Ca-lowering effect of ethanol, 2.5 g/kg, injected intraperitoneally into rats; even lower doses were also found to lower Ca and to increase PTH, as measured by a sensitive N-terminal assay for rat PTH.[11] On the other hand, Thomas et al.[12] did not find an increase in serum PTH in response to alcohol-induced hypocalcemia when rats were given ethanol at a dose of 2 g of ethanol/kg body weight. They compared their results of no change in PTH using ethanol with the increased serum PTH observed in rats given a dose of EDTA that lowered serum Ca to the same extent as the ethanol. In another study Chanard et al.[13] gave a large dose of ethanol, 6 g/kg, which resulted in both hypocalcemia and hypermagnesemia. The hypocalcemia persisted even after the administration of exogenous PTH, confirming the earlier finding of Peng and Gitelman.[9] Chanard et al.[13] also found that when ethanol was added to parathyroid glands *in vitro,* PTH secretion did not increase, but the elevation in PTH observed after adding EDTA was inhibited.

TABLE 1
Effect of Oral Doses of Ethanol on Serum Calcium and PTH in Normal Human Subjects

Dose g/kg	N	Hours Examined	Change in Serum Values: Calcium	PTH	Reference	Comments
1.2–1.5	24	16	—	– then +	14	Some females. Some controls were fasted.
0.8	12	2	None	none	15	Males, 6 controls, not fasted
0.8	11	4.5	None	+	16	Males: EtOH (6), Controls (5)
1.4	5	4	None	not measured	17	Males; no controls

2. Effects of Alcohol in Humans

Some investigators have made similar observations in humans.[14-17] For example, Laitinen, et al.[14] observed hypocalcemia in normal men and women consuming 1.2 to 1.5 g/kg of alcohol; serum levels of PTH decreased at first and then increased above controls. This study used more subjects, a more reliable assay (immunoradimetric, IRMA) for PTH, and measured levels of Ca and PTH over a more extended time interval than earlier studies in which results were not as consistent (Table 1).

The mechanism(s) leading to the hypocalcemia after the oral administration of alcohol in rats has/have not been elucidated. This hypocalcemia cannot be explained by increased urinary losses of Ca because ethanol typically decreased, rather than increased, the urinary excretion of Ca.[8] Because blood pH and total serum proteins remain unchanged, these factors are not responsible for the acute hypocalcemia, and, as already mentioned, ethanol administration also lowers serum-ionized Ca.[9] The possibility that calcitonin (CT) may be involved was ruled out when the Ca-lowering effect of ethanol was still observed in CT-deficient (thyroidectomized) rats with functional parathyroid transplants.[8] The fall in serum Ca apparently results from the inhibition of the Ca-mobilizing action of PTH, as suggested by the studies just described. Thus, a net shift of Ca from extracellular fluid into tissues, most likely bone, follows ethanol administration.[18]

Relevant to the role of the acute effects of ethanol on the subsequent loss of bone in chronic alcoholism are the results of a recent study by Laitinen et al.[19] These authors found that alcohol-intoxicated men known to be heavy users of alcohol were hypocalcemic relative to healthy male controls, whereas PTH levels in the two groups were similar. However, serum levels of cross-linked carboxyterminal telopeptide of human type I collagen, a marker of bone turnover (see Chapter 10), were significantly higher in the alcohol-intoxicated subjects, and the telopeptide marker no longer correlated with serum osteocalcin, as it did in controls. On the basis of these measurements, the authors concluded that alcohol intoxication interferes with the normal response of parathyroid glands to a hypocalcemic stimulus and that the bone formation in these subjects was uncoupled from the bone resorption.

3. Summary

High doses of ethanol administered to rats and, in some instances, to humans, result in hypocalcemia. The evidence suggests that hypocalcemia usually, but not always, causes the expected increase in levels of PTH, but for reasons not yet understood, the Ca-mobilizing action of PTH is suppressed. Ethanol may also promote increased osteoclastic activity, which is likely mediated through a direct action on osteoblasts (see later), but the inhibition of PTH action by ethanol appears primary to the inhibition of bone formation and the maintenance of the remodeling process.

B. EFFECTS OF CHRONIC ALCOHOL CONSUMPTION ON CALCIUM AND CALCEMIC HORMONES

Data from both animal and human investigations are reviewed in this section, which emphasizes the chronic effects of ethanol on Ca-regulating hormones.

1. Vitamin D

The effect of alcohol on vitamin D metabolism is not well understood.[5] Unlike the diet consumed by human alcoholics who are often malnourished and may lack sunlight, the liquid diet fed to experimental rats is vitamin-supplemented and nutritionally adequate. Although sufficient vitamin D is present in the diet, its metabolism may be altered, because it is well established that chronic alcoholics sometimes present with osteomalacia and liver cirrhosis. However, there seems to be no significant correlation between plasma levels of vitamin D metabolites and the degree of osteomalacia.[5] In rats fed an alcoholic diet for 11 months, Turner et al.[20] found that serum 25-hydroxyvitamin D (25(OH)D) was significantly increased, whereas 1,25 dihydroxyvitamin D_3 (1,25$(OH)_2$D) was decreased, compared to findings in control rats fed an isocaloric diet (dextrin:maltose, 3:1). Earlier, Turner et al.[21] did not observe changes in serum vitamin D_3 metabolites in rats fed similar diets for only 3 weeks, although in both studies ethanol decreased matrix formation and mineralization of bone tissue. Gascon-Barre[22] used rats that had been depleted of vitamin D and fed them an alcohol diet in which ethanol represented 36% of the caloric intake. Each rat also was given 92 IU of [^{14}C]vitamin D_3 intragastrically 3 times a week for $3^2/_3$ weeks of the 4-week experimental period. Under these experimental conditions, tissue reserves of vitamin D_3 in plasma, muscle, and adipose tissue were reduced in ethanol-fed rats compared to those in dextrin-fed controls. In contrast, total plasma and liver 25(OH)D_3 concentrations were increased when vitamin D_3 administration was combined with the ethanol treatment.

Alcohol is known to affect liver function, and the metabolism of vitamin D is dependent on the liver. Even without fully developed cirrhosis, liver function is generally depressed. The early effects of ethanol on bone are not likely the result of changes in vitamin D metabolism, but later effects of alcohol may be related to vitamin D deficiency as a result of suppressed production of 25(OH)D_3. The multifactorial involvement of reduced sun exposure, malnutrition, and complications of liver function make interpretation difficult.[5] On the basis of a lack of osteomalacia in alcoholics and normal levels of vitamin D metabolites, Bikle et al.[23] concluded that vitamin D deficiency is not likely to be the cause of bone disease in most of the subjects from his study in San Francisco.

2. Parathyroid Hormone

The PTH serum levels of current and former alcoholics, i.e., those who had abstained for an extended period, have been compared. In some, but not all, studies blood levels of PTH have been found to be elevated.[1] Lindholm et al.[24] found that alcoholics had both lower bone formation and turnover rates, as well as lower serum levels of PTH than abstainers. Manfredini et al.[25] also found that alcohol abusers had significant reductions in plasma PTH. On the other hand, Laitinen et al.[26] did not find any difference in serum PTH or vitamin D metabolites between 27 noncirrhotic alcoholic male patients and controls. In contrast, Bikle et al.[23] found that their alcoholic subjects had increased total resorption surfaces with high normal or elevated levels of PTH that correlated with age but not with the extent of bone loss. They concluded that, although PTH may play a role in stimulating bone resorption in alcoholics, alcohol-induced bone loss appears unrelated to the status of PTH. In a recent study of alcoholic women by Laitinen et al.,[27] PTH levels were found to be normal. Heavy drinking did not lead to a decrease of bone mass in young and middle-aged women despite marked reductions in serum concentrations of both 25(OH)D_3 and 1,25$(OH)_2D_3$. The geographical location of the study, Finland, could have influenced the findings with respect to vitamin D metabolites.

3. Calcitonin

Changes in serum CT levels in alcoholics have not been studied adequately. Williams et al.[16] measured the short-term effects of oral alcohol administration on CT levels in human subjects and found that CT levels increased over the first 3 to 4 hours, but that the levels had returned to control levels by $4^1/_2$ hours. Plasma CT also rose in rats within a few minutes after they were given a large dose of ethanol, 3.7 g/kg, by gavage, but CT levels had returned to control levels in less than 1 hour.[28]

In a study of 34 hospitalized male alcoholics and 35 age-matched controls, no difference in serum levels of CT were noted between the groups.[29]

4. Summary

The overall status of Ca-regulating hormones is difficult to summarize because of the varied results. No clear picture of the role of vitamin D metabolites, PTH, or CT has emerged from studies on human subjects. The variation in the results of the studies presented herein may result from a number of factors, including different methodologies, the geographical location of patients, and the nutritional status of subjects. Results and conclusions from rat studies, however, are somewhat more consistent. Further studies are required to establish a clear picture of the roles that these hormones play in the bone loss resulting from alcohol consumption.

C. SUMMARY

Investigations of the effects of alcohol on Ca homeostasis in humans and in animal models suggest that a large, acute dose, as well as long-term usage of alcohol at modest to high doses, have significant adverse effects on the Ca-regulating hormones, serum Ca concentrations, and bone mass. The mechanisms contributing to hormonal changes and loss of bone mineral remain to be established.

III. EFFECTS OF CHRONIC ALCOHOL USE ON BONE

Alcohol has both direct and indirect effects on bone tissue, but the evidence for a direct effect, especially in humans, is not convincing. The mechanism for the chronic effects of ethanol on bone have been speculated upon, but the current knowledge is not sufficient to provide a comprehensive understanding.

A. ALCOHOL AND HUMAN OSTEOPOROSIS

The detrimental effects of alcohol abuse on bone health are gaining increased recognition.[1-6] Previously, other deleterious and easily recognizable effects of alcoholism on gastrointestinal, hepatic, cardiovascular, hematopoietic, genitourinary, and neuromuscular functions, as well as impaired social and occupational functions, have overshadowed the recognition of a relationship between alcohol consumption and the loss of bone mass. The increased incidence of fractures in alcoholics was often ascribed to increased trauma due to impaired motor function.

In 1973, Nilsson and Westlin[30] published the results of forearm bone density measurement in a large number of alcoholic patients and compared the results with those of outpatients without a history of alcoholism. Their data (Figure 1) provide convincing evidence that the chronic consumption of alcohol is a major risk factor for osteoporosis. More recent observations suggest a cumulative dose-effect of ethanol that is inversely related to bone mineral density.[31] A relationship between dose and body weight was indicated in a study of male veterans in which the maintenance of weight, even in the presence of chronic alcoholism, was found to protect against bone loss and fracture.[32]

The mechanisms responsible for the bone loss, however, have been difficult to establish. Bone loss results, in part, from a direct effect of alcohol and, in part, from indirect effects of the abnormal clinical, biochemical and electrophysiological changes associated with chronic alcoholism. Besides the changes in the Ca-regulating hormones, i.e., vitamin D, PTH, and CT, other endocrine alterations occur as a result of alcohol abuse.[4] Hypogonadism, for one, is an important factor contributing to the development of osteoporosis in both men and women.[4] Deprivation of adequate dietary requirements for health and maintenance of bone undoubtedly plays an additional role in the bone loss. The development of effective treatment to minimize bone loss in alcoholics and to restore bone lost because of alcohol abuse will require elucidation of the mechanism(s) involved. To establish with certainty which effects are directly due to alcohol and which are indirect, as well as to determine effective therapeutic measures will continue the need for suitable animal models.

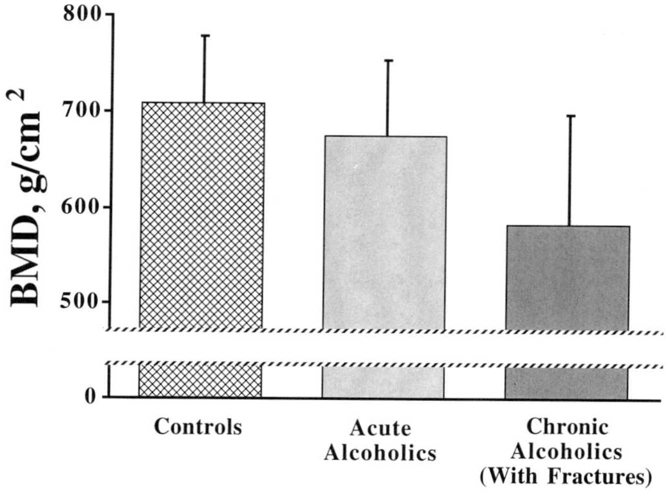

FIGURE 1. Bone Mineral Density of the Proximal Forearm of Male Controls and Chronic Alcoholics, Mean values (±)SE for BMD, mg/cm^2, are shown for 56 nonalcoholics, A: 58 patients voluntarily admitted for treatment of alcoholism to the Dept. of Alcoholism, and B: 35 patients admitted or seen as out patients in the Dept. of Orthopedics, 18 with fractures, at Malmo General Hospital, Malmo, Sweden. The alcoholic patients had significantly lower bone density, $p<0.02$, middle bar, (mean age 45), and $p<0.001$, right bar, (mean age 52), than controls (mean age 45). (Data from Reference 30).

B. RAT MODEL OF ALCOHOL EFFECTS ON BONE

The rat is the animal model most frequently used in investigations of the skeletal effects of the chronic alcohol use. Data on bone changes using several different experimental approaches are presented.

1. Diet and Alcoholism

The finding of a Ca-lowering effect of a single dose of ethanol in rats[8] stimulated investigators to study the effects of chronic administration of alcohol on bones of rats. In these studies the control rats are fed a nutritionally adequate liquid diet in which alcohol is replaced with an isocaloric amount of carbohydrate in the control diet. This experimental approach helps eliminate some, but not all, of the multifactorial components that are undoubtedly responsible for part of the human condition. The main objective in these rat studies is to identify those effects on bone that can be ascribed *directly* to the consumption of alcohol. Once the changes are identified, the mechanisms involved can be elucidated. Some early studies did not produce bone loss, apparently due to the short interval of alcohol treatment[33] or to doses insufficient to obtain bone loss.[34] As described in detail next, many studies have now been reported that show clearly that large doses of alcohol given to rats do decrease bone mass, even when a nutritionally adequate diet is provided.

2. Color, Fragility, and Morphology of Bone

Peng et al.[35] fed male and female rats liquid diets containing either 8% ethanol (w/v) or an isocaloric diet in which glucose was substituted for alcohol. The volume of the liquid diet presented to the rats was 35 ml, but, especially early in the experiment, the total volume was not always consumed. At the end of the experiment at 4 or 6 weeks, males weighed more than the females. The liquid diets were restricted so that by the end of the feeding period, control rats fed a commercial rat chow weighed more than thê experimental rats.

At the end of the experimental period, when the tibiae were removed and dried, the bones from the alcohol-fed rats were more fragile than those from the control-fed rats.[35] The greater fragility of the bones from the alcohol-fed rats was undoubtedly due to the loss of mineral easily seen by scanning electron microscopy.[36] Examination of the ultrastructure of the distal ends of femurs from rats fed the 8% ethanol diet revealed much thinner and more fragile appearing trabeculae than those from control rats (Figure 2).

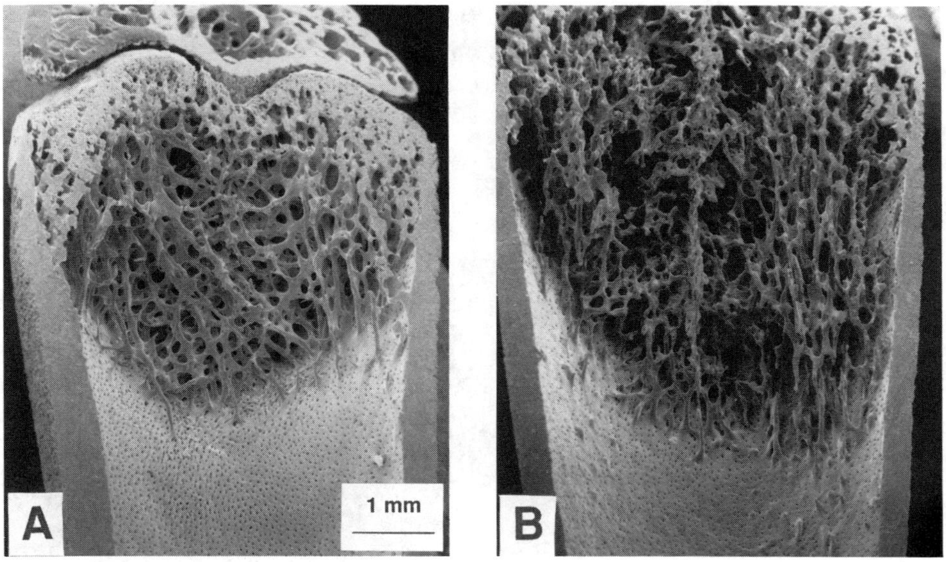

FIGURE 2. Scanning Electron Micrographs of the Distal End of Rat Femurs. Panel A is a micrograph of the femur from a rat fed the control liquid diet for 6 weeks. Panel B is a micrograph of a femur from a rat fed the ethanol liquid diet for 6 weeks. The trabeculae in the femur of the alcohol-treated rat appear thinner, more fragile, and extend much further into the diaphysis than those in the control femur. Cortical thickness also appears reduced in the femur from the ethanol-fed rats.

The dried femurs from alcoholic rats were much darker in appearance than the bones from control rats.[35,36] The color change may have been due to the thinner cortical bone through which marrow and blood vessels may be more readily seen.

3. Mechanical Properties of Bone

Measurements of mechanical properties of femurs from ethanol-fed rats were obtained by Peng and co-workers and compared with those from control-fed rats.[36,37] Femurs were removed from rats fed the liquid diets for 4 weeks, and the mechanical properties of the femurs were estimated using a three-point bending test.[36] The definitions of the mechanical properties examined are listed in Table 2.

Male and female rats were presented with 35 ml of liquid diet each day. In the early part of the study, when the rats were small, not all of the diet was consumed, and the males grew faster than the females. Although the male rats were heavier than females, no significant difference was found between the weights of the alcohol- and the control-fed rats, an indication that isocaloric intake within sexes was adequately achieved.

Examination of the results revealed a large bone loss in females administered the alcohol diet for 4 weeks. The changes in mechanical properties appeared larger with smaller rats, suggesting a relationship between body weight and dose. For this reason, the results for whole-bone properties were expressed as mechanical measurement divided by body weight. Table 3 shows the results of measurements of mechanical properties of femurs from control- and ethanol-fed female rats.[36,37] The most striking effect of chronic feeding of ethanol was on the reduced strength of femurs. Stiffness also decreased, but not all of the mechanical properties of bones from alcohol-fed rats were significantly different from those of control rats.

The mechanical measurements of femurs were also plotted against the specific dose of ethanol, i.e., grams of ethanol/gram of body weight. The relationship between femoral bone strength and dose of ethanol in male and female rats was found to be highly significant ($p < 0.001$).[36] The plot also revealed that a threshold dose existed at 0.012 g of ethanol/day/g body weight. If this dose was exceeded, the strength of the femurs would fall below those obtained from the control-fed rats.[36]

TABLE 2
Definitions of Mechanical Properties

Strength	The maximum force required for failure or to fracture
Stiffness	The slope of the force deflection curve
Ductility	The time after applying increasing force to fracture or for failure
Toughness	The area under the force deflection curve

TABLE 3
Specific Strength, Stiffness, Toughness, and Ductility of Femurs

			Specific Whole Bone Properties*			
Exper.	(No. of rats)	Diet	Strength† (N/g) × 10^2	Stiffness [N/(mxg)] × 10^{-3}	Toughness (Nxm/g) × 10^3	Ductility (m/g) × 10^5
1	(5)	CLD	38.6 ± 1.5	1.072 ± 0.046	0.151 ± 0.001	0.281 ± 0.013
	(5)	ELD	32.2 ± 1.6	0.951 ± 0.050	0.106 ± 0.012	0.237 ± 0.014
Relative change			–16.6%	–11.3%	–29.8%	–15.7%
p value			<0.025	NS	<0.025	NS
2	(6)	CLD	31.3 ± 1.2	1.023 ± 0.072	0.171 ± 0.014	0.389 ± 0.041
	(5)	ELD	24.2 ± 1.4	0.634 ± 0.079	0.164 ± 0.016	0.556 ± 0.045
Relative change			–22.7%	–38.0%	–4.1%	+42.9%
p value			<0.005	<0.01	NS	<0.05

Note: Female rats were fed either a control or an ethanol liquid diet for 4 weeks.
* Values for whole bone properties are expressed as means ±SE.
† Units for whole bone properties are N = newtons, g = grams of body weight, and m = deflection at maximum force.
Data obtained from References 36 and 37.

Plots of the other mechanical properties against the specific dose of alcohol also revealed significant relationships.[37] Table 4 shows the equations, r values, and significance levels obtained for the correlations between the four mechanical properties measured and the dose of alcohol. All of the correlations were significant.

The results of studies in rats have helped investigators gain understandings of the nature of alcohol effects. For example, when bone mineral loss occurs, declines in both strength and stiffness may follow, as the bone becomes more plastic. The resulting increase in flexibility may mean that the amount of energy required for fracture (toughness) may not be markedly affected.

Although the measurement of mechanical properties of bones from alcohol-fed animals may be useful in determining the mechanism(s) of the deleterious effects of alcohol consumption of bone strength, there are important differences between fractures in alcoholics and the *ex vivo* testing of whole-bone properties. Many fractures in alcoholics result from a sudden, although often modest, impact, in which the energy propagates rapidly and causes prompt failure. In contrast, the fractures of bones during mechanical testing (Table 3) result from a force applied at a constant rate until failure occurs.[37]

Establishing measurements of the properties of intact bone, as well as the relationship between the mechanical properties and the specific dose of alcohol, is important. Such measurements are easily obtained in experiments on rats. Because of the quantitative nature of the measurements, they will be most helpful in assessing the value of treatments employed to prevent bone loss during excessive ethanol consumption and/or to reverse the deleterious effects after withdrawal. Whereas other measurements of bone, such as biochemical changes, help to elucidate mechanisms, the purpose of therapeutic intervention is to reduce the incidence of fracture by improving the quality of bone. The improvement of the mechanical properties of bone, an objective way of assessing the

TABLE 4
Relationship between the Dose of Alcohol, Grams/Day/Body Weight and Mechanical Properties

Specific Bone Property*	Linear Relationship	r	P
Strength	Strength = 140.4–600.3 × (dose) (N/g) × 10^2	0.81	< 0.001
Stiffness	Stiffness = 344.1–13.72 × (dose) [N/(mxg)] × 10^{-3}	0.64	< 0.001
Toughness	Toughness = 49.42–1.400 × 10^3 × (dose) (Nxm/g) × 10^3	0.43	< 0.05
Ductility	Ductility = 275.6 × 10^{-3} + 39.76 × (dose) (m/g) × 10^5	0.43	< 0.05

Note: Rats were fed on ethanol-containing diet for 4 weeks, and specific strength, stiffness, toughness, and ductility of femurs were measured.

* There were 27 rat femurs obtained from three experiments with males and two with females.

Data obtained from References 36 and 37.

success of therapeutic intervention, can be approached by quantitative measurements of mechanical properties, especially strength and stiffness of femurs in the alcoholic rat model.

4. DNA, RNA, and Protein Synthesis in Bone

Preedy and Peters[38] found that chronic ethanol consumption in rats for up to 42 days had no significant effect on either DNA or RNA content, or on the bone protein synthesis of tibiae according to a comparison of these measurements with those of isocalorically pair-fed controls. However, large differences existed between the rats fed standard laboratory chow and those fed the restricted diet. These studies are important because they again point out that bone biochemical parameters can be markedly influenced by feeding restricted diets.

5. Osteocalcin and Bone

Osteocalcin (bone Gla-protein or BGP) has attracted much attention because it is a sensitive marker of bone turnover.[39] Osteocalcin, the most abundant noncollagenous protein in bone, is synthesized in osteoblasts and then secreted into the blood. Since serum osteocalcin concentrations correlate well with osteoblastic activity,[40-42] studies on the effect of alcohol on blood levels of osteocalcin have been undertaken.

Acute doses of alcohol in humans have been found to lower serum osteocalcin. For example, Rico et al.[43] found low serum osteocalcin in patients with acute alcohol intoxication. These authors concluded that the response resulted from a direct effect of ethanol on osteoblasts. In another human study a single dose of alcohol, 50 g, reduced serum osteocalcin levels significantly ($p < 0.02$) during the first two hours. Although 25 g of alcohol lowered serum osteocalcin, the change was not significant.[44] These results suggest that a dose-response relationship exists between ethanol consumption and the inhibition of osteoblastic activity.

Whether or not alcohol abuse leads to an increase in osteoclastic activity has been investigated. Examination by scanning electron microscopy of bone biopsies from alcoholic patients suggests marked defects in osteoblastic function and a lower bone formation rate that leads to a thinning of bone trabeculae.[45] Although trabecular resorption surfaces were markedly increased, the authors concluded that impaired osteoblastic activity was primarily responsible. Bikle et al.[23] reported extended and scalloped resorption surfaces in patients with many years of alcohol abuse. However, both groups of investigators concur that reduced osteoblastic activity associated with normal osteoclastic function plays a major role in the pathogenesis of the osteoporosis observed in alcoholic patients.

Thomas et al.[12] found that a single dose of ethanol (2 g/kg) given to rats intraperitoneally did not affect osteocalcin levels over the subsequent 6-hour period, even though serum Ca did fall. Serum osteocalcin has not been measured in rats receiving larger doses of ethanol, such as that given by Peng et al. (8 mg/kg), which induces significant hypocalemia.[8]

The results of studies of chronic alcoholism on osteocalcin in humans and rats appear to be similar. Peng et al.[46] fed rats an 8% ethanol diet for up to 4 weeks; serum osteocalcin was 30% lower ($p < 0.001$) at both 1 and 4 weeks than that in control rats fed an isocaloric diet. Even in rats fed only a 6% ethanol diet for 12 days, serum osteocalcin fell by over 30%.[46] A number of human studies have shown that osteocalcin levels are low in chronic alcoholics.[24,31,47-50] Evidence has also been obtained in humans showing that, after a period of alcohol withdrawal, osteocalcin levels return to normal, an indication that the effect of ethanol on osteoblasts may be reversible.[24,31,48-50]

In summary, alcohol, either directly or indirectly, inhibits osteoblastic activity as indicated by the typical decline in serum osteocalcin. This effect may represent a major reason for the bone loss in chronic alcoholics. Since the effect of ethanol on serum osteocalcin in humans is easily duplicated in rats, this biomarker offers an opportunity to examine the mechanisms involved in ethanol-induced loss of bone mass and to explore effective ways to prevent or reverse the adverse effects of alcholism on osteocalcin.

6. Bone Collagen

Preedy and collaborators have reported on the effects of ethanol on bone collagen[51,52] in rats. Urinary hydroxyproline excretion was markedly increased, 40 to 60%, by 42 days of treatment with ethanol, a finding that suggested enhanced collagen degradation.[51] However, in the second study[52] the urinary excretion of the collagen degradation markers pyridinoline and deoxypyridinoline was measured. Free, total, and conjugated pyridinoline excretion was not altered by ethanol feeding. In fact, urinary excretion of total and conjugated deoxypyridinoline was significantly reduced in ethanol-treated rats, and the excretion of free deoxypyridinoline was also lower, but these effects were not statistically significant. Urinary pyridinoline/deoxypyridinoline molar ratios of total and conjugated forms were increased.

The interpretation of these results is difficult in view of the earlier findings of increased urinary excretion of hydroxyproline in ethanol-fed rats. The authors suggest that either ethanol feeding inhibits the normal formation of the pyridinium cross-links of collagen that would lead to a decline in skeletal levels of collagen, or ethanol may have a direct effect on the synthesis of collagen in bone tissue.[52]

IV. SUMMARY AND CONCLUSIONS

Despite extensive investigations on Ca metabolism in chronic alcoholics, the available information on the mechanisms of the effects of alcohol on Ca metabolism remains rather fragmentary. Studies in rats have been helpful in delineating those effects of chronic consumption of alcohol that are not the result of malnutrition or diseases commonly found among alcoholics. Still, even when an attempt is made to maintain caloric balance, the rats fed alcohol as a liquid diet consume less food than control rats fed *ad libitum*, a factor that may contribute to the effects noted. Also, questions remain as to whether or not the changes that can definitely be ascribed to ethanol consumption are caused by direct or indirect actions.

The use of animal models such as the rat for the study of the deleterious effects of ethanol will undoubtedly play a role in elucidating mechanisms of ethanol effects. These models also can be used to test therapeutic procedures to prevent or delay mineral loss during alcohol abuse and to restore mineral previously lost by recovering alcoholics. Therapeutic trials in humans can then be designed and tested. Although we are still a long way from establishing new and effective procedures for the treatment of ethanol-induced osteporosis, recognition of the problem and the progress in understanding the mechanisms involved provide hope that therapeutic interventions will be forthcoming.

REFERENCES

1. **Spencer, H., Rubio, N., Rubio, E., Indreiko, M., and Seitam, A.,** Chronic alcoholism: frequently overlooked cause of osteoporosis in men, *Am. J. Med.*, 80, 393, 1986.
2. **Schapira, D.,** Alcohol abuse and osteoporosis, *Semin. Arth. Rheum.*, 19, 371,1990.
3. **Laitinen,K. and Valimaki, M.,** Alcohol and bone. *Calcif. Tissue Int.*, 49 (suppl), S70, 1991.
4. **Adler, R. A.,** Clinically important effects of alcohol on endocrine function, *J. Clin. Endocrinol. Metab.*, 74, 957, 1992.
5. **Bikle, D. D.,** Alcohol-induced bone disease, *World Rev Nutr Diet*, Karger, Basel, 73, 53, 1993.
6. **Moniz, C.,** Alcohol and bone, *Brit. Med. Bull.*, 50, 67,1994.
7. **Peng, T-C., Kusy, R. P., Hirsch, P. F., Liu, C-C., and Lester, G. E.,** Bone histomorphometry and mechanical properties in an alcoholic rat model, *Cells Materials*, 1, 175, 1991.
8. **Peng, T. C., Cooper, C. W., and Munson, P. L.,** The hypocalcemic effect of ethyl alcohol in rats and dogs, *Endocrinology*, 91, 586, 1972.
9. **Peng, T. C. and Gitelman, H. J.,** Ethanol-induced hypocalcemia, hypermagnesemia and inhibition of serum calcium-raising effect of parathyroid hormone in rats, *Endocrinology*, 94, 608, 1974.
10. **Shah, J. H., Bowser, E. N., Hargis, G. K., Wongsurawat, N., Banerjee, P., Henderson, W. J., Williams, G. A.,** Effect of ethanol on parathyroid hormone secretion in the rat, *Metabolism*, 27, 257, 1978.
11. **Hargis, G. K., Bowser, E. N., Henderson, W. J., and Williams, G. A.,** Radioimmunoassay of rat parathyroid hormone in serum and tissue extracts, *Endocrinology*, 94, 1644, 1974.
12. **Thomas, S., Movsowitz, C., Epstein, S., Jowell, P., Ismail, F.,** The response of circulating parameters of bone mineral metabolism to ethanol- and EDTA-induced hypocalcemia in the rat, *Bone Miner.*, 8, 1, 1990.
13. **Chanard, J., Lacour, B., Drüeke, T., Brunois, J. P., and Ruiz, J. C.,** Effect of acute ethanol loading on parathyroid gland secretion in the rat, *Adv. Exp. Med. Biol.*, 128, 495, 1980.
14. **Laitinen, K., Lamberg-Allardt, C., Tunninen, R., Karonen, S. L., Tähtelä, R., Ylikahri, R., and Välimäki, M.,** Transient hypoparathyroidism during acute alcohol intoxication, *New Engl. J. Med.*, 324, 721, 1991.
15. **Ljunghall, S., Lundin, L., and Wide, L.,** Acute effects of ethanol intake on the serum concentrations of parathyroid hormone, calcium and phosphate, *Exp. Clin. Endocrinol.*, 85, 365, 1985.
16. **Williams, G. A., Bowser, E. N., Hargis, G. K., Kukreja, S. C., Shah, J. H., Vora, N. M., and Henderson W. J.,** Effect of ethanol on parathyroid hormone and calcitonin secretion in man, *Proc. Soc. Exp. Biol. Med.*, 159, 187, 1978.
17. **Earll, J. M., Gaunt, K., Earll, L. A., and Djuh, Y. Y.,** Effect of ethyl alcohol on ionic calcium and prolactin in man, *Aviat. Space Env. Med.*, 47, 808, 1976.
18. **Talmage, R. V. and Meyers, R. A., Jr.,** Physiological role of parathyroid hormone, in *Handbook of Physiology*, Aurbach, G. D., Ed., Williams and Wilkins, 1976, 343.
19. **Laitinen, K., Tähtelä, R., Luomanmäki, K., and Välimäki, M. J.,** Mechanism of hypocalcemia and markers of bone turnover in alcohol-intoxicated drinkers, *Bone Miner.*, 24, 171, 1994.
20. **Turner, R. T., Aloia, R. C., Segel, L. D., Hannon, K. S., and Bell, N. H.,** Chronic alcohol treatment results in disturbed vitamin D metabolism and skeletal abnormalities in rats, *Alcohol. Clin. Exp. Res.*, 12, 159, 1988.
21. **Turner, R. T., Greene, V. S., and Bell, N. H.,** Demonstration that ethanol inhibits bone matrix synthesis and mineralization in the rat, *J. Bone Miner. Res.*, 2, 61, 1987.
22. **Gascon-Barré, M.,** Interrelationships between vitamin D_3 and 25-hydroxyvitamin D_3 during chronic ethanol administration in the rat, *Metabolism*, 31, 67, 1982.
23. **Bikle, D. D., Stesin, A., Halloran, B., Steinbach, L., and Recker R.,** Alcohol-induced bone disease: relationship to age and parathyroid hormone levels, *Alcohol. Clin. Exp. Res.*, 17, 690, 1993.
24. **Lindholm, J., Steiniche, T., Rasmussen, E., Thamsborg, G., Nielsen, I. O., Brockstedt-Rasmussen, H., Storm, T., Hyldstrup, L., and Schou, C.,** Bone disorder in men with chronic alcoholism: a reversible disease?, *J. Clin. Endocrinol. Metab.*, 73, 118, 1991.
25. **Manfredini, R., Bariani, L., Bagni, B., Cavallini, A. R., Gallerani, M., Salmi, R., Pasin, M., Cecchetti, E., Rosini, M., Franceschini, F., and Fersini C.,** Hypoparathyroidism in chronic alcohol intoxication: a preliminary report, *Eur. Rev. Med. Pharmacol. Sci.*, 14, 293, 1992.
26. **Laitinen, K., Lamberg-Allardt, C., Tunninen, R., Härkönen, M., and Välimäki, M.,** Bone mineral density and abstention-induced changes in bone and mineral metabolism in noncirrhotic male alcoholics, *Am. J. Med.*, 93, 642, 1992.
27. **Laitinen, K., Kärkkäinen, M., Lalla, M., Lamberg-Allardt, C., Tunninen, R., Tähtelä, R., and Välimäki, M.,** Is alcohol an osteoporosis-inducing agent for young and middle-aged women? *Metabolism*, 42, 875, 1993.
28. **Dupuy, B., Angibeau, R., Mendoza, N., Rouais, F., and Blanquet, P.,** Effet de l'éthanol sur la sécrétion de calcitonine chez le rat, *C. R. Acad. Sci. Paris*, 292, 557, 1981.
29. **Bjorneboe, G. E., Bjorneboe, A., Johnsen, J., Skylv, N., Oftebro, H., Gautvik, K. M., Hoesith, A., Morland, J., and Drevon, C. A.,** Calcium status and calcium-regulating hormones in alcoholics, *Alcohol. Clin. Exp. Res.*, 12, 229, 1988.
30. **Nilsson, B. E. and Westlin, N. E.,** Changes in bone mass in alcoholics, *Clin. Orthop. Rel. Res.*, 90, 229, 1973.

31. **Gonzalez-Calvin, J. L., Garcia-Sanchez, A., Bellot, V., Muñoz-Torres, M., Raya-Alvarez, E., and Salvatierra-Rios, D.,** Mineral metabolism, osteoblastic function and bone mass in chronic alcoholism, *Alcohol Alcohol.*, 28, 571, 1993.
32. **Crilly, R. G. and Delaquerrière-Richardson, L.,** Current bone mass and body weight changes in alcoholic males, *Calcif. Tissue Int.*, 46, 169, 1990.
33. **Saville, P. B. and Lieber, C. S.,** Effect of alcohol on growth, bone density and muscle magnesium in the rat, *J. Nutr.*, 83, 477, 1965.
34. **Baran, D. T., Teitelbaum, S. L., Bergfeld, M. A., Parker, G., Cruvant, E. M., and Avioli, L. V.,** Effect of alcohol ingestion on bone and mineral metabolism in rats, *Am. J. Physiol.*, 238, E507, 1980.
35. **Peng, T. C., Garner, S. C., Frye, G. D., and Crenshaw, M. A.,** Evidence of a toxic effect of ethanol on bone in rats, *Alcohol. Clin. Exp. Res.*, 6, 96, 1982.
36. **Peng, T. C., Kusy, R. P., Hirsch, P. F., and Hagaman, J. R.,** Ethanol-induced changes in morphology and strength of femurs of rats, *Alcohol. Clin. Exp. Res.*, 12, 655, 1988.
37. **Kusy, R. P., Hirsch, P. F., and Peng, T-C.,** Influence of ethanol on stiffness, toughness, and ductility of femurs of rats, *Alcohol. Clin. Exp. Res.*, 13, 185, 1989.
38. **Preedy, V. R. and Peters, T. J.,** Effects of chronic ethanol consumption and pair feeding on rates of protein synthesis and nucleic acid composition in rat tibia, *Alcohol Alcohol.*, 27, 29, 1992.
39. **Price, P. A., Parthemore, J. G., and Deftos, L. J.,** New biochemical marker for bone metabolism; measurement by radioimmunoassay of bone gla-protein in the plasma of normal subjects and patients with bone disease, *J. Clin. Invest.*, 66, 878, 1980.
40. **Lian, J. B. and Gundberg, C. M.,** Osteocalcin, biochemical considerations and clinical application, *Clin. Orthop.*, 226, 267, 1988.
41. **Brixen, K., Nielsen, H. K., Eriksen, E. F., Charles, D., and Moskekilde, L.,** Efficacy of wheat germ lectin-precipitated alkaline phosphatase in serum as an estimator of bone mineralization rate: comparison to serum total alkaline phosphatase and serum bone Gla-protein, *Calcif. Tissue Int.*, 44, 93, 1989.
42. **Garcia-Carrasico, M., Gruson, M., de Vernejoul, M. C., Denne, A., and Miravet, L.,** Osteocalcin and bone morphometric parameters in adults without bone disease, *Calcif. Tissue Int.*, 42, 13, 1988.
43. **Rico H., Cabranes J. A., Cabello J., Gómez-Castresana, F., and Hernandez, E. R.,** Low serum osteocalcin in acute alcohol intoxication: a direct toxic effect of alcohol on osteoblasts, *Bone Miner.*, 2, 221, 1987.
44. **Nielsen, H. K., Lundby, L., Rasmussen, K., Charles, P., and Hansen, C.,** Alcohol decreases serum osteocalcin in a dose-dependent way in normal subjects, *Calcif. Tissue Int.*, 46, 173, 1990.
45. **Chappard, D., Plantard, B., Petitjean, M., Alexandre, C., and Riffat, G.,** Alcoholic cirrhosis and osteoporosis in men: a light and scanning electron microscopy study, *J. Stud. Alcohol*, 52, 269, 1991.
46. **Peng, T-C., Lian, J. B., Hirsch, P. F., and Kusy, R. P.,** Lower serum osteocalcin in ethanol-fed rats, *J. Bone Miner. Res.*, 6, 107, 1991.
47. **Crouzet, J., Bochet-Cadiou, A., Denis, J., and Brossard, C.,** L'ost'eocalcine chez l'alcoolique chronique, *Rev. Rhum. Mal. Osteoartic.*, 58, 781, 1991
48. **Peris, P., Pares, A., Guanabens, N., Pons, F., Martinez de Osaba, M. J., Caballeria, J., Rodes J., and Munoz-Gomez, J.,** Reduced spinal and femoral bone mass and deranged bone mineral metabolism in chronic alcoholics, *Alcohol Alcohol.*, 27, 619, 1992.
49. **Jaouhari, J., Schiele, F., Pirollet, P., Lecomte, E., Paille, F., and Artur, Y.,** Concentration and hydoxyapatite binding capacity of plasma osteocalcin in chronic alcoholic men: effect of three-week withdrawal therapy, *Bone Miner.*, 21, 171, 1993.
50. **Laitinen, K., Lamber-Allardt, C., Tunninen, R., Karonen, S. L., Ylikahri, R., and Valimaki, M.,** Effects of 3 weeks' moderate alcohol intake on bone and mineral metabolism in normal men. *Bone Miner.*, 13, 139, 1991.
51. **Preedy, V. R., Baldwin, D. R., Keating, J. W., and Salisbury, J. R.,** Bone collagen, mineral and trace element composition, histomorphometry and urinary hydroxyproline excretion in chronically-treated alcohol-fed rats, *Alcohol Alcohol.*, 26, 39, 1991.
52. **Preedy, V. R., Sherwood, R. A., Akpoguma, C. I. O., and Black, D.,** The urinary excretion of the collagen degradation markers pyridinoline and deoxypyridinoline in an experimental rat model of alcoholic bone disease, *Alcohol Alcohol.*, 26, 191, 1991.

Chapter 19

EFFECTS OF PHYSICAL ACTIVITY ON BONE

Robert G. McMurray, Ph.D.

TABLE OF CONTENTS

I. INTRODUCTION

Although the potential for peak bone mass (PBM) development in an individual is determined primarily by genetic factors, much evidence supports the concept that physical activity and the strains (loads) placed on bone by regular weight-bearing exercises are essential components in realizing the genetic potential for optimal bone formation. Age has a significant effect on bone mineralization and demineralization for women (Figure 1). Dietary and other factors also contribute to PBM development. As previous chapters have pointed out, peak rates of bone growth occurs up until about 25 years of age (see Chapter 17).[1] However, bone continues to grow and mineralize at some sites up to the middle ages, with PBM usually occurring around 35 years of age.[2] This period of growth is followed by approximately a decade or two of slow bone demineralization. When menopause occurs, an increased rate of bone loss follows for a period of 5 to 10 years, and then a slow decline in demineralization continues to the end of life. The postmenopausal bone mass (and density) is significantly less than that accrued by the end of the teenage years. At this part of the life

0-8493-7845-1/95/$0.00+$.50

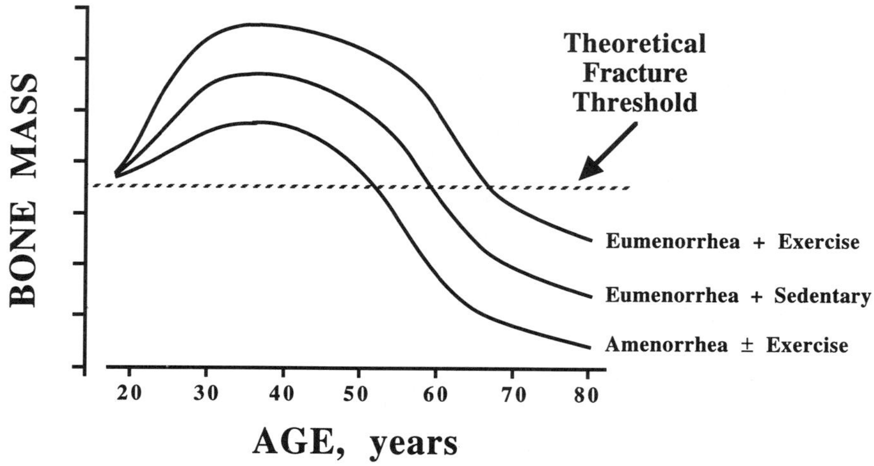

FIGURE 1. Schematic of the Effects of Premenopausal Menstrual Function and Exercise on Bone Mass with Respect to All Ages. (Adapted from Wolman.[2])

cycle, bones become osteoporotic, and they have an increased potential to fracture. Thus, to reduce the possibility of osteoporosis in late life, it is important to develop and maintain bone mass (and density) early in life. In general, bone development must be accomplished before the age of 30 years, whereas maintenance of bone is the key for a woman over the age of 35 years.

Exercise capacity and activity levels follow a similar pattern to bone development and maintenance. However, peak exercise capacity and activity levels usually occur in the early twenties and decline thereafter, even before peak bone mass is attained in most women.[3] Thus, to maintain fitness late in life, the best strategy may be to improve the fitness levels and exercise behavior patterns of children and adolescents. Concomitantly, the maintenance of fitness becomes of considerable importance during the two premenopausal decades and thereafter. Studies have shown that active individuals live longer and have a reduced risk of cardiovascular disease, the top killer in the U.S.[4] Population data are needed, however, to demonstrate that individuals who have been physically active for most of their lifetime also have reduced rates of hip fractures.

The interactions of age, bone, and exercise are complex and not well understood (Figure 1). Cross-sectional studies have shown that exercise prior to age 35 can result in peak bone densities greater than those in a sedentary population.[5-7] However, longitudinal studies have not been quite as positive. Also, some patterns of excessive exercise can result in amenorrhea, which can result in bone densities lower than those of sedentary women.[8] Thus, if the person begins the age-related demineralization process at a lower bone density, and demineralization take place at the same rate for all,[2] then the exercise pattern of the woman who was amenorrheic early in life is likely to be detrimental to bone health (Figure 1). Some forms of exercise, such as swimming, may have little or no effect on bone mineralization.[9,10] In addition, exercise may have differing effects on cortical and trabecular types of bone tissue.

Exercise increases intestinal absorption of calcium (Ca) during physical training. However, once the training stimulus ceases, this effect is lost.[11] In contrast to increased Ca absorption, Ca excretion rates may not change.[11] Thus, the source of Ca for improved bone mineralization comes from either an augmented absorption or a decline in excretory loss, or a combination of both. Thus, new bone formation as part of the remodeling of bone may be influenced by the availability of Ca from the diet, but physical activity may have an even greater effect on bone remodeling.

Research on the effects of exercise on bone is complicated by the concurrent influences of many other potential determinants of bone mass. Several factors besides genetics and age must be controlled to establish that the specific skeletal effects observed are directly related to exercise. Previous studies have implicated height, weight, Ca intake, phosphate intake, vitamin D status, caloric intake, alcohol intake, caffeine intake, smoking, endocrine dysfunction (estrogens, androgens), and birth control pills as factors affecting bone mass. The anthropometric variables of height, weight, body mass index, and body fat seem logical, because larger persons would require stronger bones to support their weight.[5,7,12,13,14] Ca intake is important as an essential element for bone mineralization.[5,12] Furthermore, individuals with limited caloric intake will generally have a diminished Ca intake.[7] For example, when caloric restriction is more severe, possible menstrual dysfunctions will follow.[15] The factors of vitamin D, caffeine, alcohol, and phosphate intake have all been shown to attenuate Ca uptake or utilization, which could diminish bone mineralization; however, the data are equivocal at this time.[7] The results of studies on smoking, alcohol intake, and the use of birth control pills are also less clear, with some studies showing an effect,[5,7,16] whereas others have found no effect.[12,17]

The purpose of this chapter is to review the effects of exercise on bone mass or density in relation to other important life-style variables such as dietary Ca. The recent literature will be highlighted, but excellent reviews of older literature are also available.[18,19]

II. EXERCISE AND BONE REMODELING

Bone remodeling requires the coordinated functions of both osteoclasts (bone-resorbing cells) and osteoblasts (bone-forming cells) to remove completely a small portion of the bone mineral and matrix and to replace it with a newly mineralized matrix that is free of any microdefects (see Chapter 7). Bone turnover has been shown to be affected by age, hormonal status, nutrition, and drugs, but more recent evidence suggests that, although the general form of the bone is genetically determined, the specific structural conformation develops and persists in response to load bearing.[20,21] Muscular contraction and gravity provide these major mechanical forces. The change in bone mass is directly related to the forces that act on the bone, the frequency of force application, and the direction of the applied force.[20] Furthermore, bone tissue will develop to the habitual level of stress placed upon it (Wolff's Law). Once adapted to that level of stress and strain, no further changes will occur unless the stress levels are modified.

Bone is composed of two types of structures, cortical bone and trabecular bone (see Chapter 7). Cortical bone usually refers to the shafts of long bones of the body, whereas trabecular bone is most prominent in the interior of flat bones, the axial skeleton (vertebrae), and the ends of long bones. Research has suggested that exercise may differentially affect these two types of bone.[22,23] Furthermore, Li et al.,[21] using rats running on a treadmill, noted that the metatarsal bone (trabecular tissue) increased in thickness, whereas the tibia (cortical tissue) did not. In addition, they observed a differential effect of exercise within the same bone. The lateral and posterior aspects of the tibia had an increase in bone cells not found in other portions of this bone. Studies have shown a differential pattern of bone development comparing the dominant and nondominant arms,[24,25] as well as legs and arms.[26] These results, taken together, suggest the importance of local strain in the maintenance and development of bone.

The exact mechanism for regulating bone turnover is not well understood, but Carter has hypothesized that stress-related fatigue may stimulate remodeling.[27] In simple terms, exercise places a strain on the bone, resulting in minor damage (stress). The osteoclasts then remove the damaged tissue, and the osteoblasts rebuild the bone with new tissue that is stronger than its previous status. Bone remodeling may be rate-limited such that the rate of osteoblastic activity may not be able to counter with an equivalent amount of bone lost via resorption if too much strain is applied.[28] Conversely, if the strain is reduced or eliminated, osteoclast activity will dominate osteoblast activity, and the bone will be resorbed and a new equilibrium of less mineral content and thereby with less strength.[18,29] The mechanism postulated for the overactivity of osteoclasts in this situation is the decreased inhibitory signal via cytokines secreted by osteoblasts. In support of this hypothesis, Malm and associates have shown that after long-distance running, an increase occurs in the urinary excretion of hydroxyproline, which is presumably derived from resorbed bone collagen matrix.[30]

Concomitantly, they also found a decrease in osteocalcin, a marker of bone formation. These markers of bone turnover returned to normal within 1–3 days, which is in agreement with the initial damage hypothesis of Carter. In another study, when women stopped exercising, their bone densities reverted to pretraining levels,[29] which is also in accordance with the above hypothesis.

Although most studies agree that exercise causes bone to grow, develop, and maintain mass, Franck and co-workers have noted that the short-term effect of exercise retards bone formation.[31] After 4 weeks of exercise, they found significant decreases in plasma levels of Ca, magnesium, and osteocalcin, and a simultaneous increase in parathyroid hormone (PTH). These changes returned to normal by the 8th week of exercise. Thus, the initial changes in the parameters measured in this study may indicate retarded bone formation followed by a long-term gain in bone mass. Other studies are needed to confirm this observation.

In summary, bone remodeling following exercise results from a complex set of regulatory mechanisms involving hormones and local factors or cytokines secreted by both osteoblasts and osteoclasts. In theory, the induction of remodeling cycles by exercise not only leads to the maintenance but to improvement of the absolute amount of bone mass.

III. EXERCISE-INDUCED HORMONAL RESPONSES AFFECTING BONE

The hormones that affect bone include growth hormone, calcitonin, parathyroid hormone (PTH), cortisol, androgens, and estrogens. Hormonal status is a significant factor in the bone mineralization process. The significance of the protective effects of estrogen cannot be neglected. Several studies have found that estrogen therapy for postmenopausal women results in better maintenance of bone mineral content.[19,32,33] In premenopausal women that have low estrogen levels, there is also a reduced bone density.[19,34-36] Chronic high cortisol levels may contribute to reduced bone density.[37] Buchanan et al. have shown a positive effect of androgens on bone mineralization in females that is independent of estrogens.[38] Similarly, the importance of androgens in bone density for males has been established.[39] Growth hormone is related to the bone mineralization process, but less is known about whether it directly influences bone formation or whether it acts indirectly through the effects of insulin-like growth factors (IGFs) on bone.

The effect of exercise on the aforementioned hormones is dependent upon the duration and intensity of exercise.[40] Short-term exercise of moderate intensity (20–30 min at 60% maximal intensity) has a minimal effect on these hormones. The effects that do occur are transient and probably would not be of sufficient duration to affect bone. Growth hormone will increase, but the increase is transient and returns to normal shortly after exercise. Cortisol and androgens may increase in an untrained individual, but are unlikely to respond in a trained person. Estrogens do not seem to be affected by this type of exercise. In contrast, prolonged exercise will cause the circulating levels of many of these hormones to rise. Growth hormone and cortisol will increase to mobilize free fatty acids. PTH will elevate to assist in maintaining circulating Ca levels. Testosterone level may fall during any type of endurance exercise. Once again, the transient nature of these hormonal responses suggest that they will not affect long-term bone development unless the activities are continued over long periods of time.

PTH increases blood Ca levels by removing Ca from bone, increasing intestinal Ca absorption (via $1,25(OH)_2D$), and reducing renal excretion of Ca.[40] In general, these effects are in opposition to improving bone mineral density. Three reports from a group of investigators led by Ljunghall indicate that exercise caused an increase in circulating PTH.[41-43] The increase in PTH occurs during high-intensity exercise or during prolonged low- or moderate-intensity exercises. Extremely prolonged periods of exercise (7 days of military exercise and maneuvers) also causes an increase in PTH.[41] Although PTH was elevated in these studies, no effects on serum Ca were observed. An interesting result of one study was that untrained individuals, such as fire fighters, had no significant increase in PTH, whereas the long-distance runners did.[43] The investigators suggested that this finding is consistent with observations that long-distance runners may have lower bone mineral densities than nonexercisers. The authors continued to state, however, that PTH has anabolic, as well as catabolic, effects on bone, and that a moderate and temporary increase in PTH, as opposed to a persistently elevated concentration, may enhance bone formation. The relationship between exercise-induced PTH elevations and bone mineral density clearly needs to be studied further.

Training does not seem to influence the resting levels of growth hormone, cortisol, or calciotropic hormones. However, training may reduce resting circulating levels of androgens and estrogens. In some women the exercise can result in amenorrhea, which is characterized by low circulating estrogens. The direction of these gonadal hormone responses is clearly in opposition to what would be expected for inducing bone mineralization. Thus, the positive effect of exercise on bone mineralization is probably unrelated to the hormonal changes.

IV. EXERCISE AND BONE IN MALES

Studies on the effect of exercise on bone mass in males are relatively rare. The bone mass of males is greater than that of females, probably related to the greater androgen levels[45] or strength of the men.[44] Although the bone mass is greater, middle-aged males are susceptible to the same environmental influences as women, e.g., cigarette smoking and alcohol.[46] Studies also suggest that males can build bone later in life. When comparing the effects of 4 months of exercise training on men and women over 60 years of age, Blumenthal et al. found an association between aerobic fitness and an increase in bone density for the men, but not for the women.[47] A study of masters swimmers (≥40 years of age) has shown that swim training increases radial and vertebral bone mass in men, but not in women.[48] Bevier et al. has also shown a direct relationship between aerobic power and bone density in older men (61–84 yr), but not in older women.[44] Thus, exercise at reasonably high intensities seems more protective for older men than women.

Williams has shown that trained male marathon runners have higher bone densities in the heel than age-matched controls; however, the bone densities of the less consistent runners was similar to that of controls.[49] In contrast, Bilanin and associates found that the bone density of the lumbar spines of male long-distance runners was lower than for nonrunners, but that the midtibia densities were similar.[50] They suggested that the differences may have been related to lower testosterone or increased cortisol levels associated with long-distance training. The conflict between Williams and Bilanin may be related to differences in the sites of measurement, or the fact that the control population used by Bilanin had a fairly high aerobic capacity, indicating a generally active lifestyle.[50]

Evidence also exists that body building exercises (weight lifting) will cause an increase in bone mineral content and bone density.[22] In support, Virvidakis et al. have found an increased bone mineral content in male weightlifters compared to that of age-matched controls.[45] These effects could not be related to the use of anabolic steroids.[22] Similarly, Colletti et al. have reported 10–15% greater vertebral, femoral, and trochanter densities in young men lifting weights compared to those of controls.[51] Hence, the data suggest that weight-resistance activities at any age may improve the bone density of men and, possibly that of women.

V. EXERCISE STUDIES OF PREMENOPAUSAL WOMEN

As indicated in the introduction, one way to maximize bone mass and decrease the potential for osteoporotic fractures is to increase bone mineral content and density early in life. Other than a genetic advantage, the limited options include optimization of Ca intake and exercise. However, the benefits of these factors may be transient unless the optimal behaviors are maintained indefinitely. Dalsky et al. have shown that when exercise is stopped, bone mineral density reverts towards normal.[29] Tylavsky et al. have shown that moderate to high levels of both physical activity and Ca intake during adolescence and early adulthood contributed to greater bone mineral content than for control females.[52] However, a low Ca intake reduces bone mineralization.[6]

Since the most rapid rate of bone growth and development occurs in the two or three years prior to puberty, one would expect that this age range should serve as a focal point for examining effects of physical activity on bone development. However, only a few research reports on the effects of exercise on bone density in children exist, primarily because of the difficulty in assessing activity levels of youngsters. The data that do exist on 5- to 14-year-old children support an interaction between bone density and total hours of weight-bearing activity, independent of gender.[53] Furthermore, McCulloch et al. have shown a positive association between childhood physical activity levels and adult bone density.[54] Thus, limited published evidence exists to support the beneficial role of increased levels of physical activity in preadolescent children as a prophylaxis for osteopenia and osteoporosis.

The onset of puberty accelerates the rate of bone growth.[52] Young women with earlier menarche seem to have greater bone densities than those with delayed onset. Women with later menarche, however, appear to benefit more from a combined effect of moderate Ca intake and physical activity.[6,52] In contrast, women that have missed 50% of their expected menstrual cycles by age 20 will have decreased bone density.[36] In spite of the lower bone density in amenorrheic adolescents, Tylavsky et al. have shown that moderate exercise can result in improved bone density and mineral content, independent of Ca intake.[52] Furthermore, Tylavsky found a dose-response effect of exercise; women who exercised less than one hour per week had 17% less bone density than those exercising over four hours per week.

A. WOMEN WITH NORMAL MENSTRUAL CYCLES

The eumenorrheic athlete presents a more positive profile than the amenorrheic athlete. The majority of studies on these women indicate that exercise will improve bone mineral density. Drinkwater has shown that active women have a 5–12% advantage in trabecular bone densities over sedentary controls.[15] Halioua and Anderson have shown that women with high levels of physical activity have increased radial bone densities compared to individuals with low levels of activity.[55] Kanders and co-workers have shown a direct relationship between average daily energy expenditure and vertebral bone density.[6] Similarly, Tylavsky and associates have shown a direct relationship between physical activity levels and radial bone density.[52] In contrast, Mazess and Barden found that daily activity levels, recorded over two 48-hr periods, had no effect on bone mineral density.[16] The conflicting results are not without precedence, but they may reflect the difficulty in obtaining an accurate assessment of physical activity, particularly when records are kept for only a brief period, as in the last study.

1. Aerobic Activities

The literature on the effect of aerobic activities on bone density in premenopausal women athletes has been conflicting because of the inadequate consideration of menstrual status and the differences in experimental designs. In addition, some studies used more active subjects as controls rather than sedentary normals. Recently, several investigators have reported that eumenorrheic runners had lumbar spine densities similar to those of controls (Snead et al.,[35] Bunt et al.,[56] and Heinrich et al.[57]) Wolman et al.[58] have found that the bone densities of the femoral (midshaft) of elite female rowers were similar to those of controls, but the midfemoral densities of runners in the same study were higher by 6–8%. Conversely, an early report by Drinkwater[8] indicated that eumenorrheic long-distance runners have higher bone densities of the lumbar vertebrae than sedentary controls. Other studies of runners have also found greater bone density and bone mineral content than in controls.[19]

The reason for the lack of consistent effects of running on BMD may be related to the cross-sectional nature of most of the reported studies. Two different cross-sectional studies reported that runners had greater lumbar BMD than controls, and that swimmers fell in between these two groups.[56,57] Conversely, another group of researchers found that runners, cyclists, and aerobic dancers had lower BMDs than control subjects.[59] Thus, both positive and negative effects of aerobic activities on BMD have been reported.

Longitudinal investigations on the effects of running on BMD in premenopausal women have not been reported. A 1-year prospective study of aerobic dancers found no difference in BMD between dancers and controls.[60] The limited results of these few studies suggest that aerobic activities per se are better for maintaining or enhancing cardiovascular fitness than for improving BMD.[15]

The data on other forms of exercise seem to be dependent on the weight-bearing properties of the exercise and the muscular strength needed to complete the exercise. Swimming exercises with different strokes seem to do little for bone densities of women, as reported studies have found little difference[48,57] or lower[61] bone densities of swimmers compared to those of controls. At present, only one study on the skeletal effects of swimming in young rats has shown positive results.[62] Thus, the data on swimming could be interpreted in two ways: (1) swimmers, due to the antigravity effects of the water, have not stressed the bone sufficiently to develop high levels of bone density, or (2) the low bone densities of some individuals may predispose them toward swimming activities because of better buoyancy in the water.

Volleyball and basketball players have been found to have bone densities that were 10–15% greater than those of sedentary age-matched controls.[61] Walking, as a form of aerobic activity, does involve sufficient intensity to enhance BMD. Mazess and Barden[16] could show no effect of walking, as measured by a pedometer, on vertebral, femoral, or radial shaft BMD. Hatori et al.[63] also found that general walking activities at low-intensity levels did not improve BMD. A recent cross-sectional study, however, suggests that high-intensity walking may have a beneficial effect on bone density.[64] The results of this study may be open to question because the investigators found no differences in BMD between subjects who walked 1 versus 7 or more miles per week. Furthermore, the authors reported a low correlation ($r = 0.16$) between miles walked per week and change in BMD. The absence of any consistent and significant effect of walking activities on BMD make it less attractive as a way to prevent bone loss compared to other aerobic activities.

The cross-sectional data reviewed herein suggest that two important factors are required if aerobic activities are to have positive effects on BMD. The first factor is that aerobic exercise must have a weight-bearing component, and the second is that, in the case of premenopausal women, moderate activities are more beneficial than high-intensity, prolonged training.

2. Resistance (Strength) Exercises

The majority of studies on weight lifting by women have shown that these individuals have greater bone densities than other athletes or sedentary controls.[57,59] In fact, muscle strength has been shown to be an independent predictor of bone density.[65] In support, data on rowers, which use considerable strength of back muscles, indicate about a 15% increase in lumbar spine bone mineral density compared to data on nonrowing controls.[66]

Prospective studies of women on weight-training regimens have resulted in mixed results. Rockwell et al. have shown that 9 months of weight training, although increasing strength by 57%, reduced lumbar bone density by about 4%.[9] The short duration, the relatively mild intensities of the exercises, and the fact that the subjects only exercised twice a week may have contributed to their findings. Two separate 1-year weight training investigations resulted in no significant improvement in bone densities.[60,67] However, Gleeson and co-workers[67] did report a trend toward improved lumbar bone density in the exercise group that was not seen in controls. On the other hand, a 6-month study by Dornemann et al.[68] showed a 1.5% gain in lumbar vertebral density in premenopausal women undergoing strength activities focused on the lower back and spine compared to control women receiving no training. The interpretation of these studies can take two directions. One is that weight-training programs do not seem to have the effects that were anticipated. The second possibility is that the programs must last much longer than 1 year to have a positive effect. Based on the results of the study of Dorneman et al.[68] and of a four-year aerobic-exercise study that will be discussed later, the second explanation seems more plausible.

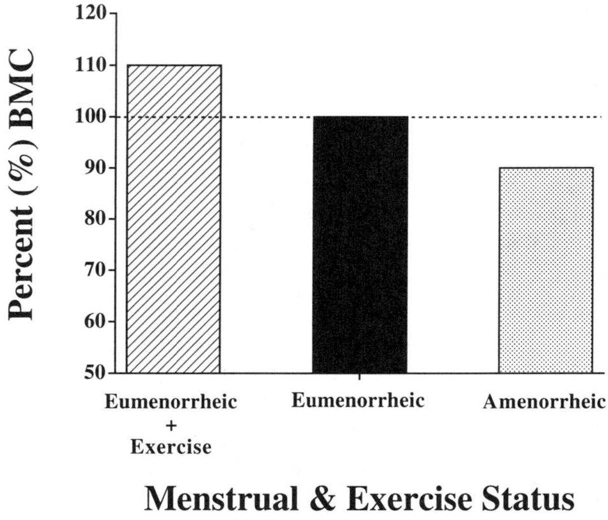

FIGURE 2. The Overriding Effect of Amenorrhea on Exercise-Induced Bone Mineralization in Premenopausal Women. (Based on data from Drinkwater et al.[8])

B. WOMEN WITH AMENORRHEA

The positive effects of normal menstrual function in the development of bone mass cannot be overlooked. Several studies of young women (ages 18–35) have noted lower bone densities in women who were amenorrheic compared to those of eumenorrheic controls (Figure 2). This finding seems consistent regardless of the cause of the amenorrhea, i.e., hypothalamic disorder,[36] exercise-induced,[1,69,70] or anorexia nervosa.[71,72]

The menstrual irregularities of most athletes have been linked to energy-restricted diets and/or strenuous, prolonged workouts. The combination of low caloric intake and high caloric expenditure results in below-normal body fat percentages. Low body fat has been associated with menstrual irregularities.[2,73] Alternatively, strenuous exercise will elevate beta-endorphin and catecholamines, either of which can block gonadotropin release from the hypothalamus and therefore contribute to menstrual irregularity.[74]

Several studies have reported lower bone mineral content and densities in amenorrheic women athletes. Since the first report that amenorrheic women long-distance runners have the bone densities of postmenopausal women,[8] more recent studies have confirmed these results.[35,69,56] The majority of research has focused on amenorrheic women runners; however, other types of athletes such as dancers and rowers have similar results.[58] Other studies, summarized by De Cree et al., have found no differences in bone density between amenorrheic and eumenorrheic athletes.[34] The seemingly conflicting results can be resolved by examining the site of the bone measurement. Those studies that have examined trabecular bone, i.e., the lumbar spine,[35,37,75,76] have consistently shown an adverse effect of amenorrhea, whereas studies that have based their results on cortical bone tissue, i.e., femoral or radial shaft,[2,35] have found no effect of amenorrhea. In contrast, when exercise activities are targeted on the spine, as in rowers, little differences in bone density have been found between amenorrheic and eumenorrheic athletes.[66]

Research has suggested that athletes with amenorrhea may be at higher risk for stress fractures.[26,69] Conclusions based on these studies, however, are difficult to draw because of differences in training durations and intensities of the eumenorrheic and amenorrheic runners. Also, the rate of stress fractures seems to be directly related to the duration and intensity of exercise. Research has indicated that women with exercise-induced amenorrhea, who subsequently reduce their running distance, gain weight, and resume normal cycling, gain some benefit,[11,69] but they will also have a residual deficit in bone density. Drinkwater has suggested that estrogen therapy may be of benefit to these women through stabilization of their bone density.[15] Clearly, the amenorrheic woman athlete illustrates the case in which exercise does not protect against bone loss.

C. SUMMARY

The cross-sectional model used by many researchers to examine the effects of exercise on bone is based on the assumption that all subjects were initially the same, and that the observed effects of exercise were directly related to the specific variable investigated. However, humans are not all genetically the same, nor do they have the same nutritional habits. The definition of being trained may to one person mean they exercise 6 days a week for 2 hours, but for another it may mean 3 times a week for 30 minutes. Thus, to examine the interaction of exercise and bone, longitudinal studies, lasting at least a year, and preferably 2 years, are necessary. Reports of studies of this duration are scarce.

Specific exercises and activities are needed to maximize bone mass in the young adult in addition to maintaining adequate nutrient intakes, including that of Ca. It is most important for female athletes, however, to avoid disruption of menstrual function, and secondly, to exercise regularly. The exercise program should be weight-bearing in nature, involving both aerobic activities and some resistance training or weight lifting to build muscle. The training stimulus should be gradually, but consistently, increased. One should start with walking or low-impact aerobics, increasing to jogging or high-impact aerobics. The same progressive resistance and overload principles apply to weight training. The weight/resistance program should not only involve the muscles of the arms and legs, but also the torso, to bring about positive changes in vertebrate. Avoid overtraining or prolonged, severe training and severe weight loss that could result in disruption of menstrual function, which is deleterious to bone mass and density.

VI. EXERCISE STUDIES OF POSTMENOPAUSAL WOMEN

The major consideration for the post-menopausal woman is to minimize or prevent the bone demineralization processes. The prescription to attenuate bone loss seems to have three components: estrogen therapy, Ca supplementation, and exercise. Ca supplements of 500 or 1000 mg a day insure that women achieve the RDA levels of intake. Estrogen treatment at the standard replacement dosage may provide the permissive effect for the other therapies (see Figure 3), as it is a strong inhibitor of bone resorption, even stronger than Ca.[19] Administration of estrogens to postmenopausal women has been shown to improve both lumbar and femoral bone densities.[32,77] The exercise component of the prescription is not as definitive, but some beneficial clues are provided in published reports.[18,19]

Exercise during the postmenopausal years has been shown by many investigators to slow the rate of bone loss.[15,73] Although the majority of studies suggest improved bone mass following the completion of an exercise program, others are less positive or even show no benefit. The lack of consistency of the study results may be related to questions of experimental design, such as failure to control for Ca and estrogen therapy, differences in life-styles of the subjects (i.e., selection bias), and other aspects that could impact on measurements of outcome variables. Additional well-designed longitudinal studies are warranted.

A. AEROBIC ACTIVITIES

A few cross-sectional exercise studies have demonstrated that postmenopausal, trained women generally have higher bone mineral densities than in nonexercising women. Nelson et al. reported that 60-year-old trained runners with no history of premenopausal amenorrhea, and not taking estrogens, have higher bone densities with respect to weight.[78] Similarly, Michel et al. reported that lumbar bone mineral content was greater in men and women over age 50 that regularly exercise up to 300 min/week.[79,80] Cross-sectional data also indicate that participation in high levels of physical

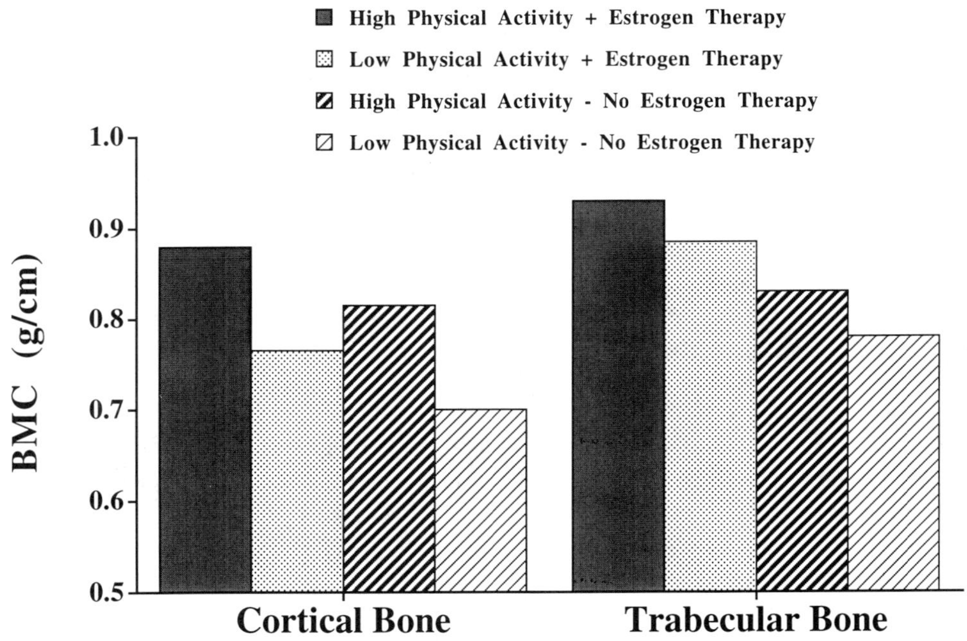

FIGURE 3. Comparative Effects of Sedentary Life-style, Exercise, and Exercise Plus Estrogen Therapy on Bone. (Based on data from Ballard et al.[81])

activity, as measured by an activity survey, reduces the risk of bone loss in postmenopausal women.[81]

The primary concern about cross-sectional studies is that they do not account for initial bone status. A woman exercising regularly throughout her life may have already established greater bone densities, whereas another woman who was sedentary may have lower bone densities. Thus, at any time during the postmenopausal period the habitual exerciser would have an advantage. The data of Cheng et al.[82] and Silbermann et al.[28] support this hypothesis. Silbermann, using a mouse model, found that the animals that exercised over a lifetime had greater lumbar bone mass and had retarded bone loss during old age.[28] Cheng and co-workers studied the bone mineral densities of Finnish women with respect to the number of times and hours per week of exercise with consideration to previous exercise experience.[82] Although the correlation was low ($r = 0.29$; $p = 0.01$), they concluded that the bone densities were directly related to the total amount of physical activity over the lifetime.

Recent studies involving forms of exercise other than weight training have produced mixed, but generally favorable, results. Prince et al. reported that aerobic exercise plus estrogen replacement was effective in increasing bone mass.[83] Other studies on short-term (6–12 months) aerobic exercise programs (jogging, cycling, aerobic dance) have also found improvements in lumbar bone density and bone mineral content.[29,47,60,77,84-86] A 4-year study by Smith et al., involving aerobic dance and strength exercises, found that the exercise significantly reduced the rate of bone mineral loss.[73] In contrast, Nelson et al. reported that 1 year of walking had no impact on bone density (and neither did Ca supplementation in their study).[87] This result suggests that the intensity of walking may not be sufficient to bring about a change in bone density. Blumenthal et al. reported mixed results from a 1-year cycle ergometry, walking, and stretching program.[47] They found that the program increased bone density in their male subjects but not in their female subjects. Dalsky demonstrated that there was no significant relationship between maximal oxygen uptake (aerobic fitness) and bone density, suggesting that aerobic fitness may not be as important as weight-bearing exercise in older women.[29]

B. RESISTANCE (STRENGTH) EXERCISES

Studies have also shown a relationship between strength and/or muscle mass and bone density. Halle et al. found that in postmenopausal women, trunk flexor and extensor strength was directly related to bone mineral densities of the lumbar spine, femoral neck, greater trochanter, and Ward's Triangle.[88] Zimmermann et al. also noted that the bone mineral densities of the lumbar spine and hip were related to torque (strength) of the extremities.[89]

The results of longitudinal training regimens have not been quite as convincing as the cross-sectional data. Simkin et al. have shown that 45–50 min of resistance training 3 times a week for 5 months resulted in a 3.8% increase in radial bone mass, at a time when control subjects were experiencing a 1.9% loss in bone mass.[90] Similarly, Pruitt and associates have found that 9 months of weight training prevented lumbar bone demineralization.[91] Notelovitz et al. examined the interaction of estrogen therapy with a 1-year weight training program and found that the addition of weights added bone density to both the axial (lumbar) and appendicular (radial) skeleton.[33] Other studies using weight training or strength exercise as part of their programs have also shown definitive results.[84,85] One study found that improvements in the radial bone mineral content could be obtained with only 6 weeks of squeezing a tennis ball.[24]

Not all the studies on weight training by postmenopausal women, however, have been positive. Smidt et al. found that 3 sets of 10 sit-ups, prone trunk extensions, and double-leg flexion exercises performed 3 times a week for 6–12 months did not modify the lumbar bone densities of the exercisers versus control subjects.[10] These results may be considered tentative, because the researchers did not account for the activity levels of the control subjects. Peterson et al. have noted that the addition of weight training to an aerobic dance program did not result in any further improvement in bone density over participation in just the aerobic dance.[60] Both groups improved, however, compared to control subjects. The problems with the Peterson study have been previously noted. Sinaki et al. found that 2 years of daily back extension exercises with weight increased back strength but did not slow bone resorption.[92] This modest program, one exercise repeated 10 times a day, may not have provided sufficient stimulus to evoke a change in bone density.

C. SUMMARY

In conclusion, the literature suggests that postmenopausal women that exercise have an advantage in maintaining BMD over nonexercisers. Although the process of bone resorption cannot be entirely prevented by exercise, the rate of loss can be slowed by participation in exercise programs. Long-term exercisers typically have entered the menopause with greater BMD than women who have not been active in exercise programs. Thus, women who have maintained high levels of physical activity throughout their lives have an additional benefit compared to novice exercisers during the postmenopause. As was found for premenopausal women, strength and weight-bearing activities that place strains on bone, such as weight lifting, seem to be the most beneficial for maintaining BMD among elderly women. If the postmenopausal woman is at high risk for osteoporosis, then estrogen therapy combined with weight-bearing exercises seems to be most beneficial.

VII. THE EXERCISE PRESCRIPTION

The preponderance of recent literature favors the use of exercise as a modality to increase bone mineral content as well as to prevent or slow bone demineralization. The questions then become what types of exercise are best and how much exercise is needed. At present no definitive answer exists, but tentative recommendations can be made based on the aforementioned literature.

The recommended activities include both aerobic and resistive (strength) exercises. The aerobic activities should be weight bearing: jogging, running, stair climbing, dance, aerobic dance, court games (basketball & volleyball), and possibly racquet sports. The present data on walking are not as convincing of a beneficial effect. The use of swimming and cycling (both nonweight-bearing activities) as the primary exercise modality is also questionable. There are no data on skiing, cross-country skiing, skating, or rope skipping. Logic would suggest that of these five sports, rope skipping and hard downhill skiing would put the most stress on the vertebral column and, therefore, would be the best choices. Participation in a variety of exercises may prove more beneficial in reducing osteoporosis, as they would produce different stresses on the bone, which would result in greater bone strength.[20] Consistent use of any of these exercises should result in improved aerobic capacity; however, this improvement is not needed to improve bone health. Dalsky reported that in postmenopausal women no significant relationship was evident between maximal oxygen uptake and bone density, suggesting that fitness may not be as important as weight-bearing activity.[29]

A portion of the exercise session should involve some resistive or weight training. This training should involve exercises that strengthen all the major muscle groups, including the back. Such exercises as leg and bench presses, upright curls, latissimus pull downs, biceps and triceps curls, sit-ups and back and leg extensions should be included.[60] Free weights may be of more benefit than weight machines because the machines may reduce the weight-bearing nature of the exercises. If weight equipment is not available, elastic bands or simply body resistance (like shoulder dips or chin-ups) could be used.

Some exercises can actually exacerbate the osteoporotic fractures. Exercising osteoporotic women should consider avoiding exercises that "compress" or "wedge" the spine.[93] Examples include toe touches, bent rowing, the plow, the cobra, straight leg sit-ups and some hip stretchers. The forces generated by these exercises could contribute to future injuries.

The amount of exercise needed to bring about changes in bone mineralization can be related to the exercise frequency, duration, and intensity. Based on the literature, 30- to 60-minute exercise sessions produce the most positive results. The standard length of weight-training sessions also seem to be sufficient. With regard to frequency, the evidence suggests that 3–5 days per week are needed. However, one study has shown improvements in as little as 2 days per week.[94] Exercising 6–7 days a week may be too much. The evidence for weight training indicates that 3 days a week is optimal. More than 3 sessions per week may not allow adequate time for adaptation to occur. Serious weight lifters can work out 6 days a week by alternating muscle groups, legs one day, upper body the next.

There is limited information regarding the optimal exercise intensity. One study has suggested that moderate-to-high levels of exercise are superior to low levels of intensity.[81] Bone tissue will accommodate to the habitual level of stress imposed upon it. Furthermore, the intensity of the exercise must be greater than the strain normally placed on the bone. These two axioms suggest that the intensity of the exercise is individually set, based on the initial status and ultimate goal of the exerciser. Sedentary individuals should start at a less strenuous level of exercise than more active persons. However, the sedentary person has more potential gains to be made in bone density. Generally speaking, the interrelationship between duration, frequency, and intensity with regard to bone density is not known. Could individuals exercise longer and more often at lower intensities, or exercise fewer times a week at higher intensities, and receive greater benefits? Studies addressing these questions need to be conducted.

Besides these factors two others should be considered. First, the exercise should become part of the life-style. Dalsky et al. have indicated that when exercise is reduced (detraining), bone mass reverts back to baseline levels.[29] Similarly, Slemenda and co-workers have shown in a 16-year study that a reduction in physical activity can contribute to bone loss in men.[46] Thus, the choice of activities that would keep the exercisers active should be based on the likes and dislikes of the participants, within their physical limitations. The second factor is that overexercising can lead to lower bone densities. Preliminary data by Michel and associates have indicated that postmenopausal women exercising more than 300 min/week have lower bone mineral content than those exercising less than 300 min/week.[79,80] In fact, the women that participated in the high levels of exercise had bone mineral contents similar to those of nonexercising controls. In premenopausal women, over-training could lead to menstrual dysfunction, which would adversely affect bone mineral content. Thus, exercise should be used in moderation.

TABLE 1
General Recommendations for Exercise

1. Follow the American College of Sports Medicine Guidelines: 3–4 days a week, for 20–40 minutes at an intensity 60–80% of maximal heart rate.
2. Start slowly and build-up.
3. Include a variety of exericses.
4. Choose exercises that are liked.
5. Choose aerobic exercises that are weight bearing: jogging, stair climbing, aerobic dance or court games.
6. Have a strength component using exercises that use major muscle groups: leg press, leg extensions, leg curls, rowing, bench press, latissimus pull down, and arm curls and reverse curls.
7. Avoid exercises that compress or "wedge" the spine, i.e., the "plow", "cobra", straight-leg sit-ups.
8. The exercise needs to become a way of life.

Low bone density has been shown to be a risk factor for stress fractures. This relationship is significant in both pre- and post-menopausal women, as well as in men [95] In premenopausal women the relationship is inversely related to menstrual function and may be reversible with a resumption of menstrual function. The relationship also seems to be contingent upon Ca status. Participation in exercise through the early 20s has been shown to reduce the risk of bone fractures after age 50 years by maximizing bone mass prior to the onset of normal bone aging.[96] With regard to postmenopausal women, the data are sparse. A study of exercising old rats has shown that concomitant with the increase in bone density there occurred an increase in the breaking force needed to cause the bone to fracture.[97] This finding would suggest that exercise has a role in reducing the potential for fractures. Lanyon has suggested that a variety of physical activities is better than only one form of activity in preventing vertebral crush fractures.[20] This comment is based on the fact that bone generally adapts best when stresses are imposed from a variety of angles. Exercise can help prevent fractures, not only by preventing bone loss, but also by improving neuromuscular coordination, strength, and reaction time, which reduce the risk of falling.[98] Exercise may also stimulate new bone remodeling cycles, which result in new bone tissue that is free of microfractures, i.e., healthy. Thus, exercise may have an important role in reducing osteoporosis-related fractures. Clearly, more longitudinal investigations are needed on this topic of exercised-induced bone formation and maintenance.

VIII. SUMMARY AND CONCLUSIONS

The increase in bone mass produced by exercise in sedentary women can be significant, up to 12% in premenopausal women. Although this amount of gain may be significant, if the bone mineral status is considerably below normal, a 12% gain may not be enough to restore bone mass to that achieved by other women with more active life-styles. However, starting menopause with 12% more bone mass could make a difference. A sedentary postmenopausal woman had a bone mineral content loss of 1–2% per year. This steady annual rate of bone loss means that there is an ever-increasing risk of osteoporotic fractures with age. Exercise can reduce the rate of bone loss and possibly increase the mineral content by as much as 6–8%. This potential benefit of exercise does not suggest that exercise should serve as an alternative to estrogen therapy, but rather that it may be an important adjunct to estrogen replacement therapy and Ca supplementation. The potential beneficial effects on bone status of exercise are obvious, but the impact will continue only as long as the person exercises. Thus, the triad of normal menstrual or estrogen status, adequate Ca, and moderate weight-bearing physical activity will optimize bone growth and development early in life, maintain bone density in midlife, and minimize the development of low bone density and fractures late in life.

In summary, the majority of research reports indicates a positive effect of exercise on bone mass or density at various skeletal sites. Furthermore, when aerobic and strength exercises are combined, along with adequate Ca intake and estrogen therapy, if needed, the optimal bone densities can be obtained, and the potential risk of bone fractures reduced. Additional prospective studies are needed to establish the appropriate types of bone-enhancing activities at the different stages of the life cycle of both females and males. Comparative studies of diverse racial or ethnic groups are also needed.

REFERENCES

1. **Sowers, M. R., Clark, K., Hollis, B., Wallace, R. B., and Jannausch, M.,** Radial bone mineral density in pre- and perimenopausal women: a prospective study of rates and risk factors for loss, *J. Bone Miner. Res.*, 7, 647, 1992.
2. **Wolman R. L.,** Bone mineral density levels in elite female athletes, *Ann. Rheum. Dis.*, 49, 1013, 1990.
3. **Astrand, P. O. and Rodahl, K.,** *Textbook of Work Physiology*, McGraw-Hill, New York, 1977, 318–325.
4. **Paffenbarger, R. S., Hyde, R. T., Wing, A. L., and Hsieh, C-C.,** Physical activity, all-cause mortality, and longevity of college alumni, *New Engl. J. Med.*, 314, 605, 1986.
5. **Fehily, A. M., Coles, R. J., Evans, W. D., and Elwood, P. C.,** Factors affecting bone density in young adults, *Am. J. Clin. Nutr.*, 56, 579, 1992.
6. **Kanders, B., Dempster, D. W., and Lindsay R.,** Interaction of calcium, nutrition, and physical activity on bone mass in young women, *J. Bone Miner. Res.*, 3, 145, 1988.
7. **Toss, G.,** Effect of calcium intake vs. other life-style factors on bone mass, *J. Intern. Med.*, 231, 181, 1992.
8. **Drinkwater, B. L., Nilson, K., Chesnut, C. H., Bramner, W. J., Shainholtz, S., and Southworth, M. B.,** Bone mineral content of amenorrheic and eumenorrheic athletes, *New Engl. J. Med.*, 311, 277, 1984.
9. **Rockwell, J. C., Sorensen, A. M., Baker, S., Leahey, D., Stock, J. L., Michael, J., and Baran, D. T.,** Weight training decreases vertebral bone density in premenopausal women: a prospective study, *J. Clin. Endocrinol. Metab.*, 71, 988, 1990.
10. **Smidt, G. L., Lin, S-Y., O'Dwyer, K. D., and Blanpeid, P. R.,** The effect of high-intensity trunk exercise on bone mineral density of postmenopausal women, *Spine*, 14, 280, 1992.
11. **Yeh, J. K., and Aloia, J. F.,** Deconditioning increases bone resorption and decreases bone formation in the rat, *Metabolism*, 39, 659, 1990.
12. **Picard, D., Ste Marie, L. G., Coutu, D., Carrier, L., Chartrand, R., Lepage, R., Fugere, P., and D'Amour, P.,** Premenopausal bone mineral content relates to height, weight and calcium intake during early adulthood, *Bone Miner.*, 4, 299, 1988.
13. **Reid, I. R., Ames, R., Evans, M. C., Sharpe, S., Gamble, G., France, J. T., Lim, T. M. T., and Cundy, T. F.,** Determinants of total body and regional bone mineral density in normal postmenopausal women — a key role for fat mass, *J. Clin. Endocrinol. Metab.*, 75, 54, 1992.
14. **Turner, J. G., Gilchrist, N. L., Ayling, E. M., Hassall, A. J., Hooke, E. A., and Sadler, W. A.,** Factors affecting bone mineral density in high school girls, *New Zealand Med. J.*, 105, 95, 1992.
15. **Drinkwater, B. L.,** Physical exercise and bone health, *J. Am. Med. Women Assoc.*, 45, 91, 1990.
16. **Mazess, R. B., and Barden, H. S.,** Bone density in premenopausal women: effects of age, dietary intake, physical activity, smoking, and birth-control pills, *Am. J. Clin. Nutr.*, 53, 132, 1991.
17. **Hirota, T., Nara, M., Ohguri, M., Manago, E., and Hirota, K.,** Effect of diet and lifestyle on bone mass in Asian young women, *Am. J. Clin. Nutr.*, 55, 1168, 1992.
18. **Snow-Harter, C. and Marcus, R.,** Exercise, bone mineral density, and osteoporosis, *Exer. Sport Sci. Rev.*, 19, 351, 1991.
19. **Dalsky, G. P.,** Effect of exercise on bone: permissive influence of estrogen and calcium, *Med. Sci. Sports Exer.*, 22, 281, 1990.
20. **Lanyon, L. E.,** The success and failure of the adaptive response to functional load-bearing in averting bone fracture, *Bone*, 13, S17, 1992.
21. **Li, K-C., Zernicke, R. F., Barnard, R. J., and Li, F-Y.,** Differential response of rat limb bones to strenuous exercise, *J. Appl. Physiol.*, 70, 554, 1991.
22. **Fiore, C. E., Cottini, E., Fargetta, C., DiSalvo, G., Foti, R., and Raspagliesi, M.,** The effect of muscle-building exercise on forearm bone mineral content and osteoblast activity in drug-free and anabolic steroids self-administerıng young men, *Bone Miner.*, 13, 77, 1991.
23. **Zylstra, S., Hopkins, A., Erk, M., Hreshchyshyn, M. M., and Anbar, M.,** Effect of physical activity on lumbar spine and femoral neck bone densities, *Int. J.Sports Med.*, 10, 181, 1989.
24. **Beverly, M. C., Rider, T. A., Evans, M. J., and Smith, R.,** Local bone mineral response to brief exercise that stresses the skeleton, *Br. Med. J.*, 299, 233, 1989.
25. **Huddleston, A. L., Rockwell, D., Kulund, D. N., and Harrison, R. B.,** Bone mass in lifetime tennis players, *J. Am. Med. Assoc.*, 244, 1107, 1980.

26. **Marcus, R., Cann, C., Madvig, P., Minkoff, J., Goddard, M., Bayer, M., Martin, M., Gaudiani, L., Haskell, W., and Genant, H.,** Menstrual function and bone mass in elite women distance runners: endocrine and metabolic features, *Ann. Intern. Med.*, 102, 158, 1985.
27. **Carter, D. R.,** Mechanical loading histories and cortical bone remodeling. *Calcif. Tissue Int.*, 36 (suppl), 19, 1984.
28. **Silbermann, M., Bar Shira Maymon, B., Coleman, R., Reznick, A., Weisman, Y., Steinhagen-Thiessen, E., von der Mark, H., and von der Mark, K.,** Long-term physical exercise retards trabecular bone loss in lumbar vertebrae of aging female mice, *Calcif. Tissue Int.*, 46, 80, 1990.
29. **Dalsky, G., Stocke, K. S., Eshani, A. A., Slatopolsky, E., Lee, W. C., and Birge, S. J.,** Weight-bearing exercise training and lumbar bone mineral content in post menopausal women, *Ann. Intern. Med.*, 108, 824, 1988.
30. **Malm, H. T., Ronni-Sivula, H. M., Viinikka, L. U., and Ylikorkala, O. R.,** Marathon running accompanied by transient decreases in urinary calcium and serum osteocalcin levels, *Calcif. Tissue Int.*, 52, 209, 1993.
31. **Franck, H., Beuker, F., and Gurk, S.,** The effect of physical activity on bone turnover in young adults, *Exp. Clin. Endocrinol.*, 98, 42, 1991.
32. **Cauley, J. A., Gutai, J. P., Kuller, L. H., LeDonne, D., Sandler, R. B., Sashin, D., and Powell, J. G.,** Endogenous estrogen levels and calcium intakes in postmenopausal women. Relationships with cortical bone measures, *J. Am. Med. Assoc.*, 260, 3150, 1988.
33. **Notelovitz, M., Martin, D., Tesar, R., Khan, F. Y., Probart, C., Fields, C., and McKenzie, L.,** Estrogen therapy and variable-resistance weight training increase bone mineral in surgically menopausal women, *J. Bone Miner. Res.*, 6, 583, 1991.
34. **De Cree, C., Vermeulen, A., and Ostyn, M.,** Are high-performance young women athletes doomed to become low-performance old wives? A reconsideration of the increased risk of osteoporosis in amenorrheic women, *J. Sports Med. Phys. Fitness*, 31, 108, 1991.
35. **Snead, D. B., Weltmen, A., Weltman, J. Y., Evans, W. S., Veldhuis, J. D., Varma, M. M., Teates, C. D., Dowling, E. A., and Rogol, A. D.,** Reproductive hormones and bone mineral density in women runners, *J. Appl. Physiol.*, 72, 2149, 1992.
36. **White, C. M., Hergenroeder, A. C., and Klish, W. J.,** Bone mineral density in 15- to 21-year-old eumenorrheic and amenorrheic subjects, *Am. J. Dis. Child.*, 146, 31, 1992.
37. **Ding, J. H., Sheckter, C. B., Drinkwater, B. L., Soules, M. R., and Bremner, W. J.,** High serum cortisol levels in exercise-associated amenorrhea, *Ann. Intern. Med.*, 108, 530, 1988.
38. **Buchanan, J. R., Myers, C., Lloyd, T., Leuenberger, P., and Demers, L. M.,** Determinants of peak trabecular bone density in women: the role of androgens, estrogen, and exercise, *J. Bone Miner. Res.*, 3, 673, 1988.
39. **Finkelstein, J. S., Klibanski, A., Neer, R. M., Greenspan, S. L., Rosenthal, D. I., and Crowley, W. F.,** Osteoporosis in men with idiopathic hypogonadotropic hypogonadism, *Ann. Intern. Med.*, 106, 354, 1987.
40. **McArdle, W. D., Katch, F. I., and Katch V. L.,** *Exercise Physiology*, 3rd Ed., Lea & Febiger, Philadelphia, 1991, 384–417.
41. **Ljunghall, S., Joborn, H., Roxin, L-E., Skarfors, E. T,. Wide, L. E., and Lithell, H. O.,** Increase in serum parathyroid hormone levels after prolonged physical exercise, *Med. Sci. Sports Exer.*, 20, 122, 1988.
42. **Ljunghall, S., Joborn, H., Roxin, L-E., Rastad, L., Wide. L. E., and Akerstrom, G.,** Prolonged low-intensity exercise raises the serum parathyroid hormone levels, *Clin. Endocrinol.*, 25, 535, 1986.
43. **Selvesen, H., Johansson, A. G., Foxdal, P., Wide, L., Piehl-Aulin, K., and Ljunghall, S.,** Intact serum parathyroid hormone levels increase during running exercise in well-trained men, *Calcif. Tissue Int.*, 54, 256, 1994.
44. **Bevier, W. C., Wiswell, R. A., Pyka, G., Kozak, K. C., Newhall, K. M., and Marcus, R.,** Relationship of body composition, muscle strength and aerobic capacity to bone mineral density in older men and women, *J. Bone Miner. Res.*, 4, 421, 1989.
45. **Virvidakis, K., Georgiou, E., Korkotsidis, A., Ntalles, K., and Proukakis, C.,** Bone mineral content of junior competitive weightlifters, *J. Appl. Physiol.*, 11, 244, 1990.
46. **Slemenda, C. W., Christian J. C., Reed, T., Reister, T. K., Williams, C. J., and Johnston, C. C.,** Long-term bone loss in men: effects of genetics and environmental factors, *Ann. Intern. Med.*, 117, 286, 1992.
47. **Blumenthal, J. A., Emery, C. F., Madden, D. J., Schniebolk, S., Riddle, M. W., Cobb, F. R., Higgenbotham, M., and Coleman, R. E.,** Effects of exercise training on bone density in older men and women, *J. Am. Geriatr. Soc.*, 39, 1065, 1991.
48. **Orwoll, E. S., Ferar, J., Oviatt, S. K., McClung, M. R., and Huntington, K.,** The relationship of swimming exercise to bone mass in men and women, *Arch. Intern. Med.*, 149, 2197, 1989.
49. **Williams, J. A., Wagner, J., Wasnich, R., and Heilbrun, L.,** The effect of long-distance running upon appendicular bone mineral content, *Med. Sci. Sports Exer.*, 16, 223, 1984.
50. **Bilanin, J. E., Blanchard, M. S., and Rusek-Cohen, E.,** Lower vertebral bone density in male long-distance runners, *Med. Sci. Sports Exer.*, 21, 66, 1989.
51. **Colletti, L. A., Edwards, J., Gorden, L., Shary, J., and Bell, N. H.,** The effects of muscle-building exercise on bone mineral density of the radius, spine, and hip in young men, *Calcif. Tissue Int.*, 45, 12, 1989.
52. **Tylavsky, F. A., Anderson, J. J. B., Talmage, R. V., and Taft, T. N.,** Are calcium intakes and physical activity patterns during adolescence related to radial bone mass of white college-age females?, *Osteopor. Int.*, 2, 232, 1992.

53. **Slemenda, C. W., Miller, J. Z., Hui, S. L., Reister, T. K., and Johnston, C. C.,** Role of physical activity in the development of skeletal mass in children, *J. Bone Miner. Res.*, 6, 1227, 1991.
54. **McCulloch, R. G., Bailey, D. A., Houston, C. S., Dodd, B. L.,** Effects of physical activity, dietary calcium intake and selected lifestyle factors on bone density in young women, *Can. Med. Assoc. J.*, 142, 221, 1990.
55. **Halioua, L., and Anderson, J. J. B.,** Lifetime calcium intake and physical activity habits: independent and combined effects on the radial bone of healthy premenopausal Caucasian women, *Am. J. Clin. Nutr.*, 49, 534, 1989.
56. **Bunt, J. C., Going, S. B., Lohman, T. G., Heinrich, C. H., Perry, C. D., and Pamenter, R. W.,** Variation in bone mineral content and estimated body fat in young adult females, *Med. Sci. Sports Exer.*, 22, 564, 1990.
57. **Heinrich, C. H., Going, S. B., Pamenter, R. W., Perry, C. D., Boyden, T. W., and Lohman, T. G.,** Bone mineral content of cyclically menstruating female resistance and endurance trained athletes, *Med. Sci. Sports Exer.*, 22, 558, 1990.
58. **Wolman, R. L., Faulmann, L., Clark, P., Hesp, R., and Harries, M. G.,** Different training patterns and bone mineral density of the femoral shaft in elite, female athletes, *Ann. Rheum. Dis.*, 50, 487, 1991.
59. **Davee, A. M., Rosen, C. J., and Adler, R. A.,** Exercise patterns and trabecular bone density in college women, *J. Bone Miner. Res.*, 5, 245, 1990.
60. **Peterson, S. E., Peterson, M. D., Raymond, G., Gilligan, C., Checovich, M. M., and Smith, E. L.,** Muscular strength and bone density with weight training in middle-aged women, *Med. Sci. Sports Exer.*, 23, 499, 1991.
61. **Risser, W. L., Lee, E. J., LeBlanc, A., Poindexter, H. B., Risser, J. M. H., and Schneider, V.,** Bone density in eumenorrheic female college athletes, *Med. Sci. Sports Exer.*, 22, 570, 1990.
62. **Swissa-Sivan, A., Simkin, A., Leichter, I., Nyska, A., Statter, M., Bivas, A., Menczel, J., and Samueloff, S.,** Effect of swimming on bone growth and development in young rats, *Bone Miner.*, 7, 91, 1989.
63. **Hatori, M., Hasegawa, H., Shinozaki, A., Hayashi, R., Okano, H., Mizunuma, H., and Murata, K.,** The effect of walking at the anaerobic threshold level on vertebral bone loss in postmenopausal women, *Calcif. Tissue Int.*, 52, 411, 1993.
64. **Krall, E.A. and Dawson-Hughes, B.,** Walking is related to bone density and rates of bone loss, *Am. J. Med.*, 96, 20, 1994.
65. **Snow-Harter, C., Bouxsein, M., Lewis, B., Charette, S., Weinstein, P., and Marcus, R.,** Muscle strength as a predictor of bone mineral density in young women, *J. Bone Miner. Res.*, 5, 589, 1990.
66. **Wolman, R. L., Reeve, J., Clark, P., Hesp, D., and McNally, E.,** Bone mineral density in elite light weight women rowers, *Br. J. Rheumatol.*, 28 (suppl), 6, 1989.
67. **Gleeson, P. B., Protas, E. J., LeBlanc, A. D., Schneider, V. S., and Evans, H. J.,** Effects of weight lifting on bone mineral density in premenopausal women, *J. Bone Miner. Res.*, 5, 153, 1990.
68. **Dornemann, T., McMurray, R. G., Renner, J., and Anderson, J. J. B.,** Effects of weight training on bone density of 40- 50-year-old premenopausal women, Master's thesis, University of North Carolina, Chapel Hill, 1994.
69. **Lindberg, J. S., Powell, M. R., Hunt, M. M., Ducey, D. E., and Wade, C. E.,** Increased vertebral bone mineral in response to reduced exercise in amenorrheic runners, *West. J. Med.*, 146, 39, 1987.
70. **Warren, M. P., Brooks-Gunn, J., Fox, R. P., Lancelot, C., Newman, D., and Hamilton, W. G.,** Lack of bone accretion and amenorrhea: evidence for a relative osteopenia in weight-bearing bones, *J. Clin. Endocrinol. Metab.*, 72, 847, 1991.
71. **Hay, P. J., Delahunt, J. W., Hall, A., Mitchell, A. W., Harper, G., and Salmond, C.,** Predictors of osteopenia in premenopausal women with anorexia nervosa, *Calcif. Tissue Int.*, 50, 498, 1992.
72. **Joyce, J. M., Warren, D. L., Humphries, L. L., Smith, A. J., and Coon, J. S.,** Osteoporosis in women with eating disorders: comparison of physical parameters, exercise, and menstrual status with SPA and DPA evaluation, *J. Nucl. Med.*, 31, 325, 1990.
73. **Smith, E. L., Gilligan, C., McAdam, M., Ensign, C. P., and Smith, P. E.,** Deterring bone loss by exercise intervention in premenopausal and postmenopausal women, *Calcif. Tissue Int.*, 44, 312, 1989.
74. **Russell, J. B., Mitchell, D., Musey, P. I., and Collins, D. C.,** The relationship of exercise to anovulatory cycles in female athletes: hormonal and physical characteristics, *Obstet. Gynecol.*, 63, 452, 1984.
75. **Drinkwater, B. L., Bruemmer, B., and Chesnut, C. H.,** Menstrual history as a determinant of current bone density in young athletes, *J. Am. Med. Assoc.*, 263, 545, 1990.
76. **Wolman, R. L., Clark, P., McNally, E., Harries, M., and Reeve, J.,** Menstrual state and exercise as determinants of spinal trabecular bone density in female athletes, *Br. Med. J.*, 301, 516, 1990.
77. **Heikkinen, J., Kurttila-Matero, E., Kyllonen, E., Vuori, J., Takala, T., and Vaananen, H. K.,** Moderate exercise does not enhance the positive effect of estrogen on bone mineral density in postmenopausal women, *Calcif. Tissue Int.*, 49 (suppl), S83, 1991.
78. **Nelson, M. E., Meredith, C. N., Dawson Hughes, B., and Evans, W. J.,** Hormone and bone mineral status in endurance-trained and sedentary post-menopausal women, *J. Clin. Endocrinol. Metab.*, 66, 927, 1988.
79. **Michel, B. A., Bloch, D. A., and Fries, J. F.,** Weight-bearing exercise, overexercise, and lumbar bone density over age 50 years, *Arch. Intern. Med.*, 149, 2325, 1989.
80. **Michel, B. A., Lane, N. E., Bloch, D. A., Jones, H. H., and Fries, J. F.,** Effect of weight-bearing exericse on lumbar bone mass after age fifty, *Ann. Med.*, 23, 397, 1991.

81. **Ballard, J. E., McKeown, B. C., Graham, H. M., and Zinkgraf, S. A.,** The effect of high level physical activity (8.5 METs or greater) and estrogen replacement therapy upon bone mass in postmenopausal females, aged 50–68 years. *J. Appl. Physiol.*, 11, 208, 1990.
82. **Cheng, S., Suominen, H., Rantanen, T., Parkatti, T., and Heikkinen, E.,** Bone mineral density and physical activity in 50–60-year-old women, *Bone Miner.*, 12, 123, 1991.
83. **Prince, R. L., Smith, M., Dick, I. M., Price, R. I., Webb, P. G., Henderson, N. K., and Harris, M. M.,** Prevention of postmenopausal osteoporosis, *New Engl. J. Med.*, 325, 1189, 1991.
84. **Chow, R., Harrison, J. E., and Notarius, C.,** Effect of two randomized exercise programmes on bone mass of healthy postmenstrual women, *Br. Med. J.*, 295, 1441, 1987.
85. **Rikli, R. E., and McManis, B. G.,** Effects of exercise on bone mineral content in postmenopausal women, *Res. Quart. Exer. Sport*, 61, 243, 1990.
86. **Jones, P. R. M., Hardman, A. E., Hudson, A., and Norgan, N. G.,** Influence of brisk walking on the broadhand ultrasonic attenuation of the calcaneus in previously sedentary women aged 30–61 years, *Calcif. Tissue Int.*, 49, 112, 1991.
87. **Nelson, M. E., Fisher, E. C., Dilmanian, F. A., Dallal, G. E., and Evans, W. J.,** A 1-yr walking program and increased dietary calcium in postmenopausal women: effects on bone, *Am. J. Clin. Nutr.*, 53, 1304, 1991.
88. **Halle, J. S., Smidt, G. L., O'Dwyer, K. D., and Lin, S. Y.,** Relationship between trunk muscle torque and bone mineral content of the lumbar spine and hip in healthy postmenopausal women, *Phys. Therap.*, 70, 690, 1990.
89. **Zimmermann, C. L., Smidt, G. L., Brooks, J. S., Kinsey, W. J., and Eekhoff, T. L.,** Relationship of extremity muscle torque and bone mineral density in postmenopausal women, *Phys. Therap.*, 70, 302, 1990.
90. **Simkin, A., Ayalon, J., and Leichter, I.,** Increased trabecular bone density due to bone-loading exercises in postmenopausal osteoporotic women, *Calcif. Tissue Int.*, 40, 59, 1987.
91. **Pruitt, L. A., Jackson, R. D., Bartels, R. L., and Lehnhard, H. J.,** Weight-training effects bone mineral density in early postmenopausal women, *J. Bone Miner. Res.*, 7, 179, 1992.
92. **Sinaki, M., Wahner, H. W., Offord, K. P., and Hodgson, S. F.,** Efficacy of nonloading exercises in prevention of vertebral bone loss in postmenopausal women: a controlled trial, *Mayo Clin. Proc.*, 64, 762, 1989.
93. **Aisenbrey, J. A.,** Exercise in the prevention and management of osteoporosis, *Phys. Therap.*, 67, 1100, 1987.
94. **Krolner, B., Toft, B., Nielsen, S. P., and Tondevold, E.,** Physical exercise as a prophylaxis against involutional vertebral bone loss: a controlled trial, *Clin. Sci.*, 64, 541, 1983.
95. **Myburgh, K. H., Hutchins, J., Fataar, A. B., Hough, S. F., and Noakes, T. D.,** Low bone density is an etiologic factor for stress fractures in athletes, *Ann. Intern. Med.*, 113, 754, 1990.
96. **Wyshak, G., Frish, R. E., Albright, T. E., Albright, N. L., Schiff, I., and Witschi, J.,** Nonalcoholic carbonated beverage consumption and bone fractures among women former college athletes, *J. Orthop. Res.*, 7, 91, 1989.
97. **Raab, D. M., Smith, E. L., Crenshaw, T. D., and Thomas, D.,** Bone mechanical properties after exercise training in young and old rats, *J. Appl. Physiol.*, 68, 130, 1990.
98. **Smith, E. L., and Gilligan, C.,** Physical activity effects on bone metabolism, *Calcif. Tissue Int.*, 49 (suppl), S50, 1991.

Chapter 20

INFLUENCE OF NUTRITIONAL FACTORS ON BONE HEALTH OF THE ELDERLY

Connie W. Bales, Ph.D. and John J. B. Anderson, Ph.D.

TABLE OF CONTENTS

0-8493-7845-1/95/$0.00+$.50

I. INTRODUCTION

Osteoporosis is an age-related disorder that affects more than 20 million older Americans, being the most common metabolic bone disease in the developed world. In the United States, this painful and disfiguring condition results in approximately 1.3 million fractures per year in older adults, escalating the cost of medical care for the aged. Hip fractures alone account for a staggering $8 billion annually in short-term medical care costs.[1]

Primary, as opposed to secondary, osteoporosis varies significantly over time. Secondary osteoporosis results from other causes or factors such as corticosteroid use or other diseases. Both types are characterized by a reduction in bone mass, also known as osteopenia, as well as an increased susceptibility to atraumatic skeletal fractures. Low bone mass is most prevalent among the elderly, but even middle-aged adults can develop this condition and sustain fractures from minimal force (strain).

Because considerable pathophysiological heterogeneity exists in cases of osteoporosis, it is often divided into subtypes, as first delineated by Riggs and Melton.[2] Postmenopausal (Type I) osteoporosis is an accelerated and disproportionate loss of trabecular bone and occurs predominantly in women. In this type of osteoporosis, increased bone resorption (and relatively constant bone formation), reduced production of parathyroid hormone (PTH), and decreased vitamin D activation lead to impaired absorption and homeostatic regulation of calcium (Ca). Type I osteoporosis is highly correlated with the decline and cessation in ovarian production and secretion of estrogens in women.

Type II or "senile" osteoporosis is common in men as well as in women; however, the onset of complications comes later in life (between the 70s and 80s for women and as much as a decade later for men). Rates of cortical and trabecular bone loss are relatively proportionate in Type II osteoporosis, and fractures of the hip are common. Both bone formation and resorption are depressed, but gradual losses in bone mass continue because resorption exceeds formation. PTH levels are frequently elevated, but both osteoblast function and calcitriol synthesis may be diminished. Bone mineral density is a good predictor of fracture risk for individuals with Type II osteoporosis, but other factors, such as loss of muscle strength, reduced body mass index (BMI), decline of coordination/balance, and increased likelihood of falls with advanced age, also contribute to fractures.

Although numerous studies have explored the relationship of environmental factors, including nutrition, to postmenopausal (Type I) osteoporosis, much less is known about the specific impact of these factors on the Type II form of this condition. This paucity of knowledge is unfortunate, because the devastating effects of senile osteoporosis on health and physical function greatly exceed that of osteoporosis in younger individuals. Despite advances in medical care, fractures of the proximal femur are persistently associated with high rates of morbidity and mortality (as high as 33%).[3] The annual rate of hip fractures in the U.S. is expected to climb in future decades because of dramatic increases projected for the elderly (over age 60 years) population (see Figure 1).[4] By the year 2040, individuals 60 years of age and older will constitute almost 25% of the population.[4] Based upon these projected population figures, the estimated annual occurrence of hip fractures will increase from the present rate of about 275,000 to more than 800,000 per year in 2040 (see Figure 2).[5]

The early prevention of bone loss and subsequent osteoporotic fractures is by far the most effective way of reducing the impact of this degenerative, incurable condition. Yet for millions of elderly individuals already affected by varying degrees of bone mineral loss, therapeutic strategies must focus on maintenance of existing bone and preservation of current levels of function, i.e., health. This chapter therefore focuses on the reported evidence of nutritional amelioration of age-related bone loss in Type II osteoporosis. Emphasis is placed on females, but males suffer the same effects of osteoporosis, except at approximately 50% of the fracture rates of females (see Chapter 22).

II. INTERACTION OF BONE METABOLISM WITH BODY COMPOSITIONAL FACTORS

Several detrimental changes in body composition occur with age. There is a definite decline in lean body mass (LBM), as well as a loss of bone mass. The fat mass increases in both absolute and

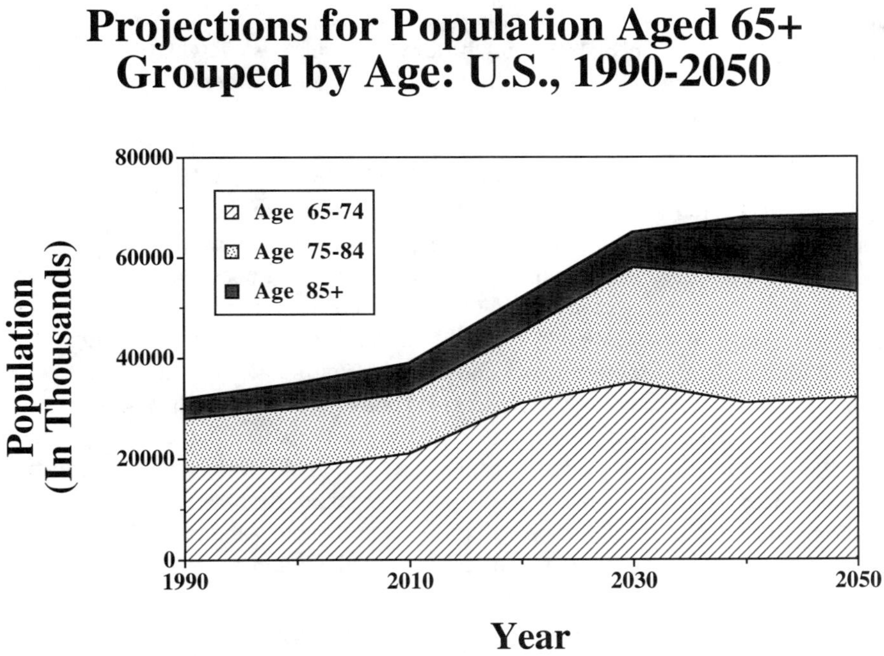

FIGURE 1. Projections for Increase in the Elderly (65 years +) in the U.S. Population through 2050.

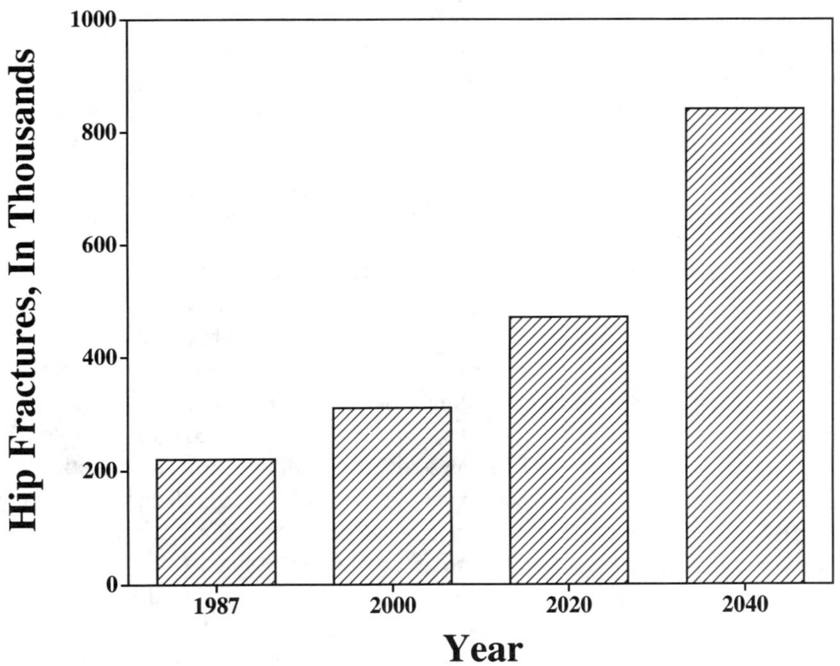

FIGURE 2. Projected Annual Rate of Hip Fractures in the U.S.

relative mass (percent). A close link exists between LBM and bone mass. In addition, fat mass has its own contribution to bone mass, i.e., the greater the fat mass, the greater the strain on the skeleton. Yet all effects of high fat mass are not detrimental to bone, since adipose tissue can contribute to the production of estrogen (see next section). For obvious reasons, it is important that the elderly try to maintain LBM and thereby bone mass whenever possible. The only documented way to maintain LBM is exercise, especially strength activities, such as weight lifting and resistance exercise. Physical activity can also be directly beneficial to the maintenance of bone density.

A. BODY COMPOSITION

A major and positive contributor to bone mass at practically any age is body weight or body mass index.[6-10] In general, the higher the mass of the body, whether from the lean compartment or from the fat mass, the greater is the bone mass. Conversely, low body weight is a risk factor for hip fractures among black and white women.[11] The advantage of greater skeletal mass conferred by higher relative or absolute increases in body fat mass, even obesity, in postmenopausal women does not apparently hold also for older men.[10-15] The reason for this gender difference apparently lies in the differential metabolism of fat tissue, but understanding of the mechanism is limited (see later).

An explanation of the protective effect of increased body mass in elderly women against fractures rests primarily on the observation that fat tissue, but not lean tissue, increases in postmenopausal women, and that the fat cells may be more responsive to adrenal hormones.[16,17] A greater fat mass contains greater activity of the enzyme, aromatase, required for the peripheral conversion of androstenedione (from the adrenal cortex) to estrone in adipocytes, and possibly in muscle cells.[18] Thus, fat cells become a significant source of estrone, which is mostly converted in these cells to estradiol, the most potent natural estrogen, via a nonenzymatic step.[19] Aromatase activity also increases with age per se in both males and females, but females have relatively more body fat at any age beyond puberty.[20] Furthermore, excessive body fat may also induce increased production of adrenal androgenic/anabolic steroids in postmenopausal women.[21]

The correlation between fat mass and bone mass is greater for females than for males, an observation made for Caucasians,[15] Asian Chinese,[22] and Japanese subjects.[17] An explanation for this difference is not available, but Felson and colleagues speculate that females have a more efficient peripheral conversion of androstenedione to estrogens after the menopause.[15] Also, because of greater numbers of estrogen receptors in bone cells of females, they may conserve bone mass more effectively than males. Thus, obese postmenopausal women with higher circulating estrogen will likely maintain greater bone mass than will lean women with basal blood levels of estrogen.

In addition to the benefits of fat tissue for the hormonal maintenance of bone mass in postmenopausal women, but not in men,[15] greater amounts of body fat are protective against hip fractures from falls, mainly backward falls.[23] Greater upper body fat mass provides greater gravitational loads, i.e., weight bearing, at the most fracture-susceptible bone sites, i.e., hips. Thus, greater amounts of body fat may influence the fracture risk of postmenopausal women in contrasting ways.

Blacks clearly differ from whites in body composition; this difference exists mainly in muscle (lean tissue) and skeletal mass, but not in fat mass.[24] An interesting report by Farmer et al. of elderly women in the NHANES Epidemiological Follow-up Study demonstrated that any anthropometric indicator of greater body mass, e.g., weight, skinfold thickness, body mass index, or midarm circumference, was inversely related to fractures.[25] This finding corresponds with the protective effect of lean body mass against hip fracture found in the National Health and Examination Survey (NHANES I, 1971–1975).[26] Farmer et al. also showed that women in the upper two quartiles for several anthropometric indicators, in addition to greater body mass index, had significantly reduced risks of hip fracture.[25] The strength of this prospective study resides in the large number of hip fracture cases (n = 84) in a cohort of 3595 white women.

Low body weight was also demonstrated by Pruzansky et al. to be an important risk factor for hip fractures in both black and white women.[11] Similar findings of low measurements of body fat in elderly Asian female populations have been associated with increased rates of hip fractures.[17,22]

Asian women with greater body mass index, weight, or fat mass as estimated by skinfolds also have greater bone mass.[22,27] Thus, body mass index or any other variable of body composition must be considered in comparative analyses of differences in bone mass of diverse ethnic groups. In a comparative study of bone measurements of adult and elderly Japanese subjects living in Japan and

Japanese descendants living in Hawaii, however, adjustments of BMC by dividing by bone width, i.e., BMD, increased the mean difference between subjects living in the two countries.[28]

In summary, several reports suggest that a greater fat mass in elderly subjects, particularly females, is protective against all fractures, and especially against hip fractures. Greater LBM, primarily skeletal muscle, would also presumably help to preserve skeletal mass.

B. PHYSICAL ACTIVITY

Physical activity remains the life-style factor most often observed to impact positively on bone mass late in life (see Chapter 19 on physical exercise). This behavior, however, must be continuously maintained in order for the bone mass to be retained over long periods of time. If these bone-positive activities cease, then the rate of loss of bone mass will increase for a period of time, perhaps as long as a year in the elderly who have slower rates of bone remodeling than in younger adults, until a new steady-state is achieved. The same phenomenon occurs after the menopause, either natural or surgical, and after the cessation of estrogen therapy in postmenopausal women. In each case, a relatively short period of rapid bone loss occurs, which lasts approximately six months, and then a period of slower bone loss occurs for a few years until the new steady-state becomes established.

An example of a gain and then a loss of vertebral bone mass in postmenopausal women placed on a controlled exercise program was reported by Dalsky et al.[29] These investigators were able to increase significantly the bone density of the lumbar vertebrae after 1 year of exercise, but when women stopped exercising, they returned to their pre-exercise bone values within 6 months. Only those women who continued exercising on their own during the next year after the program was stopped were able to retain much of the bone mass gained during the programmed exercise. This well-designed work, as well as other investigations, illustrates the great importance of keeping the same healthy behaviors for the maintenance of bone mass (or density in this case) for an indefinite period.

The natural condition of aging is for late postmenopausal women to continue to lose bone mass at a fairly steady or linear decay rate until ambulatory difficulties begin to occur.[30-32] When ambulatory problems present, or when immobility occurs, elderly individuals undergo a new phase of exponential bone loss, which lasts for a fairly long period of time, but very little information is available on this immobility-related loss in the elderly. Hospitalized patients and bed-ridden individuals are known to undergo a period of rapid bone loss until they begin to re-ambulate.

Cross-sectional data on physical activities obtained from elderly Japanese and Hong Kong Chinese women also support the concept of a positive association between diverse occupational and other activities on bone mass.[27,33]

C. SUMMARY

Daily activities requiring some exertion remain as important for the conservation of bone mass in elderly women as in premenopausal women. It appears that the consistency of patterns of activity over long periods, i.e., decades, is critical for bone mineral retention. Upper body strength exercises have been shown to benefit several skeletal sites in younger women, but similar studies have not been conducted among the elderly.

III. AGE AND NUTRIENT INTERACTIONS WITH BONE DENSITY

This section provides background on the effects, both positive and negative, of nutritional and age-associated factors on bone mass. Ca, phosphorus (P), and vitamin D are emphasized because these specific nutrients, along with energy intake (calories) have been most investigated. In particular, recent studies of vitamin D offer some promising new approaches to the treatment of osteoporosis. Newer information about the influence of or modulation by other micronutrients, such as certain trace elements and vitamin K, on bone cells in growth, development, and maintenance is also discussed, along with current interpretations of the relationships of bone density with body composition and physical activity.

A. VITAMIN D

Vitamin D has been shown to be deficient in many elderly populations. Because of its role in Ca and bone metabolism, vitamin D deficit takes on a significant role in the etiology of osteoporosis. Several recent clinical trials using supplements of vitamin D have shown positive effects on bone mass and/or fracture rates, suggesting that elderly subjects have insufficient intakes and skin production of vitamin D, and that supplements may be warranted as a way of preventing osteoporosis.

1. Potential Role of Vitamin D Deficiency in the Etiology of Osteoporosis

As noted in the preceding section, decreases in Ca intake and fractional absorption of Ca with age are thought to be important factors in the pathogenesis of osteoporosis. Dietary intakes of vitamin D_3 and exposure to sunlight are both commonly reduced with age.[34] In addition, MacLaughlin and Holick report age-related reductions in the amount of dermal precursor of vitamin D (7-dehydrocholesterol) in the skin, as well as decreases in the total quantity of previtamin D_3 produced in the epidermis and dermis of elderly subjects.[35] Aging may be related to decreased numbers of $1,25(OH)_2D$ receptors in intestinal mucosal cells.[36] Decrements in the ability to hydroxylate vitamin D in the liver[37] and kidney[38,39] with age have also been reported. Several investigators have reported lower levels of plasma calcidiol in elderly subjects,[40-42] and some have also found an age-associated decline in calcitriol concentrations.[43] In addition, evidence exists that the elderly are unable to respond appropriately to secondary hyperparathyroidism by increasing calcitriol biosynthesis.[41] Thus, whereas early postmenopausal bone loss does not appear to be associated with remarkable changes in vitamin D status, elderly individuals may have a marginal vitamin D status sufficient to compromise bone health.

To summarize, both the role of vitamin D as a primary determinant of intestinal Ca uptake and the presence of the aforementioned risk factors for vitamin D deficiency in the elderly suggest that vitamin D deficiency could be a critical factor in the development of senile osteoporosis. Elderly patients with osteoporosis commonly have subnormal blood levels of calcitriol, and many also have elevated circulating PTH concentrations.[44] PTH-mediated bone loss is a typical consequence of vitamin D deficiency and may contribute to hip fractures. In fact, several groups of investigators have reported higher rates of hip fracture in patients with vitamin D deficiency.[45-47] Lips et al. found that 60% of hip fracture patients living in Amsterdam had low (<20 nmol/L) serum levels of 25(OH)D compared with 16% of healthy controls.[48]

2. Clinical Trials Using Vitamin D Supplements to Reduce Fracture Rates

When menopause is well past, low Ca intake, decreased Ca absorption, and vitamin D deficiency become the most likely contributors to the progression of osteopenia toward osteoporosis and associated fractures. Vitamin D derivatives, such as 1,25-dihydroxyvitamin D, should help counteract age-related decreases in Ca intake and absorption by stimulating gastrointestinal uptake of Ca; these active metabolites could also stimulate osteoblastic and osteoclastic activity in the skeleton, favoring the retention of bone mineral.[49]

Although it seems logical to consider vitamin D therapy as a treatment for Type II osteoporosis, its use has been considered controversial because of its hypercalcemic effects. Moreover, until recently there has been a paucity of convincing evidence that calcitriol treatment actually reduces fracture risk. Although several studies have shown that vitamin D supplementation reduces parathyroid stimulation (thus theoretically reducing bone turnover), the results of major clinical trials concerning the long-term benefits of vitamin D therapy have been conflicting.[50] For example, Gallagher and Goldgar administered calcitriol (mean daily dose was 0.62 μg) to 50 postmenopausal women with vertebral fractures and found an increase in spine density and total body Ca at the end of the two-year study.[51] Aloia et al. also found a beneficial effect of calcitriol supplementation on bone density,[52] whereas Ott and Chesnut found bone density decreased to a similar extent in patients given calcitriol compared to those receiving a placebo.[53] Unfortunately, none of these studies had large enough numbers of subjects to show a significant effect of calcitriol on the incidence of fractures.

Recently, two fairly large intervention trials have linked vitamin D treatment with the reduction of osteoporosis-related fractures. In a prospective, randomized trial, Tilyard and co-workers studied the potential therapeutic effects of calcitriol in preventing new vertebral fractures in 622 postmenopausal women with osteoporosis.[49] These subjects ranged in age from 50 to 79 years (mean age = 63 yrs), with a postmenopause duration of almost 15 years. Those randomized to the calcitriol arm of the study received 0.25 μg of calcitriol twice daily, whereas those in the Ca-treated control group received 1000 mg of elemental Ca in the form of Ca gluconate administered twice daily. After three years, these investigators found a threefold reduction in the number of new vertebral compression fractures in the calcitriol treatment group. The number of peripheral fractures was also reduced by calcitriol therapy.

A second study has shown that the benefits of calcitriol are not limited to younger osteoporotic patients and that, indeed, the elderly may have the most to gain in bone mass from vitamin D treatment.[54] Chapuy et al. studied 3270 ambulatory, elderly women (mean age = 84 yrs) living in nursing homes in southern France.[54] Subjects in the treatment arm of the study were administered 800 IU vitamin D and 1200 mg Ca (as calcium phosphate) for 18 months. In subjects receiving this treatment, serum PTH levels were decreased by 44%, and bone density of the proximal femur was also improved. Most importantly, the rate of osteoporosis-related fractures was significantly reduced in the treatment group. These subjects experienced 43% fewer hip fractures than placebo-treated subjects.

In summary, although the benefit of vitamin D treatment for Type I osteoporosis is somewhat uncertain, recent studies provide impressive evidence that vitamin D may slow bone loss and reduce fracture rates in Type II osteoporosis. In the elderly patient with osteoporosis and low serum levels of vitamin D, combined therapy of vitamin D and Ca or therapy with vitamin D alone may significantly reduce rates of fracture.

3. Caveats Regarding Vitamin D Therapy

In the United States, vitamin D and its analogs are not commonly used as therapeutic agents for osteoporosis, except in small doses, e.g. 800 IU per day. Concern has rested on the narrow efficacy/toxicity window for these substances and, consequently, the fear of inducing toxicity. Although the potential of calcitriol to induce hypercalcemia and possibly renal stones has caused concern about its therapeutic usefulness in the past, neither Tilyard et al.[49] (who administered 0.25 μg calcitriol bid for three years) nor Chapuy et al.[54] (who gave 20 μg vitamin D_3 daily for 18 months) encountered serious side effects. Serum and urinary Ca levels, routinely monitored during administration of vitamin D supplements or derivatives, were within normal ranges.

Likewise, Fujita noted that although increased urinary Ca excretion almost invariably results from the administration of vitamin D derivatives, instances of nephrocalcinosis have been rarely reported.[36] However, this finding may be more applicable to Japan (where Ca intakes are around 500 mg/d) than to Western countries, where Ca and vitamin D intakes generally are often higher.

The development of new vitamin D derivatives, which have low potency in enhancing intestinal Ca absorption but greater effects in stimulating bone formation, could help osteoporotic patients by minimizing many of the deleterious calcemic effects of vitamin D. New clinical trials will be needed to describe the benefit/risk properties of these innovative agents.

B. CALCIUM

Although it is evident that age-associated causes of bone loss are more complex than simple Ca deficiency, Ca intakes need to meet recommended intake levels (RDAs) as a minimum in order to allow for the maintenance of tissue already present in bone. The role of Ca in maintaining bone mineral density will be addressed in detail in this section. However, Ca, it should be noted, appears to be a threshold nutrient, which means that higher intakes than that recommended (i.e., the RDA) will have little or no additional benefit to skeletal mass (and no harm either).

1. Calcium Intake and Absorption

It has been estimated that 75% of females over age 35 have Ca intakes below the RDA of 800 mg per day.[55] Ca intakes as high as 1000 to 1500 mg have been recommended by national consensus groups that have endorsed the benefits (and emphasized the minimal risks) of a high Ca diet.[56,57] The next section focuses on studies of Ca effects on Type II osteoporosis.

The absorption and utilization of Ca in the diet must be sufficiently high to promote adequate Ca status, and thus the maintenance of bone mineral mass. Ca deficiency will stimulate endogenous PTH release, which increases activation frequency of bone remodeling and, thus, accelerates bone loss because of a negative balance per remodeling cycle. Such deficiency also may increase the risk of perforations of trabecular plates, thus permanently reducing strength and biomechanical competence. Modest increments of absorbed Ca may preserve bone mass and strength by suppressing this process.[58]

2. Calcium Metabolism in the Elderly

Elderly individuals have several changes in Ca metabolism that contribute to a negative Ca balance, less efficient utilization of Ca, and continued loss of bone mass. These changes include a decline in intestinal Ca absorption, a tendency for PTH concentrations to increase with age, enhanced urinary losses of Ca, and reductions in bone formation.

Gastrointestinal function declines in most elderly subjects, and in postmenopausal women this decline is thought to begin as early as age 60 years. Part of the decrement in Ca absorption results from a reduction in gastric acid secretion,[59] i.e., hypochlorhydria, and part from the less efficient transport of Ca ions across the epithelial mucosa.[43,59-61] The latter decline may result from a poor adaptation to vitamin D deficits[62] or from a partial intestinal cell inhibition of the action of the hormonal form of vitamin D in the elderly.[63] In general, despite adequate intakes of Ca, Ca balances remain negative in the elderly.

Serum concentrations of PTH tend to be elevated in older subjects.[64-66] Most, but not all, investigators are in agreement on this point. In late postmenopausal women, PTH seems to be more effective than in premenopausal females in stimulating Ca transfer from bone to blood (extracellular fluid or ECF), whether the Ca ions are derived from bone resorption or from the increased movement of ions from the bone fluid compartment across bone-lining cells to the ECF. In part, the enhanced PTH effect is considered to result from the relative absence of circulating estrogens in elderly women.

The efficiency of renal reabsorption of Ca ions also declines in elderly individuals. In women, this decrement in reabsorptive efficiency may occur because of the loss of ovarian estrogen function, but other explanations might also be valid.[67] Males also suffer all of these system decrements in their later years, but explanatory mechanisms are not readily available, as they are, at least in part, for females. A common mechanism of bone loss may exist for both elderly females and males, but hard experimental or observational data to support any postulated mechanism in males remain sparse.

3. Calcium Effects on Maintenance of Bone Mineral

Dawson-Hughes et al. measured bone mass before and after administering Ca supplements to postmenopausal women living in the Boston area.[68] Over a two-year period of supplementation, subjects consuming lower amounts of Ca were found to show greater improvements in bone mass than those whose prestudy Ca intakes were more adequate. Elderly women living in Lyons, France, who received a combination supplement of Ca and vitamin D for two years had significantly lower nonvertebral fracture rates than placebo-controlled subjects.[54]

The intake of Ca alone, in amounts much greater than the RDA for the elderly, i.e., 800 mg per day, does not appear to be sufficient to overcome the established osteopenia and continuing loss of bone mass. Several investigators have made this finding in elderly women, and, because of the relative ineffectiveness of dietary or supplemental Ca by itself, other nutrient modalities, such as the combination of Ca and vitamin D or the use of bisphosphonates and other drugs, need to be considered in an effort to slow the rate of bone loss of elderly subjects, both female and male.

4. Summary

A reduction in the efficiency of either intestinal Ca absorption or renal Ca reabsorption will have an adverse effect on Ca balance. Furthermore, if osteoblast function declines with age, as suggested in some reports, but osteoclastic function declines less, then osteoclastic function will tend to be more effective, and a net turnover of bone will occur (as has been observed in numerous histomorphometric studies of bone tissue). The overall decline in bone mass tends to parallel the negative Ca balance, which has been found for postmenopausal women in numerous reports. Inadequate Ca intakes among the elderly generally are not accompanied by an adequate adaptation involving the vitamin D system. Therefore, any compromise of this already maladapting mechanism for absorbing and perhaps conserving Ca among elderly individuals results in the availability of less Ca for bone formation. The loss of bone mass is a continuing consequence of this maladaptation, in addition to osteoclastic domination of osteoblasts, and will eventually lead to fractures.

C. PHOSPHORUS

Dietary phosphorus (P) intakes by the typical elderly significantly exceed Ca intakes because the elderly continue to consume most foods from the basic food groups, but typically reduce their consumption of milk and other dairy products. Thus, the Ca:P intake ratios approach 0.5 to 1, which is lower than that of health-conscious individuals who have ratios of 0.70 to 0.75.[69,70] Whether low ratios, such as 0.5 or even lower, have adverse effects on the retention of bone mineral mass has not been established in long-term studies. If the possibility exists that nutritional secondary hyperparathyroidism becomes operative at these low ratios, as has been shown in short-term studies, then elderly subjects clearly would need to increase their Ca consumption or take supplements in order to reduce or eliminate the secondary hyperparathyroidism.[71] Portale and co-workers have shown in acute P intake studies that 1,25-dihydroxyvitamin D rises in response to a P challenge.[72]

Several investigations of the effects of P-supplemented foods, especially bread, on urinary Ca losses have been conducted over the last few decades. One study of elderly women by Bell et al. found increased serum PTH concentrations and decreased urinary losses of Ca over the 14-day period of study.[73] Another report using P supplements in young adult men for 60 days presented evidence of increases in urinary cyclic AMP, which suggests an elevated secretion of PTH, although the authors reported no adverse skeletal effects over this short period. These investigators, however, were able to block the effects of the high P additives by simultaneously giving a Ca supplement.[74] Data from Barger-Lux and Heaney support the concept of a low ratio of Ca to P contributing to elevations in PTH, higher urinary hydroxyproline, and increases in bone remodeling in healthy premenopausal women.[75] Furthermore, these researchers showed that low-Ca compared to high-Ca consumers had typically elevated parathyroid hormone concentrations without any P supplementation.

A recent overview of the P-Ca-bone triad by Calvo has added a new perspective by emphasizing the long-term pattern of deleterious Ca:P ratios (below 0.5:1.0) and the potential for significant losses of bone mass.[76] The question of how and where the excess P (primarily from the diet) and Ca (primarily from bone) are excreted and/or put in irretrievable storage in the body (skin, arterial walls) remains unanswered. Draper and Bell suggest that endogenous intestinal secretion and loss in the feces is the principal route of elimination of the excess P, but this has not been verified in human subjects.[77]

D. OTHER MICRONUTRIENTS

1. Vitamin K

A new role for vitamin K has been recently discovered and explored with regard to its role in bone development. It has been demonstrated that vitamin K is required for the synthesis of a bone extracellular protein (matrix) known as osteocalcin or bone GLA-protein and two other matrix proteins of bone tissue. (The GLA signifies glutamic acid residues, which are abundant in these vitamin K-dependent proteins.) This protein has Ca-binding groups inserted in the molecule similar to prothrombin. Thus, osteocalcin may be involved in the initial step of mineralization of the collagen matrix of bone, but not of the collagen in other connective tissues of the body. Osteocalcin is produced by osteoblasts in bone tissues, but not by fibroblasts or other cells in connective tissue other than bone. It is also possible that the synthesis of two additional matrix proteins may be dependent on the availability of vitamin K to bone cells.

Elderly subjects have been shown by different investigators to consume diets low in vitamin K and to have low blood levels of the vitamin as well. In addition, osteocalcin is reduced in its carboxylation under conditions of vitamin K deficiency. Two recent reports from the same laboratory include data on elderly persons, especially those living in nursing homes and related institutions, who have underdecarboxylated levels of osteocalcin in their circulating blood.[78,79] Furthermore, vitamin K replacement of elderly subjects has been shown to increase the efficiency of gamma carboxylation of osteocalcin as measured in circulating osteocalcin molecules.[78]

Vitamin K deficiency may also serve as a marker of deficiency of vitamin D, and, therefore, vitamin K deficiency is linked by complex mechanisms to osteoporosis and fractures. In a multicenter supplement study of elderly Japanese women with menatetranone (vitamin K), bone mass was shown to be increased after 24 or 48 weeks of therapy.[80] Thus, it appears that vitamin K nutriture remains important for bone health throughout life.

2. Trace Minerals

The function of other minerals in bone metabolism, specifically the trace elements copper, manganese, and zinc, has been examined by a number of groups using animal models. Copper, as a cofactor for lysyl oxidase, may affect bone via its role in collagen and elastin cross-linking, and manganese is required for the biosynthesis of mucopolysaccharides, which form part of the organic matrix of bone. The role of zinc is less well delineated, but as an enzyme activator it may be linked via effects on collagen and chondroitin sulfate synthesis and/or activity of osteoblasts. Two groups of investigators have shown that a combined deficiency of manganese and copper lowers bone mineral density in rats.[81,82] Rat studies using implantation of bone mineral powder indicate that bone formation is impaired by long-term deficits of manganese and copper.[81]

Documentation of similar interactions of these trace elements in humans is more indirect. Saltman and Strause have demonstrated that two-years of supplementation with three trace minerals, namely, zinc, copper, and manganese, along with additional Ca, contributes to improved bone mass of postmenopausal women compared to women given placebo alone.[83] Studies in Belgium[84] and Austin, Texas[85] found lower serum manganese levels in women with osteoporosis than in control subjects. In addition, Raheja and co-workers have reported results of oral manganese load tests that indicate the possibility of impaired absorption or status in women with osteoporosis.[86] This provocative evidence of an involvement of one or more trace elements in osteoporosis will likely stimulate further research in this new area of study.

E. SUMMARY

Ca and P remain the most critical nutrients required for bone maintenance among the elderly, but if dietary Ca is inadequate, vitamin D intake or skin production may become much more important. Several other minerals, especially the trace elements and vitamin K, also play important roles in bone function. Only long-term investigations have been able to determine the relative importance of each of these minerals for bone health. These studies have shown that Ca supplementation alone may improve the bone mass status of older women when they have low intakes, but that the combination of supplemental Ca and vitamin D may be even more beneficial in bone maintenance. Vitamin D alone may also be a useful adjunctive nutritional modality if dietary Ca intake is adequate. High P intakes, on the other hand, tend to have adverse effects on Ca metabolism, as manifested by elevated parathyroid hormone levels and a depressed Ca balance. Further prospective trials of the benefits of diverse nutrient supplements are needed to clarify the effects of individual minerals and of other nutrients that modulate Ca metabolism and thereby bone mass.

IV. AGE-RELATED RISK FACTORS FOR OSTEOPOROSIS

A decline in bone mineral density is in itself a risk factor for osteoporotic fractures, as several studies have reported. Hence it is important to consider factors that influence bone mass retention/loss. This section briefly reviews changes in bone mineral density late in life.

A. CHANGES IN BONE MINERAL DENSITY WITH AGE

In early childhood and adolescence, bone density can be optimized by a number of healthy life-style behaviors, including sufficient dietary intake of Ca and a regular program of physical activity, provided that girls who have achieved puberty continue to have normal menstrual cycles. Maximizing peak bone mass in early life has been demonstrated by several research groups in recent years to be enhanced through Ca supplementation. In an intervention study of 70 identical twins, Johnston and colleagues gave one twin a daily supplement of 1000 mg Ca and the other a placebo for two years.[87] All the children continued to increase their bone mass, but the supplemented group had a significantly greater gain. The biggest net gain in bone mineral density of the radius shaft of the supplemented group was observed for the prepubertal boys and girls, with much lower net accrual in the postpubertal children. Other investigators found essentially the same benefits of Ca supplementation on bone measurements of girls as Johnston et al. (1992), but with smaller numbers of subjects.[88,89] In retrospective investigations, Sandler et al.[90] and Tylavsky et al.[91] showed that a high consumption of milk or dairy products early in life contributed to improved bone mass in late adulthood.

Within a decade or so after peak bone mass is attained, i.e., by approximately 30 years of age, a new age-related trend emerges.[92] Bone mass begins to slowly diminish, at the rate of about 0.5% and 1.0% of peak bone mass per year for men and women, respectively.[93,94] In cortical bone, expansion of the marrow cavity begins to exceed periosteal growth, resulting in a decreased cortical thickness with advancing age. In a similar progressive trend, trabecular bone is also lost to the point that marked structural changes can occur. Menopause in women superimposes an additional acceleration of bone loss upon this age-related trend. In many cases bone mass and strength are sufficiently compromised by these changes that biomechanical competence is reduced and low energy strain (load) fractures begin to occur.

Bone loss rates among elderly women begin to decline at age 60, i.e., approximately ten years after the menopause. However, the cumulative loss of bone continues to significantly increase fracture risk. In a study of elderly Japanese Americans living in Hawaii, a combination of cross-sectional and prospective measurements of calcaneal bone suggests that the amount of bone lost from the midsixties on is relatively constant.[95] Thus the loss of a consistent amount of bone divided by a decreasing total bone mass may result in a greater percentage loss of trabecular bone by women in their seventies and later than in their sixties (see Figure 3). The loss of a constant proportion (percentage) of bone mineral results in a slower decrease in bone mass than the loss of a constant amount of bone mineral and will lead to a linear decrease in bone and a more rapid increase in fracture risk.

B. NUTRITIONAL RISK FACTORS FOR BONE MINERAL LOSS

The nutritional risk factors associated with age-related loss of bone mass among the elderly are numerous (see Table 1). The major known dietary risk factors include low vitamin D nutritional status linked to poor intakes and/or little exposure to sunlight for vitamin biosynthesis, secondary

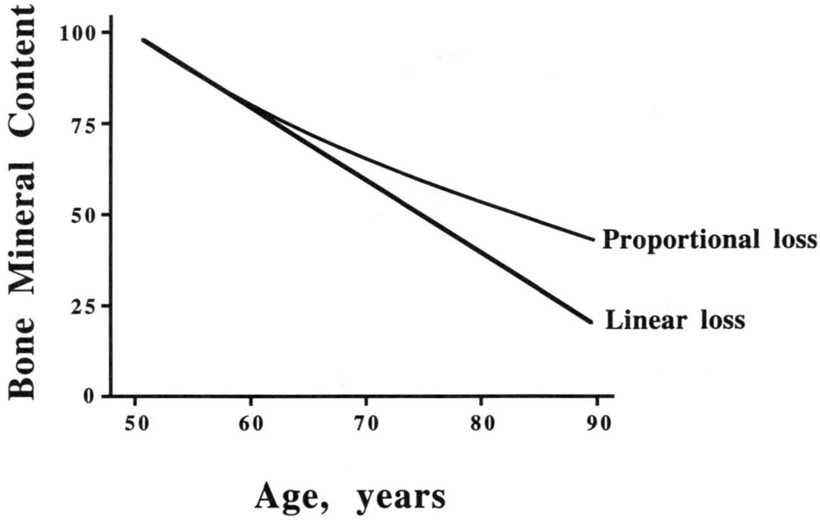

FIGURE 3. Comparison of Decrease in Bone Mineral Content when Bone Loss Is at a Proportional Rate vs. a Constant Rate. In both examples, 2% of bone mineral content (BMC) is lost in the first year. Thereafter, the line labeled "Linear" represents a continued loss of the same absolute amount of BMC. The line labeled "Proportional" illustrates the decline in bone by 2% of the remaining BMC over the course of each year.

TABLE 1
Nutritional Factors Commonly Associated with Osteoporotic Syndromes

Positive Factors	Detrimental Factors
Adequate calcium and vitamin D status	Negative calcium balance
Moderate to high physical activity	Milk intolerance/milk allergy syndrome
Adequate vitamin K and mineral intake	Petite frame/low body weight
Lacto-ovo-vegetarian diet	Lifelong high intake of:
	protein
	caffeine
	sodium
	alcohol
	phosphorus
	Anorexia nervosa
	Prolonged parenteral nutrition
	Type I diabetes mellitus

Ca deficiency, and a low consumption of Ca from foods. Changes in vitamin D status are also age-associated (see next section and Chapter 12). The role of dietary P in bone mineralization is very important, but elderly subjects, like their younger cohorts, typically obtain greater amounts of this element as phosphates relative to Ca in their foods. Proportionately higher intakes of P could potentially increase PTH concentrations and enhance bone resorption. A similar potential adverse condition may exist among the elderly who consume excessive amounts of animal proteins, especially from meats, and thereby produce hypercalciuria at the expense of bone mass (also, see Chapter 2).

Other nutrition-related changes in bone composition with age are suspected but poorly understood. General deficiencies, for example, have been found by several investigators[96-98] to be related to hip fracture among the elderly. Reduced levels of serum albumin, which reflect inadequate intakes of both protein and energy, have been linked to osteoporosis.[96-101] Furthermore, Rico et al. have shown that patients with crush vertebral fractures have lower amounts of fat free mass and body fat, as well as lower serum albumin and body mass index, than do age-matched controls.[101] Protein supplementation, either as a single nutrient or mixed with other nutrients, has been shown to improve the recovery of postfracture patients, although the specific nutrients responsible for the benefit have not been identified.[102,103] Because of well-established physical and socioeconomic risk factors for malnutrition in the elderly, particularly for the institutionalized and the very old, suggestions that sustained nutritional deficits may be related to the development of osteoporosis deserve prompt investigation.[104]

C. SUPERIMPOSED RISK OF CHRONIC ILLNESS IN THE ELDERLY

The presence of one or more chronic diseases in an elderly individual probably increases the risk for low bone mass and osteoporotic fractures. The reasons for this conjecture are based more on personal observations than published data, but Anderson et al. showed that loss of mobility among the elderly contributed to greater rates of bone loss.[30] Those disease episodes that require bedrest of the elderly appears to accelerate bone loss without any subsequent regain of the excessive loss during rehabilitation. Thus, elderly subjects who become ill and bedridden, even for short periods of a few days, will increase their risk of fracture because of the reduction of bone mass. Falls under these conditions are especially contributory events for hip fractures.

Impaired mobility is itself an important risk factor for osteoporotic fractures.[30,105] The findings of lower hip fracture rates for Asian, Hispanic, and black women compared to those for whites discharged from California hospitals suggest that genetic factors may be important in hip fracture rates, but other important factors such as better mobility due to regular physical activities cannot be ruled out.[106]

The typical modern style of living of western nations is rapidly being accepted by Asian countries and most probably contributes to low bone mass and density because it fosters inactivity and the development of many of the chronic diseases of adulthood. Thus, the limited physical activity demanded by automobile and elevator users, to name two major energy savers, limits musculoskeletal use. Modernization in Hong Kong, and potentially in other Asian countries, has been cited as the reason for the epidemic of hip fractures in recent years,[107] which is clearly associated with low bone mass in this population of Chinese women.[22]

D. SUMMARY

When partial or limited mobility occurs among the elderly of any ethnic group, it is highly probable that first, lean tissue mass, and then skeletal tissue mass will decline at increased rates. Individuals with limited mobility increase their risk for fractures, especially of the hip. Co-morbidity of other diseases, such as stroke, dementia, and heart disease, also increases the likelihood of fracture.

V. DIETARY RECOMMENDATIONS FOR ELDERLY PATIENTS WITH OSTEOPOROSIS

Osteoporosis cannot be reversed by any known drug therapy, exercise regimen, or nutritional intervention. Appropriate medical and nutritional interventions, however, have the potential to slow its progress and improve the functional quality of life in osteoporosis patients. Whereas dietary prescriptions for the management of osteoporosis will vary with the extent of bone loss, medical history, and individual needs of the patient, certain general nutritional recommendations are a part of standard care in thorough osteoporosis treatment programs.[108] This final section briefly summarizes these recommendations (see Table 2).

A. DIETARY RECOMMENDATIONS

Prescriptions for the management of osteoporosis rely heavily upon dietary modifications, including a high-Ca diet, and a reduction of behaviors likely to jeopardize Ca balance or physical

TABLE 2
Nutritional Recommendations for the Elderly

Nutrient	RDA	Special Advice for the Elderly
Protein	50, 63 g[1]	Assure adequate, but not excessive, intake.
Calcium	800 mg	Emphasize food sources or highly soluble supplemental forms.
Vitamin D	5 mg (200 IU)	Recommend 10 to 15 minutes in sun, 2–3 times/wk, alternative is 200 IU daily as supplement unless contraindicated. Supplements (400–800 IU) may be needed by institutionalized and "shut-in" individuals.
Sodium	500 mg	Avoid processed and cured foods whenever possible and limit added salt.
Dietary Fiber	—	20–30 g dietary fiber per day. Avoid taking calcium supplements with high fiber foods such as bran cereals.
Other Dietary Factors	—	Limit alcohol and caffeine-containing foods. Assure adequate vitamin K and trace element status.

[1] Females, males.

TABLE 3
Prudent Sources of Calcium

Food	Amount	Fat (g)	Ca (mg)	Energy (kcal)	Ratio of Ca/kcal
Skim milk	8 oz	Tr	302	85	3.6
Yogurt, plain	8 oz	4	415	145	2.9
Yogurt, fruit	8 oz	2	345	230	1.5
Broccoli, cooked	1 cup	Tr	177	45	3.9
Almonds	1 oz	15	75	165	0.4
Tofu, firm	4 oz	6	258	183	1.4
Salmon canned, with bones	3 oz	5	167	120	1.4

Tr = Trace amount

stamina. As mentioned earlier, Ca intakes of 800 to 1000 mg for premenopausal women and 1200–1500 for postmenopausal women (in the absence of estrogen replacement) have been recommended.

This amount of Ca may be difficult to obtain from most typical diets of older women, because Ca is present in substantial quantities in only a few foods (mainly dairy foods). It takes approximately four 8-ounce glasses (cups) of milk or 3 cups of yogurt to provide 1200 milligrams of Ca. Although some practical concerns about the fat content of a high-Ca diet may be expressed by patients, this need not be a limiting factor. As shown in Table 3, high-Ca foods, such as skim milk and yogurt, tofu, and canned salmon with bones are excellent choices for individuals following a fat-restricted diet.

The more likely limiting factor is the amount of food (and hence calories) that may be substantially restricted by individuals following weight-reduction diets. In other cases, poor appetite, food allergies, lactose intolerance, or other dietary restrictions may limit the consumption of adequate amounts of dietary Ca. In such situations, a Ca supplement may be strongly recommended. (More will be presented about this in the next section.) Other dietary recommendations in the treatment of osteoporosis include instructions to moderate the intake of diet constituents that may threaten the Ca balance when used to excess, such as alcohol, protein, sodium, caffeine, and dietary fiber.

B. RECOMMENDATIONS FOR NUTRITIONAL SUPPLEMENTS

Ca supplements are available in a variety of forms and dosages (see Chapter 2). There are slight differences in solubility, and thus absorption, of Ca compounds. Ca salts of phosphate and carbonate may, in some cases, be poorly absorbed on an empty stomach. Ca citrate has been shown to be much more absorbable than Ca carbonate when patients with achlorhydria take it without food.[109] However, the chemical form of Ca generally makes much less difference than the physical form of the salt and the tablet preparation. Fortunately, many of the problems with the solubility of Ca supplements have been remedied since this difficulty was first recognized.[110] It should be noted that Ca supplementation cannot fully compensate for bone mass loss, but the concomitant administration of Ca supplements may augment estrogen therapy, thereby reducing the necessary effective dose of the hormone.[111] However, independent verification of the Ca/estrogen trade-off is needed.

Vitamin D supplements in the range of 400 to 1000 IU per day are now being recommended by osteoporosis experts for use by elderly shut-ins and institutionalized individuals for the purpose of preventing hip and other fractures. Dosages in this range are considered safe. The rationale for this recommendation is based on studies by Chapuy et al.,[54] Heikiheimo et al.,[112] and other investigators who have demonstrated that such supplementation (along with Ca if subjects are low Ca consumers) helps to reduce the rates of hip fracture in elderly populations. Although no official body has yet made this recommendation for vitamin D supplementation when dietary intakes and sun exposures are not adequate, it has been made by researchers at recent scientific meetings.

VI. CONCLUDING REMARKS

As women proceed through the first decade following the menopause, they are already undergoing a negative Ca balance because of bone loss resulting from the cessation of ovarian estrogen production and secretion. Furthermore, parathyroid hormone may be more effective during this period while serum concentrations of estrogen are very low. During this decade, the efficiency of intestinal Ca absorption also declines, whereas renal Ca losses remain elevated. When the parathyroid hormone concentration increases, typically in the second postmenopausal decade, urinary Ca losses may continue to remain elevated because of a so-called renal leak.[67] The continuing loss of bone mass and density in the second postmenopausal decade occurs at a lower rate, but the resultant values put many women at increased risk for proximal femoral (hip) and other nonvertebral fractures.

Ca supplementation, or improvements in dietary Ca intake, during the first postmenopausal decade have little or no effect in slowing the loss of bone mass or in correcting the negative Ca balance. Physical exercise or upper body strength activities also have little effect in counterbalancing the losses of mineral (Ca) from the skeleton at this time. Only certain therapeutic drugs, such as conjugated estrogens (natural) and synthetic estrogens have been found to be effective in maintaining bone mass and Ca balance during this first decade after the menopause. In the subsequent postmenopausal decades, however, combinations of Ca and vitamin D supplements have been demonstrated to be quite effective in retaining bone mass and reducing fractures. Other micronutrients, such as vitamin K and several trace elements, have been shown in a few small investigations of elderly subjects to be beneficial to bone mass. Further experiments are needed to establish the efficacy of these other nutrients in maintaining bone and in preventing fractures. Other types of studies of elderly patients and institutionalized residents have provided evidence that elderly women and also men need to have adequate intakes of all nutrients, including energy and protein, as well as the more bone-specific nutrients detailed herein, in order to remain "bone" healthy and to avoid fractures.

Recommendations for specific nutrient intakes by the elderly are offered in comparison to the current RDAs.[113] These recommendations are based on the published reports reviewed in this manuscript. For several nutrients, intakes at the levels recommended by us from foods alone will be practically impossible, unless food fortification is drastically increased in the near future. Therefore, dietary supplements will almost certainly be needed by healthy elderly subjects if they are to meet their nutrient requirements according to the recommendations offered.

Further research using double-blinded, placebo-controlled, randomized designs will be necessary in order to establish more accurately the specific nutrient allowances of the "healthy" elderly. Our guidelines must be considered provisional at this time.

REFERENCES

1. **Kleerekoper, M. and Avioli, L. V.,** Evaluation and treatment of postmenopausal osteoporosis, in *Primer on the Metabolic Bone Diseases and Disorders of Mineral Metabolism*, Favus, M. J., ed., Second ed., Raven Press, New York, 1993, 223.
2. **Riggs, B. L. and Melton, L. J.,** Heterogeneity of involutional osteoporosis: evidence for two distinct osteoporotic syndromes, *Am. J. Med.*, 75, 899, 1983.
3. **Keene, G. S., Paker, M. J., and Pryor, G. A.,** Mortality and morbidity after hip fractures, *Br. Med. J.*, 307, 1248, 1993.
4. **Spencer, G.,** Projections of the population of the United States by age, sex, and race: 1988 to 2080, in *U.S. Bureau of the Census, Current Population Reports, Series P-25, No. 1018*, Spencer, G., ed., U.S. Government Printing Office, Washington, D.C., 1989,
5. **Schneider, E. L. and Guralnik, J. M.,** The aging of America: impact on health care costs, *J. Am. Med. Assoc.*, 263, 2335, 1990.
6. **Hassager, C. and Christiansen, C.,** Influence of soft tissue body composition on bone mass and metabolism, *Bone*, 10, 415, 1989.
7. **Bevier, W. C., Wiswell, R. A., Pyka, G., Kozak, K. C., Newhall, K. M., and Marcus, R.,** Relationship of body composition, muscle strength, and aerobic capacity to bone mineral density in older men and women, *J. Bone Miner. Res.*, 4, 421, 1989.
8. **Halioua, L. and Anderson, J. J. B.,** Age and anthropometric determinants of radial bone mass in premenopausal caucasian women: a cross-sectional study, *Osteoporosis Int.*, 1, 50, 1990.
9. **Slemenda, C. W., Hui, S. L., Williams, C. J., Christian, J. C., Meaney, F., and Johnston, C. C., Jr.,** Bone mass and anthropometric measurements in adult females, *Bone Miner.*, 11, 101, 1990.
10. **Reid, I. R., Ames, R., and Evans, M. C.,** Dietary calcium supplementation slows the decline in total body bone mineral density in post-menopausal women, *Bone Miner.*, 17 (supp 1), 73, 1992.
11. **Pruzansky, A., Turano, M., Luckey, M., and Senie, R.,** Low body weight as a risk factor for hip fracture in both black and white women, *J. Orthop. Res.*, 7, 192, 1990.
12. **Dawson-Hughes, B.,** Dietary calcium intake and bone loss from the spine in healthy postmenopausal women, *Am. J. Clin. Nutr.*, 46, 685, 1987.
13. **Ribot, C., Tremollieres, F., Pouilles, J.-M., Bonneau, M., Germain, F., and Louvet, J.-P.,** Obesity and postmenopausal bone loss: the influence of obesity on vertebral density and bone turnover in postmenopausal women, *Bone*, 8, 327, 1988.
14. **Pocock, N. A., Eisman, J. A., Gwinn, T., Sambrook, P. N., Kelly, P. J., Freund, J., and Yeates, M. G.,** Muscle strength, physical fitness, and weight but not age predict femoral neck bone mass, *J. Bone Miner. Res.*, 4, 441, 1989.
15. **Felson, D. T., Zhang, Y., Hannan, M. T., and Anderson, J. J.,** Effects of weight and body mass index on bone mineral density in men and women: the Framingham Study, *J. Bone Miner. Res.*, 8, 567, 1993.
16. **Forbes, G. B.,** Body composition of adolescent girls, *Nutr. Today*, 26, 17, 1991.
17. **Tsunenari, T., Tsutsumi, M., Ohno, K., Yamamoto, Y., Kawakatsu, M., Shimogaki, K., Negishi, H., Sugimoto, T., Fukase, M., and Fujita, T.,** Age- and gender-related changes in body composition in Japanese subjects, *J. Bone Miner. Res.*, 8, 397, 1993.
18. **Vittek, J., Altman, K., Gordon, G. G., and Southren, A. L.,** The metabolism of 7a-3H-testosterone by rat mandibular bone, *Endocrinology*, 94, 325, 1974.
19. **Grodin, J. M., Siiteri, P. K., and MacDonald, P. C.,** Source of estrogen production in postmenopausal women, *J. Clin. Endocrinol. Metab.*, 36, 207, 1973.
20. **Hemsell, D. L., Grodin, J. M., Breuner, P. F., Siiteri, P. K., and MacDonald, P. C.,** Plasma precursors of estrogen. II. Correlation of the extent of conversion of plasma androstenedione to estrone with age, *J. Clin. Endocrinol. Metab.*, 38, 476, 1974.
21. **Siiteri, P. K.,** Adipose tissue as a source of hormones, *Am. J. Clin. Nutr.*, 45, 277, 1987.
22. **Lau, E. M. C., Woo, J., Leung, P. C., and Swaminathan, R.,** Low bone mineral density, grip strength and skinfold thickness are important risk factors for hip fracture in Hong Kong Chinese, *Osteoporosis Int.*, 3, 66, 1993.
23. **Cummings, S. R. and Nevitt, M. C.,** A hypothesis: the causes of hip fractures, *J. Gerontol.*, 44, M107, 1989.
24. **Ortiz, O., Russell, M., Daley, T. L., Baumgartner, R. N., Waki, M., Lichtman, S., Wang, J., Pierson, R. N., Jr., and Heymsfield, S. B.,** Differences in skeletal muscle and bone mineral mass between black and white females and their relevance to estimates of body composition, *Am. J. Clin. Nutr.*, 55, 8, 1992.
25. **Farmer, M. E., Harris, T., Madans, J. H., Wallace, R. B., Cornoni-Huntley, J. R., and White, L. R.,** Anthropometric indicators and hip fractures: The NHANES I Epidemiological Follow-up Study, *J. Am. Geriatr. Soc.*, 37, 9, 1989.
26. **Farmer, M. E., White, L. R., and Brody, J. A.,** Race and sex differences in hip fracture incidence, *Am. J. Public Health*, 74, 1374, 1984.
27. **Lacey, J. M., Anderson, J. J. B., Fujita, T., Fukase, M., Tsuchie, S., and Koch, G. G.,** Correlates of cortical bone mass among premenopausal and postmenopausal Japanese women, *J. Bone Miner. Res.*, 6, 651, 1991.

28. **Ross, P. D., Orimo, H., Wasnich, R. D., Vogel, J. M., MacLean, C. J., Davis, J. W., and Nomura, A.,** Methodological issues in comparing genetic and environmental influences on bone mass, *Bone Miner.*, 7, 1989.
29. **Dalsky, G., Stocke, K. S., Eshani, A. A., Slatopolsky, E., Lee, W. C., and Birge, S. J.,** Weight-bearing exercise training and lumbar bone mineral content in post menopausal women, *Ann. Intern. Med.*, 108, 824, 1988.
30. **Anderson, J. J. B., Reed, J. A., Tylavsky, F. A., Laster, G. E., Talmage, R. V., and Taft, T. N.,** Lack of an effect of dietary calcium in preventing the loss of radial bone mass in high-calcium consuming elderly white women, in *Osteoporosis 1990*, Christiansen, C. and Overgaard, K., eds., Osteopress, ApS, Copenhagen, Denmark, 1990, 981.
31. **Reed, J. A., Anderson, J. J. B., Tylavsky, F. A., and Gallagher, P. N., Jr.,** Comparative changes in radial-bone density of elderly female lactoovovegetarians and omnivores, *Am. J. Clin. Nutr.*, 59 (suppl), 1197, 1994.
32. **Smith, D. M., Khairi, M. R. A., and Johnston, C. C., Jr.,** The loss of bone mineral with aging and its relationship to risk of fracture, *J. Clin. Invest.*, 56, 311, 1975.
33. **Lau, E., Donnan, S., Barker, D. B. P., and Cooper, C.,** Physical activity and calcium intake in fracture of the proximal femur in Hong Kong, *Br. Med. J.*, 297, 1443, 1988.
34. **Suter, P. M. and Russell, R.,** Vitamin requirements in the elderly, *Am. J. Clin. Nutr.*, 45, 501, 1987.
35. **MacLaughlin, J. and Holick, M. F.,** Aging decreases capacity of human skin to produce vitamin D_3, *J. Clin. Invest.*, 76, 1536, 1985.
36. **Fujita, T.,** Vitamin D in the treatment of osteoporosis, *Proc. Soc. Exper. Biol. Med.*, 199, 394, 1992.
37. **Rushton, C.,** Vitamin D hydroxylation in youth and old age, *Age Ageing*, 7, 91, 1978.
38. **Bales, C. W., Almond, J. R., Klotman, P. E., and Drezner, M. K.,** Altered renal 25-hyroxyvitamin D-1-a-hydroxylase activity: adaptation to uni-nephrectomy, *J. Bone Miner. Res.*, 2, 445, 1987.
39. **Tsai, K. S., Heath, H., III, Kumar, R., and Riggs, B. L.,** Impaired vitamin D metabolism with aging in women. Possible role in pathogenesis of senile osteoporosis, *J. Clin. Invest.*, 73, 1668, 1984.
40. **Eastell, R., Delmas, P. D., Hodgson, S. F., Eriksen, E. F., Mann, K. G., and Riggs, B. L.,** Bone formation rate in older normal women: concurrent assessment with bone histomorphometry, calcium kinetics, and biochemical markers, *J. Clin. Endocrinol. Metab.*, 67, 741, 1988.
41. **Dandona, P., Menon, R. K., Shenoy, R., Houlder, S., Thomas, M., and Mallinson, W. J. W.,** Low 1,25-dihydroxyvitamin D, secondary hyperparathyroidism, and normal osteocalcin in elderly subjects, *J. Clin. Endocrinol. Metab.*, 63, 459, 1986.
42. **Goldray, D., Miizahi-Sasson, E., Merdler, C., Edelstein-Singer, M., Algoetti, A., Eisenberg, Z., Jaccard, N., and Weisman, Y.,** Vitamin D deficiency in elderly patients in a general hospital, *J. Am. Geriatric Assoc.*, 37, 589, 1989.
43. **Gallagher, J. C., Riggs, B. L., Eisman, J., Hamstra, A., Arnaud, S. B., and DeLuca, H. E.,** Intestinal absorption and vitamin D metabolites in normal subjects and osteoporotic patients: effect of age and dietary calcium, *J. Clin. Invest.*, 64, 729, 1979.
44. **Slovik, D. M., Adams, J. S., Neer, R. M., Holick, M. F., and Potts, J. T.,** Deficient production of 1,25-dihydroxyvitamin D in elderly osteoporotic patients, *New Engl. J. Med.*, 305, 372, 1981.
45. **Aaron, J. E., Gallagher, J. C., Anderson, J., Stasiak, L., Longton, E. B., Nordin, B. E., and Nicholson, M.,** Frequency of osteomalacia and osteoporosis in fractures of the proximal femur, *Lancet*, 1, 229, 1974.
46. **Doppelt, S. H., Neer, R., Daley, M., Bourret, L., Schiller, A., Holick, M., and Mankin, H. J.,** Osteomalacia and vitamin D deficiency in patients with hip fractures — an unrecognized epidemic, *Orthop. Trans.*, 7, 512, 1983.
47. **Baker, M. R., McDonnell, H., Peacock, M., and Nordin, B. E.,** Plasma 25-hydroxyvitamin D concentrations in patients with fractures of the femoral neck, *Br. Med. J.*, 1, 589, 1979.
48. **Lips, P., Netelenbos, J. C., Jongen, M. J. M., Van Ginkel, F. C., Althuis, A. L., Van Schaik, C. L., Van der Vijgh, W. J. F., Vermeiden, J. P. W., and Van der Meer, C.,** Histomorphometric profile and vitamin D status in patients with femoral neck fracture, *Metab. Bone Dis. Relat. Res.*, 4, 85, 1982.
49. **Tilyard, M. W., Spears, G. F. S., Thomsen, J., and Dovey, S.,** Treatment of postmenopausal osteoporosis with calcitriol or calcium, *New Engl. J. Med.*, 326, 357, 1992.
50. **Lips, P., Wiersinga, A., van Ginkel, F. C., Jongen, M. J. M., Netelenbos, J. C., Hackeng, W. H. L., Delmas, P. D., and van der Vijgh, W. J. F.,** The effect of vitamin D supplementation on vitamin D status and parathyroid function in elderly subjects, *J. Clin. Endocrinol. Metab.*, 67, 644, 1988.
51. **Gallagher, J. C. Goldgar, D.,** Treatment of postmenopausal osteoporosis with high doses of synthetic calcitrol. A randomized controlled study, *Ann. Intern. Med.*, 113, 649, 1990.
52. **Aloia, J. F., Cohn, S. H., and Vaswani, A.,** Risk factors for postmenopausal osteoporosis, *Am. J. Med.*, 78, 95, 1985.
53. **Ott, S. and Chesnut, C., III,** Calcitrol treatment is not effective in postmenopausal osteoporosis, *Ann. Intern. Med.*, 110, 267, 1989.
54. **Chapuy, M. C., Arlot, M. E., Duboeuf, F., Brun, J., Crouzet, B., Arnaud, S., Delmas, P. D., and Meunier, P. J.,** Vitamin D_3 and calcium to prevent hip fractures in elderly women, *New Engl. J. Med.*, 327, 1637, 1992.
55. **Ramazzotto, L. T., Curro, F. A., Gates, P. E., and Paterson, J. A.,** Calcium nutrition and the aging process: a review, *Gerontology*, 5, 159, 1986.
56. Consensus Conference on Osteoporosis, *J. Am. Med. Assoc.*, 252, 799, 1984.
57. Consensus Development Conference, Prophylaxis and treatment of osteoporosis, *Br. Med. J.*, 295, 914, 1987.

58. **Mosekilde, L.,** Minisymposium — osteoporosis and calcium, *J. Intern. Med.*, 231, 145, 1992.
59. **Recker, R. R.,** Calcium absorption and achlorhydria, *New Engl. J. Med.*, 313, 70, 1985.
60. **Avioli, L. V., McDonald, J. E., and Lee, S. W.,** The influence of age on intestinal absorption of ^{47}Ca in women and its relation to ^{47}Ca absorption in postmenopausal osteoporosis, *J. Clin. Invest.*, 44, 1960, 1965.
61. **Bullamore, J. R., Wilkinson, R., Gallagher, J. C., Nordin, B. E. C., and Marshall, D. H.,** Effect of age on calcium absorption, *Lancet*, 2, 535, 1970.
62. **Ireland, P. and Fordtran, J. S.,** Effect of dietary calcium and age on jejunal calcium absorption in humans studied by intestinal perfusion, *J. Clin. Invest.*, 52, 2672, 1973.
63. **Eastell, R., Yeargey, A., Veiera, N., Cedel, S., Kumar, R., and Riggs, B.,** Interrelationship among vitamin D metabolism, true calcium absorption, parathyroid function, and age in women: evidence of an age-related intestinal resistance to 1,25-dihydroxyvitamin D action, *J. Bone Miner. Res.*, 6, 125, 1991.
64. **Gallagher, J. C., Riggs, B. L., Jerpbak, C. M., and Arnaud, C. D.,** The effect of age on serum immunoreaction parathyroid hormone in normal and osteoporotic women, *J. Lab. Clin. Med.*, 95, 373, 1980.
65. **Marcus, R., Madvig, P., and Young, G.,** Age-related changes in parathyroid hormone action in normal humans, *J. Clin. Endocrinol. Metab.*, 58, 223, 1984.
66. **Orwoll, E. S. and Mier, D. E.,** Alterations in calcium, vitamin D, and parathyroid hormone physiology in normal men with aging: relationship to the development of senile osteoporosis, *J. Clin. Endocrinol. Metab.*, 63, 1262, 1986.
67. **Nordin, B. E. C. and Morris, H. A.,** The calcium deficiency model for osteoporosis, *Nutr. Rev.*, 47, 65, 1989.
68. **Dawson-Hughes, B., Dallal, G. E., Krall, E. A., Sadowski, L., Sahyoun, N., and Tannenbaum, S.,** A controlled trial of the effect of calcium supplementation on bone density in postmenopausal women, *New Engl. J. Med.*, 323, 878, 1990.
69. **Tylavsky, F. A. and Anderson, J. J. B.,** Bone health of elderly lactoovovegetarian and omniverous women, *Am. J. Clin. Nutr.*, 48, 842, 1989.
70. **Hunt, I. F., Murphy, N. J., Henderson, C., Clark, V. A., Jacobs, R. M., Johnston, P. K., and Coulston, A. H.,** Bone mineral content in postmenopausal women: comparison of omnivores and vegeterians, *Am. J. Clin. Nutr.*, 50, 517, 1989.
71. **Calvo, M. S., Kumar, R., and Heath, H.,** Persistently elevated parathyroid hormone secretion and action in young women after four weeks of ingesting high phosphorus, low calcium diets, *J. Clin. Endocrinol. Metab.*, 70, 1334, 1990.
72. **Portale, A. A., Halloran, B. P., Murphy, M. M., and Morris, R. C., Jr.,** Oral intake of phosphorus can determine the serum concentration of 1,25-dihydroxyvitamin D by determining its production rates in humans, *J. Clin. Invest.*, 77, 7, 1986.
73. **Bell, R. R., Draper, H. H., Tzeng, D. Y. M., Shin, H. K., and Schmidt, G. R.,** Physiological responses of human adults to foods containing phosphate additives, *J. Nutr.*, 107, 42, 1977.
74. **Zemel, M. B. and Linkswiller, H. M.,** Calcium metabolism in the young adult as affected by level and form of phosphorus intake and level of calcium intake, *J. Nutr.*, 111, 315, 1981.
75. **Barger-Lux, M. J. and Heaney, R. P.,** Effects of calcium restriction on metabolic characteristics of premenopausal women, *J. Clin. Endocrinol. Metab.*, 76, 103, 1993.
76. **Calvo, M. S.,** Dietary phosphorus, calcium metabolism and bone, *J. Nutr.*, 123, 1627, 1993.
77. **Draper, H. H. and Bell, R.,** Nutrition and osteoporosis, in *Advances in Nutrition Research, Vol. 2*, Draper, H. H., ed., Plenum Press, New York, 1979, 79.
78. **Plantalech, L., Guillaumont, M., Leclercq, M., and Delmas, P. D.,** Impaired carboxylation of serum osteocalcin in elderly women, *J. Bone Miner. Res.*, 6, 1211, 1991.
79. **Szulc, P., Chapuy, M. C., Meunier, P. J., and Delmas, P. D.,** Serum undercarboxylated osteocalcin is a marker of the risk of hip fracture in elderly women, *J. Clin. Invest.*, 91, 1769, 1993.
80. **Orimo, H., Shiraki, M., Fujita, T., and Kushida, K.,** Clinical evaluation of menatetrenone in the treatment of involutional osteoporosis, *J. Bone Miner. Res.*, 7 (supp.1), S122, 1992.
81. **Strause, L. G. and Saltman, P. D.,** The role of manganese in bone metabolism, in *ACS Monograph Series*, Kies, C., ed., American Chemical Society, Washington, D.C., 1987, 45.
82. **Andon, M., Luhrsen, K., Kanerva, R., and Chatzidakis, C.,** Effects of dietary copper and manganese restriciton on serum mineral concentrations and femoral shaft bone density in rats, *J. Am. Coll. Nutr.*, 11, 600, 1992.
83. **Saltman, P. D. and Strause, L. G.,** The role of trace minerals in osteoporosis, *J. Am. Coll. Nutr.*, 12, 384, 1993.
84. **Reginster, J. Y., Strause, L. G., Saltman, P., and Franchimont, P.,** Trace elements and postmenopausal osteoporosis: a preliminary study of decreased serum manganese, *Med. Sci. Res.*, 16, 337, 1988.
85. **Freeland-Graves, J. H. and Llanes, C.,** Models to study manganese deficiency, in *Manganese in Health and Disease*, Klimis, D. J., ed., CRC Press, Boca Raton, FL, 1994, 59.
86. **Raheja, R., Freeland-Graves, J., and Tesar, R.,** Indicators of manganese nutriture in osteoporotic, young and elderly women, *FASEB J.*, 8, 2485, 1994.
87. **Johnston, C. C., Jr., Miller, J. Z., Slemenda, C. W., Reister, T. K., Christian, J. C., and Peacock, M.,** Calcium supplementation and increases in bone mineral density in children, *New Engl. J. Med.*, 327, 82, 1992.
88. **Matkovic, V., Fontana, D., Tomineac, C., Goel, P., and Chesnut, C. H., III,** Factors that influence peak bone mass formation: a study of calcium balance and the inheritance of bone mass in adolescent females, *Am. J. Clin. Nutr.*, 52, 878, 1990.

89. **Sentipal, J. M., Wardlaw, G. M., Mahan, J., and Matkovic, V.,** Influence of calcium intake and growth indexes on vertebral bone mineral density in young females, *Am. J. Clin. Nutr.*, 54, 425, 1991.
90. **Sandler, R. B., Slemenda, C. W., LaPorte, R. E., Cauley, J. A., Schramm, M. M., Barresi, M. L., and Kriska, A. M.,** Postmenopausal bone density and milk consumption in childhood and adolescence, *Am. J. Clin. Nutr.*, 42, 270, 1985.
91. **Tylavsky, F. A., Anderson, J. J. B., Talmage, R. V., and Taft, T.,** Are calcium intakes and physical activity patterns during adolescence related to radial bone mass of white college-age females?, *Osteoporosis Int.*, 2, 232, 1992.
92. **Halioua, L. and Anderson, J. J. B.,** Lifetime calcium intake and physical activity habits: independent and combined effects on the radial bone of healthy premenopausal Caucasian women, *Am. J. Clin. Nutr.*, 49, 534, 1989.
93. **Riggs, B. L., Wahner, H. W., Melton, L. J., Jr., Richelson, L. S., Judd, A. J., and O'Fallon, W. M.,** Dietary calcium intake and rates of bone loss in women, *J. Clin. Invest.*, 80, 979, 1987.
94. **Sowers, M. R., Clark, M. K., Hollis, B., Wallace, R. B., and Jannowski, M.,** Radial bone mineral density in pre- and perimenopausal women: a prospective study of rates and risk factors for loss, *J. Bone Miner. Res.*, 7, 647, 1992.
95. **Davis, J. W., Ross, P. D., Wasnick, R. D., MacLean, C. J., and Vogel, J. M.,** Comparison of cross-sectional and longitudinal measurements of age-related changes in bone mineral content, *J. Bone Miner. Res.*, 4, 351, 1989.
96. **Burr, M. L., Milbank, J. E., and Gibbs, D.,** The nutritional status of the elderly, *Age Ageing*, 11, 89, 1982.
97. **Older, M. W. J., Edwards, D., and Dickerson, J. W. T.,** A nutrient survey in elderly women with femoral neck fractures, *Br. J. Surg.*, 67, 884, 1980.
98. **Delmi, M., Rapin, C.-H., Bengoa, J.-M., Delmas, P. D., Vasey, H., and Bonjour, J.-P.,** Dietary supplementation in elderly patients with fractured neck of the femur, *Lancet*, 335, 1013, 1990.
99. **Orwoll, E., Weigel, R. M., Oviatt, S. K., Meier, D. E., and McClung, M. R.,** Serum protein concentrations and bone mineral content in aging normal men, *Am. J. Clin. Nutr.*, 46, 614, 1987.
100. **Rudman, D., Rudman, I. W., Mattson, D. E., Nagraj, H. S., Caindec, N., and Jackson, D. L.,** Fractures in the men of a Veteran's Administration Nursing Home: relation to 1,25-dihydroxyvitamin D, *J. Am. Coll. Nutr.*, 8, 324, 1989.
101. **Rico, H., Revilla, M., Villa, L. F., Hernandez, E. R., and Fernandez, J. P.,** Crush fracture syndrome in senile osteoporosis: a nutritional consequence?, *J. Bone Miner. Res.*, 7, 317, 1992.
102. **Bonjour, J. P., Rapin, C.-H., Rizzoli, R., Tkatch, L., Delmi, M., Chevalley, T., Nydegger, V., Slosman, D., and Vasey, H.,** Hip fracture, femoral bone mineral density, and protein supply in elderly patients, in *Nutrition of the Elderly, Nestle Nutrition Workshop Series, Vol. 29*, Munro, H. and Schlierf, G., eds., Raven Press, NY, 1992, 152.
103. **Tkatch, L., Rapin, C.-H., Rizzoli, R., Slosman, D., Nydegger, V., Vasey, H., and Bonjour, J.-P.,** Benefits of oral protein supplementation in elderly patients with fracture of the proximal femur, *J. Am. Coll. Nutr.*, 11, 519, 1992.
104. **Santora, A. C., II,** Role of nutrition and exercise in osteoporosis, *Am. J. Med.*, 82, 73, 1987.
105. **Ooms, M. E., Lips, L., Van Lingen, A., and Valkenburg, H. A.,** Determinants of bone mineral density and risk factors for osteoporosis in healthy elderly women, *J. Bone Miner. Res.*, 8, 669, 1993.
106. **Silverman, S. L. and Madison, R. E.,** Decreased incidence of hip fracture in Hispanics, Asians, and blacks: California hospital discharge data, *Am. J. Public Health*, 78, 1482, 1988.
107. **Lau, E. M. C., Cooper, C., Wickham, C., Donnan, S., and Barker, D. J.,** Hip fracture in Hong Kong and Britain, *Int. J. Epidemiol.*, 19, 1119, 1990.
108. **Bales, C. W.,** Nutritional aspects of osteoporosis: recommendations for the elderly at risk, in *Annual Review of Gerontology and Geriatrics, Vol. 9*, Lawton, P., ed., Springer Publishing, New York, NY, 1989, 7.
109. **Harvey, J. A., Kenny, P., Poindexter, J., and Pak, C. Y. C.,** Superior calcium absorption from calcium citrate than calcium carbonate using external forearm counting, *J. Am. Coll. Nutr.*, 9, 583, 1990.
110. **Carr, C. J. and Shangraw, R. F.,** Nutritional and pharmaceutical aspects of calcium supplementation, *Amer. Pharm.*, NS27, 49, 1987.
111. **Ettinger, B., Genant, H. K., and Cann, C. E.,** Postmenopausal bone loss is prevented by treatment with low-dosage estrogen with calcium, *Ann. Int. Med.*, 106, 40, 1987.
112. **Heikinheimo, R. J., Inkovarra, J. A., Harju, E. J., Haavisto, M. V., Kaarela, R. H., Kataja, J. M., Kokko, A. M.-L., Kolho, L. A., and Rajala, S. A.,** Annual injection of vitamin D and fractures of aged bones, *Calcif. Tissue Int.*, 51, 105, 1992.
113. National Research Council, National Academy of Sciences, *Recommended Dietary Allowances,* 10th Ed., National Academy Press, Washington, D.C., 1989.

Section V.

OSTEOPOROSIS

This section on osteoporosis underscores the breakdown of normal homeostatic mechanisms that operate to conserve calcium (Ca) and preserve bone. Among the old (60 and over) osteoporosis has become a dominating disorder, which becomes even more severe with increasing longevity. Chapter 21 defines the disorder in terms of two types and provides information on its differential diagnosis. Information is also provided on the prevention and treatment of osteoporosis. Chapter 22 reviews the epidemiology of osteoporosis, including information on several prospective studies, some ongoing, in various parts of the world.

Osteoporosis illustrates one end-result, and economically a massive drain, of the failure of the bone structure under minimal loads (strains) that result in fractures.

Chapter 21

OSTEOPOROSIS TYPES I AND II

Marc K. Drezner, M.D.

TABLE OF CONTENTS

I. INTRODUCTION

The osteoporoses are a heterogeneous group of disorders characterized by a decrease in mineralized tissue per unit volume of bone to a level that increases the risk of fracture. This disease state may be a primary condition that occurs in the aging population where a defined predisposition is not apparent, or a secondary disorder that occurs as a complication of a large number of naturally occurring or iatrogenic diseases in which bone loss generally occurs. The primary disease includes both postmenopausal osteoporosis (Type I) and osteoporosis of aging (Type II).

Type I, or postmenopausal osteoporosis, usually occurs in women 10 to 15 years after the menopause.[1] The incidence in women is at least 8 times higher than that in men. Most commonly, patients present with fracture of trabecular-rich bones such as the vertebrae or distal forearm. As

0-8493-7845-1/95/$0.00+$.50

related later, current hypotheses indicate that factors closely associated with the meopause, such as estrogen deficiency, cause this disorder.

Type II or senile osteoporosis occurs in both women and men over age 70 years with a female/male ratio of incidence 2:1 to 3:1.[1] Affected patients usually present with fractures of the hip or vertebrae, but fractures of the pelvis, proximal humerus, or tibia also occur. The bone loss in this disorder is likely a function of the aging process and is due to such factors as increased levels of bioactive parathyroid hormone and diminished osteoblast function. However, the hip fractures of this disease are not solely the result of diminished bone density because patients over age 80 years with and without fracture exhibit similar bone densities. Rather, falls and other trauma likely play a major role in the expression of the disease.

Occurrence of primary osteoporosis is a major public health problem in Western countries, particularly among elderly white women. Indeed, approximately 20 million people are currently affected in the aging population of the United States, and at least 1.5 million osteoporotic fractures occur each year, most frequently affecting vertebrae, hip, distal forearm, pelvis, or ribs. Indeed, by age 90 one of every three women and one of every six men will suffer a hip fracture, a catastrophic complication associated with death in 12–20% of affected subjects within the first year, and long-term nursing care in 1/2 of those who survive. The economic impact of osteoporosis and these attendant complications is estimated at $8–10 billion per year in the United States alone.

II. PATHOPHYSIOLOGY

Skeletal growth begins in utero and continues for about two decades (see Chapter 17). It is regulated by central endocrine and peripheral biophysical and biochemical processes. After longitudinal bone growth ceases, bone mass continues to increase by radial growth until age 30–35 years. The resulting skeleton contains 80% cortical bone, which forms the outer wall of all bones and constitutes most of the osseous tissue in the shafts of long bones, and 20% of cancellous or trabecular bone, which is present primarily in the bones of the axial skeleton and in the ends of long bones.

Throughout life, bone constantly remodels and reappropriates its matrix and mineral stores along lines of mechanical stress. Such activity occurs predominately in trabecular bone because this form of osseous tissue has the greatest surface area. The factors that control the bone remodeling process (resorption and formation) are not well understood. However, the relative constancy of bone mass that persists during this continuous activity indicates that the processes must be tightly coupled, resulting in a precise balance between the net bone formation and bone resorption. Indeed, both primary and secondary osteoporosis (and other metabolic bone diseases) result from an imbalance between resorption and formation.

A. BONE REMODELING

Remodeling is carried out by osteoclasts and osteoblasts on the periosteal, haversian, endosteal, and trabecular surfaces.[2] The osteoclasts serve as the cells mainly responsible for bone resorption. The resorptive activity is marked by solubilization of bone mineral, depolymerization of glycosaminoglycans in the matrix, and disaggregation of collagen fibrils and subsequent cleavage into peptide fragments.

The osteoblasts are the cells responsible for bone formation. In contrast to resorption, the formative process occurs in two discrete and easily identifiable stages: matrix formation and mineralization. Osteoblast-directed synthesis of collagen, proteoglycans, and glycoproteins results in matrix formation, which occurs at the interface between cells and the bone surface. After the initial deposition of the bone matrix, a series of changes ensues, including an increase in the cross-linking between the polypeptide chains of the collagen molecules, that prepare the osteoid for the deposition of mineral. Subsequently, calcification is initiated at the interface between the osteoid and mineralized bone. Although this discrete location is distant from osteoblasts, the (primary) mineralization appears to be under the direct control of these cells.

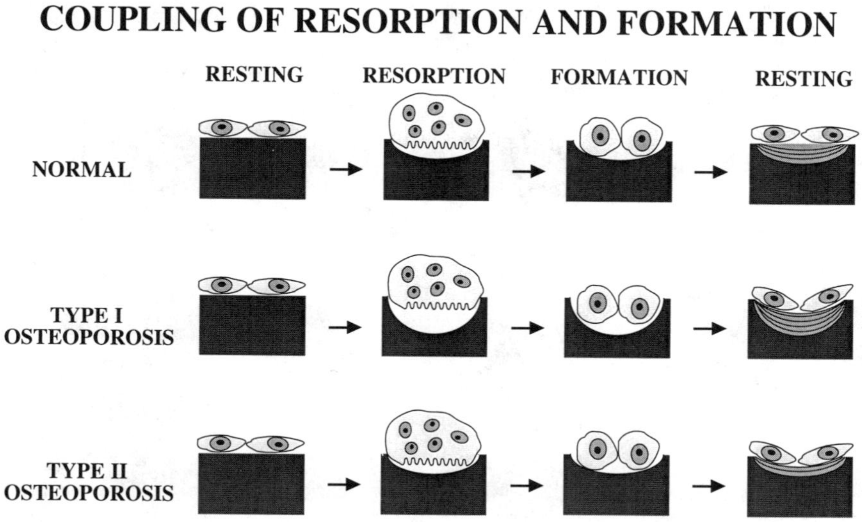

FIGURE 1. Coupling of Resorption and Formation. In normal young adults, tight coupling of resorption and formation conserves bone mass. In Type I osteoporosis, the rapid phase of bone loss results from accelerated bone turnover with a greater number of osteoclasts creating deeper resorption cavities. The osteoblasts follow by increasing bone accretion, but incomplete repair results in a net loss of bone. In Type II osteoporosis, a slow, age-dependent loss of bone occurs, and the imbalance results mainly from impaired bone formation. Osteoclasts create resorption cavities of normal depth, but osteoblasts fail to refill them completely, indicating a decline in osteoblast function.

The coupling of bone resorption and formation probably results not from the coordinated activity of randomly distributed cells, but from the integrated activity of packets of interacting cells, the basic multicellular units. In each unit, newly formed osteoclasts excavate bone to a depth that varies only between narrow limits. Thereafter, the osteoclasts disappear, resulting in a quiescent interval of variable duration. A coordinated unit of osteoblasts likely derived from different precursor cells next appears. These cells replace as exactly as possible the recently removed bone. The structural order of the bone results from the coordination of cellular activity within each of these multicellular units.

In normal young adults, tight coupling of the resorption and formation phases conserve bone mass (Figure 1). The mechanism underlying this integrated function remains unknown. Nevertheless, a variety of regulators of both bone resorption and formation, produced locally by osteoblasts, osteocytes, cartilage and marrow cells, and systemically, have been identified. In any case, after age 35 years a disequilibrium between these processes results in bone loss that occurs in both slow and rapid phases. In the slow, age-dependent phase, imbalance results mainly from impaired bone formation. Osteoclasts create resorption cavities of normal depth, and osteoblasts fail to refill them completely, indicating a decline in osteoblast function. By contrast, the rapid phase of bone loss occurs in women during the perimenopausal period and results from accelerated bone turnover. In this case an increased number of osteoclasts creates deeper resorption cavities, and although osteoblasts follow by increasing bone accretion, incomplete repair results in a net loss of bone.

The slow phase of bone loss occurs in both sexes, affects both cortical and trabecular bone, results in a decrease of bone mass of 0.3–0.5% annually, and persists late into life. With acceleration of the process in the perimenopausal period, trabecular and cortical bone losses increase to rates of 0.6–6.0% and 2–3% per year, respectively. Over the 8–10 years following menopause, the bone loss declines to the rates sustained by the slow phase process.

B. CAUSE OF ABNORMAL BONE REMODELING IN OSTEOPOROSIS

The specific mechanisms underlying the accelerated bone loss evidenced in perimenopausal women remain unclear. In general, estrogen deficiency appears central to this event. In fact, the recent demonstration of estrogen receptors within the skeleton provides the first evidence of a

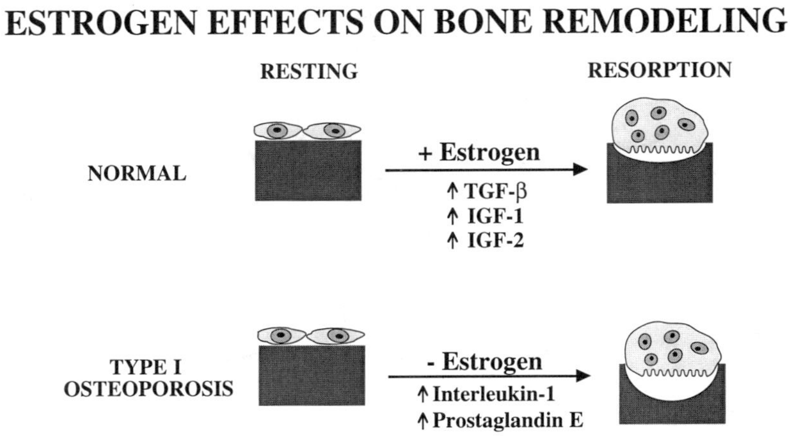

FIGURE 2. Effects of Estrogen on Bone Remodeling. Estrogen deficiency is central to the accelerated bone loss in perimenopausal women. Estrogen stimulates the production of a variety of growth factors, including transforming growth factor-β (TGF-β), insulin-like growth factor-1 (IGF-1), and insulin-like growth factor-2 (IGF-2). However, estrogen deprivation increases the production of bone resorption stimulants, such as interleukin-1 and prostaglandin E, which may be responsible for the increased osteoclastic resorption characteristic of Type I osteoporosis.

potential direct effect of sex steroids on bone cells. Indeed, data from *in vitro* studies indicate physiologic responses of bone cells to appropriate concentrations of 17-β-estradiol. In this regard, estrogen stimulates the production of a variety of growth factors, including TGF-β, IGF-1 and IGF-2 (Figure 2). Moreover, estrogen deprivation increases the production of bone resorption stimulants, such as interleukin-1 and prostaglandin E. Thus, several potential mechanisms exist within bone to account for the changes in bone remodeling that occur across the menopause.

Additional factors that undoubtedly influence the process of bone loss have been identified. Riggs and Melton[3] have proposed a metabolic defect that might provide a mechanism for bone loss occurring in both sexes with advancing age. They propose that the primary event is an age-related reduced capacity of the kidney to synthesize calcitriol in response to appropriate stimuli. Attempts to maintain production of this active vitamin D metabolite include increased circulating concentrations of parathyroid hormone, which may cause increases in bone remodeling and loss of skeletal tissue. Several studies have also identified that calcium absorption declines with age due to an increased resistance of the intestine to the actions of calcitriol. Thus, moderate calcium deficiency likely contributes to the bone loss observed in many elderly patients. In fact, other dietary factors modify the risk of osteoporosis by interacting or interfering with calcium utilization.

The outcome of the age-dependent imbalance of bone remodeling is a decrease in the trabecular wall thickness in aging individuals, a thinning and perforation of trabecular plates, conversion of the plates to rods and ultimately loss of the rods (Figure 3), accounting for the decrease in trabecular number characteristic of bone biopsies in affected patients. This complex pathological scenario renders bone weakened and subject to fracture.

III. CLINICAL PRESENTATION

The most common fractures with which patients present are those of the vertebrae, proximal femur, and wrist, but low bone mass can result in fracture of almost any bone of the body.

A. VERTEBRAL FRACTURES

A decrease in bone density, the hallmark of the osteoporotic disorders, is generally a slowly evolving process that progresses silently until fracture occurs. As a consequence, knowledge of the disease is often delayed until minimal trauma from coughing or bending, a fall, or from lifting a

Loss of Trabecular Structure with Aging

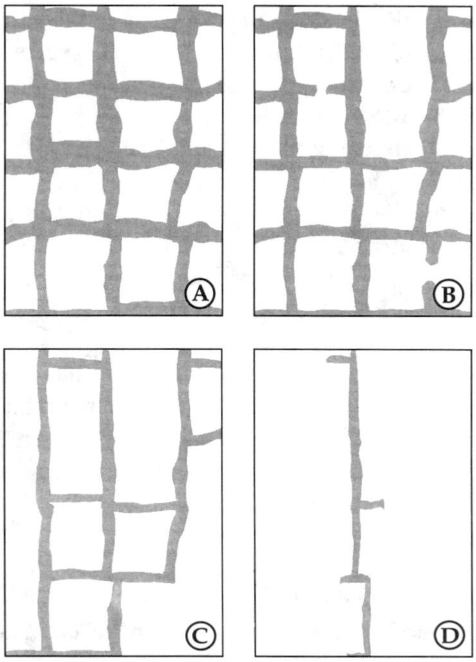

FIGURE 3. Age-Dependent Loss of Trabecular Bone Structure. The normal trabecular structure in young individual (A) consists of connected rods and plates. With aging, there is a thinning and perforation of trabecular plates (B), conversion of the plates to rods (C) and ultimately loss of the rods in advanced osteoporososis (D). This complex pathological scenario accounts for the decrease in trabecular number characteristic of bone biopsies in affected patients and renders bone weakened and subject to fracture. (Based on scanning electron micrographs of trabecular bone in Mosekilde.[13])

heavy object incorrectly precipitates a vertebral crush fracture. These osteoporotic fractures generally affect the lower thoracic and lumbar vertebrae. The pain of such a fracture is often severe and localized to the fracture site but may radiate to the abdomen or into the flanks. The pain may be sufficiently severe to cause breathlessness, pallor, nausea, and vomiting. In the acute phase, tenderness is evident over the affected vertebrae. The pain lasts from several days to 2–6 weeks and may require treatment with bed rest, analgesics, and antispasmodics.

In contrast, the majority of vertebral crush fractures cause no pain and are discovered incidentally on routine radiographs, most often of the chest. The reasons underlying the variable presence of acute pain remain unclear. However, patients so affected often chronically complain of a persistent dull low backache. The pain may be throbbing and radiate laterally, often mimicking nerve root compression. However, this backache may be explained by chronically aching muscles extended abnormally around the kyphotic deformity that results in muscular and ligamental strain.

The natural progression of the clinical problems associated with vertebral fractures is quite variable. Frequently, patients have several years between fracture episodes and may be symptom free or in the interval suffering only low back pain, as described previously. In any case, patients lose height with repetitive compression fractures and may develop kyphosis of the dorsal spine. In addition, shortening of the thoracic and lumbar vertebrae leads to relaxation of the abdominal muscles and abdominal protuberance. Fracture of multiple vertebrae often results in angulation of the ribs and ultimately resting of the ribs on the iliac crests. With such progression the chest exhibits reduced compliance, and patients complain of early satiety and regurgitation of gastric contents due to compression of the stomach. In severe forms of the disease, the loss of lumbar lordosis may produce a forward pelvic tilt, hamstring contractures, permanent hip joint flexion, stiff ankles, and pronated feet, resulting in a shuffling unsteady gait.

B. HIP FRACTURES

In the more aged population, osteoporosis may manifest as a subcapital or trochanteric fracture of the hip. Indeed, the incidence of hip fractures doubles every 6 years after the age of 40 years and by age 90 years a woman has a 32% chance of sustaining such a fracture and a man a 17% chance. From most affected patients, a history of a fall from a standing height can be elicited, although it occasionally appears that the fracture precedes the fall. The subcapital fractures occur in one-third of cases, and the trochanteric fractures in the remaining two-thirds.

Subcapital fractures occur in the femoral neck and are intracapsular (inside the ligamentous capsule of the hip joint). The common complications of this fracture type include nonunion and posttraumatic degenerative joint disease secondary to avascular necrosis or cartilage damage. A small percentage of the subcapital fractures is impacted, consequently, more stable and lead to less frequent complications.

The trochanteric fractures are extracapsular and occur in the intertrochanteric or subtrochanteric regions of the hip. Since the blood supply to these areas is abundant, avascular necrosis is not a commonly occurring late complication. However, bleeding at the fracture site, as well as instability and deformity, especially with comminuted fractures, does complicate the recovery period. Moreover, surgical repair of the trochanteric fractures is technically more difficult, most notably in older patients with subtrochanteric injury.

Not surprisingly, many of the elderly patients presenting with hip fractures have other significant health problems. Thus, careful assessment of the antecedent functional status of the patient is crucial. Indeed, if the patient was nonambulatory prior to the hip fracture, surgical intervention may be inappropriate. On the other hand, if repair may return the patient to ambulatory status, surgery must occur within the 72 hours immediately following injury in order to avoid local complications of fracture repair and, more importantly, an increased death rate. Consequently, only life-threatening coexistent conditions should delay a warranted surgical intervention.

C. COLLES' FRACTURES

Less frequently, the clinical picture of osteoporosis includes a fracture of the distal radius of the Colles' type that occurs as a patient attempts to lessen the impact of a fall by extending the wrist. As with other osteoporotic fractures, the incidence of this fracture type increases after the menopause. However, unlike other fractures, there is not an age-dependent increase, and the incidence plateaus after age 60 years. The absence of continuous increased occurrence thereafter likely reflects the changing gait pattern of the elderly. As the gait slows and becomes shuffling, falls less often occur upon the outstretched hand and more likely involve a direct trauma to the hip. In any case, these fractures result in limited morbidity and no mortality. Indeed, when reduced, the Colles' fracture usually heals completely, leaving the patient with virtually no limitation of motion in the wrist.

IV. DIFFERENTIAL DIAGNOSIS

Since the presentation of osteoporosis is most commonly back pain with or without an associated deformity or asymptomatic fractures, the differential diagnosis is that of these presenting symptoms. Kyphosis, the usual deformity, may be congenital, occurring after trauma or radiation, in inflammatory disease of the spine (such as ankylosing spondylitis) or as part of other bone disorders including osteomalacia, osteogenesis imperfecta, skeletal dysplasias, and collagen disorders (Marie-Strumpell disease).

The back pain typical of osteoporosis, when present, may mimic that of many other diseases. Osteomalacia is commonly associated with more severe long-standing pain than osteoporosis, and there is often marked bony tenderness. In this disorder newly formed osteoid tissue fails to mineralize normally, and vertebral fracture is not uncommon. The most common causes of this disorder are vitamin D deficiency and phosphate depletion from antacid use or renal phosphate wasting. When osteomalacia is considered in the differential diagnosis, a bone biopsy of the iliac crest following tetracycline labeling and histomorphometric assessment of the resulting specimen should be performed.

Neoplasia of several types may also cause osteopenia and associated back pain. Among these are multiple myeloma, lymphoma, leukemia, and carcinomatosis. These diseases, especially multiple myeloma, may be difficult to distinguish from primary osteoporosis, particularly in their early stages. Indeed, since multiple myeloma is a disorder with an age-dependent increased incidence, this diagnosis must be considered in elderly patients with vertebral crush fracture and anemia.

Back pain may also manifest as a complication of Paget's disease and may be confused with osteoporosis when presenting in the lytic phase. In fact, the bone destruction typical of this stage of the disorder resembles osteoporosis. However, an elevated alkaline phosphatase and increased urinary hydroxyproline excretion distinguish this disease. In addition, the presence of isotopic uptake in the peripheral skeleton on bone scan will favor the diagnosis of Paget's disease or neoplasia.

The diagnosis of osteoporosis may also be applied in the occasional patient with radiological evidence of diminished bone density and persistent low back pain without evidence of vertebral fracture. However, the presence of pain secondary to osteoporosis in the absence of vertebral fractures is unusual. More often such a pain syndrome is associated with other diseases such as osteoarthritis, degenerative disc disease, spondylolisthesis, or enthesopathy.

The differential diagnosis of primary osteoporosis must also include exclusion of those disorders that predispose to secondary osteoporosis. These disorders are many (Table 1) but are generally infrequent and their presence immediately apparent due to other presenting symptoms. Nevertheless, a history and physical exam should seek to exclude signs and symptoms of Cushing's syndrome, intestinal malabsorption, nephrolithiasis, thyrotoxicosis, liver disease, gastrointestinal surgery, rheumatoid arthritis, and alcohol abuse. In addition a drug history should address the use of thyroid replacement therapy, corticosteroids, and anticonvulsants.

A. LABORATORY INVESTIGATION

Laboratory tests are often used to assist in the differential diagnosis of osteoporosis because most results in patients with the primary disorders are well within the normal range. Selection of tests, therefore, is aimed at the exclusion of commonly occurring, often silent, disorders or diseases that mimic unique symptoms evident in presenting patients. In this regard, elderly patients should be routinely screened with thyroid function tests, assessment of serum calcium, and serum and urine protein electrophoresis to exclude relatively asymptomatic thyrotoxicosis, hyperparathyroidism, and multiple myeloma. In contrast, determination of serum cortisol, 25-hydroxyvitamin D and parathyroid hormone should be reserved for those occasions when there is clinical reason to suspect Cushing's disease, osteomalacia, or hyperparathyroidism. Elevations in bone-specific alkaline phosphatase levels may also prove helpful in making the diagnosis of a variety of metabolic bone diseases, including Paget's disease, hyperparathyroidism, osteomalacia, renal osteodystrophy, and hypercortisolism. Since alkaline phosphatase may increase 7–10 days after a fracture, care must be exercised in evaluating an abnormality of this measurement.

More recently, a variety of biochemical markers have been discovered that permit assessment of bone remodeling activity in patients with both primary and secondary osteoporoses (see Chapter 10). Although these measures do not always aid in the differential diagnosis of the osteopenic disorder, they often guide the choice of an appropriate therapy that may be designed to halt increased bone turnover or facilitate new bone formation. In this regard, markers of increased bone turnover now include (1) tartrate-resistant acid phosphatase, an index of osteoclast-derived enzyme activity; and (2) urinary deoxypyridinoline, a reflection of bone-specific collagen breakdown. By contrast, serum osteocalcin (bone gla-protein) likely reflects bone formation and correlates closely with the histologically derived bone formation rate in mixed patient populations.

TABLE 1
The Primary and Secondary Osteoporoses

Primary
- Type I osteoporosis, postmenopausal
- Type II osteoporosis, senile
- Idiopathic osteoporosis

Secondary
- Metabolic
  - Cushing's syndrome
  - Hyperparathyroidism
  - Hypogonadism
  - Hyperthyroidism
  - Hypercalciuria
  - Scurvy
  - Diabetes mellitus
- Drug-Induced
  - Glucocorticoids
  - Anticonvulsants
  - Aluminum
  - Heparin
  - Thyroid hormone
- Congenital
  - Wilson's disease
  - Osteogenesis imperfecta
  - Hypophosphatasia
  - Homocystinuria
- Gastrointestinal Disease
  - Gastrectomy
  - Chronic liver disease
  - Intestinal malabsorption
- Miscellaneous
  - Alcoholism
  - Immobilization
  - Rheumatoid arthritis
  - Severe calcium deficiency

B. RADIOLOGICAL EVALUATION

The radiological assessment of patients with primary osteoporosis relies on the presence of fractures that have occurred as a consequence of relatively trivial trauma. In the absence of a clinically apparent fracture, conventional radiographs are not useful as a measure of bone mass because 30–60% of the bone mineral must be lost in order to achieve detection limits. However, characteristic morphological changes affecting the vertebrae may be evident. These include loss of horizontal trabeculae and consequent creation of a more prominent appearance of the remaining vertical trabeculae. In addition, vertebral endplates may be accentuated, and biconcave depressions on the superior and inferior surfaces can occur from expansion of the intervertebral discs into the vertebrae. With continued bone loss, the vertebrae become weakened and fail to withstand force, resulting in a compression fracture. In osteoporosis, the apex of the wedge fracture in lumbar and thoracic vertebrae is usually anterior. Indeed, posterior wedging of a fracture suggests another disease such as metastatic disease or Paget's disease.

During the past two decades, new methods for the assessment of bone density have increased diagnostic efficiency in both symptomatic and asymptomatic patients.[4] At present, the most accurate and precise of these techniques is dual energy x-ray absorptiometry, which permits assessment of bone mass in the lumbar vertebrae, the hip, and the distal forearm. Recent studies indicate that vertebral bone mineral density obtained in the supine lateral position tightly correlates with the force necessary to induce compression fractures.[5] Thus, such bone mass measurements are useful for both clinical practice and research studies. Indeed, for women, starting around the age of 60 years, the relative risk of fracture increases by 1.3 for every standard deviation decrease in bone mass. Moreover, the increase in relative risk may be even greater for younger individuals. Not surprisingly, therefore, the data from several studies demonstrate that baseline bone mass measurements predict the risk of fracture and may be used as a guide to therapeutic decision making in asymptomatic patients. However, all patients do not require bone mass measurement; thus, this technique should not be used as a widespread screening technique. Rather, in clinical practice, the position of the Scientific Advisory Committee of the National Osteoporosis Foundation appears most rational. In this regard, bone mass measurements are useful in (1) estrogen-deficient women, to diagnose significantly low bone mass in order to make decisions about hormone replacement therapy; (2) patients with vertebral abnormalities or roentgenographic osteopenia, to diagnose spinal osteoporosis in order to make decisions about further diagnostic evaluation and therapy; (3) patients receiving long-term glucocorticoid therapy, to diagnose low bone mass in order to adjust therapy; and (4) patients with asymptomatic primary hyperparathyroidism, to diagnose low bone mass in order to identify those at risk of severe skeletal disease and who may be candidates for surgical intervention. Future studies may indicate that serial assessment of bone density is also reasonable for determining response to therapy.

V. PREVENTION OF OSTEOPOROSIS

Prevention of osteoporosis remains the most cost-effective means for the management of this disease. Such efforts are a combination of approaches designed to enhance the accrual of bone mass during the adolescent and young adult years, and to prevent bone loss secondary to known risks in later life.

The several strategies available to maximize bone mass include (1) maintaining dietary calcium intake at levels of 1200 mg/d in adolescents and 800 mg/d in adults beyond 24 years of age, (2) encouraging physical exercise,[6] and (3) avoiding cigarette smoking and excessive alcohol consumption. Increasing calcium intakes by using foodstuffs as the source of supply is preferable to tablets because such medications in the United States are not regulated as drugs and are not subject to rigorous quality control. Indeed, many calcium supplements are so poorly formulated that they do not disintegrate in an acid environment *in vitro,* and the calcium is not available for absorption. In contrast, calcium absorption from foods such as milk, cheese, yogurt, and most green vegetables ranges from 21–26%, whereas that from spinach is limited to only 5%.

VI. TREATMENT OF OSTEOPOROSIS

In later life, the use of estrogen is the most effective therapy to prevent postmenopausal bone loss in the vertebrae, wrists, and hips. In fact, epidemiological evidence suggests that estrogen use decreases fracture frequency in women. A low dose of estrogen is effective; higher doses provide no additional benefit and increase the incidence of complications and noncompliance. Treatment should be initiated as soon after the menopause or oophorectomy as possible and continued for at least 10 years (following menopause). Some authorities suggest that therapy should, in fact, be lifelong.

The side effects of estrogen treatment include an increase in endometrial hyperplasia and uterine cancer. Indeed, patients receiving estrogens often have abnormal vaginal bleeding, which should prompt endometrial biopsy or dilation and curettage. Estrogen therapy also may cause breast enlargement and tenderness. Less certain is the effect of estrogen administration on the incidence of breast cancer. Several studies indicate that the use of conjugated estrogens (commonly employed in the United States) is not associated with an increased risk for this disease. In contrast, more potent synthetic estrogens, such as ethinyl estradiol, do increase the risk of breast cancer. Estrogens may also increase the incidence of gallstones and venous thrombosis.

Ancillary benefits of estrogen use have also been identified. Estrogen decreases the incidence of vasomotor symptoms (hot flashes), vaginal discomfort, and vaginal and urinary tract infections. In addition, estrogen therapy likely reduces cardiovascular mortality in postmenopausal women.

For skeletal protection, the estrogen may be administered as an oral preparation or via a skin patch. Usually patients and physicians choose the oral route and a standard dose of conjugated equine estrogen (Premarin): 0.625 mg/d, or its equivalent, which is the minimum effective dose for the prevention of bone loss. For transdermal administration, current data indicate that 50 μg of 17 β-estradiol, administered twice weekly by patch (Estraderm), will reduce bone loss at all skeletal sites. The estrogens are taken continuously, and for those with an intact uterus, a progestin is added 12–14 days each month (medroxyprogesterone actetate 5–10 mg/d) or continuously (medroxyprogesterone acetate 2.5 mg/d) to reduce the risk of uterine cancer. Use of the first regimen will result in withdrawal bleeding each month, whereas the alternative program will not lead to bleeding in 60% of treated patients.

Although the treatment is somewhat controversial, most authorities agree that the ancillary use of calcium supplementation effectively contributes to the prevention of osteoporosis in the elderly population. Therefore, in 1984 a Consensus Development Conference sponsored by the National Institutes of Health recommended a calcium intake of 1500 mg/d for women who are estrogen deficient. This recommendation is a compromise to achieve a balance between the factors of achievability, compliance, efficacy, and safety.

VII. SPECIFIC THERAPIES FOR OSTEOPOROSIS

Treatment of established osteoporosis may be divided into management of the acute symptoms relative to the disease, and therapy to prevent progression and reverse the skeletal abnormalities. Physicians and other health care workers must superimpose on these therapeutic strategies efforts to minimize suffering and maximize coping with this debilitating disease. Indeed, for patients with established osteoporosis, issues surrounding quality of life are of primary importance.

A. SYMPTOMATIC THERAPY

The pain from an acute vertebral fracture is often severe, and strong analgesics, including narcotics and muscle relaxants, may be required to achieve relief. Frequently bed rest of several weeks is necessary before the pain and muscle spasm ease sufficiently for a patient to resume activities. During this period and following mobilization, a back brace may provide the support requisite to minimize spasm.

After the acute pain secondary to vertebral fracture subsides, many patients suffer chronic low back pain due to persistent muscle spasm. In the absence of relief upon the use of a brace, physical therapy, including flexion and extension exercises, may be helpful. Unfortunately, chronic pain is often the unrelenting consequence of this disorder, and patients must learn to cope with this severe debilitating complication of the disease.

The treatment of hip and Colles' fractures are discussed above.

B. THERAPY TO PREVENT PROGRESSION AND REVERSE THE BONE DISEASE

Drug treatment of established disease has become the therapy of choice as authorities better understand the pathogenesis of osteoporosis. In this regard, it is clear that progression of osteoporosis may be retarded through the use of antiresorptive drugs. These agents slow bone resorption and limit the destruction of bone that is a primary event underlying evolution of the disease. Unfortunately, these drugs lack the ability to overcome already existent, significant bone loss, and to improve deficient osteoblast function. Nevertheless, the antiresorptive agents do decrease the fracture rate by stabilizing bone mass and possibly by other speculative means. Thus, their use is common and, in fact, these agents are the only approved drugs for the treatment of osteoporosis.

Calcium, estrogen, and calcitonin are the antiresorptive agents currently in use for the management of osteoporosis. Calcium likely exerts its effects by the suppression of parathyroid hormone secretion and consequent reduction of bone loss. Current recommendations hold that this drug should be given to all patients with osteoporosis in doses of 1000 to 1500 mg/d divided into 3–4 doses.[7] The major contraindications to such treatment are hypercalcemia and nephrolithiasis. The absorption of calcium improves upon coincident administration of vitamin D, 400–1000 U/d. Some studies suggest that antiresorptive effects similar to those of calcium supplementation may be achieved with the use of calcitriol in doses of 0.25–0.75 μg/d.[8]

Estrogen therapy likewise effects its action through decreasing bone resorption, but the mechanism underlying this response remains unclear. Nevertheless, as noted previously, the use of estrogen therapy for at least 5–10 years following the menopause or for a lifetime is suggested. Although some authorities feel that once compression fractures have occurred, estrogen treatment is not useful in protecting bone mass, further study is required.

Calcitonin treatment of osteoporosis is dependent upon inhibition of osteoclast function and consequent bone resorption. Indeed, several studies suggest that this drug may prevent postmenopausal bone loss. Thus, treatment with this agent should be considered for estrogen-deficient women in whom replacement therapy is contraindicated, such as those with breast cancer. An additional positive feature of this drug is the pain relief afforded patients with acute vertebral fractures and chronic back pain. Unfortunately, the obligatory administration by injection limits the use of this agent. However, the development of a nasal spray to administer this drug may increase its attractiveness as a therapy for women in whom estrogens are contraindicated.

More recently, a new class of drugs, bisphosphonates, has been extensively tested in patients with osteoporosis.[9] The effects of these drugs are somewhat similar to those of the other antiresorptive agents, most notably estrogens and calcitonin. Experimental investigations indicate that first and second generation agents reduce the incidence of vertebral fractures in affected patients and induce a limited increase in bone mass. As with all antiresorptive drugs, the latter occurs due to filling of the remodeling space of bone, and is therefore confined to a maximum of 5–7% of bone mass. At present, the long-term effects of the bisphosphonates are unknown, and their eventual role in the management of osteoporosis is ill-defined.

Reversal of the bone lesion underlying osteoporosis remains the primary goal of treatment. Such therapy should increase existing bone mass and re-connect perforated trabecular plates, thereby reducing the chance of further fractures. Although no drug regimen has all of these properties, several have been identified that increase bone formation and, thus, bone mass. Among the better studied of such agents are fluoride and parathyroid hormone.

Fluoride, administered in doses of 40–80 mg/d orally, directly stimulates osteoblast function and increases deposition of new trabecular bone. Similar effects are not apparent in cortical bone. Coadministration of calcium, 1000 mg/d, is requisite to prevent abnormal bone formation. However, several studies indicate that bone formed in the presence of fluoride is less strong than normal bone. Nevertheless, additional studies indicate that fluoride administration does reduce the incidence of vertebral fractures. In contrast, two recent studies in which fluoride was administered at excessively high doses suggest that fluoride does not influence the incidence of vertebral fractures and may increase fractures of the peripheral skeleton. The side effects of fluoride therapy include nausea and gastric irritation, and lower extremity pain secondary to stress fractures or tendonitis. The use of this drug should be reserved for patients with marked bone loss and vertebral fractures, in whom additional bone mass may reverse the disease process. Of course, the benefits and risks of such therapy must be made clear to patients, and they should be followed closely. Indeed, at present, authorities consider this treatment experimental.

Treatment of osteoporotic patients with the amino-terminal fragment of parathyroid hormone (PTH) has also received recent attention.[10] Several reports suggest the accrual of increased bone mass in response to small doses of (1-34)hPTH administered subcutaneously to animals and humans. The results are in general impressive, with significant and potentially meaningful increments in bone mass. The mechanism underlying the effects apparently require stimulation of renal 25-hydroxyvitamin D-1α-hydroxylase activity and consequent elevation of circulating calcitriol levels. In any case, further studies are necessary to understand fully the potential impact of this drug in the management of osteoporosis.

Several additional experimental drugs have been identified that increase new bone formation. These agents, including IGF-1 and Zeolite A, stimulate osteoblast replication and/or activity and, thereby, enhance new bone formation.[11] The effects are relatively rapid, and changes in bone mass of 25–30% have been observed. Toxicity trials in humans and evaluation of the effects on fracture rate will determine if such agents may herald new forms of treatment for osteoporosis.

VIII. COPING STRATEGIES IN THE MANAGEMENT OF OSTEOPOROSIS

Since a cure for osteoporosis is not yet available, treatment options in affected individuals must focus, not only on influencing bone remodeling, but on ways in which we can improve negative disease outcomes such as pain, depression, and loss of self-esteem. Unfortunately, little is known about the ways in which osteoporosis compromises psychosocial functioning, and health-care providers have made few efforts to increase the relevant knowledge base. Nevertheless, we do know that several psychosocial limitations occur with some regularity in osteoporotic patients. These negative outcomes of established disease may be broadly classified as psychological problems, social consequences, and functional limitations. In addition, both acute and chronic pain affect the ability of a patient to cope with this disease.

The psychological effects common to many chronic diseases occur with notable frequency in patients with osteoporosis. Not surprisingly, depression is one of the primary consequences. Sleep problems, diminished appetite, and apathy about daily activities and relationships with family and friends are the most common symptoms encountered. Other aspects of psychological dysfunction in osteoporotic patients relate to the stress attendant upon failure to achieve specific expectations of themselves. Women in whom disease limits their abilities to clean house or cook meals, for example, report stress symptoms. Moreover, the lost ability to fulfill social role expectations often results in diminished self-esteem.

Changes in social behavior that result from osteoporosis also make coping with the illness difficult. These social consequences, which may include relinquishing some or all occupational responsibilities and/or receiving disability payments, make social support crucial for people with osteoporosis. Indeed, only with the assistance of others will patients successfully manage the limitations they face.

Many of the psychological and social consequences of the disease discussed above result directly from the functional limitations secondary to osteoporosis and related fractures. The range of functional loss is quite broad. Gold et al.[12] at Duke University recently compared patients with at least two 25% vertebral compression fractures to age- and gender-matched individuals with no fractures. The patients with fractures had substantially worse performances on functional reach and mobility skills. Further, affected subjects had diminished trunk extension strength and could not walk short or long distances as effectively as control patients. Clearly these functional limitations affect the success with which patients complete daily tasks such as preparing meals, cleaning house, gardening, shopping, and folding laundry as well as bathing, dressing, and general personal care.

These multiple interactive psychosocial phenomena are, in large measure, the treatment challenge for those health care providers who manage patients with osteoporosis. Unfortunately, established methods to combat these multiple problems have been inadequately developed. The experience at Duke University, however, indicates that the most effective treatment for these psychosocial problems is provided in a multidisciplinary program context, in which extended care is provided by physician, physical therapist, nutritionist, and social worker alike. Under these circumstances a support program is developed that benefits from the group dynamics encountered in a program provided by a team of professionals who work together on an ongoing basis. Indeed, in this context the social worker may develop a successful strategy of support for the patient that all professionals use to overcome treatment problems. However, regardless of the availability of a multidisciplinary team or a physician in private practice, acknowledging and treating the psychosocial consequences of this disease are paramount in long-term disease management. Undoubtedly, we can help patients cope more effectively with the problems of osteoporosis and improve the overall quality of their lives through the recognition and treatment of these psychosocial consequences of their disease.

IX. SUMMARY AND CONCLUSIONS

Osteoporosis, as a disease, represents a great challenge to societies with extended longevity because many more fracture patients are anticipated in future decades. Osteoporotic fractures have been recognized since antiquity, but until the last century, the rates have remained relatively inconsequential.

The anticipated new drug therapies, especially the bisphosphonates, should be as effective as estrogens in preserving bone mass and delaying osteoporosis, but without the unwanted side effects on reproductive tissues. They will not, however, maintain high HDL and low LDL cholesterol concentrations in blood, as oral estrogens do. Other therapies that potentially increase bone mass in elderly subjects, except for fluorides, have not yet been well tested in experimental trials, but Zeolite A and local growth factors, such as IGF-1, hold promise.

The prevention of osteoporosis through early-life development of peak bone mass should become an increasingly important societal strategy.

REFERENCES

1. **Melton, L. J., III,** Epidemiology of fractures, in *Osteoporosis: Etiology, Diagnosis and Management,* Riggs B. L. and Melton, L. J., III, eds., Raven Press, New York, 1988, 133.
2. **Eriksen, E. F., Vesterby, A., Kassem, M., Melsen, F., and Mosekilde, L. E.,** Bone remodeling and bone structure, in *Physiology and Pharmacology of Bone,* Mundy, G. R. and Martin, T. J., eds., Springer Verlag, New York, 1993, 67.
3. **Riggs, B. L. and Melton, L. J., III,** Clinical Review 8. Clinical heterogeneity of involutional osteoporosis: implications for preventive therapy, *J. Clin. Endocrinol. Metab.*, 70, 1229, 1990.
4. **Genant, H. K., Block, J. E., Steiger, P., Glower, C. C., Etinger, B., and Harris, S. T.,** Appropriate use of bone densitometry, *Radiology,* 170, 817, 1989.
5. **Myers, B. S., Arbogast, K. B., Lobaugh, B., Harper, K. D., Richardson, W. J., and Drezner, M. K.,** Improved assessment of lumbar vertebral body strength using supine lateral dual energy x-ray absorptiometry, *J. Bone. Min. Res.,* 9, 687, 1994.
6. **White, M. K., Martin, R. B., Yeates, R. A., Bulcher, R. L., and Radin, E. L.,** The effects of exercise on the bones of postmenopausal women, *Int. Orthop.,* 7, 209, 1990.
7. **Nordin, B. E. C. and Heaney, R. P.,** Calcium supplementation of the diet justified by current evidence, *Br. Med. J.,* 300, 1056, 1990.
8. **Drezner, M. K. and Nesbitt, T.,** Role of calcitriol in prevention of osteoporosis, *Metabolism,* 39, 18, 1990.
9. **Storm, T., Thamsborg, G., Steiniche, T., Genant, H. K., and Sorensen, O. H.,** Effect of intermittent cyclical etidronate therapy on bone mass and fracture rate in women with postmenopausal osteoporosis, *New Engl. J. Med.*, 322, 1265, 1990.
10. **Neer, R., Slovik, D., Daly, M., Lo, C., Potts, J., and Nussbaum, S.,** Treatment of postmenopausal osteoporosis with daily parathyroid hormone plus calcitriol, in *Osteoporosis 1990. Proceedings of the Third International Symposium on Osteoporosis,* Copenhagen, Denmark, Christiansen, C. and Overgaard, K., eds., Osteopress ApS, Copenhagen, 1990, 1314.

11. **Drezner, M. K., Nesbitt, T., and Quarles, L. D.,** Zeolite A: a potential successful therapy for osteoporosis, in *Osteoporosis: Fourth International Symposium on Osteoporosis and Consensus Development Conference, Proceedings, 1993,* Christiansen, C. and Riis, Eds., Handelstrykkereit Aalborg ApS, Copenhagen, 1993, 114.
12. **Gold, D. T., Stegmaier, K., Bales, C. W., Lyles, K. W., Westlund, R. E., and Drezner, M. K.,** Psychosocial functioning and osteoporosis in late life: results of a multidisciplinary intervention, *J. Women's Health*, 2, 149, 1993.
13. **Mosekilde, L.,** Age-related changes in vertebral trabecular bone architecture — assessed by a new method, *Bone*, 9, 247, 1988.

Chapter 22

EPIDEMIOLOGY OF OSTEOPOROSIS

Erik Allander, M.D.

TABLE OF CONTENTS

I. INTRODUCTION

Osteoporosis is defined as a reduction of bone density and strength. The epidemiology of osteoporosis can be studied by two principally different approaches: by measuring bone mineral density (BMD) and by measuring the occurrence of fractures that largely depends on the force(s) of the trauma. For both, epidemiologic methodology of some sophistication is needed. The ideal design is to elucidate the relative importance of risk factors in a large prospective study, including, among others, repeat BMD measurements. A few such resource-demanding studies are currently under way. The vast majority of fractures is easy to define and localize, and, also, it is relatively straight-forward to determine when they occurred, with the exception of vertebral fractures. The epidemiological of the latter is subject to special methodological challenges.

BMD is a continuous variable, as opposed to fracture, a discrete variable. BMD increases to a peak by age 30–35 and declines thereafter. Women have some 20% lower BMD than men. The decline in BMD in women is rapid within a few years after menopause, but then it falls more gradually with increasing age. Postmenopausal osteoporosis (Type I) is replaced by the ever rapidly increasing involutional osteoporosis (Type II) (see Chapter 21). A substantial overlap exists between

0-8493-7845-1/95/$0.00+$.50

the two forms of primary osteoporosis, i.e., postmenopausal osteoporosis (Type I), and involutional osteopenia (Type II). A small group of osteoporotic patients suffer from secondary osteoporosis related to specific diseases (e.g., Cushing's syndrome) or caused by medical treatment (e.g., cortisone).

II. MEASUREMENT OF BONE MINERAL DENSITY

The present method of choice for the measurement of BMD is DEXA (Dual-Energy X-ray Absorptiometry). A measurement takes 10 minutes for the lumbar spine and proximal femur and 20 min for a total body scan. DEXA possesses a high precision. A higher BMD typically means stronger bone, unless fluoride treatment is involved. Fluoride therapy results in higher BMD, but the bone is more brittle. BMD varies by site even within the same individual. Evidence for a defined threshold in BMD when a fracture appears is limited, but the concept of a threshold remains useful to researchers.

A recent WHO report on osteoporosis[1] adopted a previously (1991) published definition of osteoporosis: "A disease characterized by low bone mass and microarchitectural deterioration of bone tissue, leading to enhanced bone fragility and a consequent increase in fracture risk."

The measurement of BMD is expensive and results differ among regions of the body within the same individual. Therefore, changes in BMD have usually been said to be followed by an increased or decreased fracture rate. However, in follow-up studies only a lesser part of fractures could be predicted by a low BMD. On the other hand, in another study a reduction of BMD from 1.20–1.29 to 0.60–0.69 g/cm^2, that is by half, resulted in a 30-fold increase in fracture incidence.[2]

Racial differences in BMD have been found; members of the black race have more dense bone and substantially less fracture incidence than those of the white race, and to some extent than those of Chinese descent.[3,4] A long-term secular trend in BMD has been the subject of a study of femoral bone from the beginning of the 19th century into the 20th century in England.[5] BMD was shown to be definitely higher in the past than today, probably as a result of the much more physically demanding life-style in earlier times.

III. DIETARY FACTORS

The study of dietary factors and their putative relationship to osteoporosis is difficult because these factors are interwoven with energy consumption, energy expenditure in the physical workload, and variation according to age. Furthermore, the interference of coffee, tea, smoking, and alcohol with dietary habits needs to be considered. A recent study[6] showed a negative influence of coffee on BMD that, however, could be reduced by a higher milk (calcium) intake. A moderate milk consumption during adolescence might improve BMD.[7] The positive importance of vitamin D is also being more acknowledged. Smoking and alcohol are probably among the factors that negatively affect BMD.[8,9]

IV. OVERALL FRACTURE INCIDENCE

Of the fractures under epidemiological study, hip fracture has received the major focus, followed by Colles' fracture and vertebral fractures. The annual incidence rates of all fractures have been studied in Rochester, Minnesota (U.S.). Before the age of 35, males suffer twice as many distal forearm fractures as females of the same age, but the reverse is the case for age groups above 55 years of age.[10]

V. HIP FRACTURE

A hip fracture is by far more devastating to an individual than a fracture at any other site because of the total, or near total, loss of mobility. Individuals with hip fractures have increased mortality

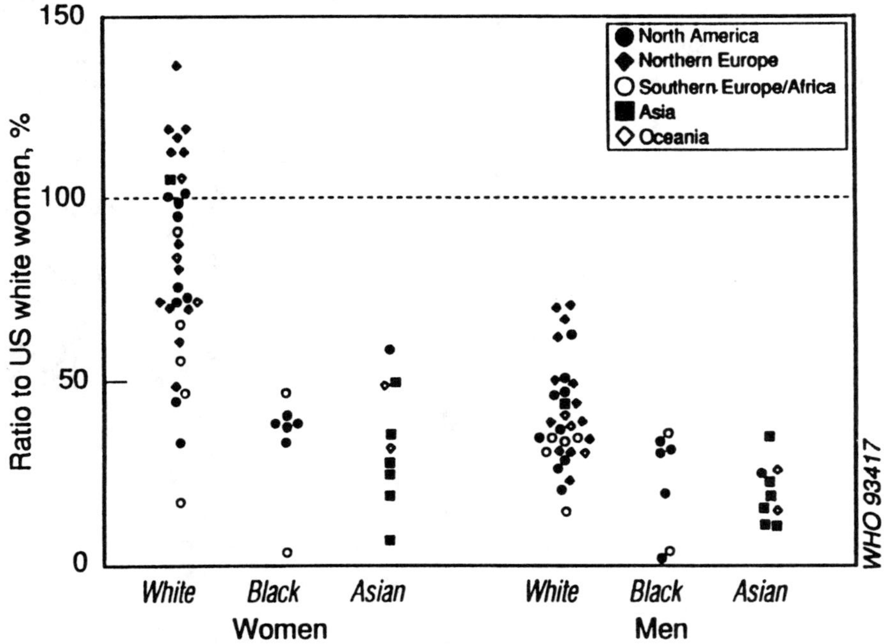

FIGURE 1. Hip Fracture Incidence Around the World as a Ratio of the Rates Observed in Various Populations to Those Expected for White Women in the U.S. (Based on Reference 31) Source: WHO Technical Report Series 843, WHO, Geneva, 1994.)

as well as other adverse health effects (morbidity). The burden this places on society, which is high, has been estimated for several countries.[1] Hip fracture incidence is a good indicator of the level of osteoporosis in a population (Figures 1 and 2).

A. AGE, SEX, AND SEASONAL VARIATION

Hip fracture incidence increases with age; a 50-fold increase for intertrochanteric fractures has been reported for women between the ages 50 and 85 years.[2] Before the age of 50, few fragility fractures, but more fractures related to severe trauma, have been recorded. In a recent study (the Mediterranean Osteoporosis Study [MEDOS] based on hip fracture incidence in 14 centers in 6 countries in Southern Europe),[11,12] the incidence for males rose from 1/10,000 for age group 50–54 to 96/10,000 for age group 90+ and for females from 1/10,000 for age group 50–54 to 170/10,000 for age group 90+. This increase was logarithmic after the age of 50, when most of the fractures found are of the fragility type. Hip fracture is around twice as common in women as in men. The female hip fracture incidence is similar to that of a male who is 10 years older. The doubling time is approximately 5.9 years (4.0–9.9) for males and 5.7 years (4.5–13.3) for females.

The lifetime incidence of risk of hip fracture has been estimated at 15% for females and 6% for males. The higher the mean age of a population, the higher the fracture risk. On the other hand, Colles' fracture does not show the steep increase in incidence with increasing age that is seen with hip fracture. Seasonal variation has been described for Colles' fracture, with more fractures occurring in the winter season; however, for hip fracture, conflicting evidence of changes in incidence with the seasons has been reported.[13]

B. GEOGRAPHY

The geographic differences in hip fracture incidence are impressive. Sweden and Norway have the world's highest hip fracture incidence rates (after age standardization). Substantial research has been devoted to exploring the background of these differences, which compose a complex mixture of ethnicity, lifestyle, and phase of demographic transition.[14]

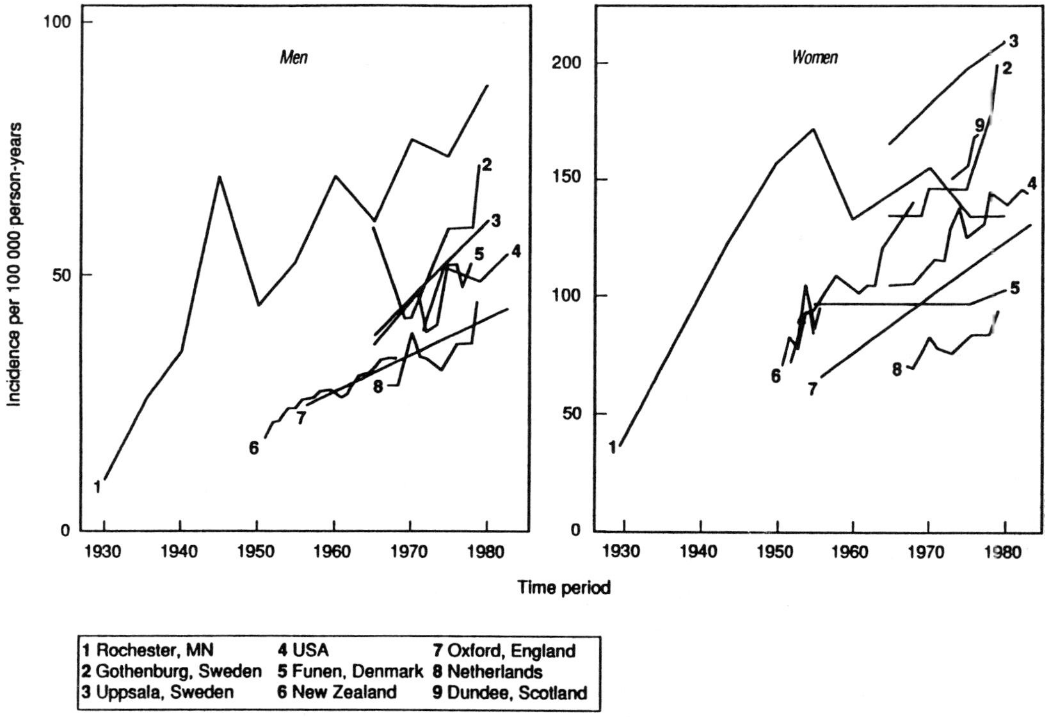

FIGURE 2. Incidence of Hip Fractures over Time as Reported from Various Centers. (Based on Reference 29) Source: WHO Technical Report Series 843, WHO, Geneva, 1994.)

If we study a country in detail, the geographical fracture pattern is also complex; this type of analysis has been carried out for the U.S.[15] Regional differences in fracture incidence were not related to activity level, obesity, smoking, alcohol consumption, or Scandinavian heritage. However, incidence was negatively correlated with latitude, water hardness, and mean hours of January sunlight, and it was positively associated with poverty, proportion of the land in farms. and proportion of the population with fluoridated water.[16]

A recent register study from Europe reported a fracture incidence for females of 504/100,000 in Sweden as against only 46/100,000 in Poland.[17] Present public data sources for hip fractures, however, show considerable methodological variation and lack of standardization in the methods of recording and reporting fracture incidence in different nations.

In the MEDOS study,[11,12] hip fracture incidence was also found to vary considerably; the incidence was high in France, Spain, and Italy, but it was considerably lower in Turkey, which had a span of 4.6 to 20/10,000 for males and 3.6 to 40.6/10,000 for females. Older studies from the black population in South Africa show very low incidence rates of hip fracture. People of Asian ancestry also had a low fracture rate. Low frequency of hip fractures exist in Japan, in spite of the bone mass in Japanese women being somewhat lower than in Caucasian women. Studies of America-born and Japan-born Hawaiians of Japanese ancestry show that the America-born Japanese had a greater bone mass.[18]

C. SECULAR TRENDS

The secular trend for hip fracture increased annually during a 30-year period by 1.6% to 3.9% for males and 1.4% to 2.3% for females beyond the aging of the population in a Swedish study.[19] For the UK, US, and other countries, similar observations have been made, and also, data are emerging from Hong Kong and Japan. Studies are ongoing in China. This increasing secular trend is currently believed to be consequential to less physically demanding life-styles, but this issue has to be explored further. Basically an osteoporotic fracture results from a truly multicausal etiology.

D. RISK FACTORS INCLUDING FALLS

A number of genetic, medical, and behavioral factors have been causally linked to increased fracture risk. Risk factors are related to environment (trauma), life-style, or physiological processes involved in aging. Several studies have shown that obesity seems to be protective against hip fracture, whereas lean women have a higher risk. It is also reasonably established that a longer fertile period means a reduced risk for hip fracture, and the inverse also holds.

If an increased BMD means a reduced risk of fracture when one is falling, then an increased intake of calcium above today's average may be protective.[20]

Parkinson's disease, stroke, and perhaps even diabetes have been shown to be risk factors for hip fracture in several epidemiological studies, but osteoarthrosis is protective by a relative risk ratio (RR) of 0.64; the effect is somewhat less for males (RR = 0.45) than for females (RR = 0.68).

Studies on circumstances around falls have shown that slipping on the same level is the most common type of accident. Six percent (6%) of falls in the elderly result in a fracture, but only 1% of falls results in a hip fracture.[21] The exponential increase of hip fracture incidence with aging is, in part, a result of an age-related increase in the risk of falling. However, it has been estimated that only 5 out of 100 falls result in a fracture.[22] One in 3 women aged 80–84 years had fallen in previous years, and this fraction rose to nearly half of the women 85 years and older.

E. MORTALITY

The natural history for hip fracture is fairly well known. Hip fracture is followed by approximately a 30% increase in mortality during the year after the fracture. In another study a hip fracture meant a 12%-20% reduction of expected survival with the highest excess mortality the year after the fracture.[23]

VI. VERTEBRAL FRACTURE

Vertebral fractures show a similar pattern of hip fracture incidence with aging. Fractures of the vertebrae show a logarithmic increase in those above 60 years of age. Vertebral fracture prevalence is 5% in the age group of 50–54 years as against 45% in the age group of 85+.

The "true" epidemiology of vertebral fracture is still fairly unknown because of measurement problems and the fact that many are asymptomatic. There is also great variation in the definition of what constitutes a vertebral deformity and fracture. The effect on disability, except for a minor proportion of cases, is not very significant. A major ongoing European study[24] involving 34 countries will hopefully shed further light on this difficult research field.

VII. HEALTH ECONOMY, PROJECTIONS AND INTERVENTION

For the U.S., total costs related to osteoporotic fractures in 1986 were 5.15 billion dollars. Approximately 35% of the costs were related to hospital inpatient days and another 18% to nursing homes.[25] The increased number of fractures, age at fracture, hospital days and disability mean that hospital health care costs increase more than other parts of the total costs per year.

The impact of hip fracture based on future projections has been studied. One estimate predicts a total incidence of 2.5 million hip fractures in the world annually by the year 2025, as compared to 800,000/year today. Another projection estimates 1,660,000 fractures in 1990 and 6,260,000 by the year 2050. The majority of "new" incidence is projected to appear in Southeast Asia (Figure 3). How much of this increase could be prevented by life-style changes, drugs, and other factors needs to be investigated further.[15]

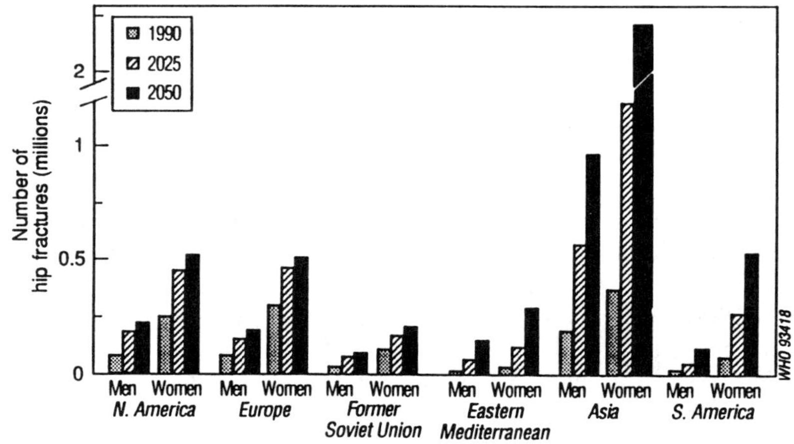

FIGURE 3. Estimated Number of Fractures for Men and Women in Different Regions of the World in 1990, 2025, and 2050. (Based on Reference 30) Source: WHO Technical Report Series 843, WHO, Geneva, 1994.)

VIII. CONCLUDING REMARKS

Reasonable scientific evidence accumulated over the past decade suggests that effective preventive treatment, including moderate lifestyle modification, could mean a reduction of hip fracture incidence. Some measures could be applied already today. One of several examples comes from the MEDOS study, in which it was found that the risk for hip fracture could be positively influenced even among those above the age of 70 years. A significant reduction (to RR = 0.75) was found in those taking estrogen, calcium, and calcitonin.[26] Estimates of effects of specific interventions are currently published.[27,28]

The World Health Organization (WHO) has taken a series of initiatives to focus on the occurrence and burden of osteoporosis, fractures, and their prevention. Gradually support is emerging on an international level to create better programs for the prevention of osteoporosis and associated fractures.

GENERAL REFERENCES

1. **Fogelman, I. and Ryan, P.,** Osteoporosis: a growing epidemic, *Br. J. Clin. Pract.*, 45, 189, 1991.
2. **Johnston, C. C., Jr., Slemenda, C. W., and Melton, L. J., III,** Clinical use of bone densitometry, *New Engl. J. Med.*, 324, 1105, 1991.
3. **Kanis, J. A.,** Hip fracture and the MEDOS Study, *Bone*, 14 (suppl. 1), 8756, 1993.
4. **McGowan, J. A.,** Osteoporosis: assessment of bone loss and remodeling, *Aging Clin. Exp. Res.*, 5, 81, 1993.
5. **Melton, L. J., III,** Epidemiology of fractures, in *Osteoporosis: Etiology, Diagnosis, and Management*, Riggs, B. L. and Melton L. J., III , Eds., New York, Raven Press, 1988, 133.
6. **Notelovitz, M.,** Osteoporosis: screening, prevention, and management, *Fertility Sterility*, 59, 707, 1993.
7. **Sattin, R. W., Huber, D. A. L., DeVito, C. A., Rodriguez, J. G., Ros, A., Bacchelli, S., Stevens,J. A., and Waxweiler, R. J.,** The incidence of fall injury events among the elderly in a defined population, *Am. J. Epidemiol.*, 131, 1028, 1990.
8. World Health Organization, *Report of the Joint WHO/EOPF/NIAMS (NIH) Consultation on Osteoporosis*, Geneva, 13–15 July, 1988.

REFERENCES

1. WHO Technical Report Series No. 843: assessment of fracture risk and its application to screening for postmenopausal osteoporosis. Report of a WHO Study Group. World Health Organization, Geneva, 1994.
2. **Melton, L. J., III, Wahner, H. W., Richelson, L. S., O'Fallon, W. M., Riggs, B. L.,** Osteoporosis and the risk of hip fracture, *Am. J. Epidemiol.,* 124, 254, 1986.
3. **Russelaulet, M., Wang, J., Thornton, J. C., Colt, E. W. D., and Pierson, R. N.,** Bone mineral density and mass in a cross-sectional study of white and Asian women, *J. Bone Miner. Res.*, 8, 575, 1993.
4. **Cummings, S. R., Cauley, J. A., Palermo, L., Ross, P. D., Wasnich, R. D., Black, D., and Faulkner, K. G.,** (for the Study of Osteoporosis Fractures Research Group), Racial differences in hip axis lengths might explain racial differences in rates of hip fracture, *Osteoporosis Int.*, 4, 226, 1994.
5. **Lees, B., Molleson, T., Arnett, T. R., and Stevenson, J. C.,** Differences in proximal femur bone density over two centuries, *Lancet*, 341, 673, 1993.
6. **Barrett-Connor, E., Chang, J. C., and Edelstein, S. L.,** Coffee-associated osteoporosis. Offset by daily milk consumption, *J. Am. Med. Assoc.*, 271, 280, 1994.
7. **Stracke, H., Renner, E., Knie, G., Leidig, G., Minne, H., and Federlin, K.,** Osteoporosis and bone metabolic parameters in dependence upon calcium intake through milk and milk products, *Eur. J. Clin. Nutr.*, 47, 617, 1993.
8. **Holbrook, T. L. and Barrett-Connor, E.,** A prospective study of alcohol consumption and bone mineral density, *Br. Med. J.*, 306, 1506, 1993.
9. **Hopper, J. L. and Seeman, E.,** The bone density of female twins discordant for tobacco use, *New Engl. J. Med.*, 330, 387, 1994.
10. **Melton, L. J., III and Cummings S. R.,** Heterogeneity of age-related fractures: implications for epidemiology, *Bone Miner.,* 2, 321, 1987.
11. **Allander, E., Lindahl, B. I. B., and the MEDOS Study Group,** The Mediterranean Osteoporosis Study (MEDOS): theoretical and practical issues of a major international project on hip fracture epidemiology, *Bone,* 14 (suppl. 1), S37, 1993.
12. **Elffors, L., Allander, E., Kanis, J. A., Gullberg, B., Johnell, O., Dequeker, J., Dilsen, G., Gennari, C., Lopes Vaz, A. A., Lyritis, G., Mazzuoli, G. F., Miravet, L., Passeri, M., Perez Cano, R., Rapado, A., and Ribot, C.,** The variable incidence of hip fracture in Southern Europe: The MEDOS study, *Osteoporosis Int.*, 4, 253, 1994.
13. **Pedrazzoni, M., Alfano, F. S., Malvi, C., Ostanello, F., and Passeri, M.,** Seasonal variation in the incidence of hip fractures in Emilia-Romagna and Parma, *Bone*, 14 (suppl. 1), S57, 1993.
14. **Maggi S., Kelsey J. L., Litvak J., Heyse S. P.,** Incidence of hip fractures in the elderly: a cross-national analysis, *Osteoporosis Int.*, 1, 232, 1991.
15. **Melton, L. J., III,** Hip fractures: a worldwide problem today and tomorrow, *Bone*, 14 (suppl. 1), S1, 1993.
16. **Cooper, C.,** Osteoporosis, in *Epidemiology of the Rheumatic Diseases*, Silman A. J. and Hochberg M. C., eds., New York, Oxford University Press, 422, 1993.
17. **Johnell, O., Gullberg, B., Allander, E., Kanis, J. A., and the MEDOS Study Group,** The apparent incidence of hip fracture in Europe: a study of national register sources, *Osteoporosis Int.*, 2, 298, 1992.
18. **Soda, M. Y., Mizunuma, H., Honjo, S. I., Okano, H., Ibuki, Y., and Igarishi, M.,** Premenopausal and postmenopausal bone mineral density of the spine and proximal femur in Japanese women assess by dual-energy X-ray absorptiometry: a cross-sectional study, *J. Bone Miner. Res.*, 8, 183, 1993.
19. **Gullberg, B., Duppe, H., Nilsson, B., Redlund-Johnell, I., Sernbo, I., Obrant, K., and Johnell, O.,** Incidence of hip fractures in Malmö, Sweden (1950–1991), *Bone*, 14 (suppl. 1), S23, 1993.
20. **Anderson, J. J. B. and Metz, J. A.,** Contributions of dietary calcium and physical activity to primary prevention of osteoporosis in females, *J. Am. Coll. Nutr.*, 12, 378, 1993.
21. **Cummings, R. G., Kelsey, J. L., and Nevitt, M. C.,** Methodological issues in the study of frequent and recurrent health problems. Falls in the elderly, *Ann. Epidemiol.*, 1, 49, 1990.
22. **Rubenstein, L. Z., Robbins, A. S., Schulman, B. L., Rosado, J., Osterweil, D., and Josephson, K. R.,** Falls and instability in the elderly, *J. Am. Geriatr. Soc.*, 36, 266, 1988.
23. **Keene, G. S., Parker, M. J., and Pryor, G. A.,** Mortality and morbidity after hip fractures, *Br. Med. J.*, 307, 1248, 1993.
24. **Cooper, C., O'Neill, T., and Silman, A.** (on behalf of the European Vertebral Osteoporosis Study Group), The epidemiology of vertebral fractures, *Bone*, 14 (suppl. 1), S89, 1993.
25. **Norris R. J.,** Medical costs of osteoporosis, *Bone*, 13, S11, 1992.
26. **Kanis, J. A., Johnell, O., Gullberg, B., Allander, E., Dilsen, G., Gennari, C., Lopes Vaz, A. A., Lyritis, G. P., Mazzuoli, G., Miravet, L., Passeri, M., Perez Cano, R., Rapado, A., and Ribot, C.,** Evidence for the efficacy of drugs affecting bone metabolism in preventing hip fracture, *Br. Med. J.*, 305, 1124, 1992.

27. **Cummings, S. R., Rubin, S. M., and Black, D.,** The future of hip fractures in the United States, *Clin. Orthop. Rel. Res.*, 252, 163, 1990.
28. **Grisso, A. J., Kelsey, J. L., Strom, B. L., Chiu, G.Y., Maislin, G., and O'Brien, L.A., Hoffman, S., Kaplan, F., and the Northeast Hip Fracture Study Group,** Risk factors for falls as a cause of hip fracture in women, *New Engl. J. Med.*, 324, 1326, 1991.
29. **Melton, L. J., III, O'Fallon, W. M., and Riggs, B. L.,** Secular trends in the incidence of hip fractures, *Calcif. Tissue Int.*, 41, 57, 1987.
30. **Cooper, C., Campion, G., and Melton, L. J., III,** Hip fractures in the elderly: a world-wide projection, *Osteoporosis Int.*, 2, 285, 1992.
31. **Melton, L. J., III,** Differing patterns of osteoporosis across the world, in *New Dimensions in Osteoporosis in the 1990s*, Chesnut, C.H., III, ed., Hong Kong, Excerpta Medica Asia, 13, 1991.

Chapter 23

FUTURE DIRECTIONS IN RESEARCH ON CALCIUM AND PHOSPHORUS IN BONE HEALTH

John J. B. Anderson, Ph.D. and Sanford C. Garner, Ph.D.

TABLE OF CONTENTS

I. INTRODUCTION

This volume covers many of the major topics of importance in the development and maintenance of bone health, particularly those issues related to nutrition. This field of scientific research, however, has expanded tremendously in recent years. As a result, many topics have not been adequately covered herein. Several topics not covered reflect on the enigmas or conundrums of calcium (Ca) and bone metabolism that require further investigation to uncover mechanistic understandings. A selected list of these topics is given in Table 1.

II. SPECIFIC AREAS FOR FUTURE RESEARCH

Four illustrative examples are briefly reviewed in this concluding chapter in order to offer young investigators potential research topics for dissertations or fellowship projects. The four topics, which represent under-researched areas of investigation in Ca and bone metabolism, are: (1) interactions of nutrients, growth factors, and hormones in peripubertal skeletal growth; (2) cross talk among bone cells via cytokines and regulation of bone resorption and formation; (3) loss of bone mass during bedrest and spaceflight — explanatory mechanisms; and (4) regulation of secretion of calcemic hormones and the relationship to pathologies of the parathyroid and thyroid glands.

A. INTERACTIONS OF NUTRIENTS, GROWTH FACTORS, AND HORMONES IN PERIPUBERTAL SKELETAL GROWTH

Skeletal growth in children prior to puberty requires an adequate supply of nutrients, especially energy and protein, in order to maximize the production of growth hormone by the anterior pituitary and tissue-specific insulin-like growth factors (IGFs) and their binding proteins (IGF-BPs), which apparently drive the local tissue growth. This sequence of events operates in a highly dominant way in prepubertal skeletal growth when the reproductive hormones are less influential; however, after

0-8493-7845-1/95/$0.00+$.50

TABLE 1
Potential Research Topics Suitable for Investigation by Young Researchers

Nutrition and Bone Health

1. What controls the development of peripubertal bone growth and closing of epiphyses?
2. How can we reverse the general nutritional inadequacy of Ca by females across the life cycle and the resulting low bone mass?
3. How is intestinal Ca absorption regulated during pregnancy and lactation?
4. What are the potential adverse effects of excessive consumption of protein (animal), phosphorus, and sodium on bone?
5. What role(s) does vitamin K play in bone metabolism?
6. What are the interactions of micronutrients and bone maintenance?
7. What role(s) does magnesium play in bone mass maintenance?
8. What are the mechanisms of intestinal phosphorus (Pi) absorption?
9. What are the mechanisms of transcellular versus paracellular Ca absorption?

Basic Physiology of Bone During Development and Aging

1. What are the roles of various local tissue factors/cytokines in the regulation of bone formation/resorption by bone cells?
2. How can we promote the building of new bone late in life?
3. How is bone mineralization regulated, i.e., the intricate steps involving matrix proteins and mineral seeds?
4. How can pathological soft tissue calcification, including renal stones, be prevented?
5. What treatments are possible for cancers of bone and the resulting increased resorption?
6. What are the fundamental roles of vitamin D receptor alleles (heredity) and osteoporosis?
7. Can the collagen cross-links in urine specific for bone Type I collagen be used as markers for bone turnover in the diagnosis and treatment of bone disorders?

Environmental Effects on Bone and Calcium Metabolism

1. What are the signals for loss of bone mass during bedrest and extended space flight?
2. What is the role of phytoestrogens as agonists and/or antagonists of estrogens in bone?

Regulation of Calcemic Hormone Secretion and Effects on Bone Health

1. What is the role of the cell-surface Ca receptor(s) in the regulation of PTH and CT secretion and in Ca sensing by other cells?
2. What are the mechanisms for the development of hyperparathyroidism (primary and secondary)?
3. How do nutrients, including dietary Ca, P, Mg, and vitamin D regulate PTH secretion?
4. What are the impacts of thyroid hormones (thyroxine and CT), corticosteroids, etc., on bone turnover?

the onset of puberty the reproductive hormones ascend in importance in the control of linear growth, and the IGFs take a role of lesser importance in governing growth.

In the case of individuals with delayed puberty, growth in height continues for additional years beyond normal because the reproductive hormones remain suppressed. In these individuals, height is typically much greater than in individuals with more normal timing of puberty, but bone mass, and especially density, are significantly lower than normal in both males and females. Whereas the mechanisms explaining the differences in height and bone mass according to the timing of pubertal development are not clear, it has been established that well-nourished individuals from affluent nations — yet having low body fat mass — are more likely to have delayed puberty. Children from families without adequate incomes for the optimal nutritional support of their offspring, on the other hand, typically have a form of delayed puberty because of nutritional imbalances and general nutrient inadequacies. These children typically are shorter in stature, more squat in physique, and have normal or slightly subnormal bone mineral content and density.

The hormones and growth factors responsible for the changes in bone mass and skeletal height in individuals with normal versus delayed puberty under conditions of adequate to optimal nutrition require further study.

B. CROSS TALK AMONG BONE CELLS VIA CYTOKINES AND REGULATION OF BONE RESORPTION AND FORMATION

All bone cells produce and secrete cytokines, which affect both cells of the same type (autocrine factors) and different cell types (paracrine factors). Recent research suggests that the signaling or cross talk among the major skeletal cell types and their precedent stem cells via cytokines may serve as major local homeostatic mechanisms controlling bone resorption, perhaps in part through the recruitment of new osteoclasts from progenitor cells. Similarly, osteoblasts may be recruited for new bone formation. Physical strains on osteocytes buried in bone tissue, especially in cortical bone tissue and less so in trabecular bone tissue, may stimulate new bone formation through transduction of the gravitational forces (strains) on osteocytes through the release of cytokines that act on osteoblasts or their precursors. Furthermore, it is generally accepted now that osteoblasts elaborate specific cytokines that stimulate osteoclasts to initiate resorption at new sites, and that the presence of estrogens, at least in females, inhibits this process, thereby preserving or maintaining bone mass.

The linkages among the three major types of bone cells via cytokines need further investigation in experimental models, perhaps mice because of the great potential for manipulating the genome in this rodent species.

C. LOSS OF BONE MASS DURING SPACEFLIGHT AND BEDREST — EXPLANATORY MECHANISMS

A vexing problem to space biologists has been the loss of bone mass (and muscle mass) under hypogravic or even zero-gravity conditions. The bone loss and muscle wasting during weightlessness is somewhat similar to that observed under forced bedrest or the immobilization of experimental subjects with total body casting, but it is not exactly the same. In the classical experiments on bedrest subjects, urinary Ca losses increased shortly after bedrest was initiated and then continued at significantly elevated rates for almost two weeks. Ca losses were accompanied by increased urinary nitrogen losses as well as increased excretions of several other metabolites.

In space or simulated space experiments with low gravity, bone loss increases to a great extent, and then it declines exponentially, essentially independently of any other modalities, such as isometric exercises and additional Ca intakes. In distinction to bedrest loss, the bone loss of spaceflight differs somewhat because greater losses occur in the trunk and upper limbs than in the legs, and it appears that trabecular bone tissue is more greatly affected than cortical tissue by spaceflight, a situation more similar to bone changes in females following ovariectomy. Astronauts also lose nitrogen and other markers of bone tissue in greater amounts during hypogravity. In-flight exercises, however, have been employed in recent long-term spaceflights by Americans and Soviets and have been partially successful in reducing both bone and muscle tissue loss.

The mechanical signal from the lack of gravity, i.e., loss of strain, is thought to be transduced in bone tissue to a chemical signal, which then activates osteoclasts to resorb bone. This strain-chemical linkage, however, has not been elucidated. Apparently in long-term space flights, the absence of loading (strain) on the skeleton cannot be overcome by any known form of exercise available on spaceships. If small centrifuges could be designed for spacecraft, astronauts could spend some time each day getting the appropriate loads to help maintain the linkage between the mechanical loading and signals that enhance bone formation via osteoblasts, inhibit osteoclastic bone resorption, or both. The administration of high amounts of dietary Ca has virtually no effect in preserving bone mass, but bisphosphonates or other drugs may be at least partially effective. These drugs, however, have not yet been used on astronauts under hypogravic space conditions.

Much investigation is needed on the mechanisms that explain the bone losses following bedrest and during extended spaceflight.

D. REGULATION OF SECRETION OF CALCEMIC HORMONES AND PATHOLOGIES OF THE PARATHYROID GLAND

The primary calcemic hormones, i.e., PTH, CT, and $1,25(OH)_2D$, have been known for many years; however, we are far from understanding all aspects of their regulation and function. The recent cloning of the "Ca receptor" protein from the cell membrane of the parathyroid cell has added to our knowledge of the means by which the changes in extracellular Ca are communicated to the intracellular environment to evoke secretion of PTH. This receptor protein is found in other tissues, including the kidney, thyroid, intestine, pituitary, and brain. Thus, the function of this Ca-sensing protein in functions of other cells will need to be elucidated in the future. Even knowing the identity of a protein that responds to changes in the extracellular Ca concentration does not define completely the regulation of PTH secretion. The cellular second messenger has been suggested to be intracellular Ca, cAMP, or PKC activation through Ca and diacylglycerol. No single pathway yet described, however, is consistent with the known regulation of PTH secretion by extracellular Ca. Either another pathway exists that is capable of transducing the signal from the Ca sensor to the secretory signal inside the parathyroid chief cell, or the interaction of several pathways already described must be involved.

In addition to the acute regulation of PTH secretion by extracellular Ca, much more needs to be learned about the mechanisms by which the generally benign adenomas of the parathyroid arise in primary hyperparathyroidism. Genetic analysis of parathyroid adenomas supports the idea that many are derived from clonal expansion of a single cell or small group of cells. Thus, a relatively small change in one or more cells of the parathyroid gland may be responsible for the development of hypersecretion of PTH. The etiology of secondary hyperparathyroidism is related to the chronic hypocalcemia that results from the hyperphosphatemia accompanying renal failure. In this condition, hyperplasia of all four parathyroid lobes with excessive secretion of PTH follows the chronic hypocalcemia. When the secondary hyperparathyroidism is present for longer periods, however, a change in parathyroid response to Ca may occur that is similar to that observed in primary hyperparathyroidism. Do these cases of tertiary hyperparathyroidism result from clonal expansion of parathyroid chief cells similar to that proposed for primary hyperparathyroidism?

Further research is needed on the role of the Ca-sensing protein(s) in the regulation of PTH and CT secretion and in the pathologies of the parathyroid and thyroid glands.

III. CONCLUDING REMARKS

Many knowledge gaps exist despite significant advances in understandings at the organ, tissue, cellular, and molecular levels of organization. The new knowledge gained from the techniques of molecular biology has been truly astounding, but linking and applying this information to the treatment of metabolic bone disorders has been disappointing. The greatest gains in this translation of fundamental genetic information to disease therapy have been made in the hereditary vitamin D-related types of rickets. It is hoped that improved treatments will follow in the future from basic research that will aid patients with osteoporosis and other metabolic bone diseases.

New understandings of PTH, CT, and vitamin D (and their analogs) have resulted from modern molecular techniques as well. Each of these molecules is available for therapeutic strategies aimed at preserving bone mass. It is anticipated that PTH will be used more in the future in intermittent therapy to improve bone mass in elderly subjects with osteopenia or osteoporosis. Other therapeutic modalities will also be used to improve or to maintain bone mass, and thereby reduce the chance of fractures. Growth hormone and anabolic steroids have already been used for this purpose. Fluoride therapy, utilizing a capsule that prevents dissolution in the stomach, will also be employed in the future to stimulate bone formation. Finally, several third-generation bisphosphonates will be available in the next few years to enhance the retention of the bone mass of elderly subjects.

The general conclusion of these current activities of widely diverse research areas in the bone field is that understandings of fundamental bone biology are too often being set aside for applied research toward the discovery of new drugs for the treatment of osteoporosis. Much more basic research needs to be directed toward generating better understandings of integrated cellular functions that maintain the integrity of bone tissue, and of nutritional problems that require long periods of study in well-designed prospective trials. New information is needed on many fronts in the broadly encompassing field of Ca nutrition and bone.

INDEX

A

B

C

D

F

G

H

I

M

Q

R

S

T

U

V

W

X

Y

Z